THE BIOLOGY OF THE FLUIDS OF THE FEMALE GENITAL TRACT
Workshop Conference in Murnau, Bavaria
June 11–13, 1979
Sponsored by ORGANON

Honorary Chairman: Richard J. Blandau
Chairmen: Fritz K. Beller and Gebhard F.B. Schumacher
Editors: Fritz K. Beller and Gebhard F.B. Schumacher
Associate Editors: Don P. Wolf and Klaus-H. Geissler

With contributions by:

H. M. Beier	J. A. Holt	G. F. B. Schumacher
F. K. Beller	P. R. Koninckx	K. W. Schweppe
R. J. Blandau	J. Kuhl	S. T. Shaw, Jr.
R. Bourdage	H. J. Lindemann	U. M. Spornitz
K. H. Broer	J. Lippes	P. F. Tauber
I. Brosens	K. S. Ludwig	H. D. Taubert
H.-W. Denker	D. H. A. Maas	A. Uettwiler
C. Ebert	L. Macaulay	G. Vasquez
C. A. Eddy	M. Mall-Haefeli	G. Wagner
A. Ferenczy	L. Mastroianni, Jr.	H. Wagner
C. E. Flowers	K. S. Moghissi	I. Werner-Zodrow
K. J. Go	D. L. Moyer	W. H. Wilborn
M. S. Guralnick	C. Oberti	D. P. Wolf
S. Halbert	C. J. Pauerstein	R. M. Wynn
W. H. Heyns	F. Reale	S. L. Yang
H. A. Hirsch	W. B. Robertson	J. Zanartu
	S. El Sahwi	

ELSEVIER/NORTH-HOLLAND
New York • Amsterdam • Oxford

© 1979 Elsevier North Holland, Inc.

Published by:
Elsevier North Holland, Inc.
52 Vanderbilt Avenue
New York, New York 10017

Sole distributors outside the United States and Canada:
Elsevier/North-Holland Biomedical Press
335 Jan van Galenstraat, PO Box 211
Amsterdam, The Netherlands

Library of Congress Cataloging in Publication Data

International Workshop on the Biology of the Fluids of
    the Female Genital Tract, Murnau, Ger., 1979.
    The biology of the secretions of the fluids of the
female genital tract.
    Bibliography: p.
    Includes index.
    1. Generative organs, Female—Secretions—Congresses.
I. Beller, Fritz K. II. Schumacher, Gebhard F. B.
III. ORGANON GmbH. IV. Title.
QP259.157   1979   612.6'2   79-19886
ISBN 0-444-00362-2

Manufactured in the United States of America

CONTENTS

Foreword

List of Participants

PART I:	VAGINA	
	Morphology of the Human Vagina A. Ferenczy and M. S. Guralnick	1
	Vaginal Fluid Constituents K. S. Moghissi	13
	Vaginal Transudation G. Wagner	25
PART II:	UTERUS (EXCEPT CERVIX)	
	Morphology of the Endometrium R. M. Wynn	37
	Cells of the Uterine Fluid D. L. Moyer, S. El Sahwi, L. Macaulay, and S. T. Shaw, Jr.	59
	Histoenzymology of Human Endometrium During the Proliferative and Secretory Phases (I) W. H. Wilborn and C. E. Flowers	73

Endometrial Secretion Proteins — Biochemistry and Biological Significance *H. M. Beier*		89
Approaches to the Analysis of Human Endometrial Secretions *G. F. B. Schumacher, J. A. Holt, and F. Reale*		115
Biochemical Components of the Human Endometrium *P. F. Tauber*		131
Inhibitors of Trophoblast Proteinases *H.-W. Denker*		151
Menstruation: Endocrine Aspects *H. D. Taubert and H. Kuhl*		163
The Histology and Proliferation Kinetics of Menstrual Endometrium *A. Ferenczy and M. S. Guralnick*		177
Ultrastructural Aspects of Human Endometrium During Menstruation *H. Wagner and F. K. Beller*		187
Histoenzymology of the Human Endometrium (II) *C. E. Flowers and W. H. Wilborn*		203
Hysteroscopic Data During Menstruation *H. J. Lindemann*		225
Review on the Biology of Menstrual Blood *F. K. Beller and K. W. Schweppe*		231
Biochemistry of Menstrual Blood *C. Ebert, F. K. Beller, K. W. Schweppe, and H. Wagner*		247
Bacteriology of Lochiae *H. A. Hirsch*		257
Ultrastructural Observations on Transformation of Decidua into Endometrium Post Partum *H. Wagner, K. W. Schweppe, and F. K. Beller*		265
Biochemistry of Post Partum Fluid (Lochiae) *C. Ebert, K. W. Schweppe, and F. K. Beller*		281
PART III:	**OVIDUCT**	
	Morphology of the Fallopian Tube *C. J. Pauerstein and C. A. Eddy*	299
	Tubal Transport *R. J. Blandau, R. Bourdage, and S. Halbert*	319
	Tubal Secretions *L. Mastroianni, Jr., and K. J. Go*	335

Tubal Secretions — Ultrastructure Related to Endocrinology *M. Mall-Haefeli, K. S. Ludwig, U. M. Spornitz, A. Uettwiler, and I. Werner-Zodrow*	345
Ultrastructural Changes in the Human Oviduct Epithelium During the Puerperium and Lactation *C. Oberti, J. Zanartu, G. Vasquez, I. Brosens, and B. Robertson*	361
Analysis of Human Oviductal Fluid for Low Molecular Weight Compounds *J. Lippes*	373
Specific Antibodies in Oviduct Secretions of the Rhesus Monkey *G. F. B. Schumacher, S. L. Yang, and K. H. Broer*	389
Studies of the Protein Content of Human Oviductal Flushings *D. H. A. Maas*	399
Mammalian Fertilization *D. P. Wolf*	407
Peritoneal Fluid in Female Fertility and Sterility *P. R. Koninckx, I. A. Brosens, and W. H. Heyns*	415

PART IV: **SUMMARY AND CONCLUSIONS**
Summary and Conclusions of the Conference   427
R. M. Wynn

Index   435

FOREWORD

This workshop conference was designed to assess the present state of knowledge about the biology of the fluids of the female genital tract. It follows a workshop organized by V. Insler and G. Bettendorf (The Uterine Cervix in Reproduction, G. Thieme Publishers, Stuttgart, 1977) which was devoted to the cervix. We therefore felt it appropriate to exclude this particular topic since the time interval was rather short.

The understanding of the biology of secretions of the female reproductive organs requires a morphological description of these organs. This is the reason that light and electron microscopy, both scanning and transmission, comprise a large section of this symposium.

A closed meeting is justified only if the new information generated is rapidly transmitted to the scientific community. This requires support from the contributors by submitting papers well in advance. Also, it requires the publisher's support and we thank Mr. Yale Altman of Elsevier North Holland, Inc., New York, for his cooperation.

Instead of printing the discussion in detail we asked Dr. Ralph Wynn to provide the participants and the readers with a synopsis of this meeting and the discussion it generated. We are grateful for his willingness to undertake this time-consuming task and for doing it so well.

The ORGANON GmbH, Oberschleissheim/Munich, deserves our greatest appreciation for the generous support which made this workshop conference possible.

We are especially indebted to Dr. Günter Weiland for his help and advice. The organization of this meeting guided by Dr. Geissler and Mrs. Hinds was outstanding. Mrs. Thrän, Münster, and the secretarial and technical staff of ORGANON were of great help in all technical matters.

We should like to express our sincere appreciation to the contributors who made this meeting a success by their expert knowledge and diligent work. The editors are proud of the acceptance by Dr. Richard Blandau to serve as an Honorary Chairman. His almost unlimited knowledge and experience were greatly appreciated by all participants.

G. F. B. Schumacher *F. K. Beller*

LIST OF PARTICIPANTS

H. M. Beier
Abteilung Anatomie und
  Reproduktionsbiologie
Rheinish-Westfälische Technische
  Hochschule
Melatener Strasse 211
5100 Aachen
Federal Republic of Germany

F. K. Beller
Frauenklinik der Westfälischen
Wilhelms-Universität
Westring 11
4400 Münster
Federal Republic of Germany

R. J. Blandau
Department of Biological Structure SM-20
School of Medicine
University of Washington
Seattle, Washington 98195 U S A

H.-W. Denker
Abteilung Anatomie
Rheinisch-Westfälische Technische
  Hochschule
Melatener Strasse 211
5100 Aachen
Federal Republic of Germany

C. Ebert
Frauenklinik der Westfälischen
Wilhelms-Universität
Westring 11
4400 Münster
Federal Republic of Germany

K. W. Eickstedt
Bundesgesundheitsamt
Stauffenbergstrasse 13
1000 Berlin 30
Federal Republic of Germany

A. Ferenczy
Department of Pathology
McGill University
Jewish General Hospital
3755 Cote Ste. Catherine
Montreal, PQ. H3T 1E2
Canada

C. E. Flowers, Jr.
Department of Obstetrics and Gynecology
The University of Alabama in Birmingham
  Medical Center
University Station
Birmingham, Alabama 35294 U S A

K. H. Geissler
Organon GmbH
Mittenheimer Strasse 62
8042 Oberschleissheim
Federal Republic of Germany

H. A. Hirsch
Universitäts-Frauenklinik
Schleichstrasse 4
7400 Tübingen
Federal Republic of Germany

D. de Jager
Organon International
Kloosterstraat 6
4202 Oss
The Netherlands

P. R. Koninckx
Academisch Ziekenhuis
Sint-Rafael
Kapucijnen Voer 33
3000 Leuven
Belgium

H. J. Lindemann
Geburtschilfliche-Gynäkologische
  Abteilung des Elisabeth-Krankenhauses
Kleiner Schäferkamp 43
2000 Hamburg 6
Federal Republic of Germany

J. Lippes
Department of Obstetrics and Gynecology
Deaconess Division
State University of New York at Buffalo
10001 Humboldt Parkway
Buffalo, New York 14208 U S A

D. H. A. Maas
Frauenklinik im Krankenhaus Oststadt
Medizinische Hochschule
3000 Hannover 51
Federal Republic of Germany

K. S. Moghissi
Division of Reproductive Biology
Department of Gynecology and Obstetrics
Wayne State University School of
  Medicine
C.S. Mott Center for Human Growth and
  Development
275 East Hancock Avenue
Detroit, Michigan 48201 U S A

D. L. Moyer
Section of Experimental Pathology
Department of Obstetrics and Gynecology
University of Southern California Medical
  Center
2025 Zonal Avenue
Los Angeles, California 90033 U S A

C. J. Pauerstein
Departments of Obstetrics and Gynecology
  and Physiology
The University of Texas
Health Science Center
7703 Floyd Curl Drive
San Antonio, Texas 78284 U.S.A

G. F. B. Schumacher
Section of Reproductive Biology
Department of Obstetrics and Gynecology
  and Divisional Committee on
  Immunology
The University of Chicago
Pritzker School of Medicine
5841 Maryland Avenue
Chicago, Illinois 60637 U S A

K. W. Schweppe
Frauenklinik der Westfälischen
Wilhelms-Universität
Westring 11
4400 Münster
Federal Republic of Germany

U. M. Spornitz
Frauenspital Basel-Stadt
Postfach 141
4000 Basel 4
Switzerland

P. F. Tauber
Frauenklinik und Poliklinik
Universitätsklinikum der
 Gesamthochschule Essen
Hufelandstrasse 55
4300 Essen
Federal Republic of Germany

H. D. Taubert
Abteilung für gynäkologische
 Endokrinologie
Zentrum für Frauenheilkunde und
 Geburtshilfe
Johann-Wolfang-Goethe-Universität
Theodor-Stern-Kai 7
6000 Frankfurt
Federal Republic of Germany

T. Vossenaar
Organon International
Kloosterstraat 6
4202 Oss
The Netherlands

G. Wagner
Institute of Medical Physiology B
University of Copenhagen
Juliane Maries Vej 30
2100 Copenhagen
Denmark

H. Wagner
Frauenklinik der Westfälischen
Wilhelms-Universität
Westring 11
4400 Münster
Federal Republic of Germany

G. Weiland
Organon GmbH
Mittenheimer Strasse 62
8042 Oberschleissheim
Federal Republic of Germany

D. P. Wolf
Division of Reproductive Biology
Department of Obstetrics and Gynecology
University of Pennsylvania School of
 Medicine
36th and Hamilton Walk G3
Philadelphia, Pennsylvania 19104 U S A

R. M. Wynn
Department of Obstetrics and Gynecology
University of Arkansas for Medical
 Sciences
4301 W. Markham
Little Rock, Arkansas 72201 U S A

Part I:
VAGINA

Copyright 1979 by Elsevier North Holland, Inc.
F.K. Beller and G.F.B. Schumacher, eds.
The Biology of the Fluids of the Female Genital Tract

MORPHOLOGY OF THE HUMAN VAGINA

A. Ferenczy and M.S. Guralnick

SUMMARY

The cytodynamics of the vaginal squamous epithelium during the reproductive period are influenced by cyclicly released ovarian sex-steroid hormones and are geared for protective, metabolic and reproductive functions.

INTRODUCTION

The term vagina taken from the Latin means sheath. In the human it is composed of three principal tissue systems: an outer fibrous layer originating from the pelvic fascia middle muscular layer and an inner mucosal membrane. The latter consists of wavy stratified squamous epithelium that is supported by a tunica propria of collagenous tissue. The vascular system and innervation of the vagina have been investigated by Krantz (1959). The cervico-vaginal artery originating from the uterine artery irrigates the upper half of the vagina, whereas the lower half is supplied by the hemorrhoidal arteries. They form a plexus around the vagina and from this plexus a median artery supplies both the anterior and posterior walls. The vagina has a rich venous plexus which communicates with the pudendal and hemorrhoidal venous plexuses which in turn empty into the internal

Departments of Pathology and Obstetrics and Gynecology, Jewish Memorial Hospital and McGill University, Montreal, Quebec, Canada

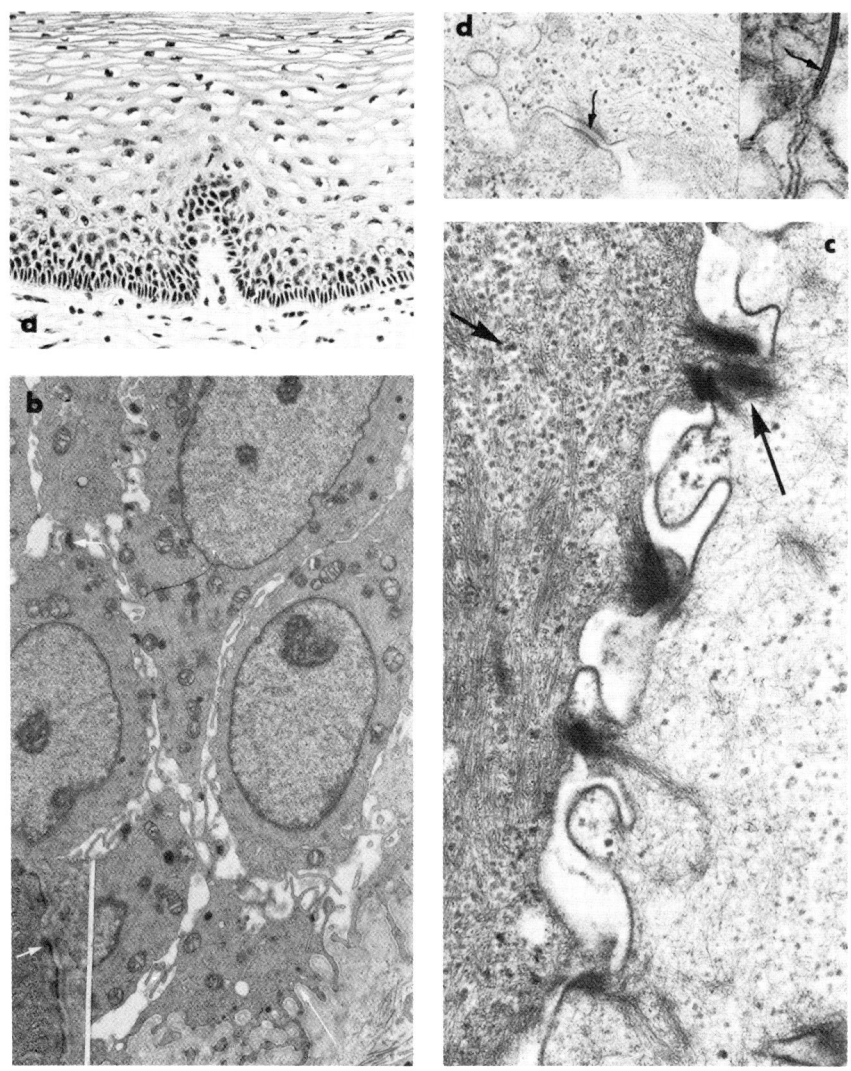

FIGURE 1. *Human vaginal epithelium.* a) Mature, non-keratinized, stratified squamous epithelium with a distinct, single basal cell layer; 2–3 cell layers thick parabasal zone; vacuolized intermediate cells; and finally flattened squamous cells with attenuated, pyknotic nuclei. Note gradual cytomegaly from the basal to the superficial cell layer (H & E × 250). b) Electron microscopy of basal cells. Prominent nuclei are associated with scant cytoplasmic substance scattered with a few mitochondria. Free ribosomes are abundant, however. Desmosomes (small arrow) are infrequent, whereas hair-like microvilli are numerous and project into the intercellular space. The cells are attached to the underlying ba-

iliac veins. The lymphatics of the vagina begin with a mucosal plexus and drain into the underlying muscular plexus. The latter drains into the external iliac, hypogastric and inguinal nodes. The innervation of the vagina is related closely to that of the uterus and both the sympathetic and parasympathetic nerve components originate from the hypogastric nerve plexuses.

HISTOLOGY

The histologic morphology of the vaginal mucosa is unique in its response to sex-steroid hormonal stimuli. Stockard and Papanicolaou (1917) and Dierks (1927) were the first to demonstrate in the guinea pig and the human, respectively that the vaginal epithelium undergoes cyclic morphologic changes that are correlated with phases of the ovarian cycle. Since that time we have learned that diagnosis of the phases can be ascertained by the microscopical examination of vaginal smears. The vaginal mucosa during the reproductive period is constantly being remodelled by proliferation-maturation-desquamation (Ferenczy and Richart, 1974). In general, estradiol (E_2) stimulates epithelial growth, maturation and desquamation, whereas progesterone (P) inhibits maturation at the upper midzone level of the epithelium. The turnover time of vaginal epithelium is about 96 hours as demonstrated by *in vitro* DNA-historadioautography and can be decreased by 50% by exogenous estrogen administration (Averette et al., 1970).

The following cell layers can be identified in the mature squamous stratified epithelium (Tubin and Novak, 1956): A basal layer composed of oval to round shaped cells with prominent nuclei, a parabasal cell layer with larger cytoplasmic substance than the basal cells, an intermediate layer of larger, flatter cells, and a superficial layer of cornified layer with pyknotic nuclei (Figure 1a). Unlike the cervical squamous epithelium, its vaginal counterpart contains narrow tongue-like buddings into the connective tissue stroma.

ULTRASTRUCTURE

The cytodynamics of the human vaginal mucous membrane have been investigated by means of electron microscopy (Ferenczy and Richart, 1974; Burgos et al., 1978; Walz et al., 1978).

The fine structural organization of basal cells is consistent with epithelial replication that is associated with active cell division. The nucleocytoplasmic ratio is in favor of the nucleus which has been shown to incorporate tritiated thymi-

---

sal lamina (long arrow) by numerous hemi-desmosomes ($\times$ 5,000). *INSET*: Detail of hemi-desmosomes (arrow) and basal lamina ($\times$ 9,000). c) High magnification of portion of a dark parabasal cell (left) and a light intermediate cell (right). Note numerous glycogen granules (short arrow) admixed with bundles of 100 Å thick tonofilaments. Cellular integrity is maintained by desmosome-tonofilament complexes (long arrow). Stubby microvilli project into the intercellular space ($\times$ 55,000). d) Detailed view of a longitudinally sectioned desmosome or macula adherens (left), ($\times$ 48,000) and a gap junction nexus (right), ($\times$ 80,000). Note central linear density (arrows) in both junctional specializations.

dine, a nucleoprotein precursor molecule (Averette et al., 1970). Although the cytoplasm is relatively poor in organelles, free ribosomes are abundant (Figure 1b). The latter increases in number during the preovulatory phase as a reflection of target cell response to estrogenic stimuli. Indeed E_2 stimulates DNA-dependent RNA-synthesis. The cytoplasm of basal cells has also been shown to contain esterase, B-glucuronidase and DPNH-diaphorase (Fishman et al., 1959). Enzymes related to glycogen systhesis are absent in basal cells, however. Basal cells are attached to the underlying basal lamina and adjacent and subjacent cells by hemidesmosomes and desmosome-tonofilaments complexes, respectively (Figure 1b). Desmosomes are comparatively more frequent in the upper parabasal and intermediate cell layers (Figures 1c, d and 2). Parabasal and intermediate cells have larger cytoplasmic substance and are involved in carbohydrate metabolism as evidenced by a massive accumulation of intracytoplasmic glycogen (Figure 1c and 2). This is associated with amylophosphorylase, amylo-1, 1-4, 6-transglucosidase and glycogen synthetase activity. The latter is considered responsible for glycogen synthesis in *in vivo* conditions (Fishman et al., 1959). The parabasal cells acquire comparatively more organelles than the underlying basal cells and produce microfilaments of about 100 Å in diameter, the so-called tonofilaments (Figure 1c). In addition to well-developed intercellular junctional attachments including macula adherences, zonula occludenses and adherences, a rare gap-junction nexus (Burgos et al., 1978) may be encountered chiefly between the intermediate cells (Figure 1d). Similar intercellular specializations are seen in the squamous mucous membrane of the portio vaginalis of the cervix. Nexuses are easier to demonstrate at the transmission electron microscopic level by using lanthanum-hydroxide impregnation or electron microscopy of freeze fractured material (McNutt et al., 1970). Nexuses are made of hollow, hexagonal microtubules and represent an open channel system between adjacent cells. Electrolytes and molecules of about 60,000 daltons can traverse through nexuses without entering the intercellular space. At this region the intercellular space is narrowed to about 20 Å in diameter. Nexuses apparently play a role in cell contact inhibition and in the formation of low resistance coupling sites between normal cells. These biophysical phenomena are responsible for the orderly arrangements and growth pattern of squamous epithelial cells.

The nuclei of parabasal cells exhibit occasional mitotic figures and radioautographic studies *in vitro* (Averette et al., 1970) demonstrates greater nuclear DNA-synthesis in the parabasal region than in the basal cells. However, exogenous estrogen treatment of premenopausal women increases DNA-synthesis in an equal proportion in both para- and basal cells (Averette et al. 1970).

The superficial zones form the most differentiated compartment of the squamous mucous membrane. The cells are flattened, have large cytoplasmic substance of about 50 μm in diameter and smaller nuclei. The latter undergo pyknosis, and DNA-synthesis is absent in superficial squamous cells. The cytoplasm is packed with PAS positive diastase labile glycogen granules (Figure 3). According to Gregoire et al., (1971), the glycogen content of the vaginal epithelium is constant during the menstrual cycle as determined by enzymehistochemistry. Similarly, no differences in glycogen content are observed between the upper and lower epithelial layers. These observations suggest that glycogen content is unaffected by circulating estrogens during the menstrual cycle. The most superficial cells are relatively poor in glycogen but are rich in intracytoplasmic microfilaments (Figure 3). These presumably provide for their

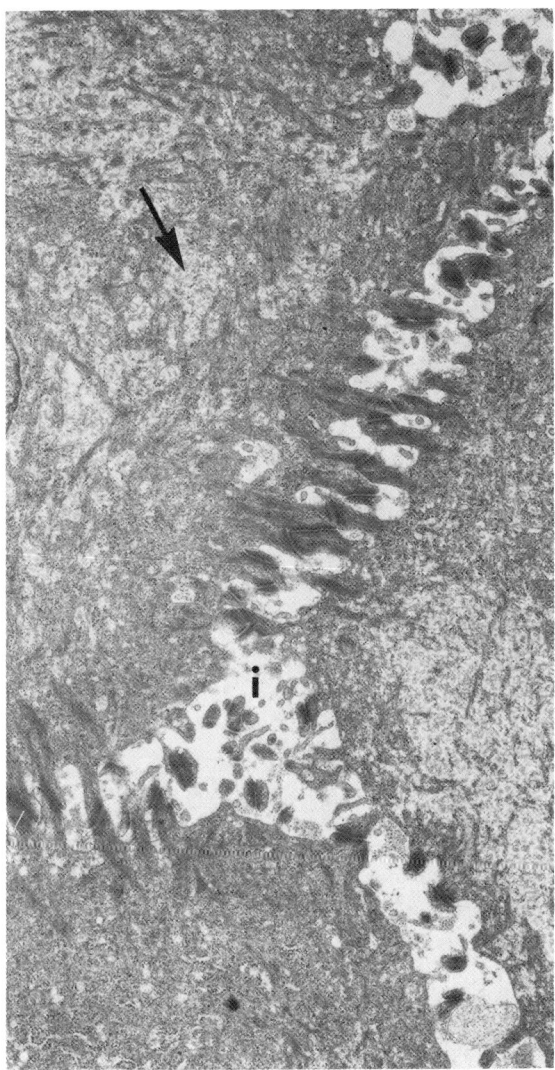

FIGURE 2. *Intermediate cells*. Note massive accumulation of electron pale glycogen granules (arrow) intermingling with bundles of tonofilaments. Desmosomes are numerous and characteristically, the intercellular space (i) is dilated (× 5,000).

rigidity and contribute to the protective role of the squamous vaginal mucous membrane. The profound decrease in desmosomes between the upper squamous cells facilitates their desquamation (Figure 3). Superficial cells of squamous mucous membranes in general contain occasional sulfur-rich keratohyalin bodies (Silverman 1971). These are responsible for both the cornification and the intricate network of microridges (Figure 4a-c). The latter are seen on the surface of the most superficial and mature squamous cells (Ferenczy and Richart, 1974; Walz et al., 1978). By contrast, the underlying intermediate cells have abundant hair-like

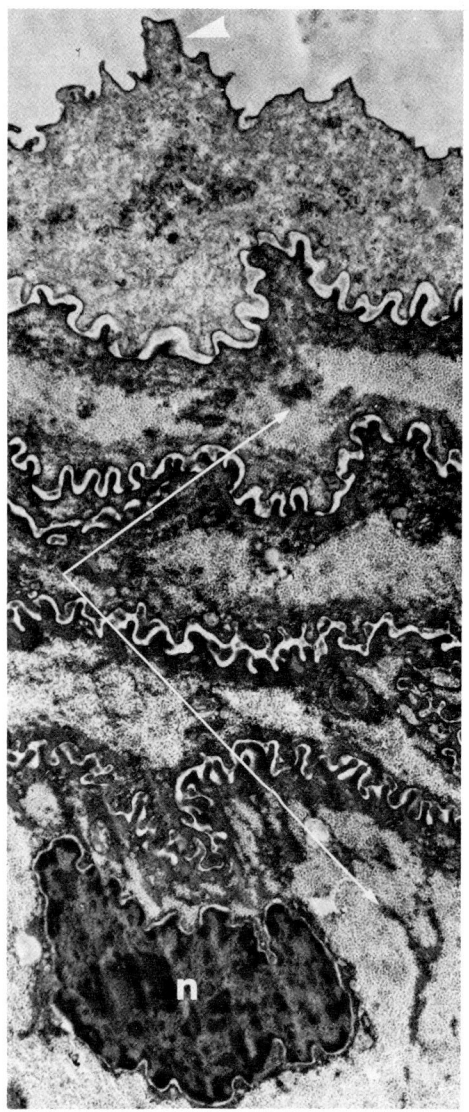

FIGURE 3. *Superficial squamous cells.* The cytoplasmic substance is packed with glycogen granules (arrows), the intercellular spaces are tight with numerous microvilli, desmosomes are rare, and nucleus (n) degenerated. The most superficial cell is rich in microfilaments and the surface membrane has irregular intraluminal projections (arrowhead) ($\times$ 7,500).

surface microvilli (Figure 4d). Surface microridges measuring 0.2 μm by 0.1 μm were not known to exist prior to using scanning electron microscopy. Microridges are a characteristic feature of all nonkeratinizing squamous mucous membranes and are believed to enhance surface adhesiveness and resistance to sideway movements. During physiologic atrophy (senescence) microridges become attenuated

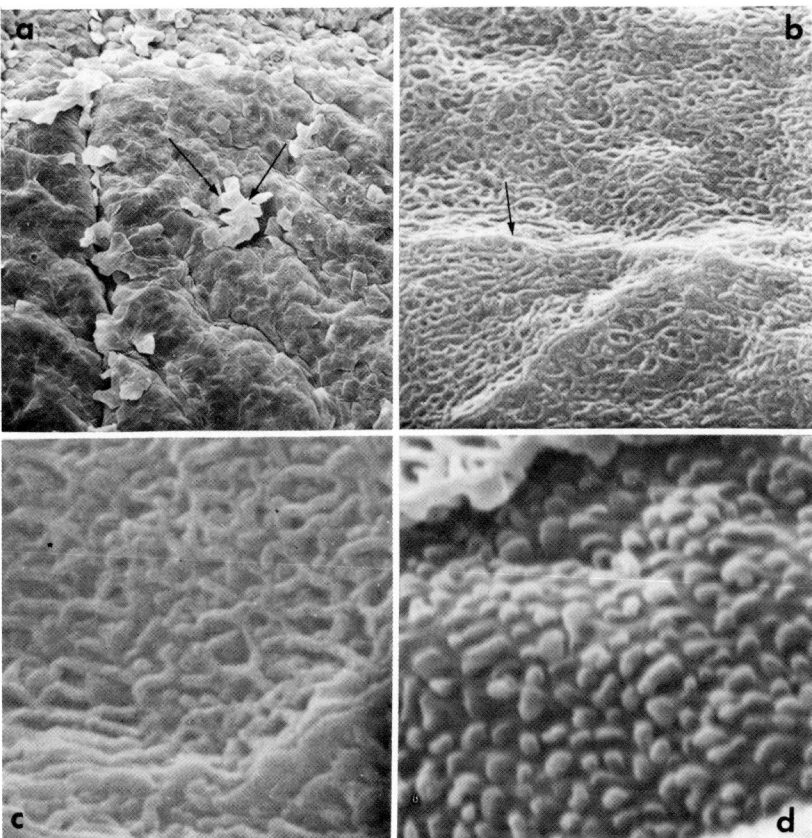

FIGURE 4. *Superficial squamous cells.* a) Scanning electron microscopy of large polygonal surface cells with a cobblestone surface pattern. Clusters of loosely attached cells are seen prior to desquamation (arrows) (× 60). b) Closer view of surface microridges and intercellular terminal bars (arrow) of the most superficial squamous cells (× 3,000). c) High magnification of surface microridges made of longitudinal elevations of the surface plasma membrane (× 28,000). d) Portion of an intermediate cell with numerous stubby surface microvilli (× 10,000).

and fragmented (Walz et al., 1978). Squamous epithelial cells in both keratinized and nonkeratinized membranes including the vagina and the cervix have been shown to contain membrane-coated granules (Grubb et al., 1968; Squier, 1977). In the nonkeratinized variety these structures are rich in acid phosphatase and mucous substances. They derive from the Golgi and are especially numerous in the upper epithelial layers. They fuse with the cytoplasmic membrane, extrude their content into the intercellular space and form a permeability barrier of the squamous epithelium (Grubb et al., 1968).

Throughout the cycle and especially during the postovulatory phase, the vaginal epithelium contains numerous migrating lymphocytes and occasionally Langerhans' cells within the intercellular spaces (Burgos et al., 1978). Their precise significance is unknown. However, they may be related to chronic

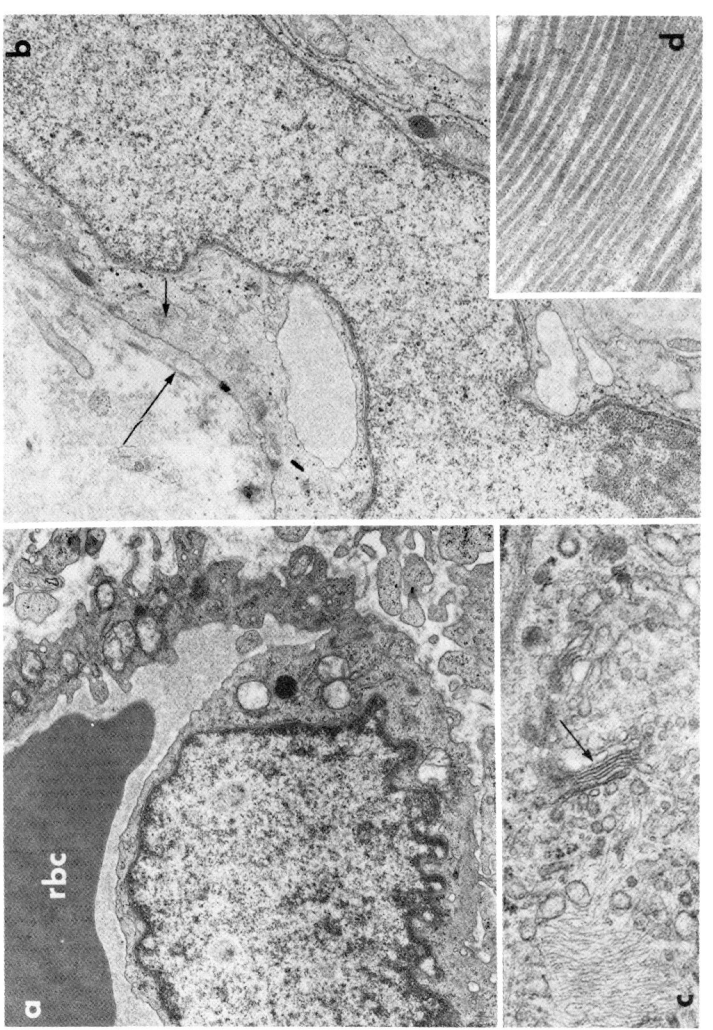

FIGURE 5. *Vaginal stroma.* a) A capillary with an intraluminal red blood cell (rbc) lined by a prominent endothelial cell (× 8,500). b) Portion of a fibroblast with peripheral condensation of procollagen microfibrils (short arrows). Scattered extracellular mature collagen fibers (long arrows) are seen near the cytoplasmic membrane (× 19,500). c) Detail of intracytoplasmic procollagen fibrils near the Golgi (arrow) and perigolgian vesicles (× 61,000). d) Extracellular mature collagen fibers with periodic cross-banding (× 49,000).

intraluminal and subepithelial stromal inflammation associated with antigen-antibody reaction. Similar phenomenon is observed in other hollow organs such as the intestines, uterus and Fallopian tube.

According to Burgos et al., (1978), the intercellular space of the vaginal mucous membrane undergoes variations in diameter during the menstrual cycle. During the follicular phase it gradually enlarges reaching a maximum diameter during the postovulatory phase. Maximum enlargement of the intercellular channel system occurs in the intermediate cell layers. In the superficial cell layer, the intercellular space remains narrowed and unchanged during the cycle. Variations in the configuration of the intercellular space are likely to facilitate bidirectional metabolic interchanges including glycoproteins, immunoglobulins and prostaglandins between the stroma and vaginal lumen (Burgos et al., 1978).

The vaginal stroma is separated from the epithelium by a well defined, continuous, 60 nm thick basal lamina (Figure 1b). Since the vessels have no direct contact with the squamous epithelium, nutrients and oxygen are delivered by diffusion. Active transport of various elements is manifested structurally by the abundance of plasma membrane micropinocytic vesicles and narrow, fenestrated cytoplasm of capillary endothelial cells (Figure 5a). Stromal fibroblasts vary from poorly developed immature to mature forms with well equipped organellar constitution (Figure 5b). These include ribosomes-Golgi-ergastoplasm-mitochondria-lysosomal complexes and are geared for synthesis and degradation of extracellular collagen fibers (Cate and Deporter, 1975). Collagen synthesis begins by the formation of intracytoplasmic, soluble, nonbanded procollagen microfibrils of about 80-100 Å in diameter (Ferenczy, 1979). They are synthesized on L-proline-rich granular endoplasmic reticulun and pass via the Golgi where they are complexed into polysaccharides (Figure 5c). They are then transported to the extracellular space where they are cleaved presumably by collagenase and elastase into 300–400 Å thick banded tropocollagen fibrils. These in turn undergo polymerization and form 900–1100 Å thick mature collagen fibers (Figure 5d). These characteristically demonstrate a 660 Å periodicity with 8 electron dense intraperiod bands. Degradation of extracellular collagen by fibroblasts and macrophages occurs by heterophagocytosis, whereby collagen fibers are engulfed into membrane-bound cytophagolysosomes and digested by hydrolytic enzymes such as acid phosphatase and cathepsin-D (Cate and Deporter, 1975; Ferenczy, 1979).

ACKNOWLEDGEMENTS

Supported in part by Grant 5137 from the Medical Research Council of Canada. The authors are indebted to Miss Rosemary De Marco for typing the manuscript.

REFERENCES

Averette, H.E., Weinstein, G.D., Frost, P.: Autoradiographic analysis of cell proliferation kinetics in human genital tissues. I. Normal cervix and vagina. Amer. J. Obstet. Gynecol. 108 (1970) 8–17.

Burgos, M.H., Roig de Vargas-Linares, C.E.: Ultrastructure of the vaginal mucosa. In: The Human Vagina. Eds.: E.S.E. Hafez and T.N. Evans, Elsevier/North-Holland Biomedical Press, New York 1978, pp. 63–93.

Cate, A.P.T., Deporter, D.A.: The degradative role of the fibroblast in the remodelling and turnover of collagen in soft connective tissue. Anat. Rec. 182 (1975) 1–13.

Dierks, K.: Der normale menstruelle Zyklus de menschlichen Vaginalschleimhaut. Arch. Gynaekol. 130 (1927) 46–69.

Ferenczy, A.: The ultrastructural cytodynamics of the human cervix. In: Dilatation of the Cervix: Connective Tissue Biology and Clinical Management. Eds.: P.G. Stubblefield and F. Naftolin, Raven Press, New York 1979, pp. 27–43.

Ferenczy, A., Richart, R.M.: Female reproductive system. Dynamics of Scan and Transmission Current concepts of the histology of oral mucosa. Eds.: C.A. Squier and J. Meyer, Charles C. Thomas, Springfield Illinois 1971, pp. 80–96.

Fishman, W.H., Mitchell, G.W., Jr.: Studies on vaginal enzymology. Ann. N.Y. Acad. Sci. 83 (1959) 105–121.

Gregoire, A.T., Kandil, O., Ledger, W.J.: The glycogen content of human vaginal epithelial tissue. Fertil. Steril. 22 (1971) 64–68.

Grubb, C., Hackemann, M., Hill, K.R.: Small granules and plasma membrane thickening in human cervical squamous epithelium. J. Ultrastruct. Res. 22 (1968) 458–468.

Krantz, K.E.: The gross and microscopic anatomy of the human vagina. Ann. N.Y. Acad. Sci. 83 (1959) 89–104.

McNutt, N.S., Weinstein, R.S.: The ultrastructure of the nexus. A correlated thin-section and freeze-cleave study. J. Cell Biol. 47 (1970) 666–688.

Silverman, S., Jr.: Non-keratinization and keratinization: The extremes of the human range. In: Current concepts of the histology of oral mucosa. Eds.: C.A. Squier and J. Meyer, Charles C. Thomas, Springfield Illinois 1971, pp. 80–96.

Squier, C.A.: Membrane coating granules in nonkeratinizing oral epithelium. J. Ultrastruct. Res. 60 (1977) 212–220.

Stockard, C.R., Papanicolaou, G.N.: The existence of a typical oestrus cycle in the guinea pig with a study of its histological and physiological changes. Am. J. Anat. 22 (1917) 225–283.

Tubin, I.C., Novak, J.: Integrated Gynecology. McGraw-Hill, New York 1956.

Walz, K.A., Metzger, H., Ludwig, H.: Surface ultrastructure of the vagina. In: The Human Vagina. Eds.: E.S.E. Hafez and T.N. Evans, Elsevier/North-Holland Biomedical Press, New York 1978, pp. 55–61.

Copyright 1979 by Elsevier North Holland, Inc.
F.K. Beller and G.F.B. Schumacher, eds.
The Biology of the Fluids of the Female Genital Tract

VAGINAL FLUID CONSTITUENTS

K.S. Moghissi

SUMMARY

Vaginal fluid is a composite of cervical mucus, transudate from vaginal mucosa, desquamated cellular debris and leukocytes. During sexual excitation the production of vaginal secretion is increased. Among electrolytes contained in the vaginal fluid, Na^+, K^+, and Cl appear to play an important role in the regulation of transudation across the vaginal mucosa and lubrication. This process is also responsible for an elevation of vaginal pH which may have a protective effect on the ejaculated sperm in the vagina.

Volatile fatty acids, particularly acetic and lactic acids, are normal constituents of human vaginal fluid. No specific function in women, however, has been attributed to these substances. Free amino acids and serum type proteins are found in normal vaginal fluid. The mean amount of protein is 18 μg/ml. Albumin, α_1-antitrypsin, α_2-haptoglobin, α_2-macroglobulin, β-lipoprotein, orosomucoid, ceruloplasmin, γ-chains, γ-G.K. (Bence Jones) and immunoglobulin G,A, and M are present in vaginal fluid. These proteins are also found in cervical mucus. Fibrin and C-reactive protein are not found in the vaginal fluid but are identified in cervical mucus. α_2-haptoglobin, α_2-macroglobulin, β-lipoprotein, orosomucoid,

Department of Gynecology and Obstetrics, Wayne State University School of Medicine and The C. S. Mott Center for Human Growth and Development, Detroit, Michigan

and immunoglobulin M are absent in the vaginal fluid of hysterectomized women, indicating that their presence in the vaginal secretion of normal women may be due to contamination from cervical mucus. Immunoglobulins whether transudated from the blood or synthesized by vaginal mucosa are probably part of an immune mechanism protecting the vagina against bacterial organisms.

INTRODUCTION

The human vagina is lined by a stratified, squamous, nonkeratinizing epithelium which is identical in origin, histology, and fine structure with that covering the portio externa of the cervix. The epithelium rests on a lamina propria of mixed collagenous and elastic connective tissue which is rich in both blood and lymphatic vessels. The lamina propria intrudes into the basal layer of the epithelium in the form of papillae similar to the dermal papillae of the skin. Lymphocytes, singly or in aggregates, are common in the lamina propria and may occasionally be observed migrating through the epithelium. Polymorphonuclear leukocytes are also observed in the epithelium and vaginal lumen at certain stages of the cycle. There are no glands in the vaginal mucosa with the exception of the Skenes and Bartholin glands, which are located in the vestibule near the urethral meatus. The vagina is kept moist predominantly by the transudation of fluid through the vaginal epithelium and by cervical secretion. Therefore, vaginal secretion is a mixture of cervical mucus, transudate from the vaginal mucosa, desquamated cellular debris, and leukocytes.

Vaginal Fluid Production

Despite the absence of glands vaginal epithelium is usually covered with a surface film of moisture resulting presumably from transudation.

Attempts to quantitate the amount and production rate of vaginal fluid have been made by several investigators using a variety of techniques.

Table I shows a summary of these studies. In the presence of the uterus the mean amount of vaginal secretion varied between 0.76 and 2.7 g/24 hours. In hysterectomized women who had also had oophorectomy the mean amount of vaginal fluid was 1.56 g/24 hours. This was increased when ovarian function was maintained or estrogen supplementation was provided (Perl et al., 1959).

During sexual excitation an increase in the production of vaginal fluid has been observed. Masters and Johnson (1961, 1966) found that within 10–30 seconds of commencement of sexual stimuli brought about by masturbation or artificial coitus an increase in the production of fluid on the surface of vaginal mucosa occurred. This phenomenon named vaginal lubrication appeared like a sweating reaction. Individual droplets of the transuding fluid suddenly appeared over the rugae making the epithelium look like a perspiration-beaded forehead. With continued stimulation, these droplets coalesced to form a glairy glistening coat over the entire vaginal wall. The lubricating material is probably the result of a marked dilatation of the vaginal venous plexus and congestion. In women with artificial vaginas made from skin where there is no possibility of cervical or Bartholin's glands secretion contributing to vaginal fluid, vaginal lubrication still takes place.

TABLE I. Production Rate of Vaginal Fluid

References	No. of Cases	Method of Collection	Amount mean ± SD (g/24h)	Uterus Present
Stone and Gamble 1959	113	Swab with cotton wad	0.76 ± 0.004	yes
Dusitsin et al., 1967	35	Vag. tampon cervical cap	2.7	yes
Perl et al., 1959	6	Cotton and tampon	1.89 ± 0.12	no
Perl et al., 1959	10	"	1.56 ± 0.05	no (+BSO)
Perl et al., 1959	5	"	1.97 ± 0.05	no (+BSO +EST)

BSO: Bilateral salpingo-oophorectomy
EST: Estrogen

Composition of Vaginal Fluid

Electrolytes. Vaginal fluid contains inorganic and organic substances. Inorganic constituents investigated include Na^+, K^+ and Cl^- (Table II.) The concentrations of K^+, Na^+ and Cl^- show marked variation from those of plasma. The K^+ is some 6.6 times greater, while the Na^+ and Cl^- are approximately 46 and 61% of the plasma levels. Wagner and Levin (1978) have postulated that the production and modification of vaginal fluid in the basal and sexually excited states appears to involve a number of mechanisms. In the basal (sexually unstimulated) state both Na^+ and Cl^- continuously enter the vaginal lumen from the cervical secretion and by transudation from the blood through the vaginal epithelium.

The vaginal epithelium, however, actively reabsorbs Na^+ ions back into the interstitial fluid generating a transvaginal electrical potential difference (p.d.). Chlorides presumably follow passively. This p.d. creates an electrical force for the movement of plasma K^+ into the lumen. Thus under basal conditions the vaginal epithelium is bathed by a fluid which has a Na^+Cl^- concentration usually well below that of plasma but with a K^+ concentration many times greater than plasma. It is possible that the high K^+ levels may come about partly from cell exfoliation and subsequent disruption and liberation of their intracellular K^+. During sexual stimulation the blood flow to the vagina is greatly increased by vasodilatation.

These hemodynamic changes cause an increase in the formation of a NaCl-rich fluid from the plasma which transudes through the vaginal epithelium and saturates its reabsorbtive capacity for Na^+. The fluid finally emerges modified as the glairy lubricating fluid on the surface of the vagina which facilitates coital activities. As vaginal fluid emerges from the plasma it will initially have a pH of 7.3. It will thus partially neutralize the acidity of the basal vaginal fluid increasing the surface pH of the vaginal wall and protecting the ejaculated sperm from the acid environment of the unstimulated vagina.

Urea. The mean urea concentration of the basal vaginal fluid is nearly twice that of the plasma (Table I). Urea is present in the vagina of all women and its level is highest in the midluteal phase. Preti and Huggins (1978) found concen-

TABLE II. Urea and Electrolyte Constituents of Vaginal Fluid

Constituents	Vaginal Fluid Mean ± SE	Plasma Mean ± SE
Urea mg %	49 ± 8 (5)	25 ± 2 (5)
K^+ mmol/L	23 ± 2 (12)	3.5 ± 0.1 (16)
Na^+ mmol/L	61 ± 7 (11)	132 ± 0.6 (14)
Cl^- mmol/L	62 ± 5 (12)	102 ± 0.7 (15)

trations of 10, 14, 21, and 11 mg/g of secretion during the follicular phase, midcycle, midluteal and late luteal phases, respectively.

Fatty Acids. The volatile fatty acids responsible for the sex attractant properties of vaginal secretion in the rhesus monkey are normal physiological constituents of the vaginal fluid of healthy young women (Preti and Huggins, 1978; Bonsall and Michael, 1978). All women produce some acetic and lactic acids in their vagina. About one third of women also produce samples that contain more than 10 Mμg of other volatile acids.

The content in acids in vaginal fluid increases dramatically with estrogen treatment and decreases with progesterone administration. Acetic acid is present in considerable amounts throughout the menstrual cycle and shows less variation than the C3–C6 acids. A preovulatory increase in both acetic acid and total aliphatic acid content of vaginal fluid during the menstrual cycle has been observed (Figure 1).

Michael and Bonsall (1977) have shown that aliphatic acids are produced in relatively large amounts in the vagina of some women (Producers). The mean acid content in these women consisted of acetic acid 183.1, propanoic 82.9, methylpropanoic 6.1, butanoic 34.1 and methyl-butanoic 14.1 ug%. According to Preti and Huggins (1978) the aliphatic acids consistently found in acid producers are acetic, propranoic, isobutyric, n-butyric, isovaleric and 2-methyl butyric.

Human olfaction is apparently able to discriminate samples of vaginal fluid obtained from producers and nonproducers (those who produce only small amounts of volatile acids).

Subjects using oral contraceptive preparations have significantly lower acid content than the nonusers. This difference is particularly well marked in the C3–C6 acids. In oral contraceptive users the preovulatory rise of volative fatty acids is also absent (Figure 2).

Aliphatic acids in the human vagina probably originate from carbohydrates. Human vaginal fluid contains carbohydrates derived from epithelial glycogen. The aerobic lactobacillus Döderlein's bacillus ferments the carbohydrate to aliphatic acids.

The precise role of volatile acids of human vaginal fluid is not known. In lower animals, however, the part played by olfaction in the reproductive process is well established. In rhesus monkeys, males made anosmic by insertion of a nasal plug do not respond to changes in the attractiveness of females brought about by the administration of hormones until their nasal plugs have been removed. In other studies it has been shown that vaginal fluid collected by lavage from ovariectomized estrogen treated females when applied to the sexual skin area of

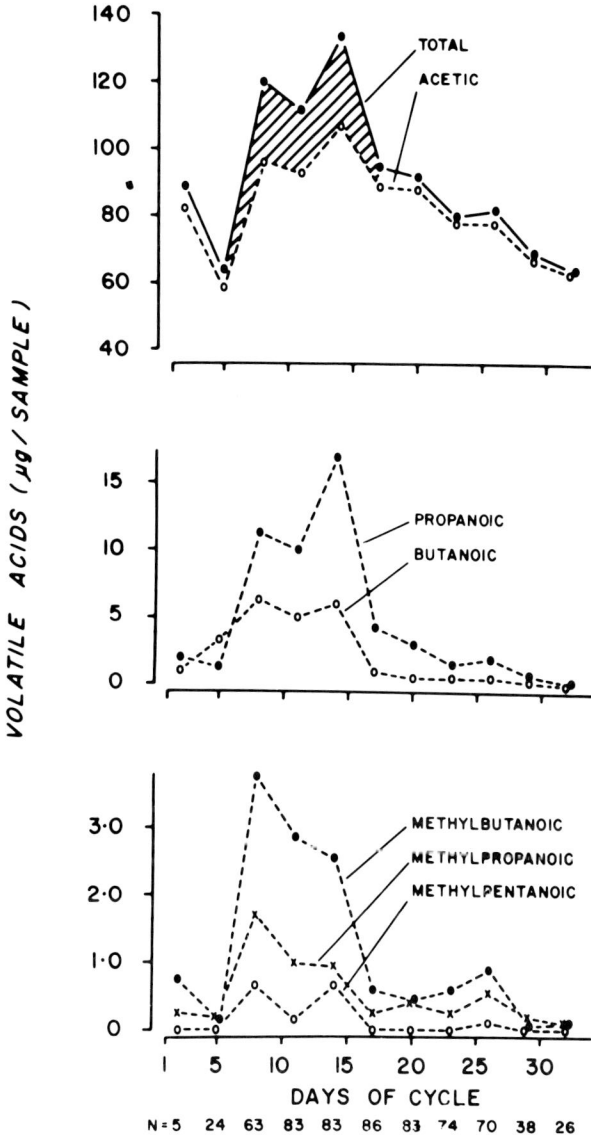

FIGURE 1. Changes in the total aliphatic acid and in the acetic acid contents of vaginal fluid during the menstrual cycle. Data from 47 women have been combined using successive 3-day means. The hatched area represents the contribution of C3–C6 acids to the increase seen near midcycle.
Middle: changes in the individual straight chain acid content.
Bottom: changes in the individual branched chain acid content.
The more odoriferous C3–C6 acids increase conspicuously near midcycle.
Day 1: first day of menstruation on which the cycles are aligned
N = number of samples
From Michael et al., 1975.

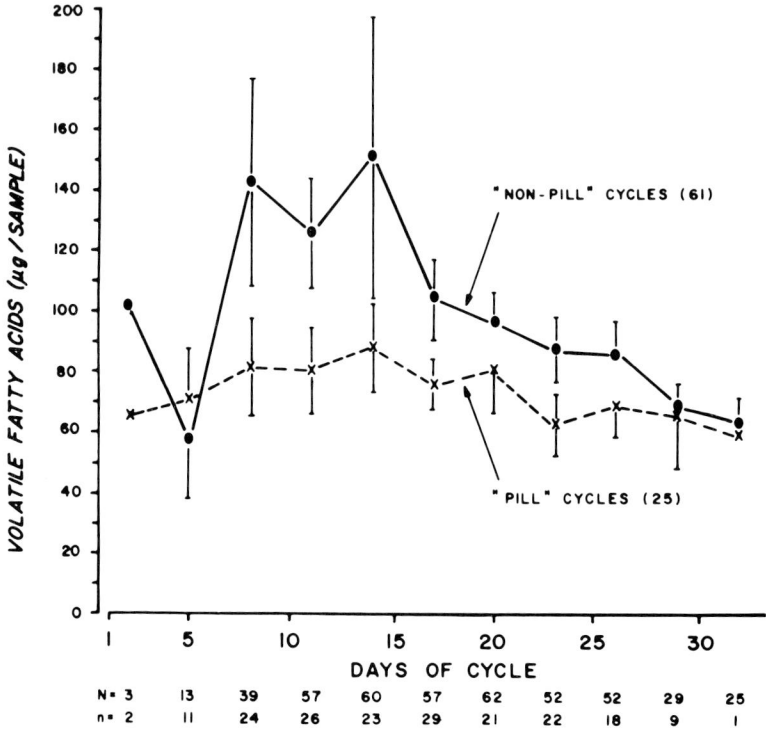

FIGURE 2. Changes in the content of volatile fatty acids in the vaginal fluid of women using oral contraceptives compared with that of women with normal cycles arranged according to successive 3-day periods of the menstrual cycle. The rise before midcycle is abolished in women taking oral contraceptives and levels are generally lower.
  N = number of nonpill samples
  n = number of pill samples
  Vertical bars = standard errors of the mean
  From Michael et al., 1974.

ovariectomized females stimulate the sexual interest and activity of the males. The substances in the vaginal fluid responsible for this effect have been identified to be C2–C6 aliphatic acids (Bonsall and Michael, 1978). Whether or not the odoriferous acids of the vaginal fluid have any influence in human reproduction remains to be explored. It is possible however that in the process of evolution this particular function has been lost in homo sapiens.

Amino Acids and Proteins. Fourteen amino acids have been identified in vaginal fluid. They are alanine, arginine, aspartic acid, glycine, histidine, isoleucine, leucine, proline, serine, taurine, threonine, tryptophan and valine (Gregoire et al., 1959; Hunter and Nicholas, 1959). Among these, only histidine has been quantitatively assayed. Histidine content of human vaginal fluid ranged between 2.2 and 9.9 mg%. Mean histidine levels were higher in late luteal phase compared to other phases of the menstrual cycle (Dusitsin et al., 1967). Amino acid constituents of hysterectomized subjects have not been investigated. It is, therefore, not known whether amino acids found in the vaginal fluid of normal women originate from the vagina or from contamination by cervical mucus which is known to contain free amino acids.

Proteins of vaginal fluid have been investigated in our laboratories. In these studies samples of vaginal secretion and cervical mucus were collected from healthy adult women between day 10 and day 20 of the menstrual cycle. Vaginal fluid was also obtained from hysterectomized (premenopausal) women. Those who showed evidence of vaginitis and/or cervicitis were excluded from the study. To obtain vaginal fluid or cervical mucus, an unlubricated speculum was inserted into the vagina. The cervix was cleansed with a dry cotton swab and the mucus aspirated from the cervical canal into a tuberculin syringe (without needle). The individual mucus samples were centrifuged at 27,000 x g for 90 minutes, and the supernatants were collected, lyophilized, and stored frozen at $-20°$ C until used. The lyophilized materials were reconstituted by dissolving them in 0.2 ml of deionized water. Vaginal fluid was collected by gently scraping the mucosa with a metal spatula. Samples were obtained only from the lateral wall of the vagina to avoid contamination by cervical mucus. Scrapings were dissolved in 1.0 ml of 0.2 M $(NH_4)_2 HCO_3$ buffer (pH 7.2) and centrifuged at 1085 X g for 30 minutes to remove cellular debris; the supernatant was then collected. A portion of each supernatant was analyzed for total protein by a modification of the technique of Lowry et al. (1951); the remainder was lyophilized and stored frozen at $-20°$ C until used. Samples were reconstituted in 0.2 ml of deionized water.

The protein composition of the vaginal and cervical supernatants was analyzed by microimmunodiffusion and immunoelectrophoretic techniques (Ouchterlony, 1958; Scheidegger, 1955). Specific antihuman sera were used to develop protein arcs.

The total protein content of 40 individual samples of vaginal secretion obtained from normal and hysterectomized women ranged from 15 to 26 $\mu g/ml$, with a mean of 18 $\mu g/ml$. No significant difference in total protein content was apparent when samples obtained from normal subjects were compared with those from hysterectomized women.

Immunoelectrophoretic and immunodiffusion analyses performed on vaginal fluid obtained from 29 normal (nonhysterectomized) women using the specific antihuman sera demonstrated the presence of albumin, α_1-antitrypsin, α_2-haptoglobin, α_2-macroglobulin, transferrin, immunoglobulin IgA, and IgG in the majority of samples tested. β-Lipoprotein, $\gamma G(K)$ (Bence Jones) orosomucoid, ceruloplasmin, and IgM were also detected in some samples, but C-reactive protein and fibrin were never observed (Table III).

The results of immunoelectrophoretic and immunodiffusion analyses using vaginal secretion obtained from 11 hysterectomized women are summarized in Table IV. Albumin, α_1-antitrypsin, ceruloplasmin, transferrin, IgA, IgG, and $\gamma G(K)$ were present in the majority of samples tested. Fibrin and C-reactive protein were again absent. α_2-Haptoglobin, α_2-macroglobulin, β-lipoprotein, orosomucoid, and IgM—which were present in vaginal fluid from nonhysterectomized women— were not detectable in samples obtained from hysterectomized subjects.

All proteins identified in the vaginal secretion were also found in cervical mucus. However, C-reactive protein and fibrin were present in cervical mucus but were not observed in the vaginal fluid (Table V).

TABLE III. Protein Content of Human Vaginal Secretions Obtained from 29 Normal Women (Nonhysterectomized)

Protein	Reaction			% Positive
	$-^a$	$+^b$	$++^c$	
Albumin	0	4	25	100
Immunoglobulin (IgG, IgA, IgM)	1	15	13	96.5
γ Chain	2	17	10	93.1
Transferrin	2	21	6	93.1
γG	3	16	10	89.6
$α_2$-Haptoglobin	3	23	3	89.6
$α_1$-Antitrypsin	3	21	5	89.6
γA	4	18	7	86.2
$α_2$-Macroglobulin	8	15	6	72.4
β-Lipoprotein	25	4	0	13.7
γ G(K) (Bence Jones)	26	3	0	10.3
Orosomucoid	26	3	0	10.3
Ceruloplasmin	28	1	0	3.4
γM	28	1	0	3.4
C-reactive protein	29	0	0	0
Fibrin	29	0	0	0

[a] $-$, Negative precipitin reaction (no precipitation bands present).
[b] $+$, Positive precipitin reaction.
[c] $++$, Strongly positive reaction (according to the density of the precipitin bands).

From: Raffi, Moghissi, and Sacco, Fertil. Steril. (1977).

DISCUSSION

Since vaginal secretion consists primarily of a transudate from the vaginal mucosa, the presence of a large number of serum type proteins in vaginal fluid is to be expected. Contamination of vaginal fluid by cervical mucus is possible and makes the precise assessment of specific vaginal fluid proteins difficult. Many serum proteins, including the immunoglobulins, are normally present in cervical mucus and may become mixed with vaginal secretion (Schumacher, 1973; Moghissi, 1973).

The results of immunoelectrophoretic and immunodiffusion studies demonstrate a different pattern of proteins in vaginal secretion collected from normal and hysterectomized women. $α_2$-Haptoglobin, $α_2$-macroglobulin, β-lipoprotein, orosomucoid, and IgM are present in vaginal fluid of nonhysterectomized women but are not observed in samples obtained from hysterectomized subjects. Since these proteins were also detected in cervical secretions, their presence in vaginal secretion is likely to be the result of contamination by cervical mucus. It is also possible that the amount of these proteins in vaginal fluid of hysterectomized women is so small as to be undetectable by the assay methods used in our studies.

The precise source of vaginal fluid protein is, at present, a matter of speculation. However, it is likely that the bulk of these proteins are diffused from serum through the mucosa into the vagina.

The absence of certain proteins ($α_2$-haptoglobin, $α_2$-macroglobulin, β-lipo-

TABLE IV. Protein Content of Human Vaginal Secretions Obtained from 11 Hysterectomized (Nonmenopausal) Women

Protein	Reaction			% Positive
	$-$[a]	$+$[b]	$++$[c]	
Albumin	0	4	7	100
γG (IgG)	0	9	2	100
α_1-Antitrypsin	0	3	8	100
Transferrin	0	7	4	100
γA (IgA)	1	7	3	90.9
γ Chain	1	8	2	90.9
γ G(K) (Bence Jones)	2	6	3	81.8
Ceruloplasmin	2	5	4	81.8
C-reactive protein	11	0	0	0
Fibrin	11	0	0	0
γM (IgM)	11	0	0	0
α_2-Haptoglobin	11	0	0	0
β-Lipoprotein	11	0	0	0
α_2-Macroglobulin	11	0	0	0
Orosomucoid	11	0	0	0

[a] $-$, Negative precipitin reaction (no precipitin bands present).
[b] $+$, Positive p recipitin reaction.
[c] $++$, Strongly positive reaction (according to the density of the precipitin bands).

From: Raffi, Moghissi, and Sacco, Fertil. Steril. (1977).

TABLE V. Comparison of Protein Contents of Vaginal Secretions and Cervical Mucus Obtained from the Same Individual

Protein	Cervical Mucus[a]			Vaginal Secretions[a]		
	Subj. 1	Subj. 2	Subj. 3	Subj. 1	Subj. 2	Subj. 3
Albumin	+	+	+	+	+	+
Ceruloplasmin	+	−	+	+	−	−
C-reactive protein	+	−	−	−	−	−
Fibrin	−	+	−	−	−	−
γA	+	−	+	−	+	+
γ Chain	+	+	+	−	+	+
γG	+	+	+	+	+	+
γG(K) (Bence Jones)	+	+	−	−	+	+
γM	+	−	+	−	−	−
α_2-Haptoglobin	−	+	+	−	−	−
β-Lipoprotein	+	+	−	−	−	−
α_2-Macroglobulin	+	−	+	−	−	−
Orosomucoid	+	+	−	−	−	−
Transferrin	+	+	+	+	+	+
α_1-Antitrypsin	+	+	+	+	+	+

[a] +, Positive precipitin reaction; −, negative precipitin reaction (no precipitation bands present).

From: Raffi, Moghissi, and Sacco, Fertil. Steril. (1977).

protein, and orosomucoid) in the vaginal fluid of hysterectomized women indicated that they may originate from cervical mucus. There is also a distinct possibility that some proteins, particularly the immunoglobulins, may be synthesized locally by the vaginal mucosa. In fact, biosynthesis of IgG and IgA in the vaginal tissues of the rabbit has been reported (Behrman and Lieberman, 1973).

The presence of immunoglobulin in the vaginal fluid demonstrated in our studies and those of Roig de Vargas-Linares (1978) indicate that the vagina has an immune function. Immunocomponent cells including plasma cells have been demonstrated in the vaginal mucosa. It appears then that in the human vagina a secretory immune system exists under physiological conditions serving as a mucous barrier which is controlled by estrogen. In the normal organ this nonspecific immune response is probably part of a defense mechanism which may be responsible for the production of naturally occurring antibodies present in the vaginal fluid.

REFERENCES

Behrman, S.J., Lieberman, M.E.: Biosynthesis of immunoglobulin by the human cervix. In The Biology of the Cervix, edited by R.J. Blandau and K.S. Moghissi. Chicago, University of Chicago Press, 1973, p. 235.

Bonsall, R.W., Michael, R.P.: Volatile odoriferous acids in vaginal fluid. In The Human Vagina, edited by E.S.E. Hafez, T.N. Evans. Holland, Elsevier, 1978, p. 167.

Dusitsin, N., Gregoire, A.T., Johnson, W.D. and Rakoff, A.E.: Histidine in human vaginal fluid. Obstet. Gynecol. 29 (1967), 125.

Gregoire, A.T., Lang, W.R. and Ward, K.: The qualitative identification of free amino acids in human vaginal fluid. Ann. N.Y. Acad. Sci. 83 (1959), 185.

Hunter, C.A. and Nicholas, H.J.: A study of vaginal acids. Am. J. Obstet. Gynecol. 78 (1959), 282.

Lowry, O.H., Rosebrough, N.J., Farr, A.L. and Randall, J.: Protein measurement with the Folin phenol reagent. J. Biol. Chem. 193 (1951), 265.

Masters, W.H., Johnson, V.E.: The physiology of the vaginal reproductive function. West. J. Surg. Obstet. Gynecol. 69 (1961), 105.

Masters, W.H., Johnson, V.E.: Human Sexual Response. Boston, Little, Brown and Company, 1966.

Michael, R.P. and Bonsall, R.W.: Chemical signals and primate behavior. In Chemical Signals in Vertebrate, edited by D. Muller-Schwarze and M. Mozell, New York, Plenum Press, 1977, pp. 251–271.

Michael, R.P., Bonsall, R.W. and Jutner, M.: Volatile fatty acids "Copulins" in human vaginal secretions. Psychoneuroendocrinology 1 (1975), 153.

Michael, R.P., Bonsall, R.W. and Worner, P.: Human vaginal secretions: volatile fatty acid content. Science 186 (1974), 1217.

Moghissi, K.S.: Composition and function of cervical secretion. In Handbook of Physiology, edited by R.O. Greep, Sect. 7: Endocrinology, Vol. 2: Female Reproductive System, Part 2. Washington, D.C., American Physiological Society, 1973, p. 25.

Ouchterlony, O.: Diffusion in gel methods for immunological analysis. 2. Prog. Allergy 5 (1958), 1.

Perl, J.I., Miller, G. and Shimonzato, Y.: Vaginal fluid subsequent to panhysterectomy. Am. J. Obstet. Gynecol. 78 (1959), 285.

Preti, G. and Huggins, G.R.: Organic constituents of vaginal secretions. In The Human Vagina, editors E.S.E. Hafez, T.N. Evans. North Holland, Elsevier, 1978, p. 151.

Raffi, R.O., Moghissi, K.S. and Sacco, A.G.: Proteins of human vaginal fluid. Fertil Steril 28 (1977), 1345.

Roig de Vargas-Linares, C.E.: The vagina as a source of immunoglobulins. In The Human Vagina, editors E.S.E. Hafez, T.N. Evans. North Holland, Elsevier, 1978, p. 193.

Scheidegger, J.J.: Gel immunoelectrophoresis technique. Int. Arch. Allergy Appl. Immunol. 7 (1955), 103.

Schumacher, G.F.B.: Soluble proteins of human cervical mucus. In Cervical Mucus in Human Reproduction, edited by M. Elstein, K.S. Moghissi and R. Borth. Geneva, World Health Organization, Scriptor, Copenhagen, 1973, p. 93.

Stone, A., Gamble, C.J.: The quantity of vaginal fluid. Am. J. Obstet. Gynecol. 78 (1959), 279.

Wagner, G., Levin, R.J.: Vaginal fluid. In The Human Vagina, editors E.S.E. Hafez, T.N. Evans, North Holland, Elsevier/North-Holland Biomedical Press, 1978, p. 121.

VAGINAL TRANSUDATION

G. Wagner

SUMMARY

The assessment of production rate of vaginal fluid in fertile women is discussed using the literature and our own results. Collection of fluid in tampons and direct gravimetric measurements gave an estimate of a daily production of vaginal fluid of around 5 g.

The electrolyte content as well as transvaginal electrical potential differences showed that passive transudation and active resorption of electrolytes and water was taking place.

Methods to assess vaginal blood flow are presented and a new technique of applying radioactive Xenon is introduced.

The above mentioned methods have been used for study of the mechanism of increase in vaginal fluid during sexual arousal.

The fluid production rate increases by at least three times and the flow rate on the order of 5-6 times.

A theory of the mechanism of this phenomenon is put forward and is based on the assumption of a flow increase brought about by precapillary vasodilation increasing capillary pressure and surface thereby facilitating transcapillary fluid transport.

INTRODUCTION

Since 1973 a course of medical sexology for undergraduate students at the University of Copenhagen has been given. As this field is reaching into various

Institute of Medical Physiology B Panum Institute, University of Copenhagen, Denmark disciplines many specialties have been involved in the teaching. The inspiration of such a teamwork has been of great value and the outcome of interdisciplinary teaching and discussions has to a great extent revealed the gaps in our understanding of human sexuality. One specific area where great ignorance existed (and still exists) is in the function of the sex organs during sexual arousal and climax. The physiology of the female and male genital organs has received little attention by the medical researcher.

ration of such a teamwork has been of great value and the outcome of interdisciplinary teaching and discussions has to a great extent revealed the gaps in our understanding of human sexuality. One specific area where great ignorance existed (and still exists) is in the function of the sex organs during sexual arousal and climax. The physiology of the female and male genital organs has received little attention by the medical researcher.

In 1976 we started a programme to investigate basal phenomena in sexual arousal partly to illuminate the physiology and partly to find ways by which improvement of diagnoses in sexual disorders could be undertaken. After three years there has been a gain in understanding in the function of the vagina but not enough to improve diagnosis or treatment of sexual dysfunctions. This has however been the case in the simultaneous male studies.

The studies of the functions of the vagina have been undertaken at the Institute of Medical Physiology in Copenhagen in conjunction with visiting collaborators, namely Roy J. Levin, Ph.D., Univ. Sheffield, James P. Semmens, M.D., University South Carolina and Bent Ottesen, M.D., Univ. of Copenhagen.

This paper will present and discuss the circumstantial and methodological problems in assessment of whether a transudation of fluid across the vaginal wall in the human female exists. It will further present data on the influence of estrogen upon the vaginal function as well as on estimates of blood flow rate of the vaginal wall under basal conditions and during sexual excitement.

One well recognized problem in clinical gynecology and sexology is that of dryness of the vagina. Sexual intercourse with penile intromission may be painful or even impossible. The condition is well known in diabetic women, in postclimacteric and in puerperal women. The moisture of the vaginal wall normally seen at inspection may be absent and this may be the only objective finding in such cases.

The fluid normally seen in the vagina may derive from many sources as fluids from the ovarian follicles, peritoneal cavity, oviducts, endometrium, cervix and the vestibular glands as well as from an ejaculate. The vaginal wall however does not contain any glandular elements, still it is known and documented that women who have had total hysterectomy and who do not receive intravaginal ejaculates may have a completely normal moisture of the vagina as well as they may be able to produce an increase in the vaginal fluid volume when sexually aroused.

The increase in fluid on the vaginal wall was described as vaginal lubrication (Masters 1959) and was found to occur during simultaneous sexual stimulation. The phenomenon was verified by filming and later confirmed under similar conditions (Wagner 1974).

The Production Rate of Vaginal Fluid

Different approaches have been tried to measure the "normal" amount of fluid in the human vagina (Odeblad 1964, Dusitsin et al., 1967, Wagner and Levin 1977, Wagner and Levin 1978a). Odeblad placed tampons at different levels of the vagina and separated these areas by rubber diaphragms including one that closed off the cervix. The average volume produced was in 12 normal women (each examined a single day) 4.5 g per 24 hrs plus 1.25 g from the cervix. The day before collection and the following day the external discharge was collected and measured to be about 1.5 g per 24 hrs. Dusitsin and collaborators used female prisoners and inserted tampons after a cervical cap had been fitted during various phases of the cycle but as the aim of the study was to measure amino acids the volume given in the paper has not been related to the phases of the menstrual cycle or to the number of participants in the various phases.

A mean value close to 3 g per 24 hrs was found.

In order to measure the total vaginal fluid during the menstrual cycle a group of women all within medical or paramedical profession was selected and carefully instructed about the insertion of a tampon into the vagina each day for a period of 4 hours at the same time of the day during the period between two menstruations. The tampons were pre-weighed and each was placed in a separate airtight numbered vial. After removal the subject placed the tampon into the vial which was kept frozen until examination. Table I indicates the findings in 165 samples collected during 8 menstrual cycles in seven women. The range is from 2.9–16.8 g/24 hours, the average of 7.5 g/24 hrs. Only 10% of the samples were above 10 g/24 hrs and these samples were scattered throughout the intermenstrual period with no correlation to supposed ovulation time. Similarly no pattern of increase or decrease in fluid production during the period could be observed in the individual cases, nor when when the results were pooled.

A direct approach has been tried as well by applying a commercially available probe on the surface of the vagina (Evaporimeter, Ep 1, Servo Med, Sweden). The probe and its placement in the vagina is shown schematically in Figure 1. The measuring principle (Nilsson et al., 1975) consists of measuring the relative humidity by two sensors placed at constant distance from each other and close to the surface to be measured. The evaporation from the surface and thereby the water transport through the cylindrical wall is then electronically calculated following the law of diffusion and read out as water evaporation in $g/m^2/hour$.

The vaginal measurements were undertaken in seven women. Before this the evaporation of the subject's non sweating palm and the dorsum of her hand was measured. The evaporation from the posterior vaginal wall at a distance of some 5 cm from the introitus was then measured. The values obtained had a range from

TABLE I

No of Samples Intermenstr. Period	Calculated Range	Production Rate (g/24hrs) Average
23	6-12	7.4
22	4.8-16.8	9.6
21	4.8-9.6	9.1
23	4.3-16.8	7.6
19	3.6-12	6
21	3.6-10	6
16	2.9-15.6	6.7
20	4.8-12.6	7.6
n = 165	2.9-16.8	7.5 ± 1.3 s.d.

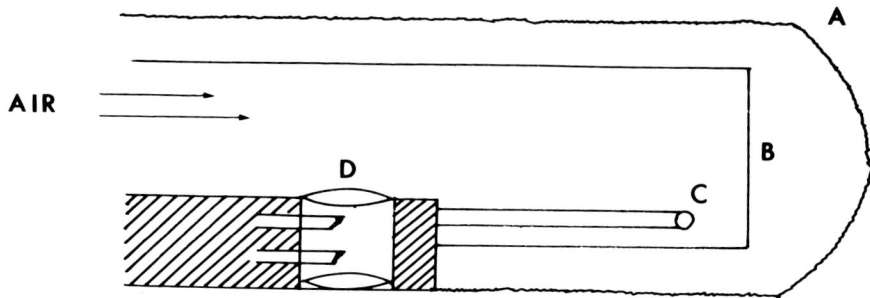

FIGURE 1. Schematic drawing of measure of evaporation from the vaginal wall.
A. Vaginal Wall.
B. Cylindrical holder to create free space around the measuring probe.
C. Hole through which slight suction is applied.
D. Probe with cylindrical well in which the two sensors are placed in fixed distances to the vaginal surface.

82 to 97 g/m^2/hour. These figures were close to those obtained from the subjects' palms, but from 6–10 times higher than the values of the dorsum of the hand. Assuming that the vaginal surface is about 50 cm^2 the calculated fluid production from the vaginal wall would be in the range of 9–11 g/24 hours. The set-up outlined here cannot be said to be ideal as a slight suction had to be applied to the inner space of the spacing tube to avoid condensation of water. The suction may have influenced the measurements and the calculated figures therefore may be too high. Further work to improve this direct measurement is thus needed.

From the results presented it would be reasonable to conclude that an average daily production of fluid from the vaginal wall would be around 5 g. Assuming that an extra 1–3 g of cervical fluid joins this volume a total volume of 7–8 is produced, but only about 1.5 g is leaving the vagina through the introitus. The concept of an internal vaginal water circulation has been proposed (Odeblad 1964). He demonstrated that by placing a tube in the lower third of the vagina it was possible to collect almost the same amount as that normally produced. Further studies of this resorption phenomenon are not to be found in the literature.

Electrolytes in Vaginal Fluid

Before considerations of the resorptive mechanisms of the vaginal wall can be given it is necessary to obtain information on the electrolyte concentrations of the most dominant ions in most biological transport mechanisms as well as on the orientation of any electrical potential on the two sides of the vaginal epithelium.

By placing pre-weighed filter papers in the vagina in the supine lying woman it was found (Wagner and Levine 1978a) that sodium concentration in vaginal fluid was considerably lower than that found in the plasma 60 mM versus 132 mM/1. In subjects fitted with tampons for 4-hour periods somewhat higher figures were found possibly due to cervical fluid influence. The range was 60–100 mM/kg vaginal fluid with a mean of 82 mM ± 21.9 s.d. The low sodium concentration was always accompanied by a chloride concentration lower than that of the plasma. In the tampon samples a mean of 76 ± 15 s.d. mM/kg vaginal fluid. Opposed to these low values the potassium concentration was inevitably found to be very much higher than that of plasma, namely 29 ± 10 mM. Although these concentrations are not corrected for dry weight of the vaginal fluid they are obviously different from the findings in plasma therefore supporting the concept that an active handling of the ions must take place in order to account for their uneven distribution. To further assess ionic movement two dialysis sacs, each containing 1 ml of the subject's own freshly drawn serum, were placed in the vagina of five women. Before the placement of the sacs the vaginal wall had been swabbed dry and no free fluid was visible. In all cases the concentrations of sodium and chloride had fallen when the sacs were analyzed after removal. On the average a fall in sodium concentration by 17 mM/l in 4-5 hours and by 32 mM in 15-21 hours was noted. The fall in chloride concentration was by 8 and 21 mM during the same period while the potassium concentration increased by 6 and 9 mM. The ion exchange during the 15-21 hour period had brought Na^+ and Cl^- close to equilibrium while a $K+$ equilibrium had still not been obtained (Levin and Wagner 1978).

The Transvaginal Potential Difference

In 1976 a study showed that a transvaginal potential difference with a negative luminal polarity existed (Duncan and Levin 1976). They found in a cross-sectional study of 39 women a potential difference of 25.4 ± 1.9 mV (millivolt) in the follicular phase and 25.2 ± 1.4 mV in the luteal phase.

Applying the same technique a plastic cannula filled with 0.9% NaCl is inserted subcutaneously into the forearm and used as a reference electrode assuming that an isopotential condition exists in the extracellular volume of the body. The vaginal electrode is a plastic catheter fitted with a cotton wick and filled with physiological saline. Into the saline of each electrode an agar-KCl bridge is placed leading to a calomel cell that is connected to the high-impedance electrometer (Figure 2).

In these studies we have found consistently higher values 44 ± 7 mV in a larger group of women than Duncan and Levin but consistent with these investigators no pattern related to the menstrual cycle was seen. The potential measurement at one given spot has a high degree of reproducibility. If the vaginal electrode is placed on the cervix the potential drops to 8–10 mV and to 12–15 mV just outside the introitus.

The findings of high potassium and low sodium concentrations in relation to plasma and a negative lumen potential may well indicate an active transporting mechanism of the vaginal epithelium. A passive distribution of K^+ according to the measured potential difference can only account for about 50% of the luminal K^+. Cell shedding or active secretion are two possible explanations for the rest of the potassium. The Na^+- concentration in the lumen is clearly against its electrochemical gradient and Na^+ therefore has to be actively transferred from the lumen into the subepithelial tissue. As a consequence of this water may pass passively from the lumen and back to the intracellular space. A precise account of the handling of Cl^- cannot be given as the movement of this ion may be linked to Na^+ and/or K^+ in a yet unpredictable way. The creation of fluid in the vagina therefore seems to be going on during the whole intermenstrual period as well as the absorption of fluid. It is well known that substances may pass from the blood into the vagina and that absorption of compounds from the vagina takes place (Hartmann 1959). The magnitude of the fluid fluxes could well be influenced by haemodynamic changes in the subepithelial tissues and methods of evaluation of the blood flow through the vaginal wall therefore have been tested.

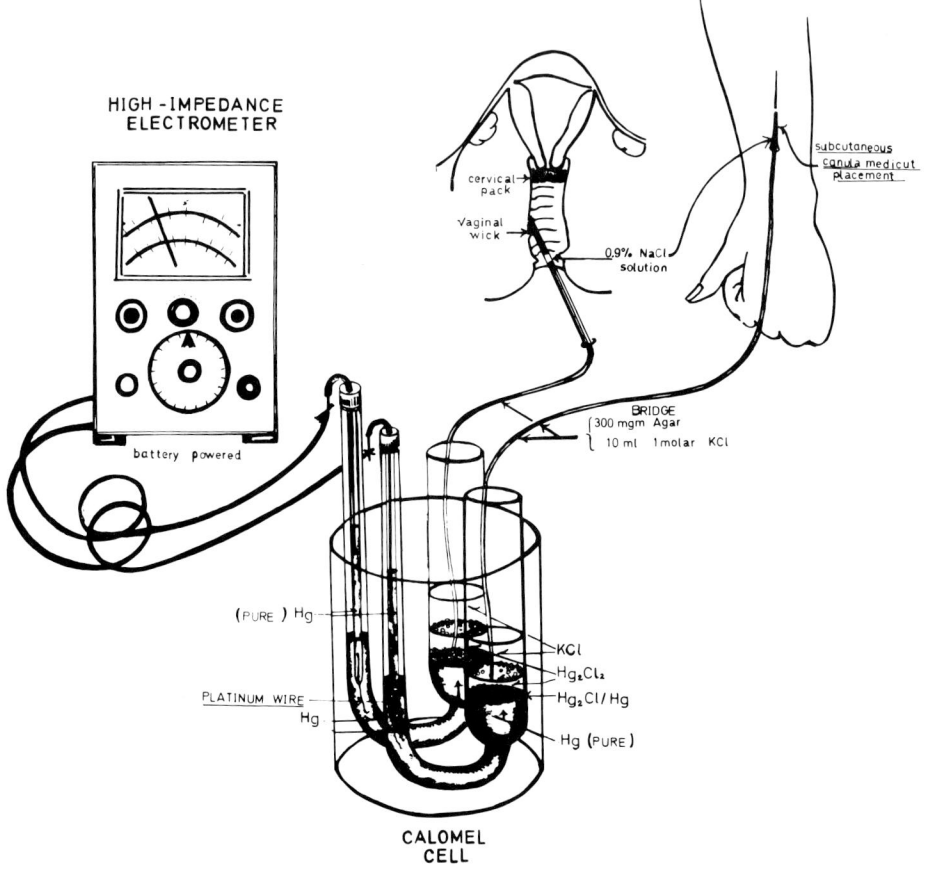

FIGURE 2. The arrangement and equipment needed to measure transvaginal potential difference.

Vaginal Photopletysmography

The principle of this measurement is based on the fact that infra-red light shown into the tissue will be scattered by the red blood corpuscles. The more scatter the less reflection occurs. The reflection is registered by a photocell. Thus it is possible with a small time lag to follow the phasic changes in the amount of blood that occurs as a consequence of each heartstroke within the region explored. For detailed discussion of the use and technical considerations see Hoon 1978 or Gillan and Brindley 1979. The amplitude of the recorded 'volume pulse' will be related to the local stroke volume. Whether the phasic or the mean reflectance of the cardiac cycle is measured the problem of artifacts occurring due to movements of the vagina still exists. In the resting 'basal' phase this may be of less importance. But during sexual stimulation the vaginal movement (i.e. tenting effect) or pelvic floor contractions may interfere in an unpredictable way. Over long periods the vaginal 'volume pulse' in the lying and resting female did not show changes. The method does not provide any quantitative measurement in blood flow but may provide information about increase or decrease of stroke volume which when compared to the heart frequency may indicate changes of flow.

Heat Method

Applying heat to a metal disc and keeping the temperature at the probe constant was first introduced in vaginal measurements by Cohen and Shapiro 1971. They measured the rate at which heat had to be supplied to the thermistor in order to keep a set temperature. In our studies a commercially available electrode has been applied (TCM 1, Radiometer, Copenhagen). This probe contains an oxygen electrode, a heating element and temperature sensor and is used to assess transcutaneously the pO_2 of the blood underlying the area to be measured upon, assuming that the heat (43°) will dilate vessels to such a degree that the blood contained therein is fully arterialized. As the heat conduction of the tissue in part will be due to removal by the blood an increase in heat consumption will be positively correlated to an increase in flow or temporarily to an increase in blood pooling of the area. To apply the method a suction device keeping the electrode in close apposition to the surface was constructed (Wagner and Levin 1978b). Figure 3 shows schematically the system described. When the electrode is applied time for equilibration (15-20 minutes) has to be allowed for. The basal heat consumption in mW (milliwatts) to keep the temperature constant may differ from subject to subject and within the same subject. There is no relation to the period in the menstrual phase. When two electrodes are placed in the same individual simultaneously they may or may not differ from each other in their basal readings but if any change occurs it will be parallel at the two sites.

In a group of postclimacteric women who were not oestrogen treated the average heat value of the group was found to increase significantly when they had

FIGURE 3. Schematic drawing showing suction device attached to the vaginal wall and heated oxygen electrode in the center.

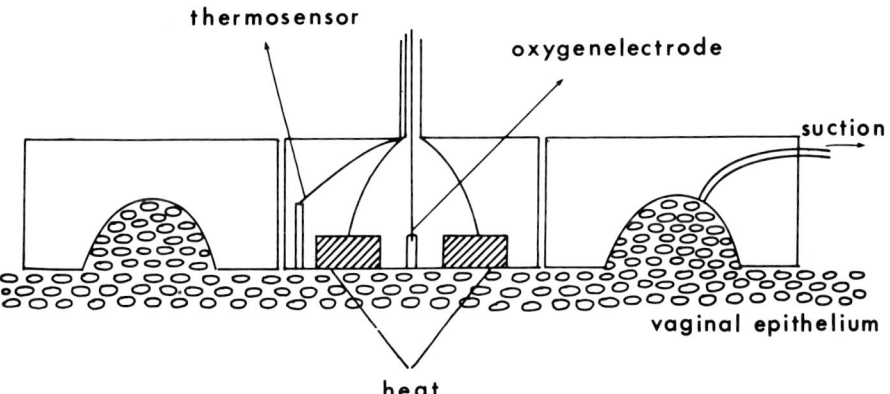

been given oestrogen as soon as three weeks after initiation of oral premarin either 0.625 or 1.25 mg daily. After three months this increased blood flow rate was still observed when on medication. So far other groups of women have not been examined by this method.

Xenon Method

The technique of measuring the washout of a small quantity of radioactive Xenon applied to a given tissue and from the slope of the curve calculate the blood perfusion rate (usually in ml/min/100 g tissue) has been extensively used in various organs and tissues in physiological and clinical work. The method was introduced by (Lassen et al., 1964) and has been used to measure blood flow of the skin as well (Sejrsen 1968).

In a few cases we have applied 3–400 μCi of Xenon^{133} dissolved in sterile saline in a volume of about 0.03 ml injected intraepithelially. The γ-detector was placed close to the mons pubis and the woman was lying on her back with bended knees. Two to three minutes is allowed for equilibration and the slope then obtained showed a straight line when plotted logarithmically thus indicating a monoexponential one-compartment system allowing for calculation of blood perfusion rate. Resting values from 5–10 ml/min/100 g have been found in the follicular as well as in the luteal phase. This is within the range of other resting tissues. This method therefore seems to be promising especially as it should be possible to apply this and one or both of the above mentioned methods simultaneously and thereby obtain values of calibration, as there are obvious advantages using the non-invasive techniques.

Changes in Vaginal Function During Sexual Stimulation

To measure and collect data in subjects during sexual arousal is obviously hampered by technical difficulties. A carefully programmed protocol cannot easily be followed as the mood of the subject at that particular session is influencing the course of the experiment. Over the years about forty women have participated in the project and close to twenty of these have worked regularly as experimental subjects. Their ages range from 21 to 42 years and they are without any known somatic or psychic diseases as well as they have no sexual dysfunctions. All are socially well adapted, have higher than average intelligence and are generally in higher education.

To assess the *fluid production* during sexual arousal the insertion of three pre-weighed filterpapers was done after the vagina had been swabbed. The amount of fluid retained in the paper after 8–10 minutes was then compared with the amount obtained from initiation of clitoral self stimulation until orgasm. This period may vary from 3 to 25 minutes. The amount of fluid collected in this way increased on the average from about 100 mg to 190 mg. Although the average time of collection in the stimulation period is longer a second collection period always will give a lower amount in the basal condition because the filterpapers dry out the area more completely than the swabbing. The time required to produce the fluid in the stimulation period is however unknown but it may very well be a few minutes. If we assume that 190 mg is produced in the 20–25% area covered by the filterpapers it would mean that the production rate has increased from 0.3 to 1.2 mg/h, supposing the fluid was produced over a 20 minute period. This is obviously a cautious calculation and this rate of production can thus be taken as a minimum rate.

In four women the *direct measurement* of evaporation performed immediately after orgasm showed increases by 2.5, 2.3, 2 and 1.8 times that of the basal evaporation. It must be noted that this was done during the restitution phase of the sexual response cycle after the period when the vaginal lubrication is supposed to take place. Yet it gives evidence of increased transudation. When the sodium concentrations in the basal and the stimulation periods were compared an increase was always found in the range of 12–50 mM/kg fluid. This clearly indicates an influx of fluid from the intercellular space. pH was occasionally measured on the wall before and after stimulation and increases from 0.2 to 1.7 pH-units were found.

If *vaginal photopletysmography* is performed and clitoral stimulation starts an immediate rise in the amplitude can be noted. This is even more evident when vibration (40 to 60 Hz) is applied to the clitoris. This clitoral-vaginal vascular response may already be noticed by increases in the first stroke volume after initiation of vibration. This may well indicate a short looped reflex via sacral centers as the first response. It means that more blood per cardiac cycle is passing the vaginal wall but does of course not tell whether more capillaries are open or whether the same vessels are more distended. After a while no further increase in amplitude will occur even when stimulation continues.

The heat measurement will show an increase in milliwatts needed to keep the set temperature. This also occurs very sudden and the increase may continue long after the maximum increase in amplitude of the photopletysmographic registration has been reached. The explanation is to be found in an increase of the heart rate. At orgasm the heat consumption drops concomitantly with the heart rate, while the amplitude of the photopletysmography is still elevated.

In a part of the study the oxygen electrode was applied to the wall of the vagina at ambient temperature. During sexual stimulation an average increase of three to four fold in oxygen tension was recorded clearly indicating that the blood perfusing the capillaries contained more oxygen during sexual stimulation (Wagner and Levin 1978b).

Not until we applied the *Xenon-method* did we have an indication of the magnitude of the already established increase in blood perfusion rate. In cases where we studied the Xenon washout at rest and during sexual stimulation leading to orgasm we were able to calculate values in the range from 30 to 50 ml/min-/100 g. This is a five fold increase in flow.

CONCLUSION

From this information we may conclude that a sudden drop in arterial (precapillary) resistance brings about an increase in flow rate, an increase in intracapillary pressure and an increase in oxygenated blood. The degree of increase in capillary surface is not possible to estimate, although it must exist. This fact and the increased pressure gradient across the capillary wall will facilitate a transcapillary flux of fluid into the extracellular space underlying the vaginal epithelium. As this epithelium contains intercellular channels (Burgos and de Vargas-

Linares 1970) as well as pores, demonstrated on the surface by scanning electron microscopy (Ludwig and Metzger 1976), it makes sense to believe that these pathways may be a low resistant area for forced fluid transportation into the vaginal lumen during sexual stimulation thus explaining the rapid and large increase in vaginal fluid production rate in this situation.

ACKNOWLEDGEMENTS

This study has been supported in part by the Novo Fund, Copenhagen and IPPF (Intern. Planned Parenthood Federation, London).

REFERENCES

Burgos, M.H., de Vargas-Linares, R.: Cell junctions in the human vaginal epithelium. Am. J. Obstet. Gynec. 108 (1970) 565–571.

Cohen, H.D., Shapiro, A.: A method for measuring sexual arousal in the female. Psychophysiology 8 (1971) 251–252.

Duncan, S.L.B., Levin, R.J.: Transuterine, transendocervical and transvaginal potential differences in conscious woman measured in situ. J. Physiol. 259 (1976) 27–28P.

Dusitsin, N., Gregorire, A.T., Johnson, W.D., Rakoff, A.E.: Histidine in human vaginal fluid. Obstet. and Gynec. 29 (1967) 125–129.

Gillan, P., Brindley, G.S.: Vaginal and pelvic floor responses to sexual stimulation. Psychophysiology (1979), in press.

Hartmann, C.G.: The permeability of the vaginal mucosa. Ann. N.Y. Acad. Sci. 83 (1959) 318–327.

Hoon, P.W.: The assessment of sexual arousal in women. In: Progress in behaviour modification, vol. 7. Academic Press. Inc., N.Y. 1978, pp 1–61.

Lassen, N.A., Lindbjerg, I.F., Munck, O.: Measurement of blood flow through skeletal muscle by intramuscular injection of ^{133}Xenon. Lancet 1 (1964) 686–689.

Levin, R.J., Wagner, G.: Mechanisms for vaginal ion movements in women. J. Physiol. 284 (1978) 172–173P.

Ludvig, H., Metzger, H.: The human female reproductive tract—a scanning electron microscopic atlas. Springer-Verlag, Berlin, 1976, p. 14.

Masters, W.: The sexual response cycle of the human female: vaginal lubrication. Ann. N.Y. Acad. Sci. 83 (1959) 301–317.

Nilsson, G., Sedin, G., Öberg, Å.: A transducer for measurement of evaporation from the skin. Int. Conf. Biomed. Transducers, Paris, 1975.

Odeblad, E.: Intracavitary circulation of aqueous material in the human vagina. Acta obst. et gynec. scand. 43 (1964) 360–368.

Sejrsen, P.: Atraumatic local labelling of skin by inert gas: epicutaneous application of Xenon–^{133}. J. Appl. Physiol. 24 (1968) 570–572.

Wagner, G.: Physiological responses of the sexually stimulated female in the laboratory, 16 mm colour film, Preisler Film Product., Copenhagen, 1974.

Wagner, G., Levin, R.J.: Human vaginal fluid, pH, urea, potassium and potential difference during sexual excitement. In: Progress in Sexology, ed. by R. Gemme, C.C. Wheeler. Plenum Publ. Comp., N.Y. 1977, pp 335–344.

Wagner, G., Levin, R.J.: Vaginal fluid. In: The human vagina, ed. by E.S.E. Hafez, T.N. Evans. Elsevier/ North-Holland Biomedical Press, Amsterdam 1978 a, pp 121–137.

Wagner, G, Levin, R.J.: Oxygen tension of the vaginal surface during sexual stimulation in the human. Fertil. Steril. 30 (1978 b) 50–53.

Part II:
UTERUS (EXCEPT CERVIX)

Copyright 1979 by Elsevier North Holland, Inc.
F.K. Beller and G.F.B. Schumacher, eds.
The Biology of the Fluids of the Female Genital Tract

MORPHOLOGY OF THE ENDOMETRIUM

R. M. Wynn

HISTOLOGY

The normal cyclic changes in the endometrium are closely correlated with those in the ovary. The proliferative, or preovulatory, phase of endometrial development corresponds temporally to the follicular phase of the ovarian cycle. The postovulatory, or secretory, phase of the endometrium corresponds to the ovarian luteal phase. Teleologically, these cyclic alterations may be considered preparation of the endometrium for nidation of the ovum. In a cycle in which fertilization does not occur, the endometrium sloughs; that is, menstruation ensues.

Dating of the endometrium refers to the classic 28-day cycle, in which ovulation is assumed to occur on day 14. Because the postovulatory phase is constant (14 days ± 36 hours), it is appropriate to designate the third postovulatory day, for example, as day 17. The day immediately preceding menstruation is day 28 and the first day of bleeding is day 1. Because the range of the normal menstrual cycle is from 21 to 35 days, the preovulatory phase may vary in length from 7 to 21 days. Because of this variation, it is inappropriate to designate the days of the preovulatory phase of the cycle by numbers. Instead, the terms "early," "mid," and "late," proliferative are used. For example, in a 28-day cycle with a 14-day

Department of Obstetrics and Gynecology, University of Arkansas College of Medicine, Little Rock, Arkansas, USA

preovulatory phase, days 1–4 would coincide with the menstrual period; days 5–7 would be early proliferative; days 8–10 would be midproliferative; and days 11–14 would be late proliferative, ovulation occurring on or very near day 14.

The first half of the endometrial cycle, before ovulation, is concerned with growth or proliferation; the second half is concerned with epithelial and stromal differentiation. During the first half of the postovulatory phase, or the third week of a typical 28-day cycle, specific synchronized changes occur in the endometrial epithelium, particularly the glands of the zona spongiosa. During the second half of the postovulatory phase, or the fourth week of a 28-day cycle, the histological changes affect primarily the stroma, leading to a predecidual reaction. If fertilization fails to occur, the stromal reaction regresses and menstruation ensues. If pregnancy occurs, the endometrial changes progress to formation of true decidua.

The early preovulatory (proliferative) endometrium measures only 1–2 mm in thickness. The superficial epithelium, composed of cuboidal cells, appears to be regenerating. The glands are short, straight, narrow, and partially collapsed (Figure 1). Mitotic figures frequently are seen in both epithelium and compact stroma, which consists of stellate cells with scanty cytoplasm. During the midproliferative phase, the epithelial cells become columnar. The glands elongate and become more tortuous. Stromal edema may appear at this stage, although it is inconstant and soon regresses. Mitotic figures are most obvious at this time. During the late proliferative phase, the glands continue to increase in length and tortuosity. Individual columnar epithelial cells achieve their greatest height, and pseudostratification of nuclei is maximal (Figure 2).

FIGURE 1. Early proliferative endometrium, showing short, narrow, straight glands.

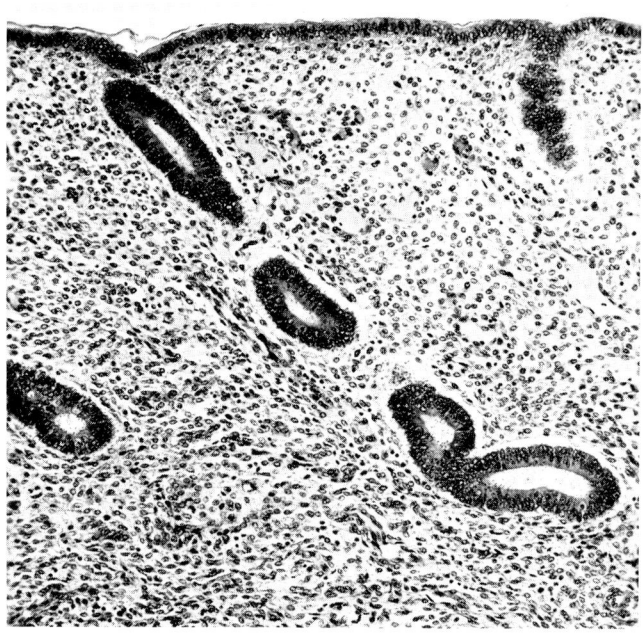

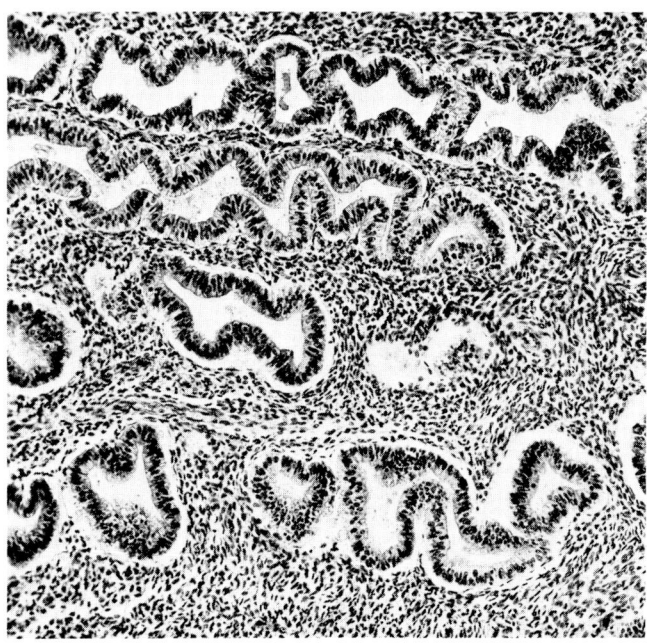

FIGURE 2. Late proliferative endometrium, showing long, dilated, tortuous glands.

The first distinct histological change in the postovulatory (secretory) phase occurs about 48 hours after ovulation (day 16), when subnuclear vacuolation of the glandular epithelium becomes prominent. Initially, these large, regularly distributed vacuoles displace the nuclei upward to create a pattern of pseudostratification. After all the vacuoles have passed the nuclei, the pseudostratification disappears, with nuclei returning to the bases of their cells. Increases in diameter and tortuosity of the glands accompany these changes.

On day 17, the glandular epithelium shows an orderly row of nuclei with homogenous cytoplasm above them and large vacuoles below (Figure 3). By day 18, the vacuoles push past the nuclei, decreasing in size and entering the cytoplasm nearer to the glandular lumen. By day 19, most of the nuclei have returned to the base of the cells and most of the vacuoles have discharged their contents. Day 19 may resemble day 16 with its early vacuolation or may even resemble the late proliferative phase, but it is distinguished from the earlier phases by intraluminal secretion and absence of pseudostratification and mitotic figures. By day 20, acidophilic intraluminal secretion reaches its peak. Thereafter, it becomes inspissated and more darkly stained (Figure 4).

Dating of the second half of the postovulatory phase (days 21–28) depends largely on stromal characteristics. Edema is rather constant in the midsecretory period, abruptly increasing on day 21 and reaching its peak on day 22. The stromal cells at this stage appear as small, dense, nearly naked nuclei with only a rim of cytoplasm. On day 23, the spiral arterioles become more prominent because of en-

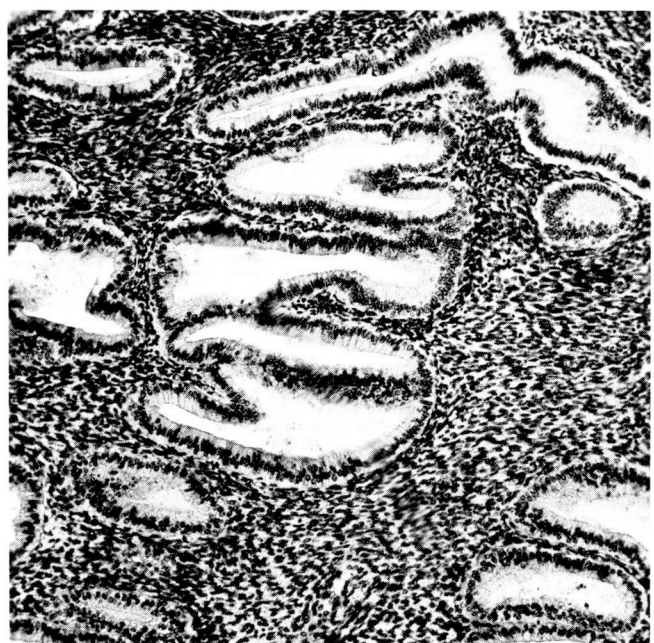

FIGURE 3. Early secretory (day 17) endometrium, showing regularly aligned subnuclear vacuoles.

largement of the nuclei and increase in the cytoplasm of the periarteriolar stromal cells. This cuff of stromal cells around the arterioles of the zona compacta is the earliest predecidual change. By day 24, distinct collections of periarteriolar predecidual cells may be identified.

Similar predecidual cells begin to differentiate beneath the epithelium of the surface on or about day 25. During the next 48 hours, patches of these cells begin to coalesce, forming solid sheets of well-developed decidua-like cells by day 27. Around day 24 of a cycle in which pregnancy does not occur, glandular epithelial involution begins. The epithelium of the dilated and tortuous glands is thrown into tufts, creating the serration that is characteristic of the last week of the cycle. The previously tall columnar epithelium diminishes in height. Its nuclei appear shrunken and its cytoplasmic borders become ragged and indistinct (Figure 5).

A few lymphocytes may be scattered throughout the stroma in the proliferative and early secretory phases, but the differentiation of predecidua is accompanied by a sharp increase in lymphocytic infiltration. Polymorphonuclear leukocytes, which first appear in large numbers on day 26, are obvious by day 27. Microscopic areas of focal necrosis and hemorrhage appear a few hours before the onset of menstruation.

In the second half of the secretory phase, the three strata, or zones, of endometrium can be distinguished. The zona compacta is the uppermost layer, so named because it consists of broad fields of compact hypertrophied stromal cells between the rather narrow necks of glands. The zona spongiosa is the middle

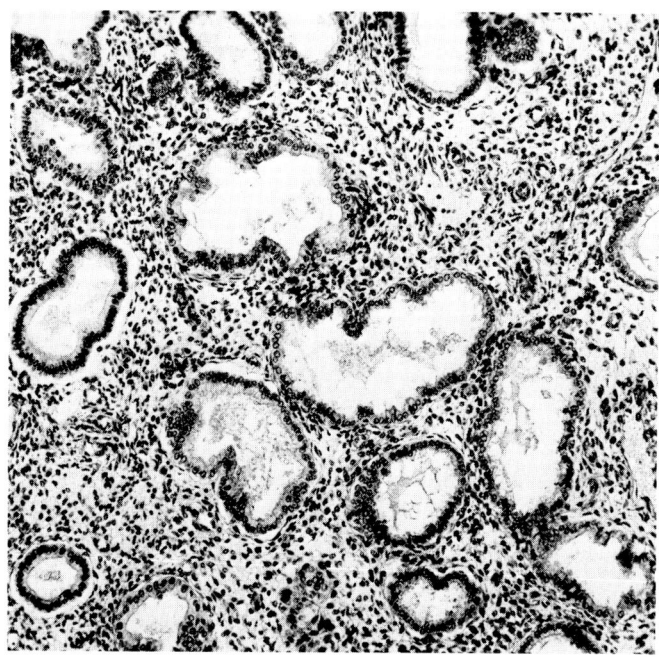

FIGURE 4. Midsecretory (day 21) endometrium, showing low glandular epithelium and inspissated intraluminal secretion.

zone, so called because of the lacy, labyrinthine appearance caused by the large numbers of dilated, tortuous glands with little intervening stroma. The zona basalis, the deepest layer, is in contact with the myometrium, because there is no uterine submucosa. The basalis is composed of bases of glands surrounded by dense stroma. The compacta and spongiosa form the zona functionalis. Part of the endometrium regenerates from the basal layer; by the time bleeding ceases, the endometrial surface is normally restored. During pregnancy, the zona compacta and zona spongiosa are converted into decidua compacta and decidua spongiosa, respectively (Figure 6).

TRANSMISSION ELECTRON MICROSCOPY

Because the endometrium is a highly sensitive target tissue for the ovarian hormones and because its morphological changes are critical in the investigation of infertility, it has been studied by electron microscopy more extensively than has any other tissue of the human female genital tract. The following description is based on earlier writings of Wynn (1977), to which the reader is referred for further details and references.

Examination of endometrial ultrastructure reveals cytoplasmic secretion into the glandular lumina throughout the cycle. The terms "secretory" and "proliferative" therefore do not accurately reflect the histological pattern. Because various

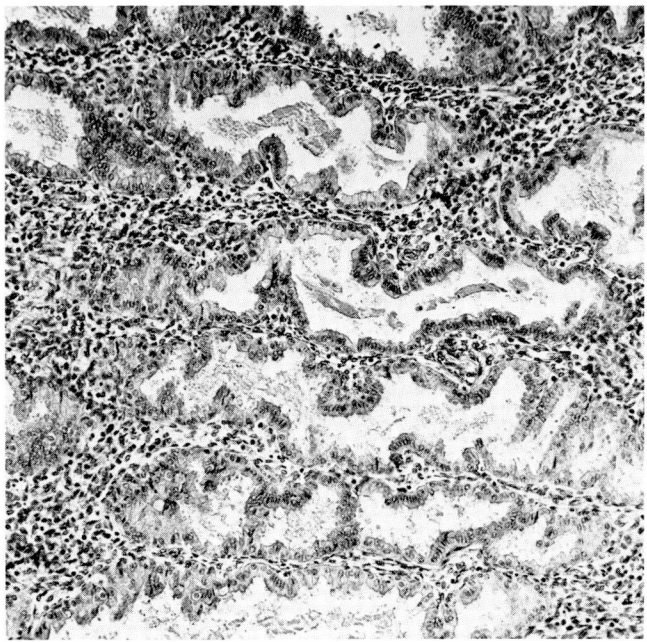

FIGURE 5. Late secretory (day 25) endometrium, showing serrated glands with ragged cytoplasmic borders (secretory exhaustion) and sparse intervening connective tissue.

degrees of differentiation may occur in the same endometrium from area to area and even from cell to cell, ultrastructural dating is based on the most advanced consistent pattern in the specimen, as with histological classification. The basal endometrium remains essentially unchanged throughout the proliferative phase, whereas cyclic changes affect primarily the glands in the zona spongiosa. The superficial epithelium undergoes less obvious cyclic alteration. The pseudostratification noted with the light microscope is not seen in thin sections if tangential cuts are avoided. Endometrial nuclei during the preovulatory period are large, regular, and oval, with prominent nucleoli (Figure 7). Mitotic figures are seen throughout the proliferative phase, most prominently in glandular epithelium and most frequently in midproliferative nuclei. The epithelial cytoplasm is poorly differentiated, containing numerous ribosomes but relatively few extensive channels of endoplasmic reticulum or elaborate Golgi complexes.

The mitochondria are scattered randomly throughout the cytoplasm in the early proliferative phase. Around the time of ovulation they are located primarily near the base of the cell. They then enlarge, forming prominent cristae and developing in relation to polyribosomes and perinuclear patches of glycogen. Shortly before ovulation the small accumulations of glycogen coalesce to form large deposits between the nucleus and the basal plasma membrane, resulting in well-defined structures that may be detected with the electron microscope about two days before the appearance of the typical "subnuclear vacuole" noted with the light microscope.

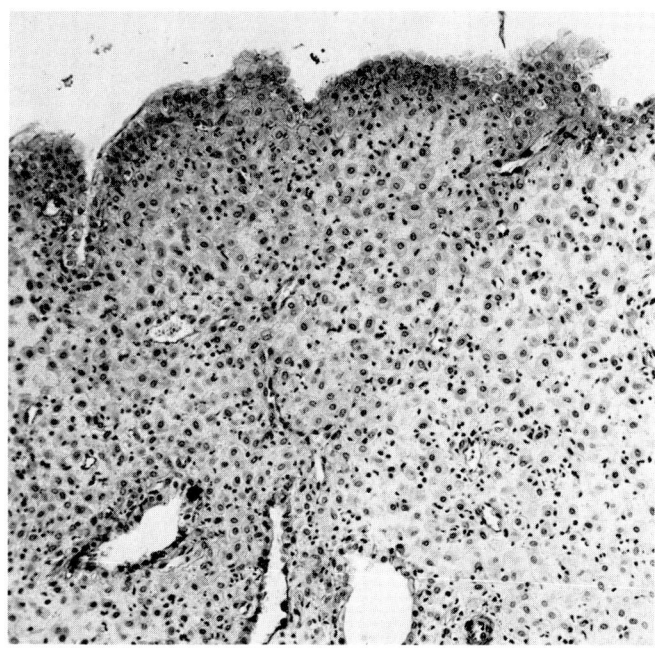

FIGURE 6. Decidua parietalis of early pregnancy, showing transformation of stromal cells in compact zone into large rounded and polygonal elements.

The Golgi apparatus increases in size during the midproliferative period, with the addition of tubules and vesicles. Microvilli are found on all epithelial cells. Endometrial cells with typical cilia are found throughout the cycle, but they are much more common in the lower uterine segment and endocervix. Extensive pinocytosis is not evident. Large cytoplasmic projections from the glandular epithelial surfaces into the lumina may be seen throughout the proliferative phase (Figure 8). The changes in endometrial organelles during the proliferative phase appear to reflect a pattern consistent with growth and endogenous metabolism rather than elaboration of proteins for export. The end of the proliferative phase is characterized by cessation of development of these organelles, possibly a "braking" effect of progesterone.

Ultrastructural features confined to the secretory phase have been identified. Confluent subnuclear patches and large mitochondria can first be detected by electron microscopy on or about day 14, or approximately 36–48 hours before subnuclear vacuolation can be recognized by light microscopy (Figure 9). The mitochondria that first appear about the time of ovulation are several times larger than the typical organelles of the proliferative phase and they have prominent crests. Not more than a few of the giant mitochondria are found in any individual cell. By day 17, deposits of glycogen are scattered diffusely throughout the cytoplasm, and supranuclear Golgi complexes are dense and well developed. Smaller mitochondria are distributed prominently between convolutions of the plasma membranes.

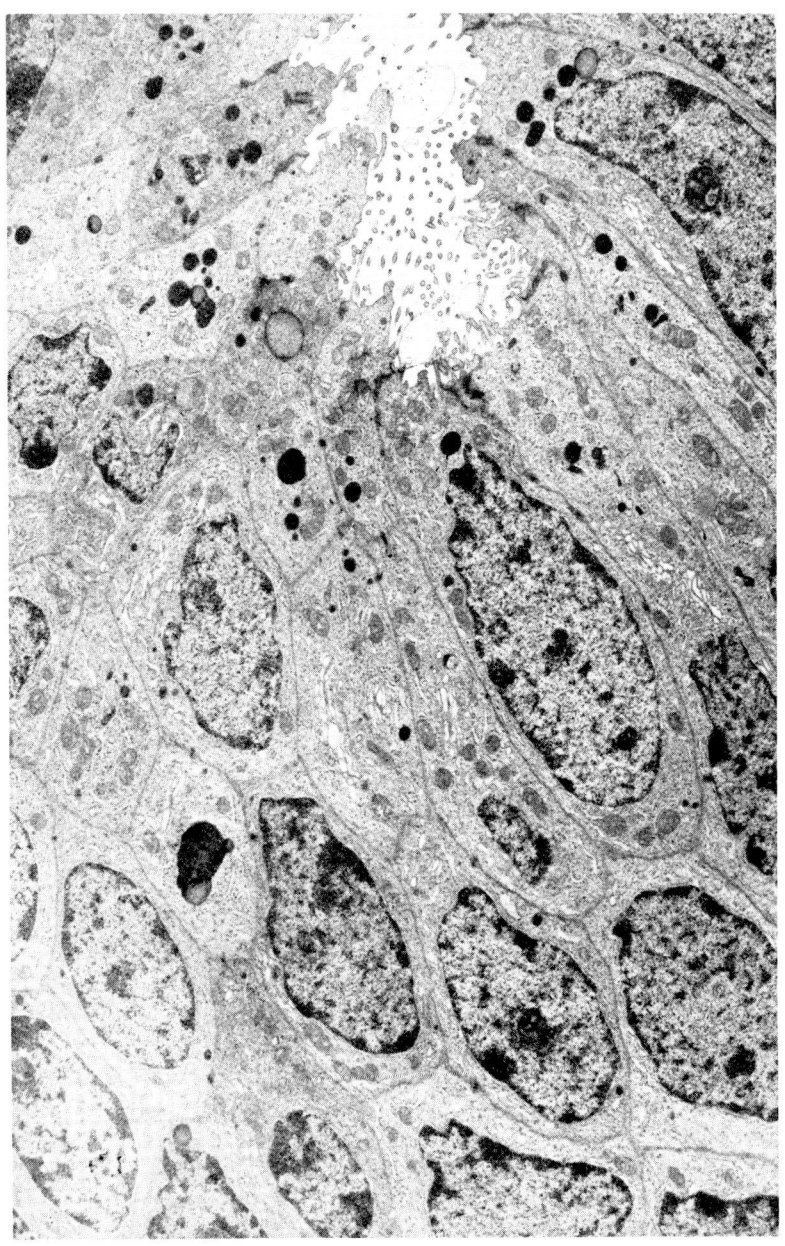

FIGURE 7. Survey transmission electron micrograph of early proliferative endometrium, showing large, dense nuclei.

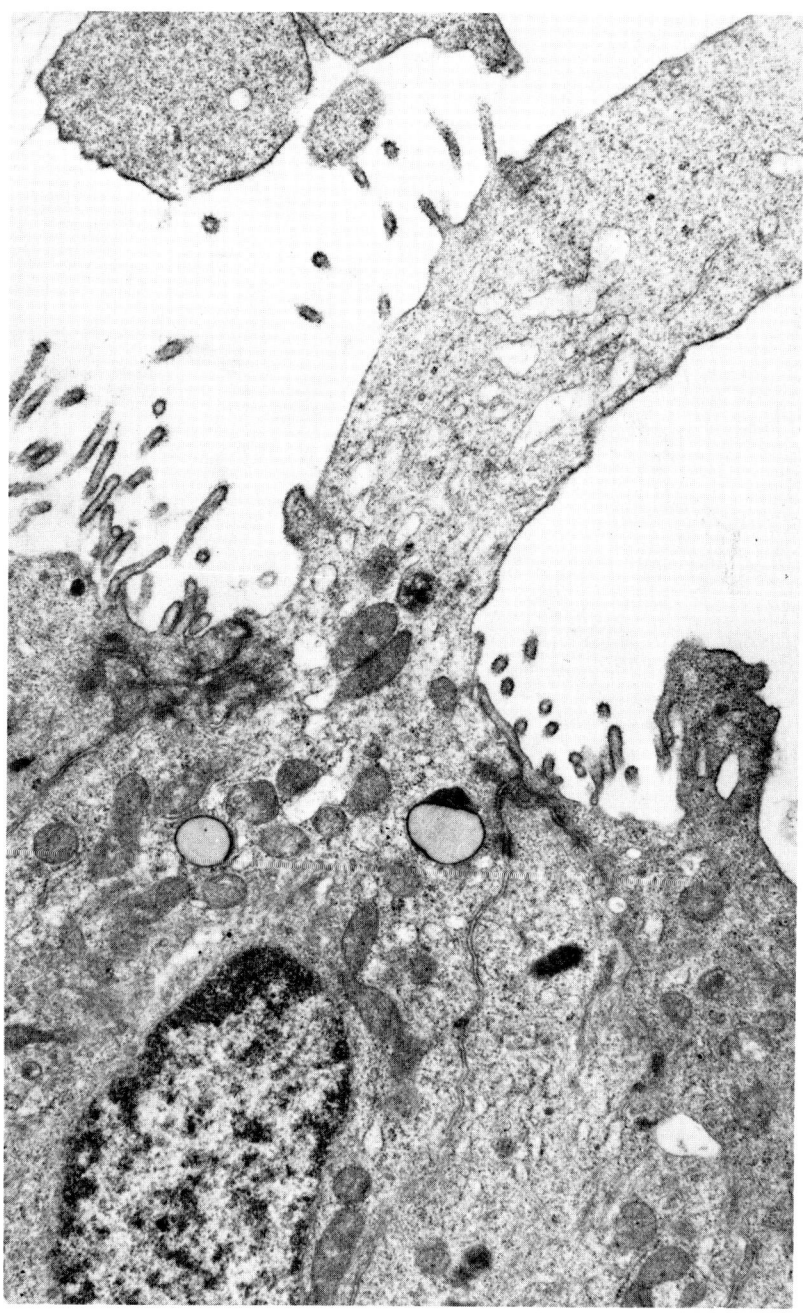

FIGURE 8. Midproliferative endometrium, showing large cytoplasmic projection into glandular lumen.

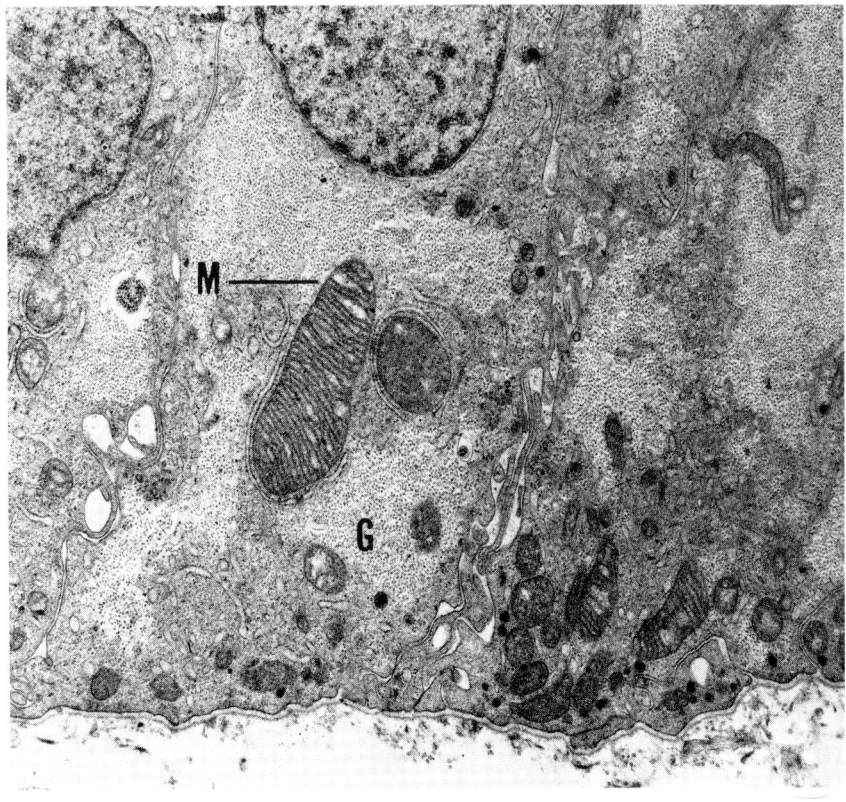

FIGURE 9. Endometrium shortly after ovulation (day 15), showing giant mitochondrion (M) and glycogen (G) between nucleus and basal lamina.

Between days 17 and 20, a characteristic nucleolar channel system is maximally conspicuous (Figures 10–11). This structure was first described by Dubrauszky and Pohlman (1960), although its discovery is often credited to other investigators who reported it in the English literature several years later. More and coworkers (1974) described a three-dimensional reconstruction of the nucleolar channel system. From the inner nuclear membrane arise two tubules, which form a nine-turn spiral to terminate bluntly at the apex. The nucleolar channel system then develops at the apex of an invagination of both inner and outer nuclear membranes. It is an ordered, hollow spherical stack of interdigitating membrane-bound tubules, 600–1000 Å in diameter, embedded in a dense matrix surrounding a core of lightly granular material. Toward the end of the cycle the nucleolar channel system appears as a dense disordered mass of tubules lacking a central core, often occurring as a protrusion of the nucleus. More and coworkers (1974) suggest that the nucleolar channel system may be extruded and possibly incorporated into giant lysosomes. They concluded that this structure may be contiguous with the true nucleolus or separate from it. In assessing the function of the nucleolar channel sys-

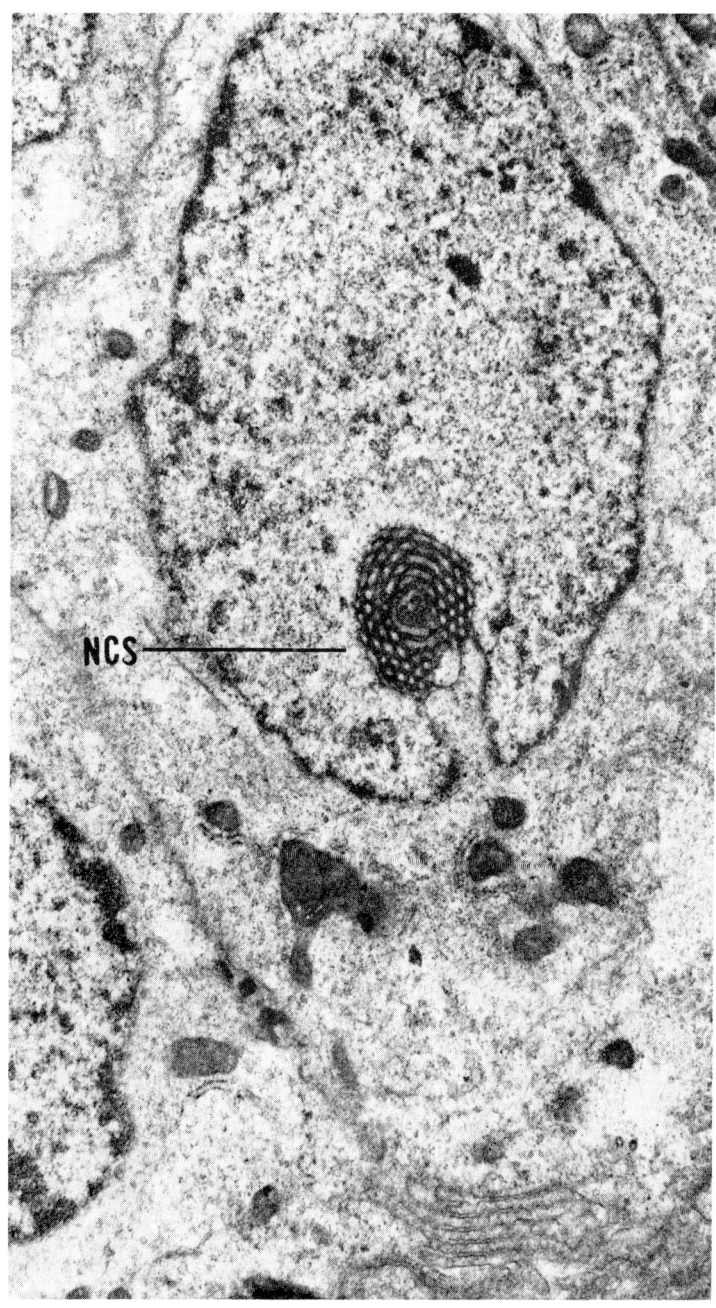

FIGURE 10. Early postovulatory (day 17) endometrium, showing prominent nucleolar channel system (NCS).

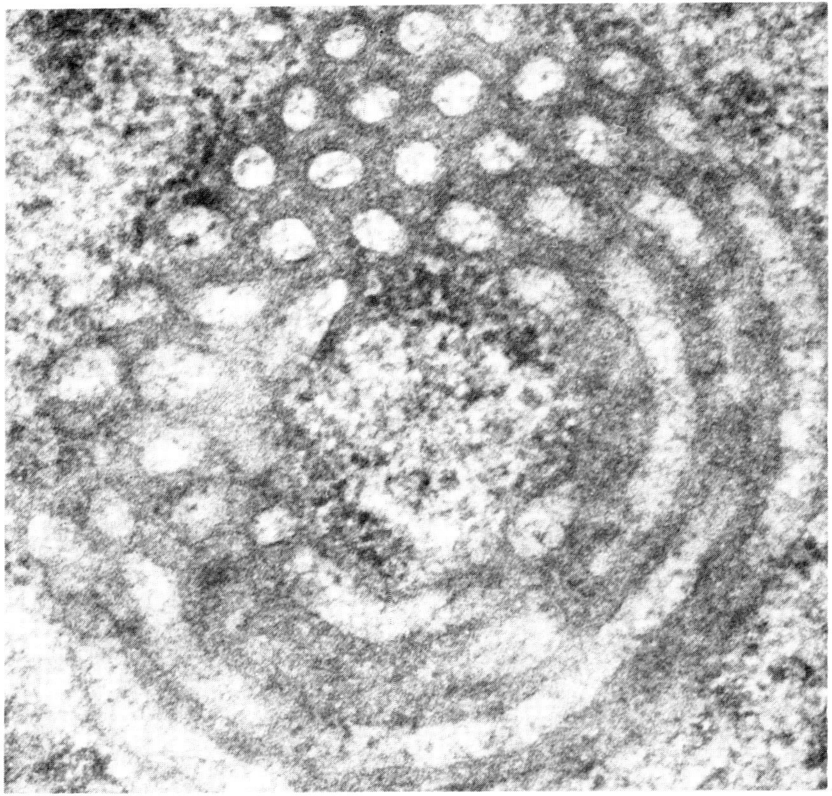

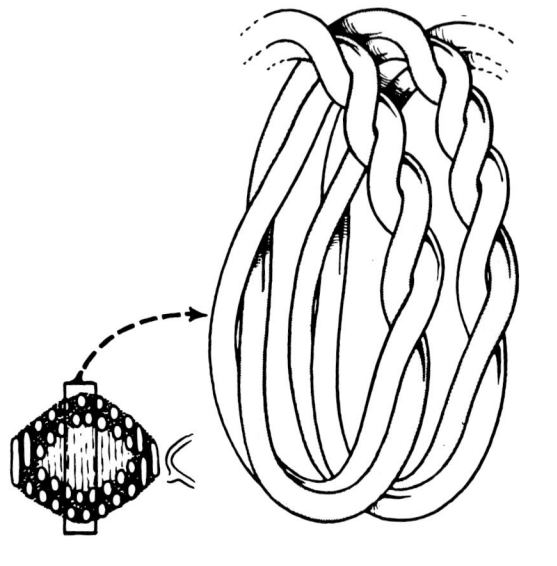

FIGURE 11. Higher-power electron micrograph of nucleolar channel system (with diagram of the system).

tem, they postulate that progesterone causes derepression of the genome, with the production of new varieties of messenger ribonucleic acid (mRNA). Several enzymes, such as acid phosphatase and phosphorylase, which increase during the secretory phase, require the mediation of mRNA. Thus the nucleolar channel system is thought to provide the pathway for rapid transport of new mRNA into the cytoplasm to act as a template for new protein.

By day 19 or 20, large projections from the surfaces of the glandular epithelial cells are found in association with extensive intraluminal secretion (Figure 12). Organelles are sparse within the cytoplasmic promontories, although ribosomes, glycogen, and occasional mitochondria and fragments of endoplasmic reticulum may be seen. These irregular protrusions from the apical surfaces of the luminal epithelial cells have been reinterpreted by Parr and Parr (1974) as being involved in the formation of endocytotic vacuoles rather than apocrine secretion. We, among others, however, have suggested that these protrusions, after being pinched off, degenerate to form nutritive material for the embryo before implantation.

By about day 19 or 20, the cytoplasm has ceased to differentiate further. The Golgi apparatus, however, remains fairly complex and the nuclei have returned from luminal to basal positions. By day 22, intraluminal secretion is prominent and the cells contain fewer intracytoplasmic secretory granules. There is little suggestion of pseudostratification. The microvilli are somewhat shorter and the epithelial cells themselves are lower. By day 23, the granular endoplasmic reticulum has become less prominent and the number of nucleolar channel systems has decreased greatly. Occasional Golgi complexes still appear well developed, and deposits of glycogen and lipid are scattered throughout the epithelial cells. The slender, elongated mitochondria resemble those of decidual cells, and the plasma membranes are highly convoluted. Mitochondria are distributed basally and peripherally and small patches of glycogen are seen apically. On day 24, isolated deposits of glycogen, large Golgi complexes, fragments of endoplasmic reticulum, and numerous small mitochondria are seen. The plasma membranes remain maximally convoluted, and complex intercellular spaces develop. Basal laminae of capillaries and epithelium may be separated by only wisps of connective tissue.

During the last few days of the cycle, the epithelial nuclei are basal; the apical surfaces are irregular; and the convolutions of the plasma membranes remain extensive. There are no consistent changes in size or number of microvilli. Nucleolar channel systems and giant mitochondria are not found. In a cycle in which pregnancy does not occur, signs of cytoplasmic degeneration appear by day 25. The decidual cell of pregnancy does not regress, but maintains its numerous characteristic slender mitochondria and short fragments of endoplasmic reticulum. The fibrillar connective tissue is condensed to form a ''capsule'' around the cell and the characteristic epithelioid pattern is established (Figure 13).

SCANNING ELECTRON MICROSCOPY

Scanning electron microscopy has confirmed the findings of transmission electron microscopy, added details about the luminal epithelial surface and its cilia, demonstrated apocrine secretion, and provided new data to explain the dynamics of endometrial regeneration (Ferenczy, 1976). Several studies by transmission electron microscopy had earlier demonstrated the persistence of cilia throughout the endometrial cycle (Figure 14), although in numbers smaller than those in

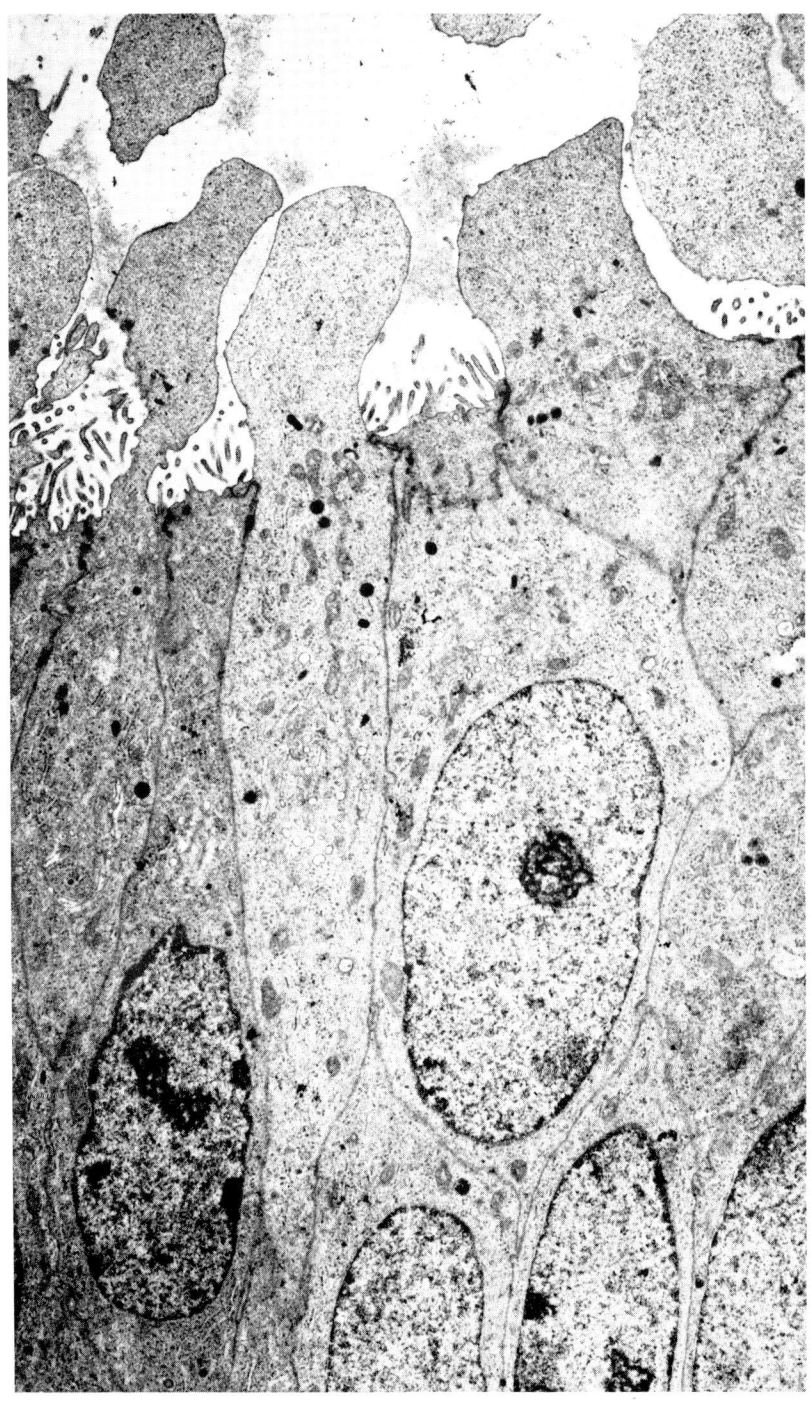

FIGURE 12. Midsecretory (day 20) endometrium, showing apical secretion into glandular lumen.

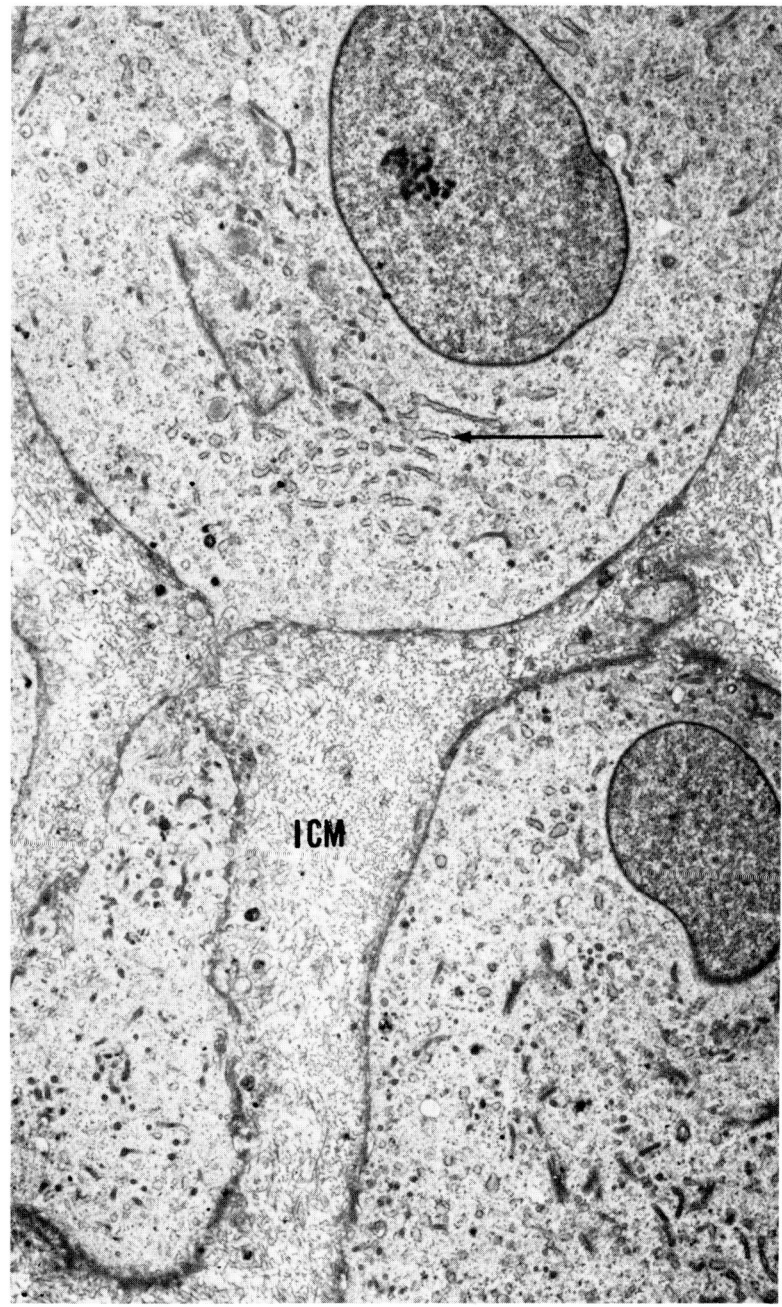

FIGURE 13. Parietal decidua from early pregnancy, showing rather poorly differentiated cytoplasm with numerous slender mitochondria (arrow), extensive intercellular matrix (ICM), and typical small, ovoid nucleus.

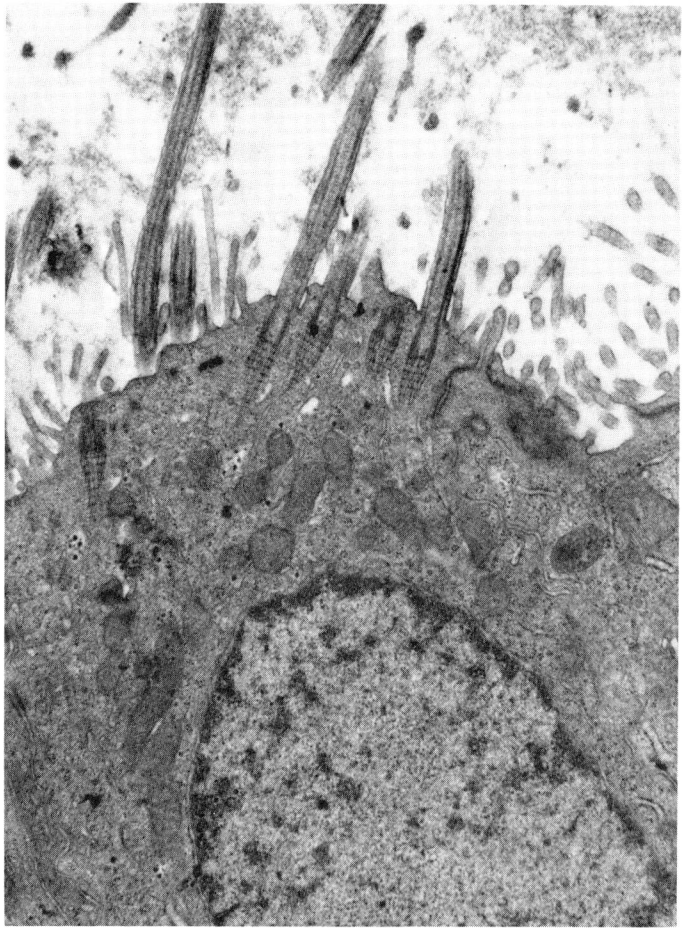

FIGURE 14. Early postovulatory (day 17) endometrium, showing persistence of ciliated and nonciliated, microvillous cells.

the oviduct and endocervix (Wynn, 1977). With the use of scanning electron microscopy, Ferenczy and coworkers (1972) found changing proportions of dome-shaped, nonciliated to ciliated cells during the endometrial cycle. In the early proliferative phase (Figure 15), the ratio of nonciliated to ciliated cells was about 30:1, whereas in the late proliferative (Figure 16), the ratio fell to 15:1. From day 21 on, the proportion of ciliated cells decreased to about 40 or 50 nonciliated cells to one ciliated cell, but ciliated cells were always readily identified throughout the postovulatory phase. Apocrine secretion is most obvious with the scanning electron microscope between days 20 and 24 (Figure 17). Masterson and coworkers (1975) suggested that the precursors of ciliated cells are sensitive to estrogen and

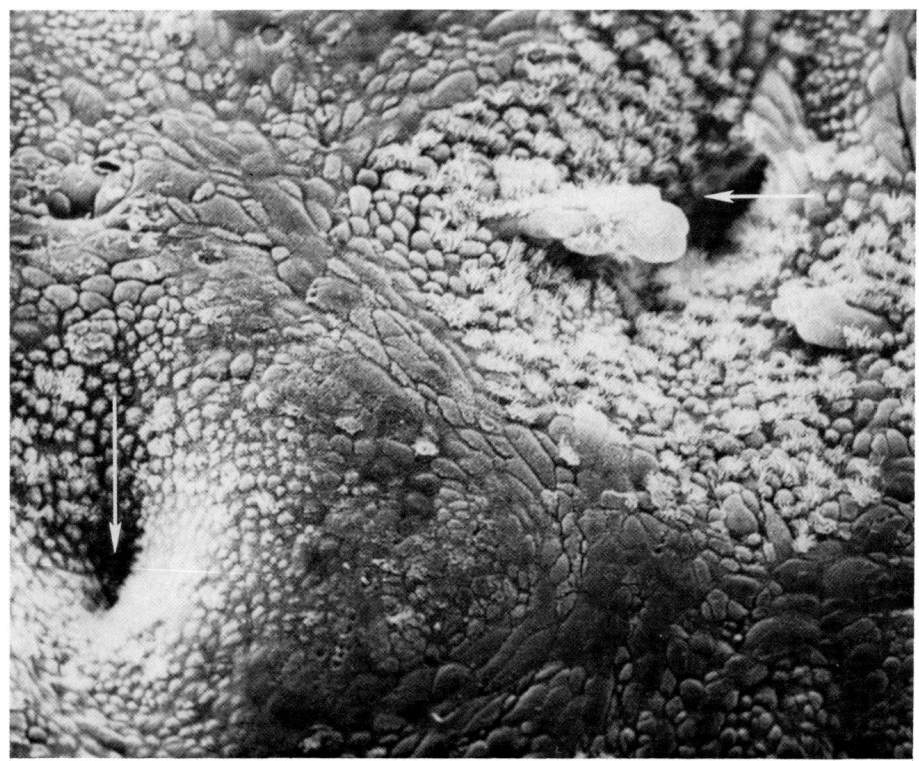

FIGURE 15. Scanning electron micrograph of early proliferative endometrium, showing glandular orifices (arrows) surrounded by ciliated cells. Courtesy of Dr. Alex Ferenczy.

that the fall in their numbers during the secretory phase reflects negative influence of progesterone.

Scanning electron microscopy confirms that the epithelium of the endometrial surface undergoes less cyclic change than does that of the glands. Perhaps the steadier rate of synthesis of ribonucleoprotein results in the greater number of ciliated cells and the earlier and more sustained appearance of cytoplasmic glycogen. With respect to the morphological response to the changing hormonal milieu, as exemplified by ciliogenesis, the epithelium of the superficial endometrium resembles that of the oviduct more than that of the endometrial glands.

ULTRASTRUCTURAL LOCALIZATION OF ENZYMES

Finally, ultracytochemical studies of the human endometrial cycle have suggested yet another means of correlating morphological changes with metabolic functions. According to Sawaragi and Wynn (1969), alkaline phosphatase is found on epithelial plasma membranes throughout the proliferative phase and into the

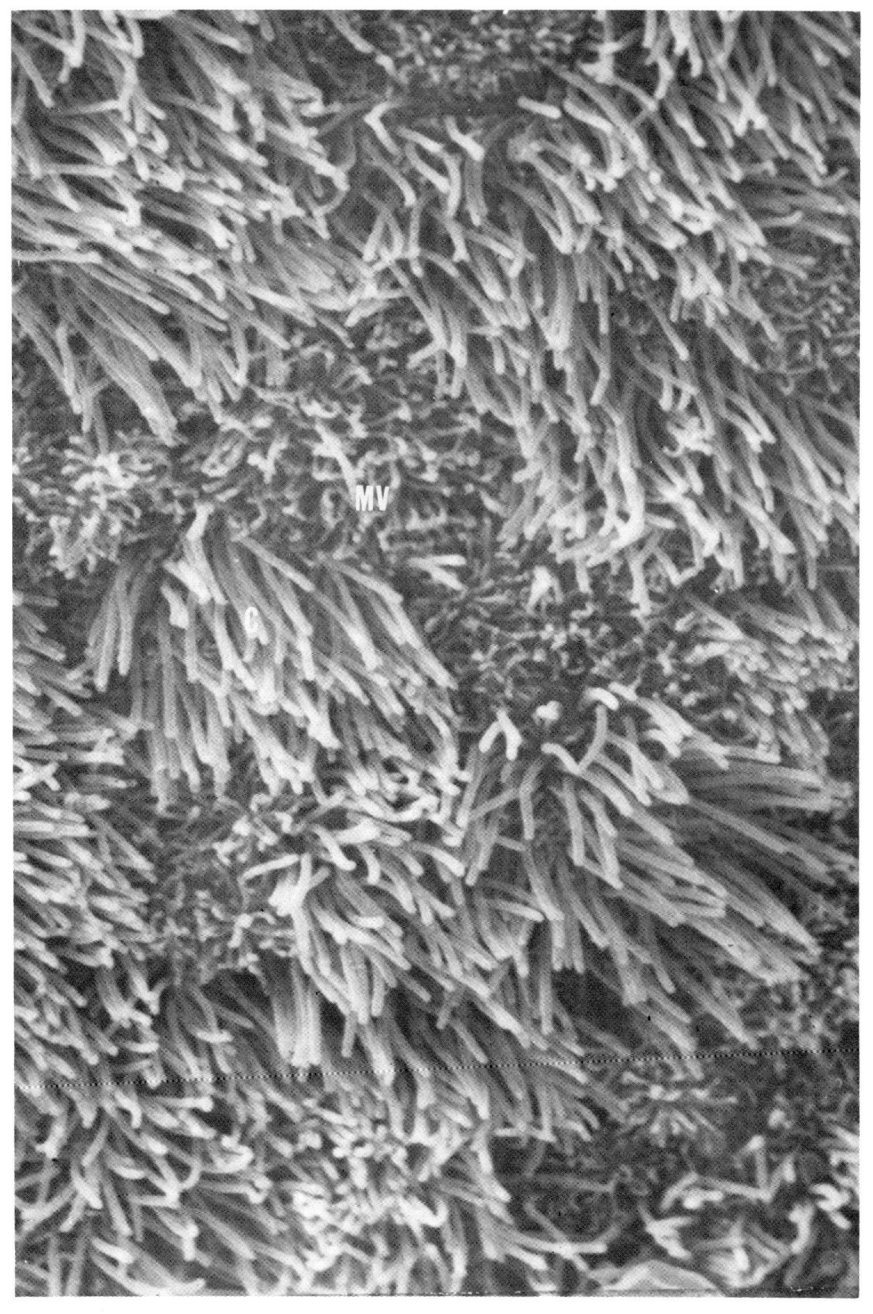

FIGURE 16. Late proliferative endometrium, showing clusters of ciliated (C) and microvillous, nonciliated (MV) cells. Courtesy of Dr. Alex Ferenczy.

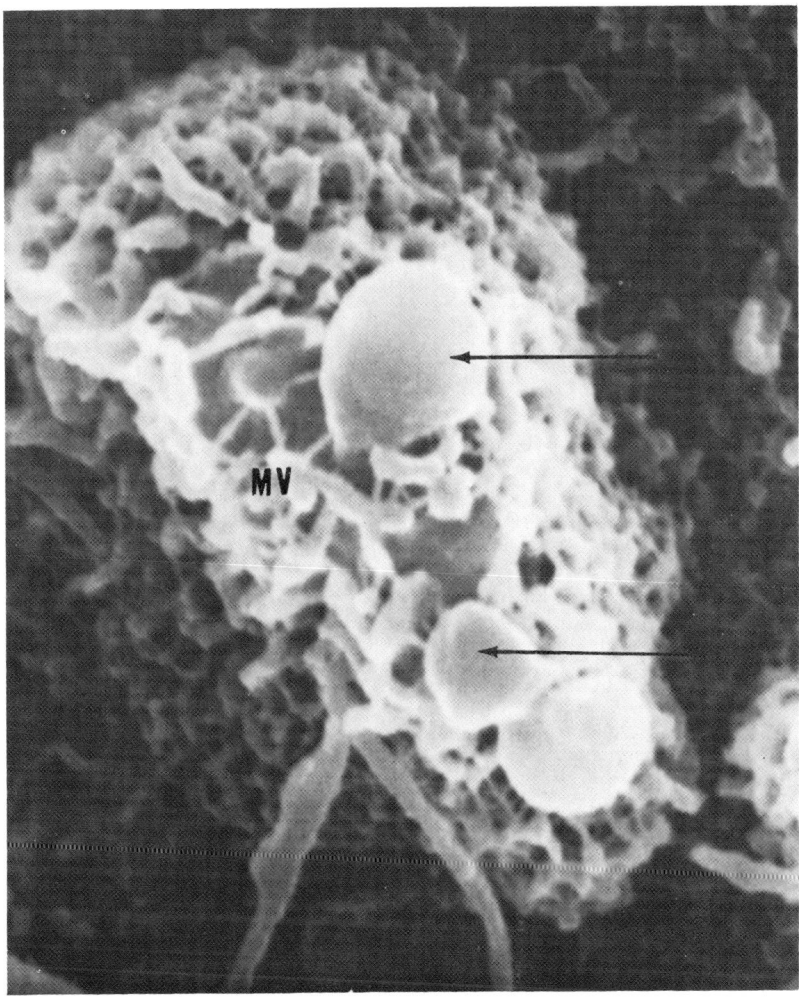

FIGURE 17. Midsecretory (day 22) endometrium, showing apical cytoplasmic projections (arrows) that resemble apocrine secretion. Microvilli (MV) are shorter and less abundant than those of the proliferative endometrium. Courtesy of Dr. Alex Ferenczy.

midsecretory phase (Figure 18). Acid phosphatase is observed in lysosomes of glandular epithelium after day 21. The release of lysozyme from these structures may be an immediate precursor of menstruation. Glucose-6-phosphatase is most evident around the time of ovulation and in the early secretory phase, localized mainly within cisternae of endoplasmic reticulum (Figure 19). The timed appearances of these enzymes during the endometrial cycle suggest that they are biochemical determinants of the events leading to menstruation, on the one hand, or implantation, on the other.

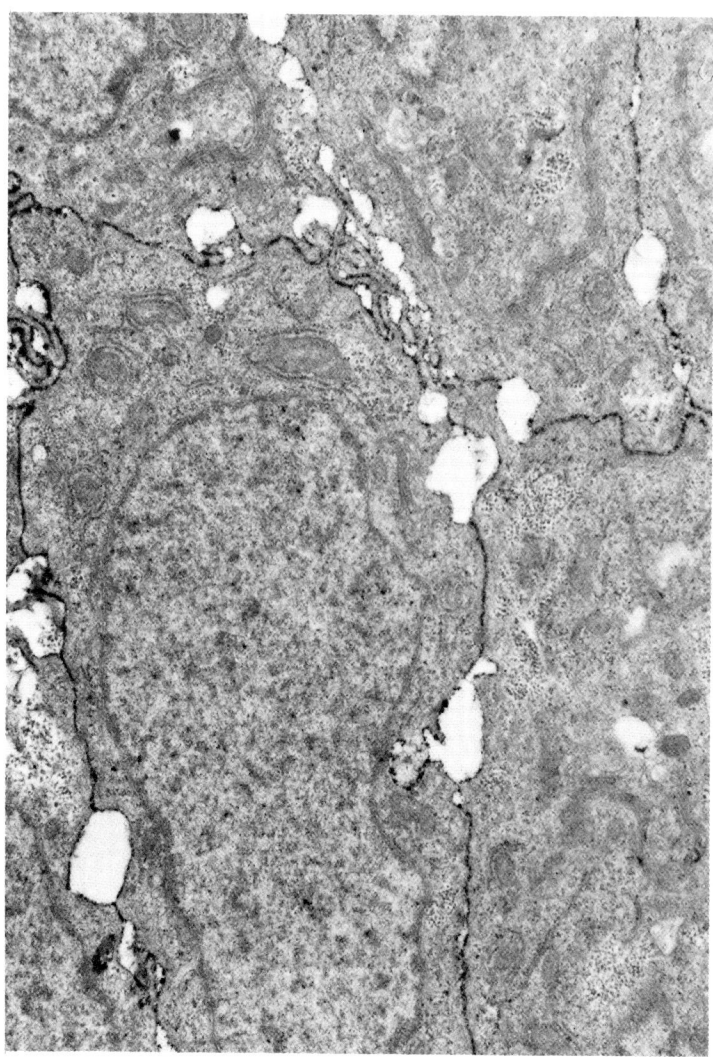

FIGURE 18. Midsecretory (day 21–22) endometrium, showing persistence of reaction for alkaline phosphatase along plasma membranes.

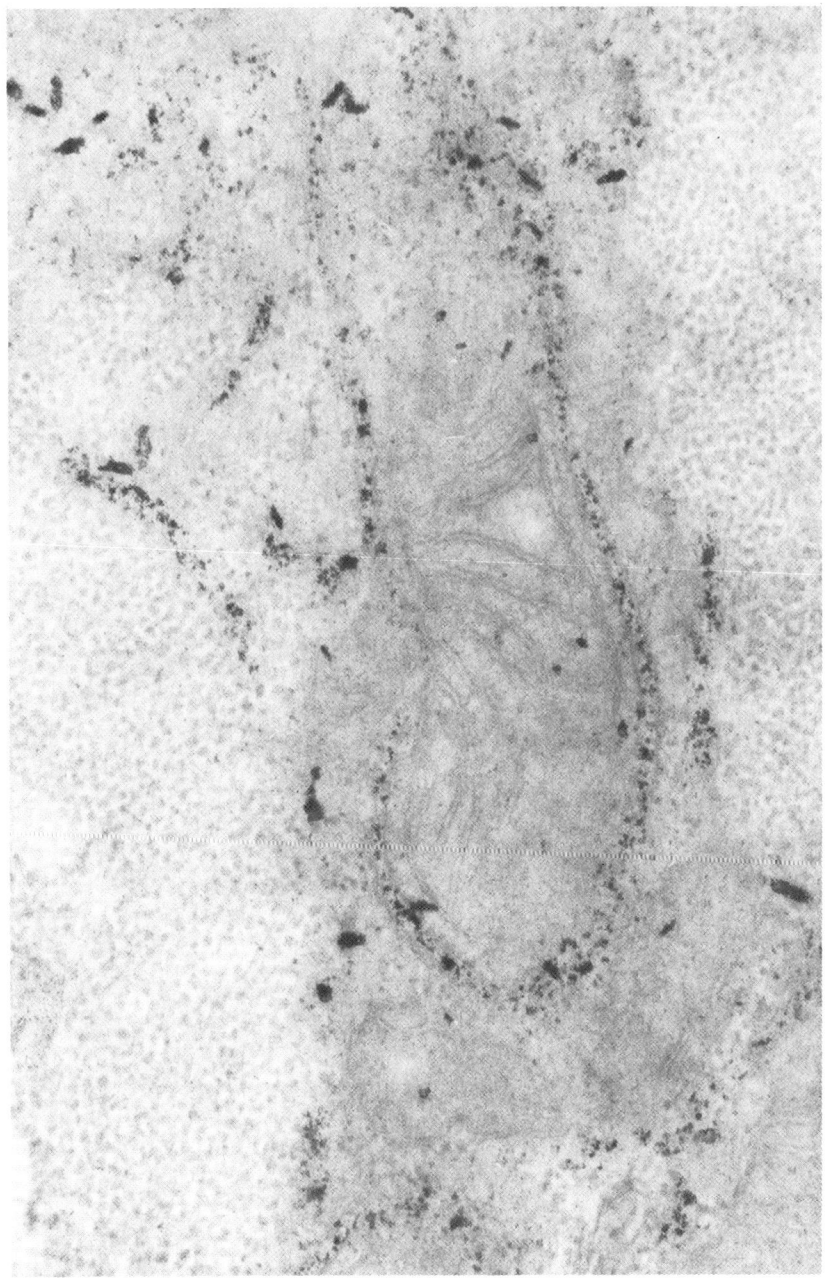

FIGURE 19. Early secretory (day 18) endometrium, showing reaction for glucose-6-phosphatase in endoplasmic reticulum in proximity to mitochondria and deposit of glycogen.

REFERENCES

Dubrauszky, V., Pohlman, G.: Strukturveränderungen am Nukleolus von Korpusendometriumzellen während der Sekretionsphase. Naturwissenschaften. 47 (1960) 523–524.

Ferenczy, A.: Studies on the cytodynamics of human endometrial regeneration. I. Scanning electron microscopy. Amer. J. Obstet. Gynecol. 124 (1976) 64–74.

Ferenczy, A., Richart, R. M., Agate, F. J. Jr., Purkerson, M. L., and Dempsey, E. W.: Scanning electron microscopy of the human endometrial surface epithelium. Fertil. Steril. 23 (1972) 515–521.

Masterson, R., Armstrong, E. M., and More, I. A. R.: The cyclical variation in the percentage of ciliated cells in the normal human endometrium. J. Reprod. Fertil. 42 (1975) 537–540.

More, I. A. R., Armstrong, E. M., McSeveney, D., and Chatfield, W. R.: The morphogenesis and fate of the nucleolar channel system in the human endometrial glandular cell. J. Ultrastructure Res. 47 (1974) 74–85.

Parr, M. B., Parr, E. L.: Uterine luminal epithelium: protrusions mediate endocytosis, not apocrine secretion in the rat. Biol. Reprod. 11 (1974) 220–233.

Sawaragi, I., Wynn, R. M.: Ultrastructural localization of metabolic enzymes during the human endometrial cycle. Obstet. Gynecol. 34 (1969) 50–61.

Wynn, R. M.: Histology and ultrastructure of the human endometrium. In: Biology of the Uterus. Ed.: R. M. Wynn, Plenum Press, New York, 1977, pp. 341–376.

CELLS OF THE UTERINE FLUID

D.L. Moyer, S. El Sahwi,* L. Macaulay, S.T. Shaw, Jr.

INTRODUCTION

Our interest in the cells of the uterine fluid originates with the use of the high surface area intrauterine devices, such as, the Marquiles spiral and the Lippes loop during the 1960's. In an early study we observed large accumulations of neutrophils and mononuclear cells present in the endometrial fluid (Moyer, D.L., and Mishell, D.R., Jr., 1971). It was unusual for us to see large quantities of inflammatory cells in the uterine fluid in patients who were not wearing an IUD. This observation led to a study which measured the numbers of free floating cells in the uterine fluid. Each patient had a uterine flushing prior to and after the insertion of an IUD. The results showed that there was a significant increase in the number of inflammatory cells in uterine fluid washings during the 6 to 12 weeks after insertion of an IUD. Both neutrophils and mononuclear cells were increased during this time.

A study of the cells of uterine fluid involves the identification of the cell types, their relative quantities in uterine fluid and the possible significance of these cells to the physiological events occurring in the uterine fluid. The cells found in the uterine fluid are a mixture of cells which migrate into the cavity,

Department of Pathology, Section of Experimental Pathology, University of Southern California Medical Center, Los Angeles, California
  * Present Address: Department of Obstetrics and Gynecology, University of Alexandria, School of Medicine, Alexandria, Egypt

cells which are exfoliated from the superficial epithelium and glands, and cells which enter through the cornua as well as the endocervical canal. We have divided the cells of the uterine fluid into the following groups:

A. Migrating Cells—Cells which have the ability to migrate by ameboid movement across the capillaries into the endometrial tissues and across the basement membrane of the superficial and glandular epithelium into the uterine cavity. Example—neutrophils, macrophages and lymphocytes.
B. Exfoliated Cells—Cells which enter the uterine cavity by exfoliation from the superficial and glandular epithelium. Example—superficial epithelial cells. This also may include cells pushed into the cavity through epithelial interspaces or defects. Examples—stromal cells and red blood cells from damaged endometrial surfaces (Shaw, S.T., Jr., and Macaulay, L.K., 1979).
C. Non-nucleated Portions of Epithelial Cells—Cell particles are formed by budding off of the apical portions of the glandular or superficial epithelium. These may be surrounded by a cell membrane. Example—glandular cells give rise to apical secretions which consist of portions of non-nucleated cytoplasm surrounded by a cell membrane.
D. Cells Containing Foreign Protein—Cells which contain protein which is foreign to the host and which enter the uterine cavity from the fallopian tubes or through the endocervical canal. Example—preimplantation embryo, spermatozoa, bacteria.
E. Cells of Menstrual Tissue—Menstrual products which contain viable cells, degenerating cells, portions of cells. The proportions of these cells mirror the constituents of the endometrial tissue with the addition of numerous red and white blood cells within the menstrual discharge.

QUANTITIES OF CELLS IN THE UTERINE FLUID

The number of cells in uterine fluid varies under different conditions. The mean total number of cells present in the uterine fluid is in the range of 10,000 to 100,000 cells during the proliferative or luteal phases. The presence of a foreign body or an acute endometritis may increase the total cell count in the uterine cavity to well over a million cells (Moyer, D.L., and Mishell, D.R., Jr., 1971). During the flushing procedure, even though much care is taken to avoid contamination with cervical mucus, the cell count will be slightly increased by a small amount of remaining cervical mucus after the cleansing and drying of the cervical canal prior to flushing of the cavity.

Different stimuli may increase the number of inflammatory cells in the endometrial fluids and tissues. A variety of bacteria enter the uterine cavity from the vaginal fluid and cervical mucus when inert objects such as an intrauterine device or a curet is passed through the cervical canal (Mishell, D.R., Jr., Bell, J.H., Good, R.G., and Moyer, D.L., 1966).

The presence of foreign protein elicits an inflammatory cell response which has a characteristic rate for both neutrophils, lymphocytes and macrophages (Spector, W.G., 1968). The number of neutrophils, is markedly increased during the early phase of an inflammatory reaction and following this, the rapid migration subsides to much lower levels. The increase in mononuclear cells is less rapid but reaches a steady but lower plateau.

In our laboratory we studied the early cellular response to a foreign body, the Lippes loop D (Moyer, D.L., and Mishell, D.R., Jr., 1971). The preinsertion concentration of total cells was 316 white cells per mm^3 (Table I). Approximately 50% of the cells were neutrophils and the remainder were mononuclear cells (macrophages and lymphocytes). In an early study 89 patients served as their control by flushing the uterine cavity prior to an IUD insertion. These patients had a uterine flushing 6 weeks later and a third uterine flushing 12 weeks after the insertion. There was a marked increase in the number of inflammatory cells during the period of study after insertion of the IUDs. This increase was approximately 6 and 10 times higher than the preinsertion flushings. Both neutrophils and mononuclear cells were increased but there was a significantly greater increase in the number of neutrophils.

In a later study, patients wearing a Lippes loop D were studied prior to and after insertion of an IUD for up to 48 months after insertion (Table II). During one through 12 months postinsertion there was approximately a six-fold increase in the total number of inflammatory cells. During the 13 through 48 month postinsertion period there was approximately a three-fold increase in the number of inflammatory cells when compared to the preinsertion values. The percentage of mononuclear cells was increased (64%) during the 12–48 month phase of the study when compared to the preinsertion value (49%).

In a study using rabbits in our laboratory a small silastic IUD was implanted into one uterine horn and there was no IUD in the opposite horn. The uterine horns were flushed 10 days later. The control and IUD uterine horns were flushed with 10 ml of physiological saline and processed through a millipore filter. Photomicrographs of the comparative flushings from each uterine horn showed a marked difference in the quantity of inflammatory cells present in each. In addition to the large number of neutrophils noted on the filter there were mononuclear cells and a rare large multinucleated macrophage. There was approximately a six-fold increase in the number of inflammatory cells flushed from the IUD horns.

CELL TYPES ENTERING UTERINE FLUID

Exfoliated Cells

The exfoliation of epithelial cells from the surface and glandular epithelium occurs throughout the menstrual cycle and during the peri- and post menopausal years. Desquamation of epithelial cells from surface epithelium is most common during the early proliferative phase when the tissues are stimulated by estrogen. Cellular samples collected from the cervical canal or the posterior vaginal fornix have shown normal endometrial cells to be present more frequently during the several days following menses than during the remainder of the cycle (Ng, A.B.P., 1975). The presence of endometrial cells is least frequent during the secretory phase of the cycle. In a study which identified normal appearing endometrial cells in cervical cytology smears, patients who were less than 40 years of age showed exfoliated endometrial cells at different times of the menstrual cycle. A small percentage of these cells were associated with benign endometrial abnormalities, such

TABLE I. Mean Intrauterine Leukocytic Concentration Before and After IUD Insertion in the Same Patient

Uterine Flushings	Number of Patients	Mean Conc. of Total Leukocytes Per mm³	Mean Conc. of Total Neutrophils Per mm³
Preinsertion	89	316	168
6 Week Return Visit	30	2205	1708
12 Week Return Visit	10	3434	2444

as, polyps or hyperplasia. In the over 50 age group, a small percentage of the patients with endometrial cells in the cervical smear were associated with an endometrial adenocarcinoma while the vast majority of patients showed endometrial cells which were benign. In our own experience, approximately 5 to 10 percent of the patients in the peri- and post menopausal age groups show benign endometrial cells on the cervical smear. Exfoliation of benign epithelial and stromal cells occurs under physiological conditions and this phenomenon is greatest during the phase of estrogen stimulation. It is likely that large numbers of these exfoliated endometrial cells may undergo degeneration and lysis prior to entering the cervical canal.

Detachment of epithelial cells from both glandular and superficial epithelium occurs as the intercellular spaces widen and the desmosomes separate (Figure 1). Exfoliated epithelial cells show an increase in the number of cytoplasmic vesicles and a decrease in the number of pseudopods on the cell membrane. Whole cells with nuclei and non-nucleated cell portions are frequently seen in gland lumens. These cells and cell portions circulate into the uterine cavity as the result of ciliary action of the glandular epithelium (Figures 2 and 3). Cilia present on the cells of the superficial epithelium create circulatory movements with eventual migration of the cells and cell products through the endocervical canal.

TABLE II. Mean Intrauterine Leukocytic Concentration Before and After IUD Insertion in Different Patients

Uterine Flushings	Number of Patients	Mean Conc. of Total Leukocytes Per mm³	Percent of Neutrophils
Preinsertion	38	316	53
1 Day to 12 Months	81	1841	47
13 Months to 48 Months	39	921	36

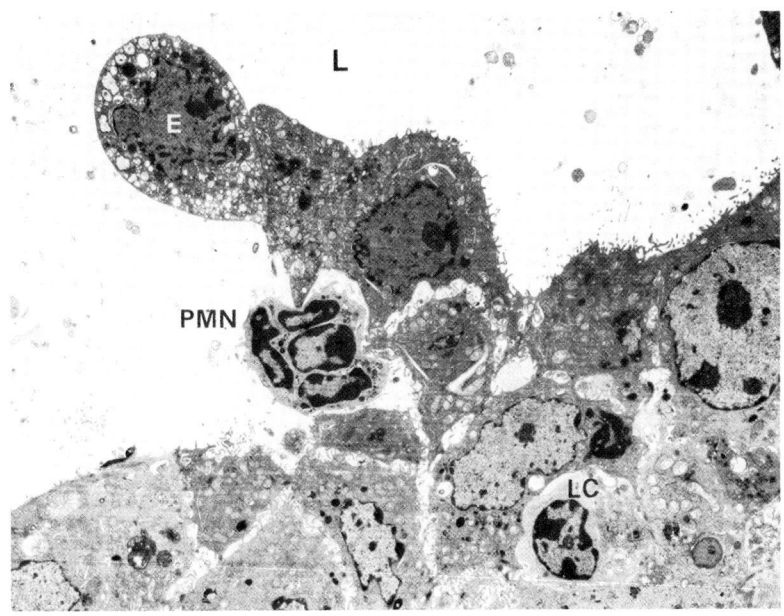

FIGURE 1. Micrograph showing active exfoliation of gland epithelium (E) into the lumen (L) as well as a migratory neutrophil (PMN) and a lymphocytes (LC). X 3,150.

FIGURE 2. Electron micrograph of degenerate cells (DC) and cell debris in the gland lumen which is surrounded by some healthy appearing glandular epithelium (E) X 4,950.

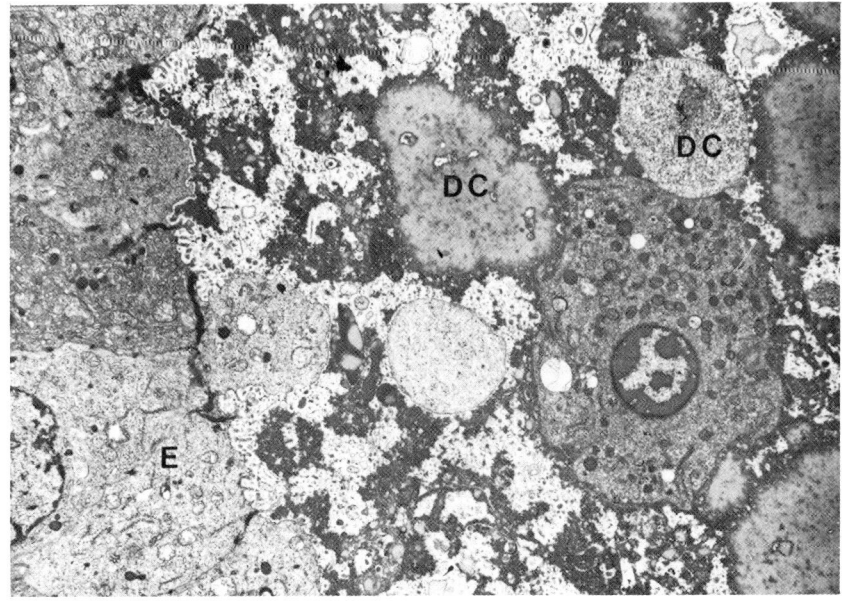

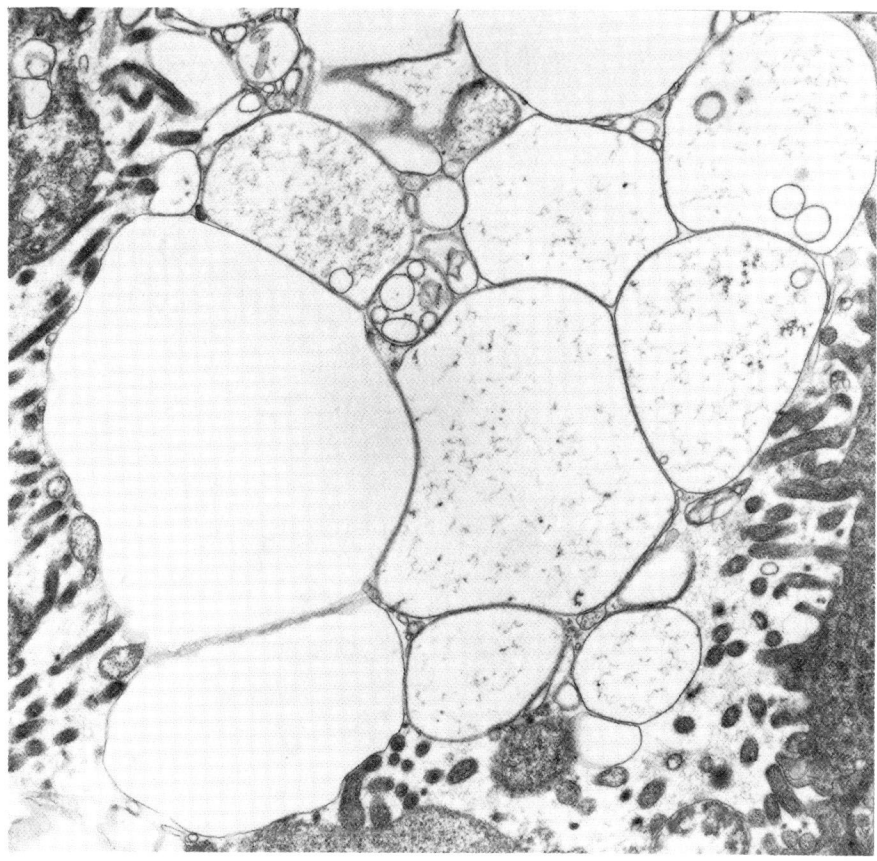

FIGURE 3. Electron micrograph of a gland lumen containing numerous exfoliated portions of cells or whole cells (which have apparently inbibed fluid) X 20,540.

Our studies (Shaw, S.T., Jr., and Macaulay, L.K. 1979) have shown that some cellular elements from the endometrial stroma and its interstitium, i.e., red blood cells in hemorrhagic stroma, may be forced under high pressure into the endometrial cavity (Figure 4). This observation was made on IUD exposed endometrium. In the tissues studied the stromal elements passed through the spaces between the surface or glandular epithelium or were extruded through defects in the surface epithelium.

MIGRATING CELLS

During the menstrual cycle, neutrophils, lymphocytes and macrophages, eosinophils and basophils may migrate through the glandular or surface epithelium entering the uterine fluid. When a foreign body is introduced into the uterine cavity, such as an IUD or bacteria residing in cervical mucus, the chemotactic re-

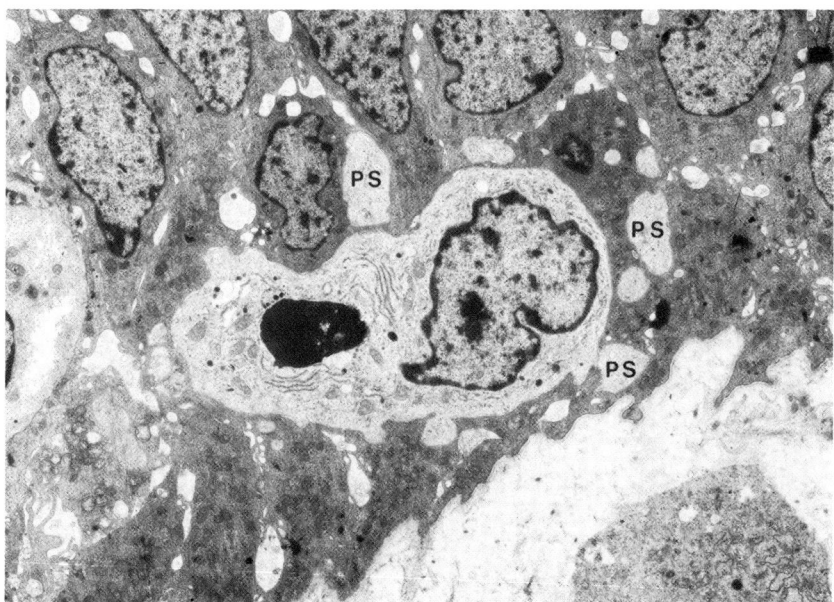

FIGURE 4. Electron micrograph of a red cell containing macrophage migrating through the endometrial surface epithelium. Note the pseudopods (PS) within the epithelial interstices X 5,720.

sponse to the foreign body produces migration of wandering cells into the uterine cavity (Moyer, D.L., Mishell, D.R., Jr., and Bell, J. 1970). These cells circulate through the bloodstream, marginating on the endothelial surface of superficial vessels and subsequently penetrating their walls to migrate into endometrial tissue. These migrating cells may then penetrate through the glandular or superficial epithelium to enter the uterine fluids. Large quantities of such cells may be seen in the uterine fluid during the first few months after IUD insertion. Chemotactic substances for wandering inflammatory cells include bacterial products (alive and dead), cellular components of leukocytes, damaged tissue products, activated components of complement and other plasma proteins, and prostaglandins. Several photomicrographs (Figures 5, 6) illustrate the process of transmigration of different types of cells (leukocytes, macrophages, and lymphocytes) through the surface or glandular epithelium. The extrusion of red cells is seen through the surface epithelium (Figures 7a, b, c).

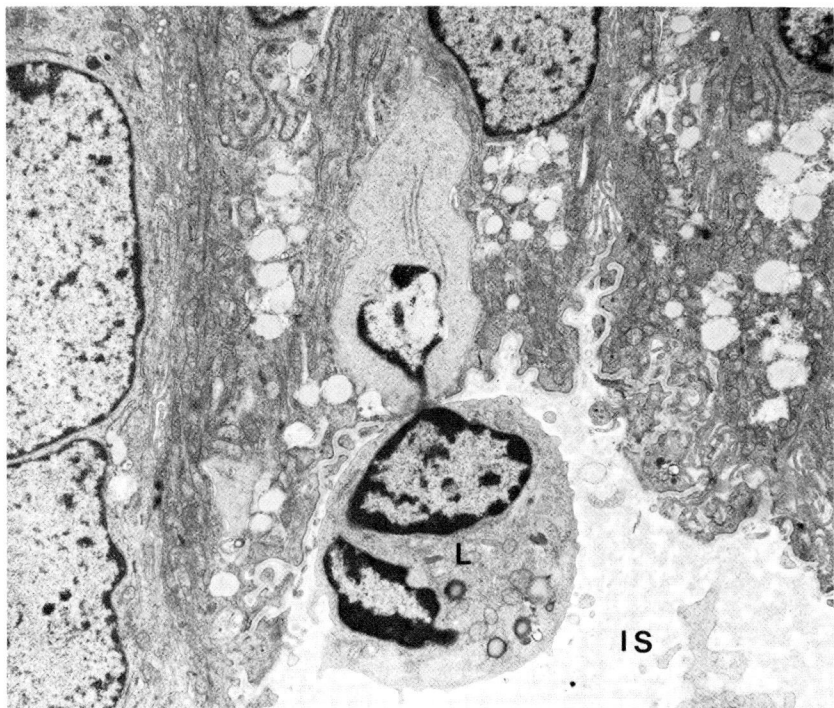

FIGURE 5. Electron micrograph of a leukocyte (L) migrating through basal lamina into a glandular epithelial interspace. Most likely it is migrating from the stromal interstitium (IS) of the endometrium to the gland lumen and eventually to the uterine cavity X 8,280.

FUNCTION AND FATE OF WANDERING CELLS IN THE UTERINE FLUID

Both the wandering cells as well as exfoliated cells show evidence of dissolution within the uterine fluid and these cells may undergo cytolysis within the uterine cavity. The cellular contents of the lysed cells are dispersed throughout the mucus-like environment of the uterine fluid. Much of the fluid volume is probably reabsorbed back through the superficial epithelium, and the remainder may exit through the cervical canal during circulation through the uterine cavity. A remote possibility is that some uterine fluid escapes in retrograde fashion into the fallopian tubes. During menses cells and tissue components reflux into the fallopian tubes giving rise to a "physiological salpingitis" (Nassberg, S., McKay, D.G., and Hertig, A.T., 1954). This condition occurs during menses and is the result of menstrual endometrial products present within the lumen of the fallopian tubes producing a sterile inflammatory reaction.

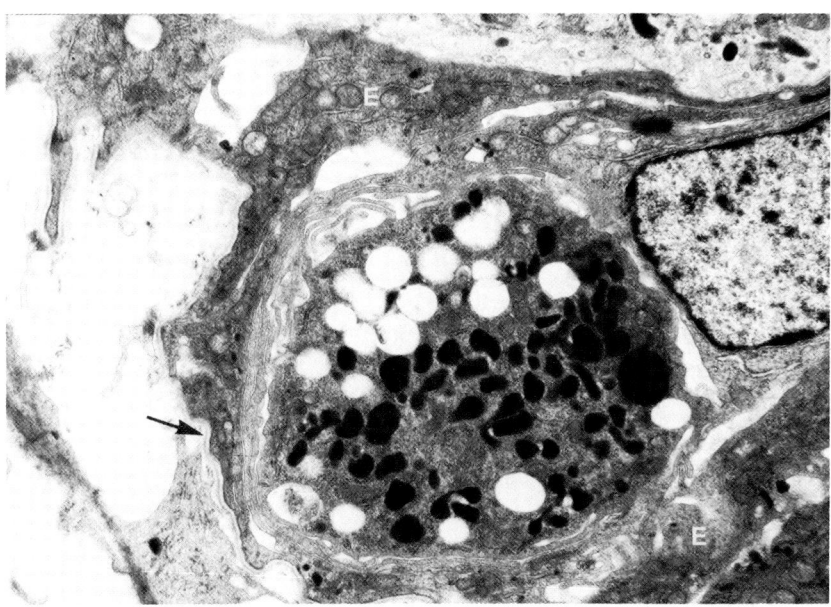

FIGURE 6. Electron micrograph of a basophil or mast cell between epithelial cells (E), above the basal lamina (arrow) of the surface epithelium X 12,825.

PHAGOCYTOSIS OF SPERMATOZOA

The phagocytosis of intrauterine and intracervical spermatozoa occurs in all species thus far studied. In our laboratory, uterine flushings from monkeys have shown the phagocytosis of a sperm head by a neutrophil (Moyer, D.L., and Maruta, H., 1967). In this study, we instilled into the uterus, monkey spermatozoa 24 hours before flushing and this in turn stimulated an inflammatory reaction. Sperm parts were phagocytized and a phagosome enclosed the sperm head (Figure 7). Degranulation of the cytoplasm occurred during the process of phagocytosis. The phagocytosis of spermatozoa occurs in humans (Moyer, D.L., Rimdusit, S. and Mishell, D.R., Jr., 1970). Human sperm parts (middle piece and principal piece) have been observed to be engulfed by a macrophage in the cervical mucus of a patient 12 hours following coitus (Figure 8). A phagosome membrane surrounds several sperm parts in addition to a small amount of debris. It is not known whether these spermatozoa were phagocytized in the uterine cavity with subsequent migration into the cervical mucus or whether the phagocytosis of sperm took place in the cervical mucus of this patient.

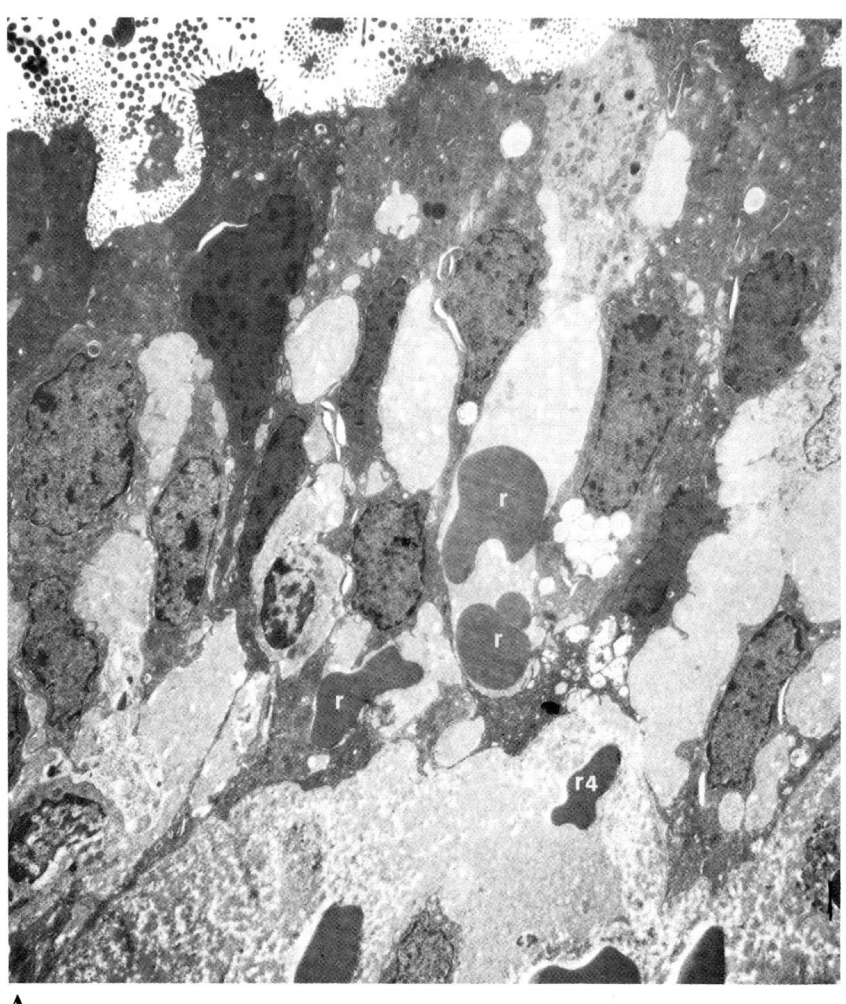

A

FIGURE 7A. Electron micrograph showing three red cells passing between surface epithelial cells which are spread apart by fluid from the underlying stroma. A fourth red cell (r4) may be about to pass through a wide defect in the subepithelial basal lamina. X 3700.
FIGURE 7B. Micrograph of a group of erythrocytes (arrow) pushing from hemorrhagic stroma through basal lamina and surface epithelium into cavity (C). Toluidine blue 1μ section, X 800.
FIGURE 7C. Micrograph showing a wide defect in surface epithelium and basal lamina with red cells (arrows) and other stromal elements pushing into the uterine cavity (C). Toluidine blue 1μ section, X 250. Figures 7a–c are from Shaw, S.T., Jr., and Macaulay, L.K.: Contraception 19:47, 1979. (Published by permission from Geroa-X Publishers.)

B

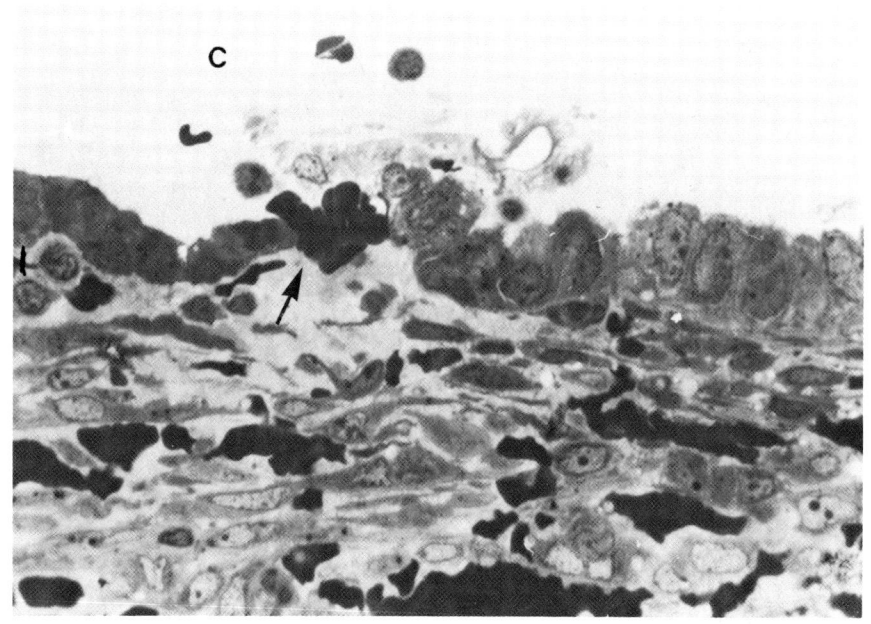

C

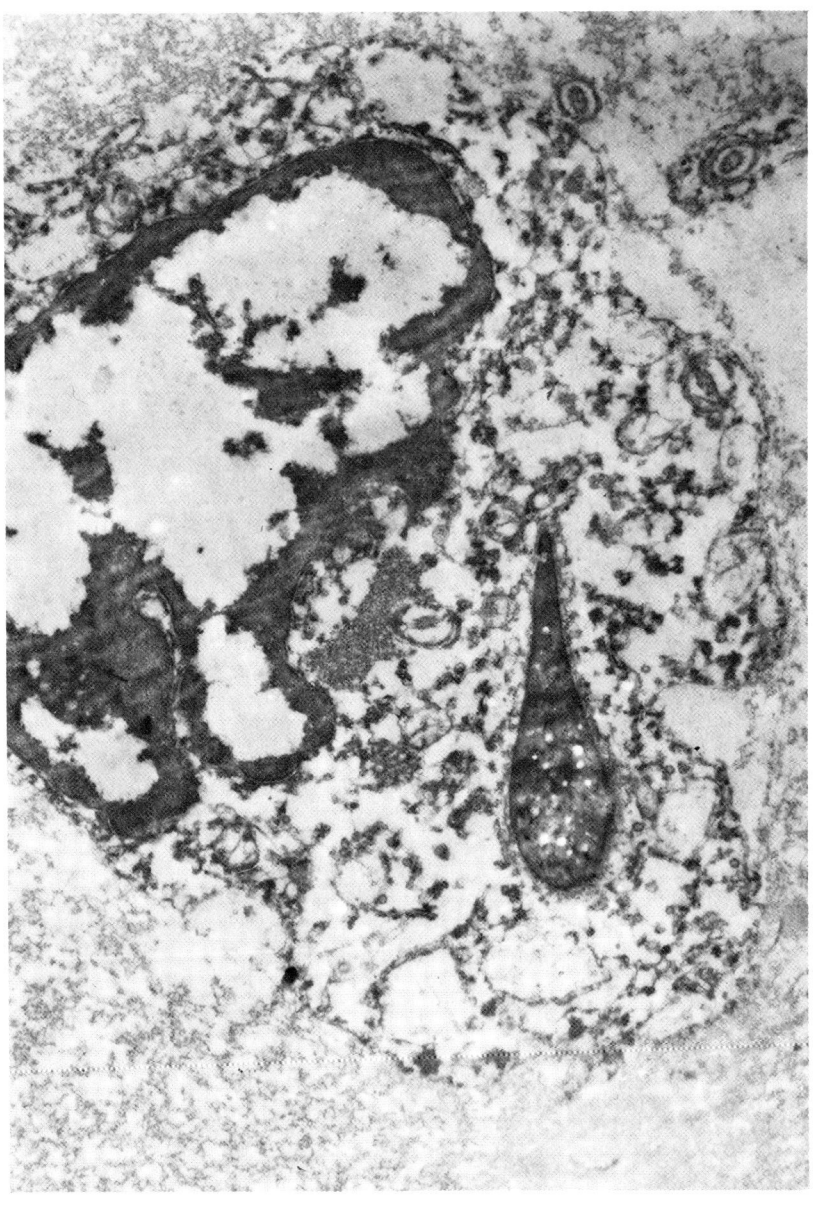

FIGURE 8. Sperm head and principal piece in cytoplasm of a degenerating neutrophil. X 18,800.

REFERENCES

Nassberg, S., McKay, D.G., and Hertig, A.T.: Physiological salpingitis. Am. J. Obstet. and Gynec. 67:130, 1954.

Ng., A.B.P.: Diseases of the uterine corpus in Manual of Cytotechnology, Eds. Keebler and Reagan, Am. Soc. Clin. Path. 4th ed, p 103, 1975.

Mishell, D.R., Jr., Bell, J.H., Good, R.G., and Moyer, D.L.: The intrauterine device: A bacteriologic study of the endometrial cavity. Am. J. Obstet. Gynec. 96:119, 1966.

Moyer, D.L., Mishell, D.R., Jr., and Bell, J.: Reactions of human endometrium to the intrauterine device. I correlation of the endometrial histology with the bacterial environment of the uterus following short-term insertion of an IUD. Am. J. Obstet. & Gynec. 106:799, 1970.

Moyer, D.L., and Mishell, D.R., Jr., Reactions of the human endometrium to the intrauterine foreign body. II—Long-term effects of the endometrial histology and cytology. Am. J. Obstet. and Gynec. 3:166, 1971.

Moyer, D.L., and Maruta, H. Induced antibody to homologous seminal and spermatozoal antigens in female monkeys. Fertil. Steril. 18:497, 1967.

Moyer, D.L., Rimdusit, S. and Mishell, D.R., Jr.: Sperm Distribution and Degradation in the Human Reproductive Tract. Obstet. Gynec. 35: 831, 1970.

Shaw, S.T., Jr., and Macaulay, L.K.: Morphologic studies of IUD-induced metrorrhagia. II. Surface changes of endometrium and microscopic localization of bleeding sites. Contraception. 19:47, 1979.

Spector, W.G.: In: Inflammation, Aetiopathogenic, clinical and therapeutic problems. Excerpta Medica Foundation, Amsterdam, 1968.

Copyright 1979 by Elsevier North Holland, Inc.
F.K. Beller and G.F.B. Schumacher, eds.
The Biology of the Fluids of the Female Genital Tract

HISTOENZYMOLOGY OF HUMAN ENDOMETRIUM DURING THE PROLIFERATIVE AND SECRETORY PHASES (I)

W. H. Wilborn* and C. E. Flowers**

SUMMARY

The endometrium completes a complicated life cycle each month that is designed to culminate in a pregnancy. The precise histological and enzymatic processes associated with the proliferative and secretory phases and the early weeks of pregnancy were studied with the periodic acid-Schiff, alcian blue, ribonucleoprotein, acid phosphatase, alkaline phosphatase, and succinate dehydrogenase techniques. These studies were correlated with the histological changes observed with light microscopy and with the transmission and scanning electron microscopes.

INTRODUCTION

Human endometrium is an interesting and dynamic tissue with the ability to reconstruct itself rapidly after menstruation and to initiate the implantation of an embryo within 21 days after the onset of clinical bleeding. This unique ability is related to the histoenzymology of the endometrium.

Both ovarian steroids stimulate enzymes and coenzymes by an intricate process. These biological catalysts play an integral part in protein, lipid, and car-

---

* Department of Anatomy, University of South Alabama, Mobile, Alabama
** Department of Obstetrics and Gynecology, The University of Alabama in Birmingham, Birmingham, Alabama

bohydrate metabolism of the endometrium. The metabolism of all these components must take place in an orderly fashion to prepare the endometrium for implantation and for the dynamic growth of the tissue after implantation. Menstruation occurs only if there is reproductive failure.

The present study focuses upon the histoenzymology of normal proliferative, secretory, and early gestational endometrium. Although somewhat similar studies are available, they are widely scattered in the literature and sometimes disparate. Furthermore, this study is the first to combine and correlate in a single source observations on the histology, histochemistry and cytochemistry, transmission electron microscopy (TEM), and scanning electron microscopy (SEM) of proliferative, secretory, and pregnant endometrium. The reader is referred to several published works related to one or more areas of the present correlative study (Schmidt-Matthiesen, 1963; Dallenbach-Hellweg, 1971; Boutselis, 1973).

MATERIALS AND METHODS

Materials

Biopsies of proliferative, secretory, and gestational human endometrium were used for this study. Observations on non-pregnant endometrium were made on approximately 100 biopsies obtained from 20 normal, ovulating patients who ranged in age from 20–42 years. Radioimmunoassays for FSH, LH, and progesterone were performed during multiple cycles on three of the patients. Biopsies from these patients were compared histologically with those from patients on which no radioimmunoassays were performed. Only those biopsies which corresponded to those from patients with known gonadotrophin and progesterone levels were used. These were dated according to the criteria of Noyes et al., (1950).

Methods

All samples were handled according to standard, previously described, techniques (Flowers et al., 1974; Flowers and Wilborn, 1978; Wilborn and Flowers, 1978).

Hematoxylin and eosin. Part of each biopsy was fixed in 10% calcium-formol, dehydrated in alcohol, cleared in xylene, embedded in paraffin, and sectioned at 6 μm. Some of these sections were stained with hematoxylin and eosin (H&E) and served to date the biopsies and as standards for the correlation of histochemical and ultrastructural data. The remaining sections were used to demonstrate carbohydrates and ribonucleoprotein.

Carbohydrates. The periodic acid-Schiff (PAS) technique was used to demonstrate glycogen and glycoprotein. PAS staining which remained after diastase digestion was interpreted as glycoprotein.

The classic alcian blue (AB) technique performed at pH 2.5 and pH 0.5 was employed to demonstrate the two types of mucins, sialomucins and sulfomucins, which are commonly associated with epithelial tissues. Despite efforts for standardization of terminology, several terms are used loosely in the literature to refer to these two mucins. Such terms include acid glycoproteins, mucopolysaccharides, glycosaminoglycans, and protein-carbohydrate complexes. The terms sialomucins and sulfomucins are still used histochemically to refer to carboxylated and sulfated mucins.

Any AB staining after nuraminidase digestion was considered in the present study to be due to sulfomucins. Sulfomucins were further identified by the AB critical electrolyte concentration method (Scott and Dorling, 1965).

Ribonucleoprotein (RNP). To demonstrate RNP, sections were stained with eosin-methylene blue (EMB) at controlled pH (4.1) in 0.2M sodium acetate buffer. Control sections were left 1 hour at room temperature in 0.1% ribonuclease (purified). Basophilia removed by ribonuclease was interpreted as RNP.

Enzymes. Part of each biopsy was frozen – 20°C. without prior fixation and sections were cut with a cryostat at 10 μm. These sections were placed on glass slides and incubated at 37°C. in the appropriate substrate to demonstrate sites and degrees of activity of several enzymes, including alkaline phosphatase, acid phosphatase, and succinate dehydrogenase. Sections incubated without substrate served as controls.

Sites of phosphatase enzymes were shown according to the technique of Gomori (1952) and the napthol-AS-phosphate azo-coupling procedure (Burstone, 1962). Both techniques gave comparable results. Succinate dehydrogenase activity was revealed by the technique of Nachlas et al., (1957). Phenazine methosulfate was added to the incubation solution (0.5 mg/ml) to enhance the reduction of Nitro-BT to diformazans at sites of enzyme activity.

Transmission electron microscopy. Tissues for TEM were fixed in 2.5% glutaraldehyde adjusted to pH 7.3 with Clark's, Millonig's collidine, or cacodylate buffer. The details of initial fixation with glutaraldehyde and postfixation with osmium tetroxide have been described elsewhere (Flowers et al., 1974; Flowers and Wilborn, 1978). Ruthenium red was added to the buffered fixatives to reveal sites of extracellular carbohydrates (Wilborn and Flowers, 1978).

Osmicated tissues were dehydrated through graded alcohols and infiltrated with propylene oxide and Epon 812 prior to embedding in Epon. Thin sections cut with diamond knives were placed on copper grids, and stained with uranyl acetate and lead citrate before viewing in a Philips EM 301 transmission electron microscope.

Scanning electron microscopy. Some of the postosmicated tissues from the various biopsies was used for SEM. Following ethanol dehydration, these tissue specimens were critical point dried with liquid CO_2, mounted on aluminum stubs, and coated with approximately 250 angstroms of gold-palladium with a Polaron sputtercoater. The specimens were examined in an Etec Autoscan scanning electron microscope.

RESULTS

Hematoxylin and Eosin

Sections stained with H&E showed the small, mitotically active glands of the proliferative phase which became hypertrophic and secretory under the influence of progesterone. Stromal cell hypertrophy accompanied that of the glands.

Periodic Acid-Schiff

The PAS method demonstrated that glycogen first appeared in gland and surface epithelial cells as small, infranuclear, PAS-positive, diastase-labile granules. These granules became visible in the early proliferative phase. Some epithelial and stromal cells contained unusually large amounts of glycogen during the early proliferative phase. They represented cells which had not expelled their secretory products during the previous menstrual cycle.

By the mid-proliferative phase, a zone of PAS-positive, diastase resistant material was present near the luminal surface of gland and surface epithelial cells (Figure 1). This material was glycoprotein which was also demonstrable by the AB(pH 2.5) technique. Less glycoprotein was present in the surface epithelial cells than in the gland cells.

The subnuclear zone of glycogen indicative of ovulation was present by the 19th day of the cycle. Most of the glycogen moved to the supranuclear region by the 21st day where it was expelled during the remainder of the cycle.

Glycoprotein increased in the epithelial cell apices during the secretory phase. The quantity of diastase-resistant glycoprotein suggested that it plays an important role in the reproductive process.

Pregnancy stimulated the production of even more glycogen and glycoprotein than observed in the secretory phase.

Alcian Blue

Sulfomucins predominated during the proliferative phase, and sialomucins in the secretory phase. Mucins were most abundant in the apices of epithelial cells and in the lumina of glands. The apical location corresponded to the PAS-positive, diastase-resistant zone of glycoprotein.

Sulfomucins were not present in large amounts even during the proliferative phase when they were at their maximal concentration. They decreased further as the secretory phase progressed.

Sialomucins were present during the proliferative phase and increased to their maximal level about the time of implantation (Figure 2). AB staining of the stroma was weak in both the estrogenic and progestational phases. It increased slightly during the late secretory phase.

Ribonucleoprotein

Epithelial RNP increased from the early proliferative to the late proliferative phase, diminished during the progestational phase, and was low in pregnancy. In contrast, RNP in stromal cells increased during pregnancy in a manner which paralleled the hypertrophy of the decidual cells. These differences in RNP levels were related to periods of maximal growth of the epithelial and decidual cells.

Alkaline Phosphatase

Enzyme activity in the epithelial cells was greatest during the proliferative phase, reached its peak shortly before ovulation, and fell during the secretory phase. Although activity was highest during the proliferative phase, many glands showed considerable activity at the time of implantation (Figure 3). Only the vas-

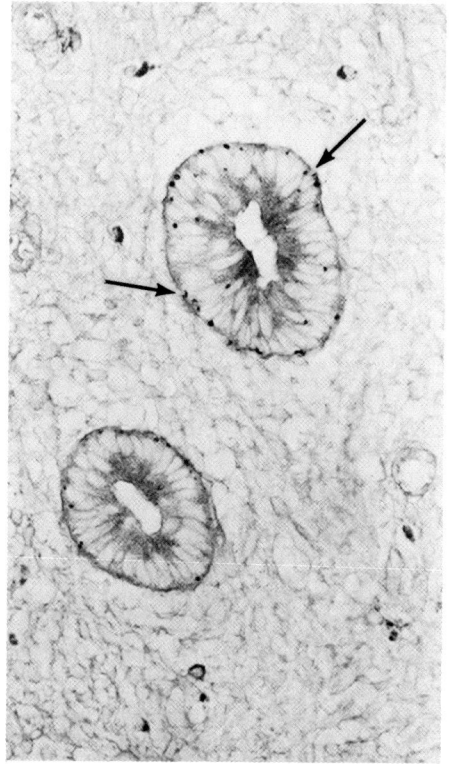
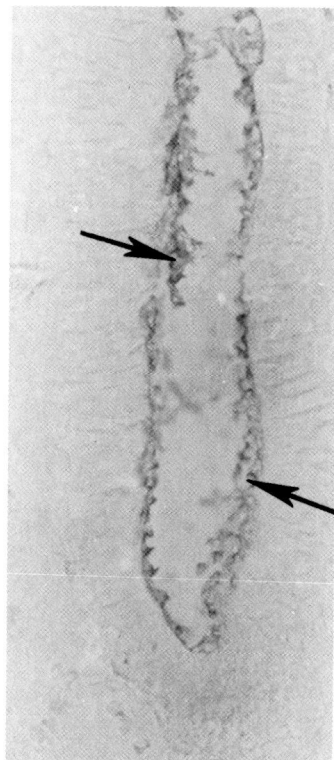

FIG. 1 **FIG. 2**

FIGURE 1. Middle proliferative phase. PAS. Two glands are shown. Each has a PAS-positive zone adjacent to the lumen and a few PAS-positive granules (arrows) in the basal zone. Nuclei are unstained. X380

FIGURE 2. Middle secretory phase. AB, pH 2.5. A gland is shown in longitudinal section with AB-positive material (arrows) at the apex and in the lumen. The remainder of the gland and the surrounding stroma is AB-negative. X480

cular endothelium retained intense enzyme activity in the event that pregnancy did not occur. Stromal cells were consistently weak in enzyme activity.

The finding of a moderate amount of alkaline phosphatase activity during the secretory phase is at variance with much of the literature concerning this enzyme. However, these histochemical studies were carefully done and consistently showed variation in the activity of alkaline phosphatase with some glands exhibiting intense activity.

Acid Phosphatase

The activity of acid phosphatase was opposite that of alkaline phosphatase. It was lowest during the proliferative phase, moderate during the mid-secretory phase, and highest immediately before menstruation (Figures 4, 5).

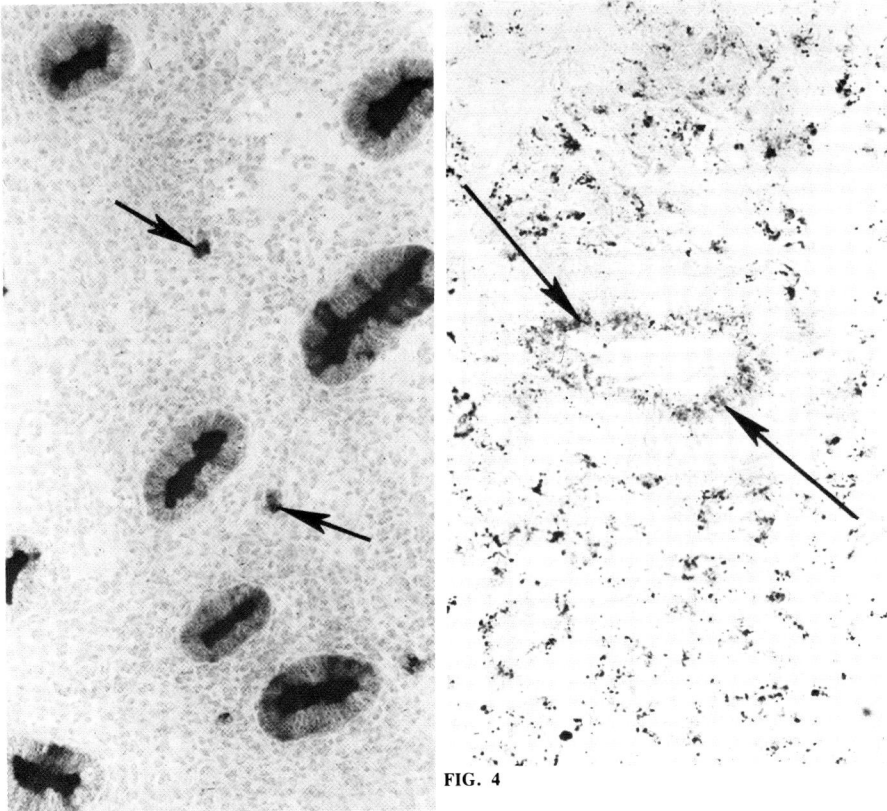

FIG. 4

FIG. 3

FIGURE 3. Middle proliferative phase. Alkaline phosphatase (Gomori). Intense enzyme activity is shown in the apical cytoplasm of the gland cells and in the vascular endothelium (arrows). X120

FIGURE 4. Middle proliferative phase. Acid phosphatase (Gomori). The gland illustrated has enzyme activity in the apical cytoplasm (arrows). Enzyme activity is also present in the stroma. X480

Essentially all investigators of the enzymes of the endometrium have reported low levels of acid phosphatase during the proliferative phase, high levels during the secretory phase, and high levels in the first trimester of pregnancy. There has also been general agreement that acid phosphatase and the other lytic enzymes of the endometrium are contained within lysosomes. There have been few explanations for the variation of this enzyme in the two phases of the menstrual cycle.

Succinate Dehydrogenase

Succinate dehydrogenase activity was low during the proliferative phase and high at the time of implantation (Figure 6). Enzyme activity decreased during the late secretory phase if pregnancy did not occur.

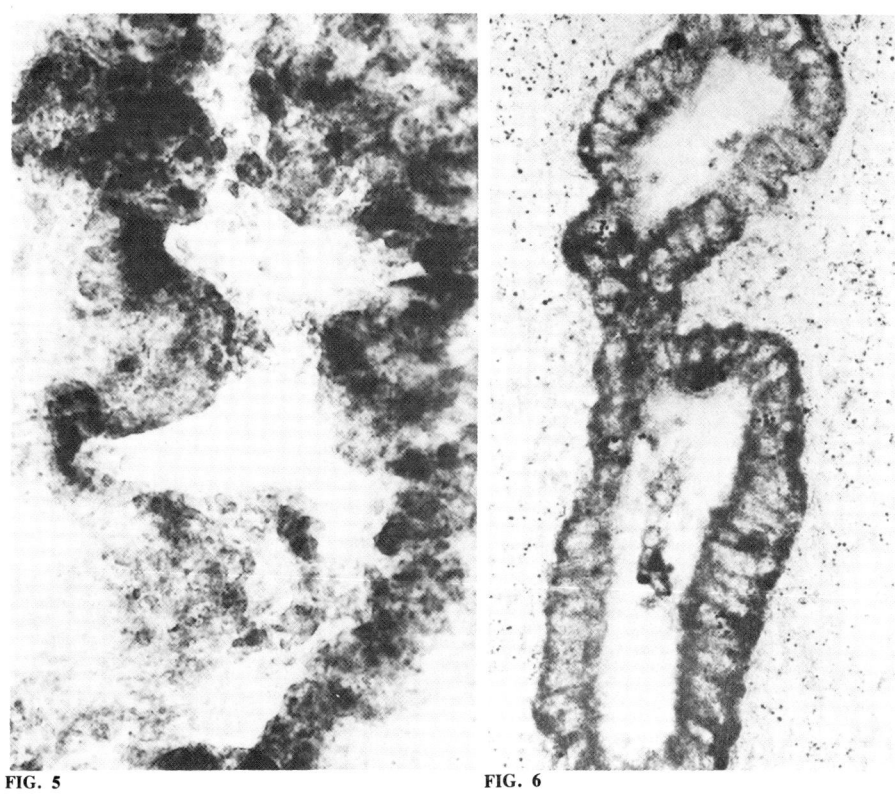

FIG. 5   FIG. 6

FIGURE 5. Late secretory phase. Acid phosphatase (Gomori). Most of the gland cells have intense enzyme activity. X480

FIGURE 6. Middle secretory phase. Succinate dehydrogenase. Note the density of diformazan particles in gland cells. Pale areas are occupied by nuclei. Sites of mitochondria in stromal cells are indicated by diformazan granules. X480

Enzyme activity was concentrated in the apical portions of the gland cells during the proliferative phase. It was rather evenly distributed throughout the cells during the secretory phase. The enzyme is found within mitochondria. Its activity and localization within the cells corresponded to the quantity and distribution of these organelles.

Scanning Electron Microscopy

SEM provided a three dimensional view of the surface epithelium and gave added importance to the histochemical findings. Since the SEM of the human endometrium has been dealt with in detail (Ludwig and Metzger, 1976), only the SEM features related to the histoenzymology of the endometrium will be emphasized here.

The proliferative phase was characterized by growth of the microvilli and an increase in number of ciliated cells. Small droplets of secretory material were present on the microvilli and cilia. The droplets corresponded to the AB-positive sialomucins and sulfomucins observed by light microscopy. The microvilli were also alkaline phosphatase–positive.

The number of cells engaged in the expulsion of secretory products and their degree of secretory activity increased through the middle secretory phase. Furthermore, the cellular method for extrusion of secretory products differed from that observed during the proliferative phase or early secretory phase. By the 21st day, large masses of secretory products distended the cell apices and extended far into the lumen (Figure 7). The greatly distended apices were lined by few or no microvilli and had a "bald" appearance. Since alkaline phosphatase is associated with microvilli and its activity falls during the secretory phase, the decrease in enzyme activity may be related to the disappearance of the microvilli. The variation

FIGURE 7. Middle secretory phase. SEM illustrating cell apices (arrows) distended with secretory products. Some secretory material has been discharged. X6,000

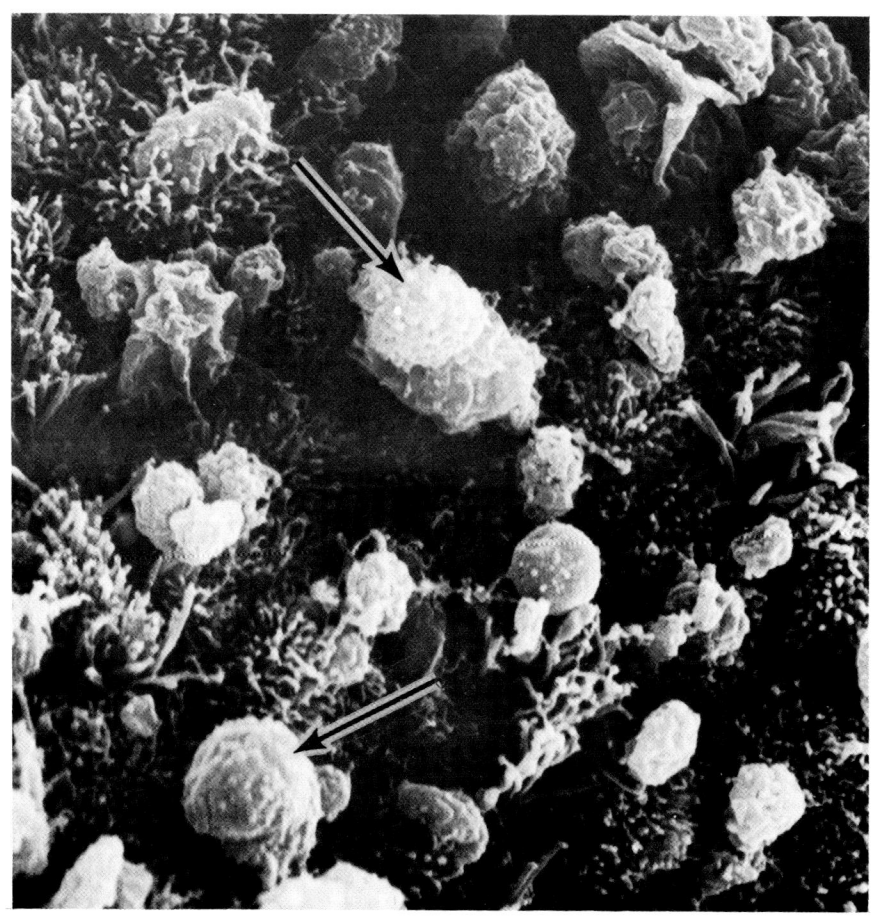

in the activity of this enzyme noted by light microscopy is possibly due to the reappearance of microvilli after the cells empty their secretory products.

The principal method for expulsion of the large masses of secretory products was by the microapocrine method. With this mode of secretion, a portion of the cell apex was shed into the lumen. Most of the glycogen was released by this method. Further degradation of the expelled secretory products occurred and this was apparently elicited by the hydrolytic enzymes in the lysosomes released concomitantly with the microapocrine secretion. This idea agrees with the histochemical data which showed that lysosomal acid phosphatase activity was highest during the secretory phase.

Microvilli attained their greatest length during the secretory phase after the expulsion of the secretory products. The growth of microvilli in response to progesterone contrasted with the growth stimulus for cilia which responded to estrogen. More droplets of secretory material were associated with the microvilli than during the proliferative phase. These droplets corresponded to the sialomucins demonstrated by the AB technique. Their presence on the microvilli would seem to add significantly to the ability of the ovum to adhere to the endometrial surface.

Transmission Electron Microscopy

Findings by TEM agreed with the histological, histochemical, and SEM observations and provided further insight into the functional significance of the various types of data. Emphasis is placed on ultrastructural features of enzymological importance and on correlating the results obtained by the various techniques.

Functionally, rough endoplasmic reticulum (RER) is associated with the synthesis of proteins for export whereas free ribosomes are concerned with the synthesis of proteins for intracellular use. During the early and middle proliferative phases, epithelial cells differed considerably in quantity of RER and free ribosomes in their basal and apical regions (Figure 8). This type of variation was also noted by the EMB technique for demonstrating cytoplasmic basophilia attributable to ribosomal RNP. The fact that EMB staining was uniform and intense by the early secretory phase correlated with the heavy concentration of free ribosomes and RER in the basal and apical regions of the epithelial cells observed by TEM (Figure 9). Decreased EMB staining intensity of the epithelial cells in the secretory phase and early pregnancy corresponded with the observation by TEM which showed the cells contained less RER and fewer free ribosomes than during the late proliferative phase. These findings indicated that protein synthesis peaked during the late proliferative phase. The cells then took on other major activities.

The epithelial cells began to accumulate glycogen as they decreased their rate of protein synthesis. Although epithelial cells contained some glycogen particles during the early and middle proliferative phases, glycogen accumulation clearly began in the late proliferative and early secretory phases where it first appeared at the cell base and then in the cell apex (Figure 9). Factors which initiate glycogen accumulation are probably related to the decline in protein synthesis and the requirement for less ATP. Consequently, glycogen particles previously used for energy requirements accumulated in the cytoplasm.

Large lakes of glycogen granules were present in the basal and apical cytoplasm by the middle secretory phase (Figure 10). Glycogen granules were well

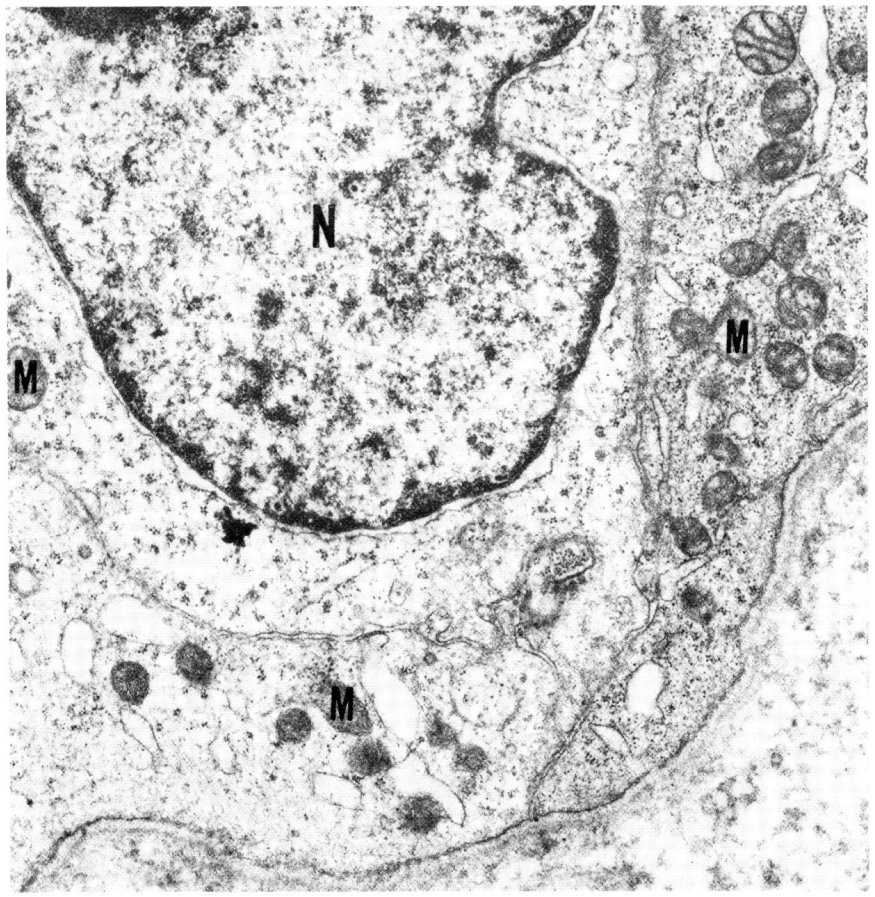

FIGURE 8. Middle proliferative phase. TEM, gland base. Note nucleus (N), mitochondria (M), and variation in the quantity of RER and free ribosomes in the cell on the right with the more electron dense cytoplasm in comparison to the cells on the left with the more electron lucent cytoplasm. X24,750

preserved by fixation in Millonig's phosphate buffer. Fixation in other types of buffer often resulted in electron lucent glycogen within large vacuoles.

It should be emphasized that glycogen accumulation was indicative of ovulation and related temporally to the appearance of the nucleolar channel system. This system of channels and tubules made a brief appearance within the epithelial cells during the early secretory phase. The system connected with the perinuclear space, which in turn connected with the RER. Thus, it provided a means for the exchange of information, via messenger RNA or ribosomal RNP, between the nucleus and cytoplasm.

Glycogen elaboration occurred in close association with mitochondria, RER, and free ribosomes. Glycogen synthesis was not intimately associated with smooth endoplasmic reticulum.

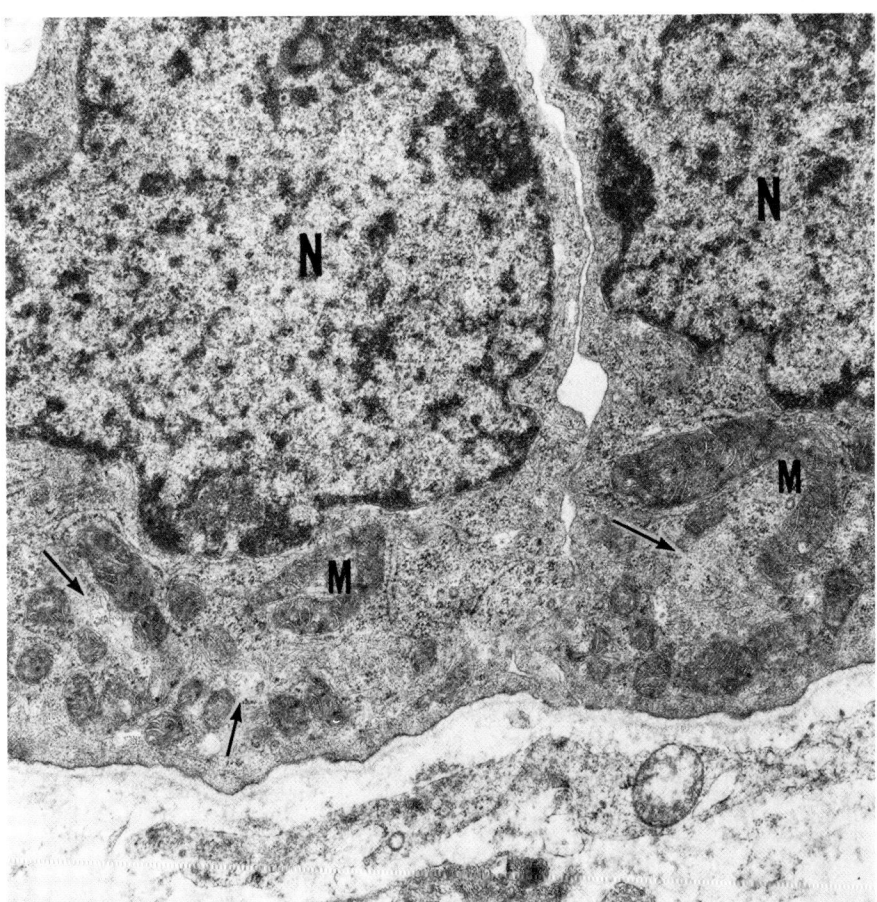

FIGURE 9. Early secretory phase. TEM, gland base. GER and free ribosomes are abundant below the two nuclei (N). Some mitochondria (M) in the basal region are large and pleomorphic. The early stage of glycogen accumulation is shown in the more electron lucent areas (arrows). X18,200

Mitochondria increased in size and number during the period of glycogen accumulation and this was accompanied by an increase in the density of their cristae. Some mitochondria reached the size of the so-called "giant" mitochondria. These mitochondrial changes paralleled the increase in succinate dehydrogenase activity shown histochemically to become dramatically enhanced during the period of glycogen synthesis. Since glycogen synthesis is initiated by the action of hexokinase, an enzyme found chiefly in mitochondria, the need for additional mitochondria in zones of glycogen synthesis is apparent.

By the 21st day of the cycle, apical protrusions rich in glycogen extended into the lumen and were released by the microapocrine method. This mode of secretion was also observed by SEM. TEM contributed additional information by illustrating that a layer of microfilaments extended across the constricted base of

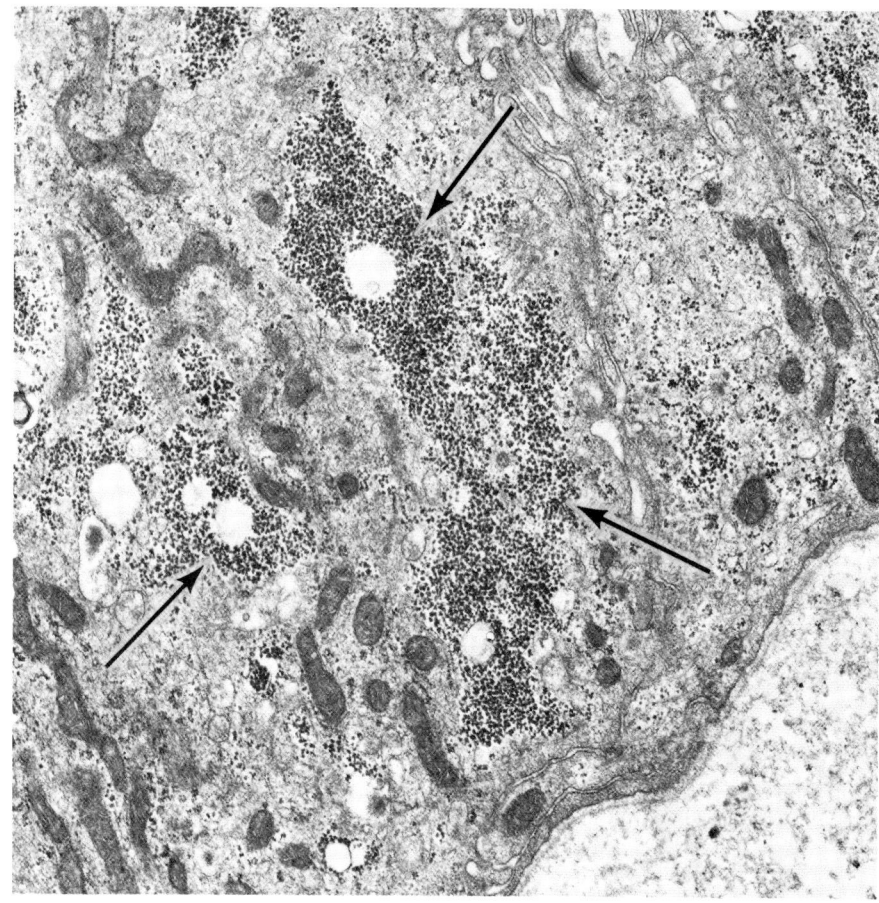

FIGURE 10. Middle secretory phase. TEM, gland base. Note large lakes of glycogen granules (arrows). Less RER and fewer ribosomes are present than in the early secretory phase. X19,800

the projection (Figure 11). The microfilaments retained constituents within the cell upon decapitation of the projection.

The Golgi appartus, which was relatively small during the proliferative phase, reached its greatest size in the secretory phase.

Golgi hypertrophy is related to the increased elaboration of secretory products which begins in the early secretory phase. The function of the Golgi in concentrating and packaging enzymes and glycoprotein secretory products is well established. Enzymes are made on the ribosomes and channeled to the Golgi through the cisternae of the RER where they are selectively packaged. The hydrolytic enzymes of lysosomes, for example, are packaged into membrane-bound vacuoles which detach from the Golgi as primary lysosomes. The Golgi also participates in the synthesis or assembly of the carbohydrate moieties of glycoproteins.

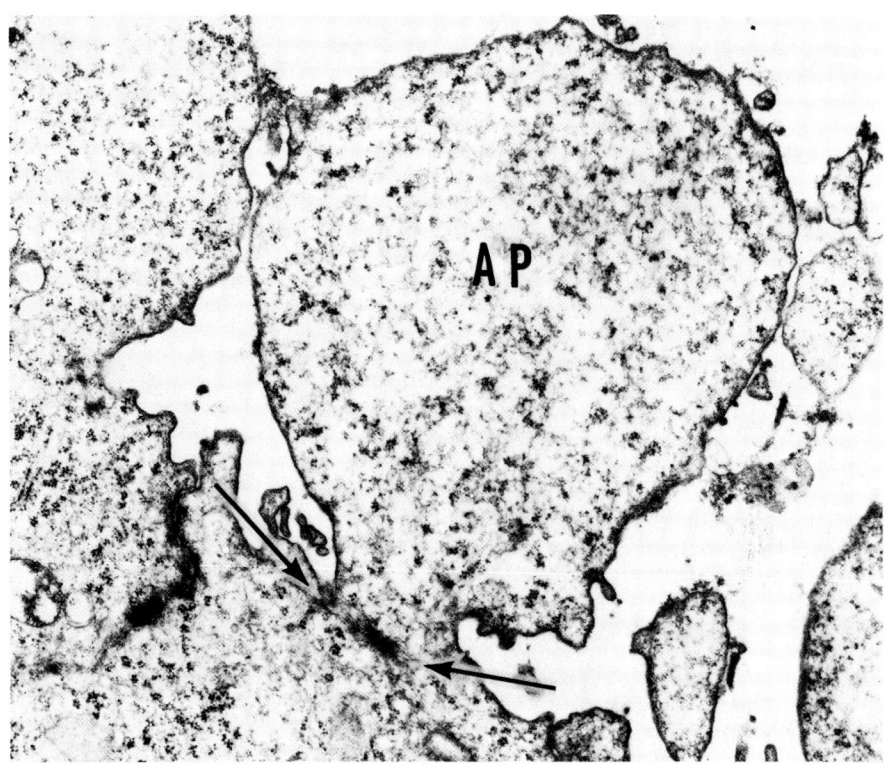

FIGURE 11. Middle secretory phase. TEM, gland apex. An apical protrusion (AP) is shown before release by the microapocrine method of secretion. Note the layer of microfilaments (arrows) at constricted base of protrusion. X22,500

The rise in lysosomal acid phosphatase activity, which was demonstrated histochemically to take place during the early secretory phase, paralleled the hypertrophy of the Golgi. The enlargement of the Golgi was also accompanied by an increase in histochemically demonstrable AB-positive material at the luminal surface. TEM showed that much of the glycoprotein-rich, AB-positive material at the luminal surface originated from the Golgi and participated in the production of the ruthenium red-positive cell coat (Figure 12). The cell coat consisted of filamentous material on the external surface of the plasma membrane. The coat was thick at the time of implantation and remained through the late secretory phase and early pregnancy.

To this point, only epithelial features of enzymological importance have been emphasized. Interestingly, many features observed by TEM in epithelial cells were also present in the predecidual stromal cells at corresponding times of the cycle. Stromal cells accumulated large amounts of glycogen, underwent pronounced hypertrophy during the secretory phase, and became true decidual cells if pregnancy occurred. They accumulated lipid after the cessation of glycogen production in a manner similar to the epithelial cells. They also exhibited a ruthenium red-positive surface coat which became especially prominent during the late secretory phase.

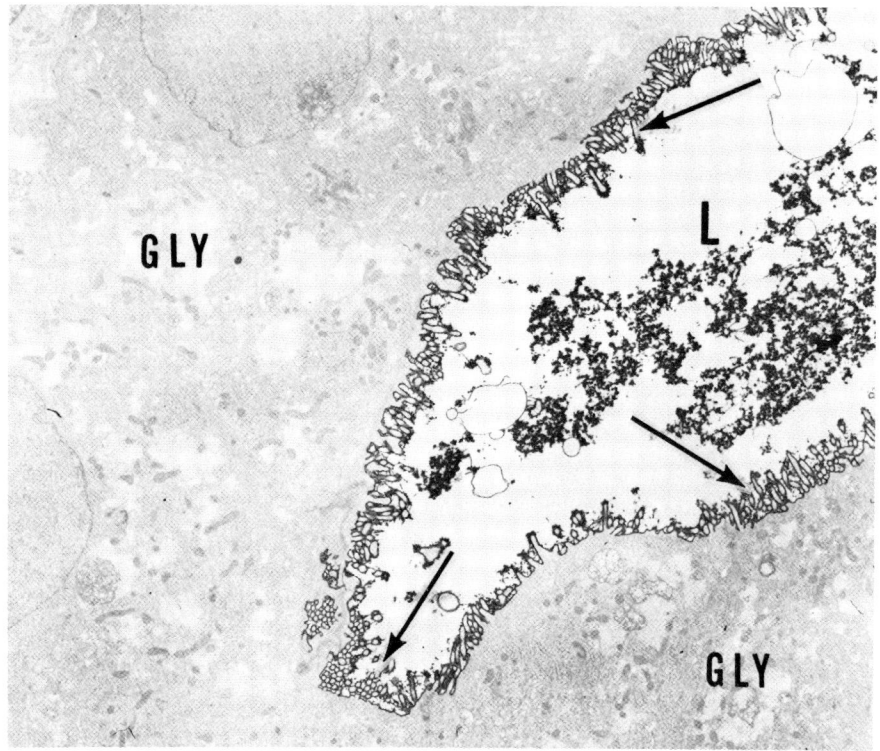

FIGURE 12. Late secretory phase. TEM, gland apex. The tissue was immersed in a solution of ruthenium red, but no other stains were used. Observe the ruthenium red-positive surface coat on the microvilli (arrows) and the positive material in the lumen (L). Areas of glycogen (GLY) and other cytoplasmic constituents are unstained. X5,100

A remarkable feature of the predecidual and decidual cells was their close proximity to the epithelial cells during the secretory phase and early pregnancy. Even closer apposition was attained by the extension of cell processes between the two cell types. Pinocytotic vesicles of cytoplasmic products passed from the predecidual and decidual cells into the epithelial cells. This mechanism of cytoplasmic exchange appeared to serve as a means for clearing the stroma of secretory products. Further passage of these products through the epithelial cells and into lumina of glands and the uterine cavity greatly increased the amount of material available for histotrophic nutrition of the embryo.

DISCUSSION

The menstrual cycle is a physiologic span of time that is designed to initiate primate reproduction. The process of menstruation is an event indicating reproductive failure; it is associated with the rapid expulsion of the catabolic products of the unsuccessful cycle and the remodeling of the endometrium to initiate an implantation in the next cycle.

Menstruation is associated with and followed by a frenzy of activities designed to initiate histoenzymatic reactions. These reactions provide the endometrium with sufficient energy, protein, and carbohydrate to quickly mature. Maturation permits the endometrium to fulfill its biologic role of providing appropriate nutrition and blood supply for implantation and the growth of the products of conception in an ensuing cycle.

Each of the various enzymatic processes which have been described occur in concert at precisely the correct time and in precisely the appropriate anatomical milieu to allow implantation to begin on or about the 21st day of the reproductive cycle. At this exact period of time every process is perfectly coordinated and geared to increase in intensity and efficiency if the corpus luteum is stimulated by HCG. If this stimulus occurs, there is an intensified secretory and enzymatic activity of the gland cells and a remarkable metamorphosis of the stromal cells. Each of these events occurs to biological perfection so that the process of implantation has more than adequate energy through coordinated enzymatic activity. However, when implantation is completed and the fetus has developed independent nutritional control, the secretory activity of the gland cells is discontinued and the metamorphosis of the stromal cells to true decidual cells occurs.

The true decidual cells seem to actually nurse the endometrial vessels and the developing trophoblast by maintaining extremely close proximity to them. In this manner they can efficiently transfer glycoprotein and other nutrients in precise physiological amounts to maintain optimal nutrition, function, and assistance in clearing catabolic products.

REFERENCES

Boutselis, J.G.: Histochemistry of the normal endometrium. In: *The Uterus*. Eds.: Norris, H.J., Hertig, A.T., and Abell, M.R., The Williams and Wilkins Co., Baltimore, MD 1973, pp. 175–184.

Durstone, M.S.: *Enzyme Histochemistry and its Application in the Study of Neoplasms*. Academic Press Inc., New York, N.Y., 1962.

Dallenbach–Hellweg, G.: *Histopathology of the Endometrium*. Springer-Verlag, N.Y., 1971.

Flowers, C.E., Wilborn, W.H.: New observations on the physiology of menstruation. Obstet. Gynecol. 51 (1978) 16–24.

Flowers, C.E., Wilborn, W.H., and Enger, J.: Effects of quingestanol acetate on the histology, histochemistry, and ultrastructure of human endometrium. Am. J. Obstet. Gynecol. 120 (1974) 589–612.

Gomori, G.: *Microscopic Histochemistry*. University of Chicago Press, Chicago, IL, 1952.

Ludwig, H. and Metzger, H.: *The Human Female Reproductive Tract: A Scanning Electron Microscopic Atlas*. Springer–Verlag, New York, 1976.

Nachlas, M.M., Tsou, K.C., De Sousa, K., Cheng, C.S., and Seligman, A.M. Cytochemical demonstration of succinic dehydrogenase by the use of a p-nitrophenyl substituted ditetrazole. J. Histochem. Cytochem. 5 (1957) 420–436.

Noyes, R.W., Hertig, A.T., and Rock, J. Dating the endometrial biopsy. Fertil. Steril. 1 (1950) 3–25.

Schmidt–Mattiesen, H.: Histochemistry. In: *The Normal Human Endometrium*. Ed.: Schmidt–Matthiesen, H., Blakiston Division of McGraw-Hill Book Co., New York, 1963, pp. 135–207.

Scott, J.E. and Dorling, J.: Differential staining of acid glycosaminoglycans (mucopolysaccharides) by Alcian Blue salt solutions. Histochemie 5 (1965) 221–233.

Wilborn, W.H. and Flowers, C.E.: Mechanisms of uterine bleeding with oral contraceptives. Transactions Amer. Assoc. Obstet. Gynecol., 1979 (in press).

ENDOMETRIAL SECRETION PROTEINS—BIOCHEMISTRY AND BIOLOGICAL SIGNIFICANCE

H. M. Beier

SUMMARY

The history of research efforts on the description and analysis of genital tract fluid is briefly reviewed. Mammalian endometrial secretion has been studied and biochemically analyzed in many small laboratory animals and also in large domestic animals. Comparatively few data are available from human uterine secretions. Two types of protein secretion patterns are recorded: the one is the production of a whole mixture of uterus characteristic protein bands, appearing dependent on certain oestrogen/progestagen ratio (cf. mouse, rat, sheep), the other type is characterized by the release of a few predominant protein fractions as a consequence of progesterone actions (cf. rabbit).

The mammalian embryonic development depends on extrinsic support by the maternal organism. During preimplantation, the growing blastocyst needs favourable environmental conditions, which are provided by endometrial transformations and secretion. The macromolecular composition of uterine secretion at different times before implantation is characterized by a spectrum of protein patterns which change daily. In an attempt to shed light on the significance of the uterine secretion proteins, particularly uteroglobin in the rabbit, in the establish-

---

Abteilung' Anatomy und Reproductions Biologie, Rheinisch-Westfälische Technische Hochschule, Aachen, FRG

ment of early pregnancy, analyses are reported which demonstrate the origin and endocrine control of synthesis and release of these proteins.

In a further comparative study of *in vivo* and *in vitro* blastocyst development, the significance and consequences of asynchrony between the embryonic and maternal reproduction phases are investigated. Within this study, particular attention has been drawn to uterine influences on the rabbit blastocyst coverings, and how embryonic development can be retarded by abnormal structural transformation of the zona pellucida and the mucin coat. The convenient experimental systems of advanced and of delayed uterine secretion in the rabbit will permit an approach to the question of whether the uterine macromolecular components constitute a maternal response to the presence of the blastocyst.

Preliminary investigations on human endometrial secretion are reported and discussed with regard to comparative conclusions, last not least because of the relevance to the synchronization problems for the egg and the maternal system in human egg transfer.

INTRODUCTION

The fluids of male and female genital tracts have been considered by the scientists of the 16th and 17th centuries to represent the male and female "semen". These scientists believed that the fusion of both male and female semen resulted in the formation of an embryo, obviously emerging from the semen pool within the cavity of the uterus. Ham and Leeuwenhoek detected in 1677 that the male semen fluid contained spermatozoa, which immediately were referred to as the male germ cells. However, the female gamete was lacking, and consequently A. von Haller, the leading physiologist of his time, taught that a fluid was delivered from the ovary into the Fallopian tube, flooding the uterine cavity and giving rise to the oocyte by a process of coagulation (von Haller, 1757, 1766). In 1827, K.E. von Baer finally detected and described properly the mammalian oocyte and its ovulation from the ovary. This discovery finalized the theories of "uterine oocytes". At the same moment, however, the old question was reopened whether or not the genital tract fluids, and in particular the uterine secretion, have a certain biological significance. K.E. von Baer extended his studies on early mammalian development to the search for human early embryonic stages. When dissecting the cadaver of an unmarried woman, who had committed suicide because of fear of pregnancy, von Baer investigated the uterus at eight days after supposed conception. He described the contents of the opened uterus as being a viscous, mucous fluid, most likely containing protein. From the recent biochemical point of view this was an assumption, however, we know by now that von Baer was right, and that with this observation the "modern history" of the scientific analysis of the female genital tract fluids, in particular the uterine fluid, began. Several investigators of the early years of our century have recognized the physiological dependency of the genital tract secretions on the stages of the reproductive or menstrual cycles (Bond, 1898, 1899, 1906; Gerlinger, 1922; Hartmann, 1923), however, it was not before sophisticated physico-chemical methods were developed that a detailed analysis was possible (Bishop, 1956; Homburger et al., 1955; Junge and Blandau, 1959; Lutwak-Mann, 1960, 1962). Finally, when high resolution electrophoretic and chromatographic means become available, particularly polyacrylmide gels, the first informative macromolecular component patterns of uterine secretions were demonstrated (Schwick, 1963; Beier, 1966, 1967, 1968 a; Kirchner, 1969).

Endometrial Secretion

At the same time when morphological and cytological transformations are preparing the endometrium for implantation of the blastocyst, we find physicochemically alterations of the uterine secretions, the characteristics of which can be shown by quantitative and qualitative means. Volume and viscosity of the secretions are dependent on the chronological stage of the reproductive cycle and the endocrine background of the maternal system. Homburger et al., (1957) and Harpel et al., (1968) demonstrated this by data on preovulatory uterine fluid, Lutwak-Mann, Boursnell and Bennett (1960) were able to show that the viscosity of uterine fluid increased after ovulation, thereby increasing the protein concentration. Even higher secretion rates were triggered by postovulatory progesterone.

As our knowledge of the biochemistry of uterine secretion components accumulates, new advances are attained concerning the origin of these molecules and the various ways in which these components (proteins) are released into the lumen of the genital tract. Analytical evidence from qualitative and quantitative studies, employing acrylamide gel electrophoresis, Ouchterlony double immunodiffusion, and other immuno-electrophoretical combinations, suggests that, whereas many genital tract fluid proteins are identical to those of the blood serum, several are only found in uterine secretion. As shown earlier (Beier, 1967), a selective transport of serum proteins into the uterine luminal fluid occurs. Serum-identical proteins are not lined up within a certain category of small molecular sizes, but there are, on the contrary, rather diverse molecular weights, disregarding any preference for small protein components that would suggest a simple sieve effect by the blood-uterine secretion barrier. The partial disparity in the relative amounts of these few identified serum proteins in uterine secretion, compared to their serum proportions, further emphasizes the selectivity of transudation process. The albumin/globulin ratio has been calculated for blood serum (1:32) however, for rabbit Day 6 uterine secretion a significant relative albumin decrease was observed. In addition, serum contains normally 15–17 rel.% of immunoglobulins, whereas uterine pre-implantational secretion has not more than 2 rel.%.

Comparative Animal Data

Changes in the nature of uterine secretion proteins have been extensively studied in several species. It was found that endometrial secretion patterns are hormone dependent and develop time specific characteristics according to the oestrogen/progesterone ratio. The following references provide basic information:

rabbit: Schwick, 1963; Beier, 1966, 1967 a, b, 1968 a, b, 1973, 1976, 1978; Kirchner, 1969; Krishnan and Daniel, 1967; Urzua et al., 1970; Shapiro et al., 1971: Johnson, 1972; Feigelson et al., 1977; Bullock, 1977; Beato, 1977;
mouse: Mintz, 1971; Aitken, 1977; Fishel, 1979;
rat: Kunitake et al., 1965; Surani, 1976;
roe deer: Aitken, 1974;
cow: Roberts and Parker, 1974; Laster, 1977; Dixon and Gibbons, 1979;

pig: Squire, Bazer, Murray, 1972; Murray et al., 1972;
sheep: Roberts, Parker and Symonds, 1976;
maccaque and baboon: Mastroianni et al., 1969, 1970; Joshi et al., 1972; Peplow et al., 1973;
man: Beier, Petry, Kühnel, 1970; Moghissi, 1970; Bernstein, Aladjem, Chen, 1971; Daniel, 1971 a; Shirai et al., 1972; Beier and Beier–Hellwig, 1973; Wolf and Mastroianni, 1975; Noske and Feigelson, 1976; Voss and Beato, 1977; Beier, 1978; Aitken, 1979.

The characteristic uterine protein patterns of some of the various species are demonstrated in Figures 1 (rabbit), 2 (mouse), 3 (rat), 4 (sheep), 5 (man). Selective transudation of serum proteins into the uterine cavity evidently occurs irrespective of the size of the protein molecules. This could be shown by immunoelectrophoretic means using available antibodies. More relevant information, however, on the synthesis and transudation of macromolecules into the uterine secretion would be gained by the use of labelled precursors. Studies of the uterine luminal proteins of the rat have been carried out using ^{3}H–leucine and ^{3}H–fucose (Surani, 1977). There is little protein synthesized and secreted when progesterone alone is dominating the spayed animal, however, when progesterone is administered together with oestradiol–17β, a substantial increase in the amounts of radiolabelled proteins was found in uterine secretion (Surani, 1977). The nature of the proteins released into the uterine cavity depends on the correct balance of oestradiol and progesterone. Similar findings are made in the mouse (Aitken, 1977; Fishel, 1979). By contrast, the most pronounced changes have been found in the endometrial secretion of the rabbit where uteroglobin represents the major fraction (50%–70%) of all proteins, and where this protein is produced in response to progesterone (Beier, 1968; Beier, Petry, Kühnel, 1970). Interestingly, no clear evidence is available that uteroglobin is more than a unique rabbit protein. Similar protein fractions have been described in human uterine fluids (see Table I), however, no immunological identity could be demonstrated.

Endocrine Regulation of Uteroglobin Synthesis and Release

It has been an interesting question since the first observations on the effects of progesterone on uteroglobin appearance in uterine secretion, whether this steroid acts directly on the synthesis, on the release, or on both processes together. By now, evidence has been attained that progesterone and also several other progestagens are capable of stimulating synthesis and release. Uteroglobin synthesis is mainly activated by progesterone, although this protein is produced in detectable amounts in the uterus of oestrogen treated castrated does. Under such experimental conditions uteroglobin is present in the epithelial cells, but it is not extruded into the cavum uteri in amounts which could be detected by immunohistochemical means, as work by Kirchner (1976) indicates. However, within the uterus we never could obtain any uteroglobin release under the influence of oestrogens, even if considerable dosages of 17β-oestradiol were used (Beier, 1974). The release response to progesterone is dose-dependent, the most effective dosage being in the range of 0.6–3.0 mg/day/animal (average weight of 2.5–3.0 kg). Higher doses do not effect an increase of uteroglobin concentrations in uterine secretion.

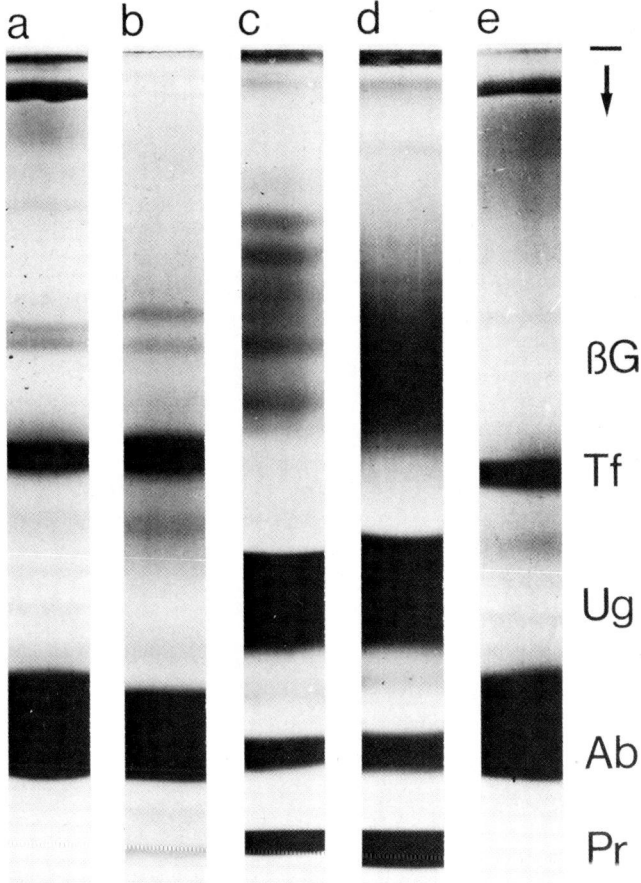

FIGURE 1. Uterine secretions of the rabbit. Polyacrylamide gel electrophoretic separation of rabbit uterine flushings during oestrous (b) and early pregnancy, compared to blood serum (a). The early pregnancy protein patterns characterize dynamic pictures which change daily (c = Day 6, d = Day 7, e = Day 9 post coitum). Note the prominent fractions of prealbumins (Pr), albumin (Ab), uteroglobin (Ug), transferrin (Tf), and β-glycoproteins (β-G). Tris-glycine-buffer pH 9.0, Amidoblack-10B-staining.

Doubtless, progesterone is required to establish the characteristic secretion pattern of uteroglobin during preimplantation *in vivo*. But, Beato and Arnemann (1975) have shown that this secretion is intact when the uterus is removed from the mother, isolated, and perfused under defined experimental conditions.

The production of uteroglobin as the major endometrial protein required identification of synthesis by demonstration of the appropriate messenger RNA (mRNA). The endometrium of progesterone stimulated rabbits has been used as a source for the isolation of uteroglobin mRNA. The translation of poly(A)-containing mRNA for uteroglobin has been demonstrated in different systems

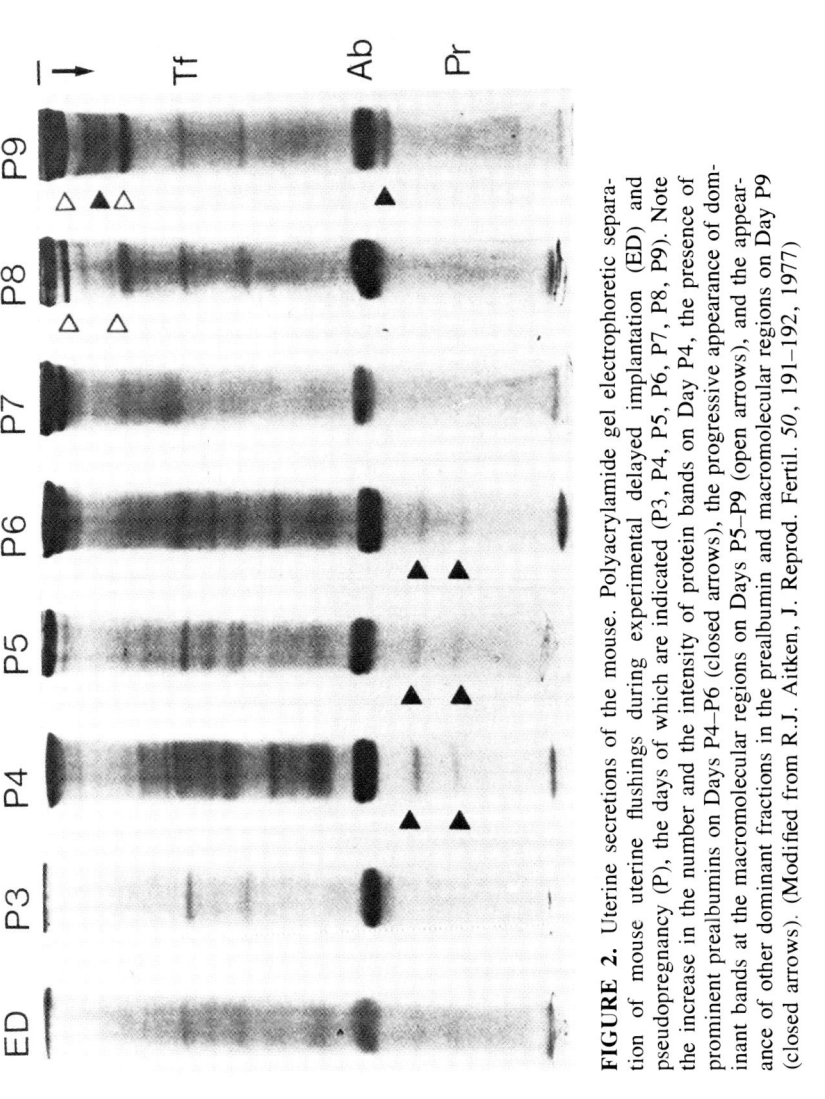

FIGURE 2. Uterine secretions of the mouse. Polyacrylamide gel electrophoretic separation of mouse uterine flushings during experimental delayed implantation (ED) and pseudopregnancy (P), the days of which are indicated (P3, P4, P5, P6, P7, P8, P9). Note the increase in the number and the intensity of protein bands on Day P4, the presence of prominent prealbumins on Days P4–P6 (closed arrows), the progressive appearance of dominant bands at the macromolecular regions on Days P5–P9 (open arrows), and the appearance of other dominant fractions in the prealbumin and macromolecular regions on Day P9 (closed arrows). (Modified from R.J. Aitken, J. Reprod. Fertil. *50*, 191–192, 1977)

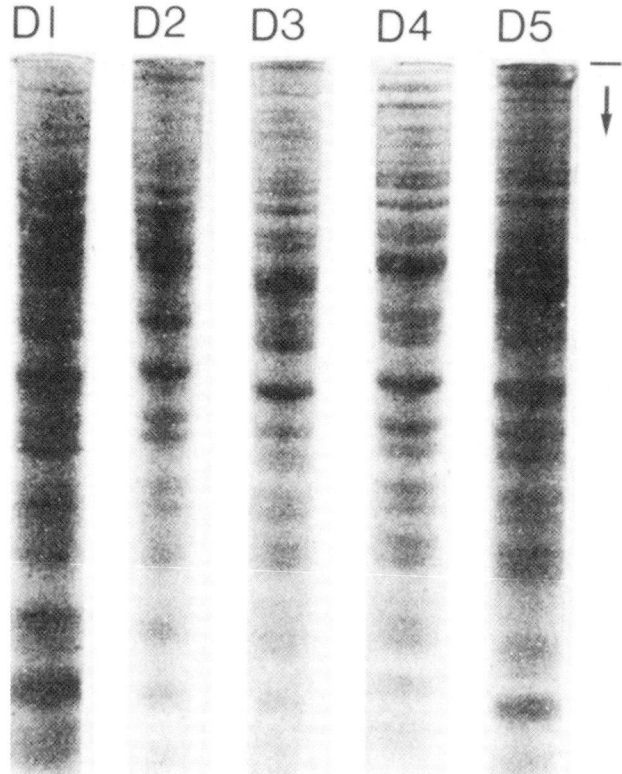

FIGURE 3. Uterine secretions of the rat. SDS acrylamide gel electrophoretic separation of rat uterine flushings. The samples are taken from normal pregnant preimplantational animals and during implantation: Days 1 to 5 (D1, D2, D3, D4, D5). Changes are appearing in the macromolecular region, where a whole "family" of bands changes from day to day. (Modified from M.A.H. Surani, J. Reprod. Fertil. *48*, 141–145, 1976).

(Beato and Rungger, 1975; Bullock, Woo and O'Malley, 1976). Identification of newly synthesized uteroglobin was presented by means of monospecific antibodies. These results definitely point out that uteroglobin is synthesized de novo in the uterus and that progesterone stimulates this synthesis. Bullock et al., (1976) have demonstrated that the specific mRNA for uteroglobin accounts for an increasing proportion of the poly(A)-rich endometrial mRNA during the preimplantation period, reaching a maximum at Day 4 post coitum in normal pregnancy. The pattern of change in uteroglobin mRNA during the preimplantation period reaches a maximum at Day 4 post coitum in normal pregnancy. The pattern of change in uteroglobin mRNA is similar to the pattern of secretion of uteroglobin during normal preimplantation and reflects the changing endocrine control mechanisms of the maternal system.

So far, it is unclear what process terminates uteroglobin presence in the secretion. It may well be that the progesterone/oestradiol ratio is more important than the level of one or both steroids alone. Since the protein pattern observed

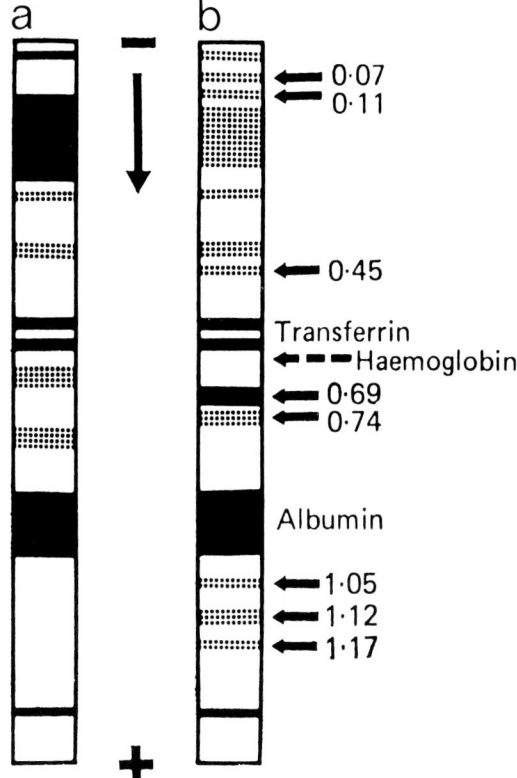

FIGURE 4. Ovine uterine secretion. Comparison of polyacrylamide gel electrophoretic patterns of ovine blood serum (a) and uterine wash fluid (b) from a 15-day pregnant sheep. The characteristic bands are indicated by the solid arrows and their migration rates relative for albumin shown by the numbers. Interestingly, a prealbumin group and as well pre- and posttransferrins appear, which were not detected in blood serum. (Modified from G.P. Roberts et al., J. Reprod. Fertil. *48*, 99–107, 1976).

during pseudopregnancy suggests that implantation itself terminates uteroglobin release or synthesis, there may be a specific "message" delivered from the blastocyst or from the decidual tissue, as has been proposed by Johnson (1974). The perfusion experiments on isolated uteri and their uteroglobin production (Beato and Arnemann, 1975) indicate that the "switch-off" *in vivo* is a termination of the synthesis rather than release, since these studies show no long-term accumulation of uteroglobin within the cytosol of the endometrial cells.

Approaches to Study Uteroglobin Function

Some biochemical and biological parameters of uteroglobin are compiled in Tables II and III. Approaches to analyze uteroglobin physiology concentrate on studies of its biochemical properties, including binding and transport func-

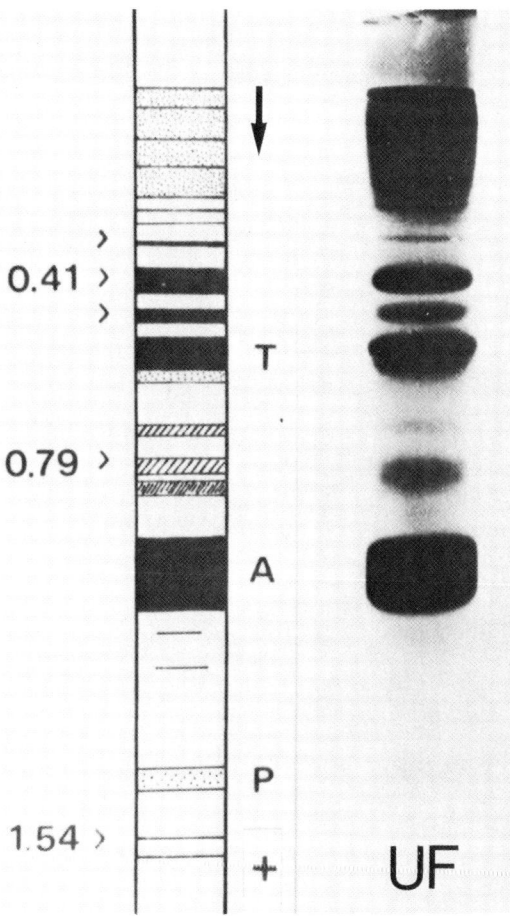

FIGURE 5. Human uterine secretion. Polyacrylamide gel electrophoretic separation of human uterine flushing (UF) collected during the early luteal phase of the cycle. The proteins which are not obviously not appearing in the paired blood serum sample are indicated by arrows. Dense bands, characteristic for uterine secretions, are the postalbumin in position 0.79 (relative migration rate to albumin) and the posttransferrin in position 0.41. A = albumin, P = prealbumin, T = transferrin. (Modified from R.J. Aitken, J. Reprod. Fertil. 55, 247–254, 1979).

tions, as well as enzyme-inhibitor activities. Additionally, a differential analysis of uteroglobin and the homologous molecules of the male reproductive tract and the lung is necessary and will be useful.

The uteroglobin-like protein from the seminal plasma and from the bronchial secretion are immunologically identical antigens, as has been confirmed by several independent investigators (Beier, Bohn and Müller, 1975; Beier, 1977; Beier, Kirchner and Mootz, 1978; Noske and Feigelson, 1976; Bullock and Bhatt, 1976). The most challenging questions arise from comparative studies on uteroglobin and the uteroglobin-like antigens. Does this "ectopic uteroglobin" show similar or

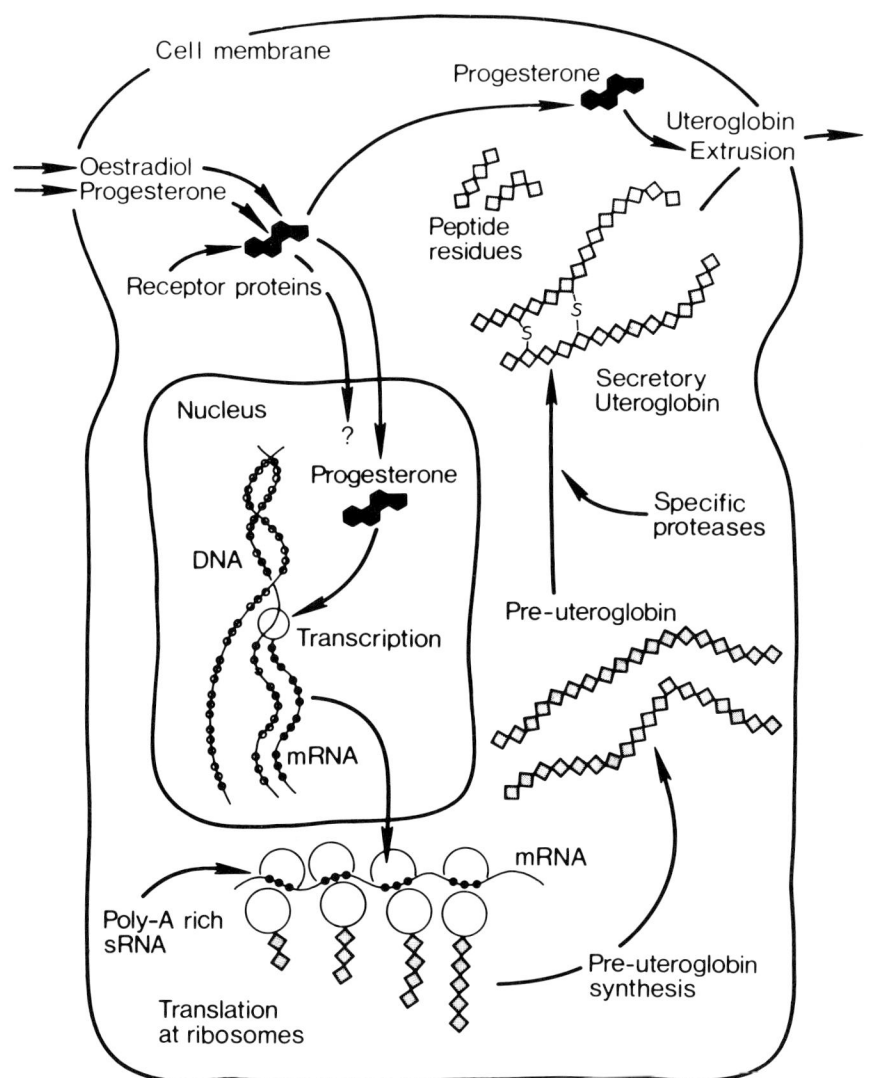

FIGURE 6. Schematic illustration of uteroglobin synthesis and release in an endometrial epithelial cell. Oestradiol and progesterone may enter the epithelial cell at any site, then being carried by receptors to the cell nucleus. Progesterone surely induces transcription of specific uteroglobin messenger RNA; however, this is not yet clear with oestradiol. Translation of uteroglobin precursor molecule. This has to be converted by some exopeptidases or other specific proteases and could be dimerized into the secretory uteroglobin. Extrusion of uteroglobin via the apical membrane of the epithelial cell is controlled by progesterone alone, the extrusion type being rather unclear yet; however, no "secretory granules" are involved in this process. For detailed informations on the biochemistry of uteroglobin and the uteroglobin molecular structure, recent publications are available: Ponstingl et al., 1978; Popp et al., 1978; Malsky et al., 1979. (Courtesy Georg Thieme Publ., Stuttgart: Human Fertilization, H. Ludwig and P.F. Tauber, Eds., 1978).

TABLE I. Uteroglobin Analogues in Various Species

Species	Criterion for similarity with rabbit uteroglobin			References
	Chromato-graphic	Electro-phoretic	Immuno-logical	
Wallaby		+		Renfree, 1973
Opossum	−	−	−	Renfree, 1975
Mouse	−	−		Mintz, 1971; Aitken, 1977; Fishel, 1979
Rat	−	−	−	Kunitake et al., 1965; Surani, 1976
Hamster		−	−	Noske and Daniel, 1974
Guinea-pig	−	−	−	Bullock, pers. comm.
Roe deer		+	−	Aitken, 1974
Cow	−	+(?)		Roberts and Parker, 1974; Laster, 1977; Dixon and Gibbons, 1979
Pig	+	+	−	Squire, Bazer and Murray, 197?
Mink	+(?)	−	−	Daniel, 1968; Daniel and Krishnan, 1969
Ferret	−	−		Daniel, 1971 a
Black bear	−	−		Daniel, 1968; Daniel and Krishnan, 1969
Dog	+		−	Daniel and Krishnan, 1969
Fur seal	+(?)	+	−	Daniel, 1971 b, 1972 a
Armadillo	−	−		Daniel, 1968; Daniel and Krishnan, 1969
Baboon		+(?)		Peplow et al., 1973
Man		+	−/+(?	Beier, Petry, Kühnel, 1970; Shirai et al., 1972; Daniel, 1973: Beier and Beier-Hellwig, 1973; Wolf and Mastroianni, 1975; Noske and Feigelson, 1976; Voss and Beato, 1977; Maathius and Aitken, 1978; Beier, 1978; Aitken, 1979.

This table was corrected and extended after a table of Daniel (1976).

identical properties, particularly with regard to the most intriguing features of steroid binding and trypsin inhibition? Purified proteins have been used in recent studies on progesterone binding to authenticate uteroglobin and the uteroglobin-like antigen from the lung (Beato and Beier, 1978). There is an identical progesterone binding to both proteins. However, synthesis and secretion are controlled by ovarian steroids within the uterus only, since lungs from ovariectomized animals, male and newborn rabbits contained the uteroglobin-like protein.

Rather surprisingly, we have found quite different results by means of fibrin-agar-electrophoresis to test the trypsin inhibitory activity of uteroglobin and the homologous antigen from bronchial secretion. Preliminary results, which need further confirmation, show that the uteroglobin fraction of endometrial secretion does inhibit trypsin whereas the uteroglobin-like protein fraction of the lung tissue does not (Beier, 1977). It remains to be clarified whether an unknown factor

TABLE II. Biochemical Properties of Uteroglobin

(a) Separation from other uterine secretion proteins by acrylamide gel electrophoresis and identification as postalbumin fraction (Beier, 1966, 1967)

(b) Identification of uteroglobin, the postalbumin fraction as identical antigen to the β_1-U-globulin from classical agar-immunoelectrophoresis performed by Schwick (1965), by means of a direct acrylamide-agar-immunoelectrophoretical combination (Beier, 1966, 1967)

(c) Sedimentation in analytical ultracentrifugation (Svedberg units analysis) $S_{c=1.0\%} = 1.38$ (Beier, 1968 a)

(d) Molecular weight around 14,000–15,000 (Murray et al., 1972; Bullock and Connell, 1973)

(e) Composition of two identical subunits of approximately 7,000–8,000 MW, linked by S-S-bonds and composed of 70 amino acids (McGaughey and Murray, 1972; Beato and Baier, 1975, Beato, 1977; Ponstingl, Nieto and Beato, 1978)

(f) Isoelectrofocussing reveals an isoelectric point of 5.4 (McGaughey and Murray, 1972)

(g) Globular "glycoprotein", only small amount of carbohydrate components attached; sialic acid is missing among the identified carbohydrate components (Beier, 1967, 1968 b, Krishnan and Daniel, 1968; Kirchner, 1969)

(h) Binding of progesterone with high affinity, in a reaction which does not involve the sulfhydryl groups, requires the opening of the disulfide bridges (Beato, 1977). Affinity for progesterone has been reported with different association constants:
5.95×10^8 M^{-1} (Arthur, Cowan and Daniel, 1972)
3.00×10^6 M^{-1} (Beato and Baier, 1975; Beato, 1977)
very much lower than these (Rahman et al., 1975)
not calculated, but estimated as low (Urzua et al., 1970)

(i) Inhibition of trypsin, tested in fibrin-agar-electrophoresis (Beier, 1970; Johnson, 1974; Beier, 1976)

(j) Uteroglobin is synthesized by endometrial cells, as indicated by isolation of mRNA for uteroglobin from this tissue, and translation of this mRNA in Xenopus laevis oocytes (Beato and Rungger, 1975), mRNA isolation by Bullock, Woo and O'Malley, 1976.

(k) Uteroglobin amino acid sequence analyzed: the molecule is composed of two identical polypeptide chains of 70 amino acids linked by 2 disulfide bonds. The sequence is not homologous to any known primary protein structure, except for a small acidic region (residues 22–29) resembling a sequence found in somatotropin (Ponstingl, Nieto, and Beato, 1978)

The larger size of pre-uteroglobin is accounted for by a 21-amino acid leader sequence, containing 15 hydrophobic residues, at the NH$_2$ terminus (Malsky, Bullock, Willard, Ward 1979)

(molecule) is involved in this proteinase inhibition, since the highest activities are always found, in our system, when total uterine flushings are tested and compared to purified or isolated fractions. Another possible difficulty may arise from the chemical purification procedure itself by alteration of the biological activity of the uteroglobin molecule. Regardless of further studies and results on the comparison of uteroglobin and the uteroglobin-like antigen, it should be pointed out here, that we cannot accept the dogma that immunological identity is proof for the total identity of two antigen molecules. Biological activities of a protein may not be localized or dependent on the immunologically determinant parts of the molecule.

Studies on Biological Systems, Where Uteroglobin May Act: The In Vivo and the In Vitro Growing Blastocyst

Injections of 17β-Oestradiol benzoate at 6 hrs and 30 hrs after mating reveal a significant delay in the secretory pattern sequence of the rabbit uterus (Figure 7).

TABLE III. Biological Features of Uteroglobin

(a) Significant and predominant protein in rabbit uterine secretion during preimplantation in normal pregnancy and in equivalent stages of pseudopregnancy (Beier, 1966, 1967, 1968 b; Krishnan and Daniel, 1967; Kirchner, 1969; Urzua et al., 1970; Beier et al., 1970, 1971; Daniel, 1971)
(b) Predominant protein of blastocyst fluid (Beier, 1966, 1967; Hamana and Hafez, 1970; Petzoldt, 1974)
(c) Uteroglobin is not detectable in cultured blastocysts, when development is accomplished from the 2-celled stage up to the large expanded blastocyst stage in BSA supplemented *in vitro* culture media (Beier and Maurer, 1975)
(d) Release from uterine epithelial cells is stimulated and controlled by progesterone (Beier, 1968 a; Beier et al., 1970; Urzua et al., 1970; Arthur and Daniel, 1972)
(e) Release can be stimulated by Chlormadinone acetate and Norgestrel (Beier and Beier-Hellwig, 1973)
(f) Release from uterine epithelial cells is delayed by postcoital oestrogen injections (17β-oestradiol benzoate) (Beier et al., 1971)
(g) Release into uterine lumen is terminated mainly by oestrogen after implantation (Bullock and Willen, 1974)
(h) Uteroglobin is antigenic in mice (Beier, 1966), rats (Schwick, 1965), guinea pigs (Beier, 1966, 1968 b; Kirchner, 1972; Johnson et al., 1972), goats (Noske and Feigelson, 1976), sheep (Beier et al., 1975)
(i) Antigenic cross-reactions can be attained under certain conditions by means of all highly potent antiserum preparations with antigens from seminal vesicle secretion, seminal plasma (Beier et al., 1975), from lung tissue extracts (Noske and Feigelson, 1976), and from lung lavage (Beier, Kirchner and Mootz, 1978)

Additional studies on rabbit esophagus tissue and flushings, jejunal flushings, and also human endometrium, human oviduct, and human seminal plasma indicate uteroglobin cross-reacting antigens to be present there (Feigelson, Noske, Goswami and Kay, 1977)

Compared to the normal preimplantation patterns, there is delay of 2–5 days, dependent on the stages compared. At earlier stages, the delay is less extended (2–3 days) than in later developmental stages (4–5 days delay). This feature is not only true for the protein patterns, but also for the histology of the endometrium and the enzyme histochemistry of the endometrial epithelia. We have claimed that these asynchronous protein patterns contribute particularly to an unfavourable uterine environment for blastocyst development (Beier, 1970; Beier, Kühnel and Petry, 1971; Beier, 1974). Subsequent egg transfer experiments have shown that normally developed blastocysts require a normally developed uterine environment to accomplish implantation and further development (Beier, Mootz and Kühnel, 1972; Adams, 1974). We transferred normal Day 4 blastocysts into Day 8 pregnant, post-coitally oestrogen treated animals. These transferred blastocysts implanted around Day 12 (recipient's reproductive stage) and developed in an experimental series circa 40% normal fetuses. Several of these fetuses were allowed to develop to viable young rabbits. In conclusion, we are convinced that the clearly synchronized uterine environment, particularly the secretion protein patterns, is an essential part in early mammalian embryogenesis. The model of Delayed Secretion has not been studied merely to demonstrate a questionable growth-inhibition effect on the native blastocysts. One particular item, however, is very important: the asynchronous egg transfer in delayed secretory uteri provides biological evidence for the necessity of a proper uterine environment to blastocyst development.

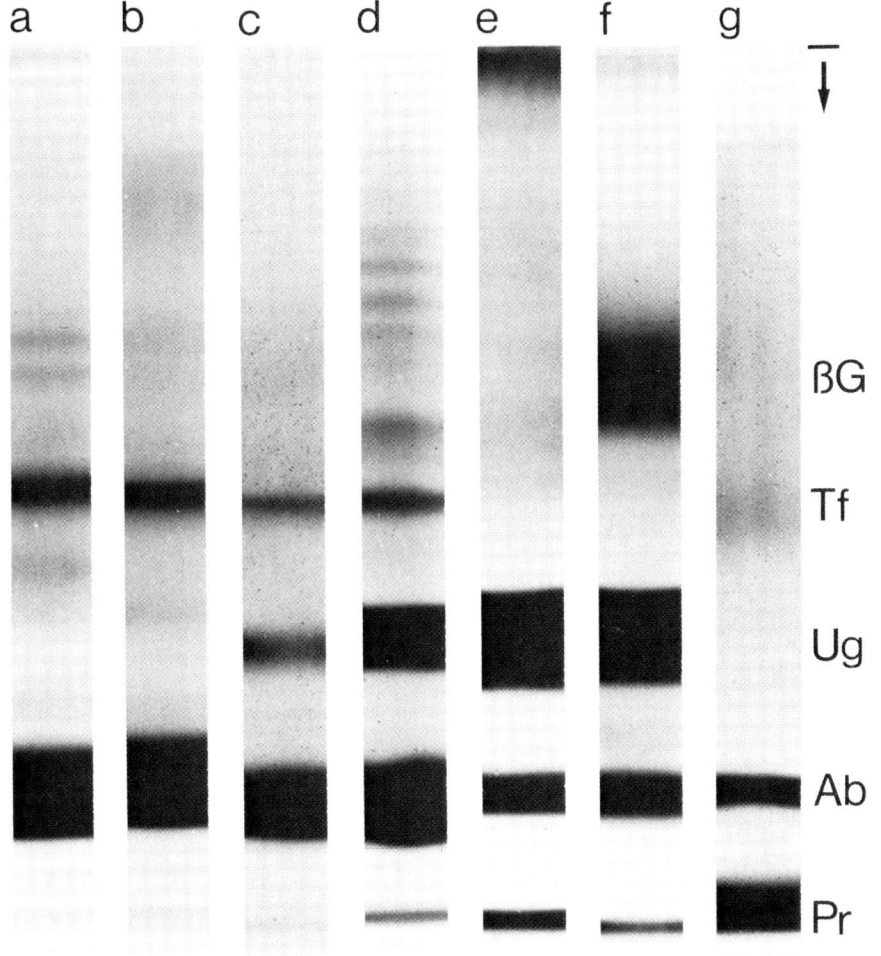

FIGURE 7. Uterine fluid protein patterns of the rabbit at delayed secretion. Polyacrylamide electrophoretic separation of protein fractions from oestrous (a), oestrogen treated controls after two injections of 100 and 150 μg, respectively, oestradiol-17β (b) and from delayed secretion stages at Day 4 (c), Day 6 (d), Day 8 (e), Day 12 (f), and Day 16 (g). Note the delay of the release of prominent protein fractions uteroglobin and β-glycoproteins. (Pr = prealbumin, Ab = albumin, Ug = uteroglobin, Tf = transferrin, β-G = glycoprotein) Tris-glycine-buffer pH 9.0, Amidoblack-10B-staining.

Consequently, the essential protein environment for normal blastocyst development is composed of a considerable number of macromolecules. Within this, uteroglobin obviously is the major component, so characteristic that it represents a specific marker molecule for the ovarian hormonal status of the animal.

Interestingly, the experimentally induced delay of uterine secretion is not the only way to desynchronize the maternal and embryonic systems. Prefertilization treatment of oestrous rabbits with progesterone (up to 2 mg/day/animal) for 8 days

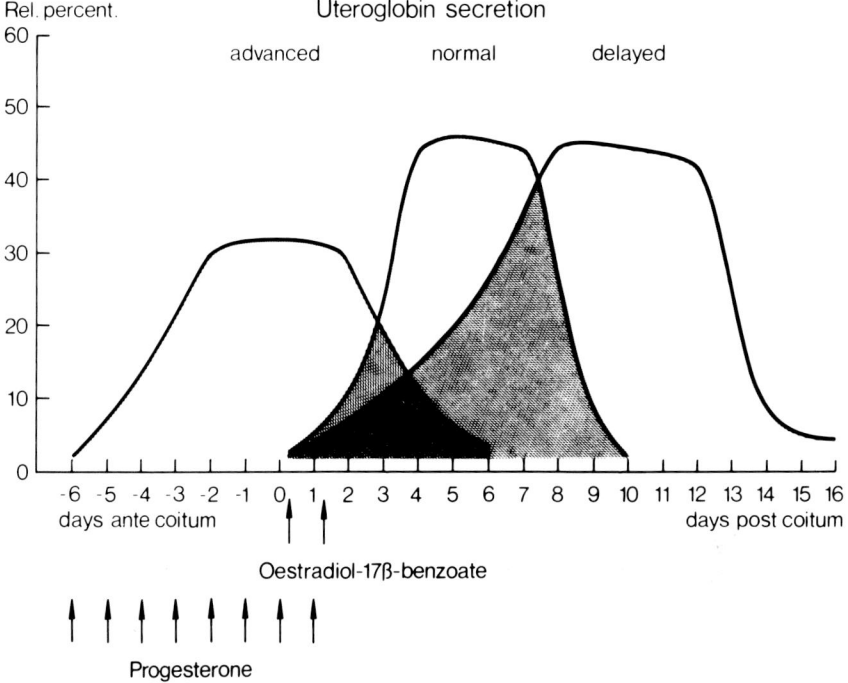

FIGURE 8. Desynchronization of uteroglobin secretion. This diagram shows the profiles of relative percentages of uteroglobin in uterine secretion protein during normal and desynchronized endometrial secretion. By two different experimental regimens, either delayed or advanced secretory activity can be triggered. Oestradiol-17β-benzoate, applied in two injections postcoitally (6 h and 30 h p.c., 100 μg and 150 μg per animal respectively) induces delay of uterine secretion. Progesterone, injected on eight consecutive days (2 mg/animal/day), designated Day−6 until Day+1 according to artificial ovulation induction by HCG on Day 0, stimulates advanced uterine secretion. Desynchronized uteroglobin profiles are consistent with retarded blastocyst development and inhibition of implantation. Experiments on advanced uterine secretion have been performed by de Visser (1976), experiments on delayed uterine secretion by Beier (1973). (Courtesy Georg Thieme Publ., Stuttgart: Human Fertilization, H. Ludwig and P.F. Tauber, Eds., 1978).

(Day−6 to +1) and induction of ovulation (by HCG-injection on Day 0) with subsequent artificial insemination results in normal egg development during oviductal passage, however, degeneration of blastocysts appears after their arrival in the uterus, mostly within 2 days of exposure to the uterine secretion environment (De Visser, 1976). If this treatment is applied, the intrauterine milieu is changed in so far as the protein patterns are advanced compared to the normal preimplantation. The exogenous progesterone induces uteroglobin synthesis and release before ovulation and fertilization. There is a maximum of uteroglobin secretion from Day−1 until Day +2, designated consequently as an *Advanced Secretion*. Comparable observations are reported by Kendle and Telford (1970) and by McCarthy, Foote and Maurer (1977). This phenomenon leads as clearly to failure of implantation as it appears during *Delayed Secretion*.

We have paid particular attention to the presence of uterine secretion proteins in blastocyst fluid. In a recent investigation on the protein patterns of rabbit blastocyst fluid and blastocyst homogenates after development *in vivo* and *in vitro*, we have tried to present evidence for the origin of the blastocyst fluid proteins (Beier and Maurer, 1975). Special emphasis was directed to the protein patterns of *in vitro* grown blastocysts, since these embryos developed from the 2- and 4-cell stages to expanded blastocysts without any rabbit protein in the culture medium. There, bovine serum albumin was used as the only protein source. Patterns from *in vivo* and *in vitro* development differ significantly, as judged by means of acrylamide gel electrophoresis and by several immunochemical test methods. These results demonstrate that blastocysts grown *in vitro* do not contain uteroglobin or β-glycoprotein in detectable amounts. Compared to the *in vivo* developed blastocysts, this is a striking difference, because uteroglobin and β-glycoprotein have been demonstrated in fluids of *in vivo* expanded blastocysts in considerable amounts, at least in such quantities that our routinely applied immunochemical tests are positive. However, our study indicates that the *in vitro* developing blastocyst cannot synthesize uteroglobin. It may well be true that the *in vivo* blastocysts also do not synthesize molecules identical to the uterine secretion proteins. All evidence now agrees with the concept that uterine secretion proteins permeate into the blastocyst fluid (Beier, 1967; Kulangara and Crutchfield, 1973; Schlafke and Enders, 1973), into the blastocyst cells, particularly trophoblast cells on the 7th day p.c. (Kirchner, 1976), and into the blastocyst coverings (Kirchner, 1972). It seems that the blastocyst utilizes these environmental proteins. Our eperiments suggest, that under the conditions of *in vitro* culture, other proteins supplemented to the culture medium pass into the blastocyst compartments in comparable quantities. This in turn indicates that the environmental proteins under *in vitro* conditions seem not to enfold a specific embryotropic activity. If we extrapolate these conclusions from the *in vitro* situation to the normal physiological situation in utero, it appears conceivable that the uterine secretion proteins act as integrated parts of a maternally- embryonically linked molecular system, the function of which is more a protective activity for the embryo (Beier, 1974), than a direct embryotropic role as suggested by Krishnan and Daniel (1967).

In addition, uteroglobin may play an important role in the biochemical reactions and the "metabolism" of the blastocyst coverings, particularly, when the blastocyst enters the uterine cavity on Day 4. Striking evidence for the involvement of uteroglobin in the physico-chemical conditioning of the blastocyst coverings, the zona pellucida and the mucin coat (mucoprotein layer), has been obtained from the comparison of two experiments on rabbit blastocysts. Blastocysts flushed from the isthmic part of the oviduct or from the upper uterine segment (approximately 70 hrs p.c.) during Delayed Secretion show herniations of the trophoblast. The same pictures of trophoblast herniation can be obtained easily by culturing early cleavage stages up to the blastocyst stage *in vitro*, using a defined medium (Maurer and Beier, 1976) with or without BSA as the only protein source. Both blastocysts are faced with an unfavourable environment, on the one hand to a desynchronized uterine secretion and on the other hand to an unnatural medium, also "desynchronized" by lack of uteroglobin or other uterine proteins.

It is likely that in consequence of this disproportion of uterine proteins, in particular of uteroglobin, the mucin coat does not show the elasticity and flexibility that is usual on Day 4, when the normally developing blastocysts start expansion. This expansion cannot take place when the rigid coverings under desynchronized conditions act as a straitjacket for the blastocyst. We have presented evidence for the influence of the uterine proteins on the coverings and their physico-chemical alternation by supplementing *in vitro* protein-free culture media with uterine secretion proteins (Maurer and Beier, 1976). Expansion does appear frequently, however, the overall development of the embryonic system occurs more slowly than normal. Since uteroglobin acts like a protease-inhibitor (Beier, 1976, 1977), it may be regulating proteases which control the structural metabolism of the blastocyst coverings. These proteases can be of uterine or embryonic (trophoblast) origin, and may be controlled by uteroglobin or other uterine secretion components (cf. Denker, 1977, 1978).

Secretory Proteins of the Human Endometrium

We have subjected human female genital tract secretion to acrylamide diskelectrophoresis (Figure 9) and several immunochemical tests, expecting an answer to the long standing question, as to whether the human uterine secretion follows the same principles as our animal model, the rabbit. Follicular and oviductal fluids, uterine and cervical secretions do not contain a predominating postalbumin component comparable to rabbit uteroglobin. However, rather surprising results have been obtained on cross-reactions of human uterine proteins with anti-uteroglobin sera from the goat and the sheep, antibodies that had been raised against authentic endometrial uteroglobin from the rabbit. Several patients' (4 out of 12) uterine secretions samples did contain a uteroglobin-like antigen, which was cross-reacting with the antibodies against rabbit uteroglobin, demonstrated by means of the acrylamide-agar-immunoreaction. The appearance of a human uterine protein, that cross-reacts with antibodies to uteroglobin is challenging, since the bulk of data from animal experiments (rabbit) awaits clarification, whether these results could be "transferred" to the human reproductive physiology or not. Even samples obtained during the midsecretory phase of the human menstrual cycle, when implantation is normally expected, do not always contain a typical uteroglobin band or a protein with the same electrophoretic mobility that stains well with amido-black. To date, we could not isolate by chromatography a predominant postalbumin fraction that shows the parameters of uteroglobin. Such results indicate that the immunological cross-reactions are probably not highly specific. By contrast even totally nonspecific reactions cannot be excluded. Since there is no immunological cross-reaction of antiuteroglobin sera with any of the uterine flushings from the well known laboratory animals, such as the mouse, rat, guinea pig, hamster, mink, and also the larger animals e.g. goat, sheep, pig, cow or baboon, we may conclude that the interspecies cross-reactions with human uterine wash-fluid or endometrial tissue homogenate are exceptional reactions. For the immediate research, it is an essential question to biochemically identify uteroglobin-like protein or analogous molecules in the human uterine secretion. The quantitative aspects of such components may differ totally from the concentrations known in the rabbit uterus, because the type of implantation of the human blastocyst differs remarkably from that in the rabbit (interstitial vs. superficial type). However, we have no reason to deny uteroglobin-like protein in the human uterus, unless this assumption has not been ruled out by convincing research data.

There are characteristic oviductal and uterine proteins in the human being,

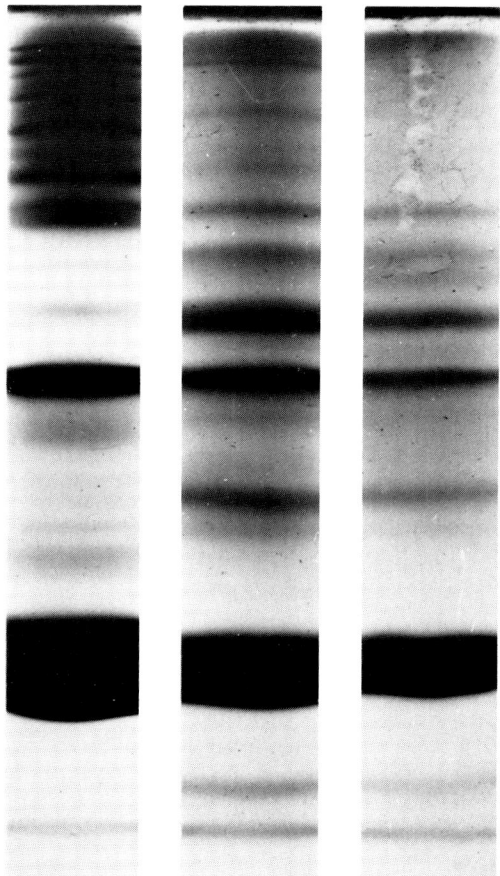

FIGURE 9. Human genital tract secretions. Polyacrylamide electrophoretic separation of uterine flushing (b) and oviductal flushing (c) from the 14th day of the cycle (Pat. H.R., 38 years, no pathological reproductive parameters), compared to the paired blood serum (a). Note the similarity of protein patterns of uterine and oviductal secretions. Pr = prealbumin, Ab = albumin, Pa = Postalbumin, Tf = Transferrin, Pt = posttransferrin. Tris-glycine-buffer pH 9.0, Amidoblack-10B-staining. (Modified from H.M. Beier and K. Beier-Hellwig, Acta endocronologica (Kbh.) Suppl. *180*, 404–423, 1973).

which we could, though not yet directly, demonstrate immunologically by specific antisera. We have observed several remarkable fractions, among which one prealbumin and one posttransferrin seem to lack any equivalent fraction in blood plasma from the same patient. Comparable posttransferrin bands have been reported by Mastroianni et al., (1970) in oviductal fluid of the rhesus monkey, by Moghissi (1970) in the human oviduct and by Wolf and Mastroianni (1975) in the human uterine washing. The prealbumin and the posttransferrin fractions both show a clear PAS-positive reaction indicating their glycoprotein nature.

Lactoferrin was initially described as the iron-binding protein in bovine and human milk. Now, we have found it in uterine and cervical secretions, as reported earlier by Masson et al. (1968). In contrast, we were not able to show its presence in follicular and oviductal fluid. The occurrence of lactoferrin in uterine and cervical secretions in addition to transferrin may indicate that it has a wider physiological role than the binding of iron and copper. Possibly these proteins protect the mucosae against poisoning by heavy metal ions as well as against infections, since bacteriostatic activities, dependent on the chelation of ionized iron and copper from the substrate fluid, could be demonstrated for both lactoferrin and transferrin (Masson and Heremans, 1967; Schade, 1967).

Among the plasma protein components, special attention has been paid to the immunoglobulins in the genital tract secretions. In contrast to other body secretions (milk, saliva, intestinal fluid) where IgA is the major immunoglobulin, the ratio of IgA/IgG in uterine and cervical mucus is approximately the same as in the blood plasma. Both immunoglobins are present in similar proportions in follicular and oviductal fluid. Interestingly, IgM occurs only in uterine secretion as a permanent component (Beier and Beier-Hellwig, 1973; Beier et al., 1976).

CONCLUSIONS

During the periovulatory time of all species so far investigated, including man, a voluminous, protein-rich uterine secretion of low viscosity is produced. By contrast, the endometrium delivers a second type of secretion which serves to induce and maintain blastocyst growth and development over the implantation period. In species with facultative or obligatory delayed implantation, such as the roe deer, the wallaby, fur seal, mouse and rat, the reactivation of the dormant blastocyst at the end of the diapause is temporally associated with an increase in uterine protein secretory activity. In the rabbit, we find a particular situation since there uteroglobin dominates the uterine proteins when enough progesterone is present. In most species investigated, the progestational endometrial secretions consist of a complex mixture of proteins (Surani, 1977; Aitken, 1979), many of which may have a transport function.

In the mouse, wallaby, rabbit and pig, evidence suggests that the implanting or the expanding blastocyst may exert local stimulatory effects on protein *synthesis*. The evidence further suggests that the implanting blastocyst may have a local stimulatory effect upon the *secretory* activity of the endometrium and on the protein *transsudation* from blood plasma (Renfree, 1973; Wyatt, Heap, Perry, 1976; Aitken, 1977, 1979). Since the progestational transformations of the secretory patterns are rather species specific, as evident by the diverse reactions of release of one or only a few major proteins on the one hand, and of the release of a whole group (rather a "family") of higher molecular weight proteins without any predominant fraction on the other hand, it may well be true that implantation or attachment stimulating (facilitating) protein fractions are only appearing in endometrial secretion in the presence of a blastocyst. Such an activating unit, trophoblast cells and probably also embryoblast cells, may be particularly important in human beings, because all results of our own laboratory and that of Maathuis and Aitken (1978) indicate that during the luteal phase of the menstrual cycle the quantity of released uterine protein is rather low. Two consequences have to be discussed therefore: It could be necessary to have the interaction of a blastocyst to trigger real preimplantational uterine protein secretion in women, or

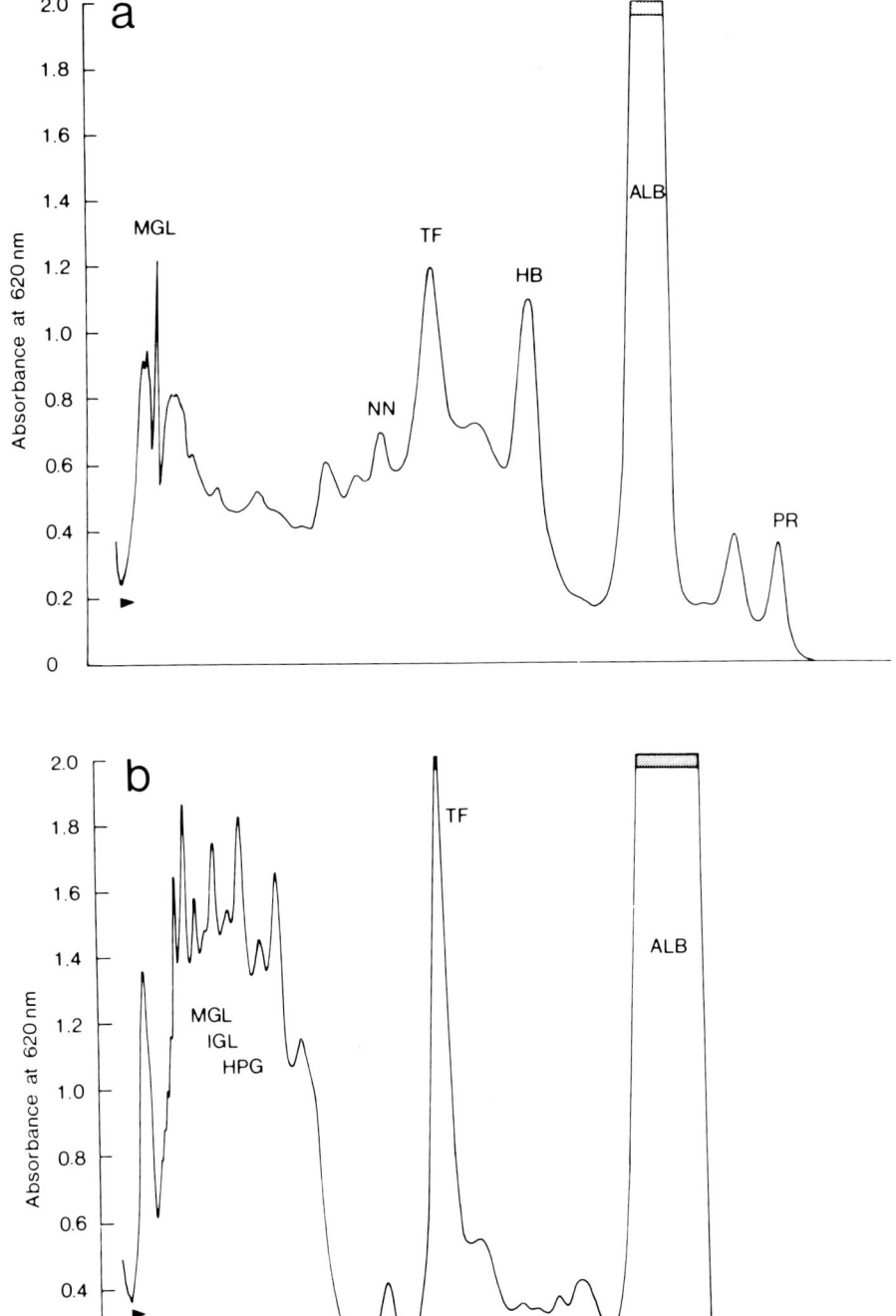

FIG. 10

FIGURE 10. Human uterine secretion protein patterns. Densitometric curves of polyacrylamide electrophoretic separation of uterine flushing (a) from the 28th day of the cycle (Pat. M.J., 47 years, no pathological reproductive parameters, cycle length usually 30 days). The blood serum pattern is shown for comparison (b). Note that uterine secretion of this premenstrual stage shows contamination by haemoglobin (HB). The possibly uterine specific prealbumin fraction is migrating next to the fast prealbumin (PR) and does not appear in serum. The posttransferrin band characteristic for uterine secretion is present (NN). ALB = albumin, TF = transferrin, MGL = macroglobulins, HPG = haptoglobins, IGL = immunoglobulins. (Modified from H.M. Beier and K. Beier-Hellwig, Acta endocrinologica (Kbh.) Suppl. *180*, 404–423, 1973).

---

it could well be that the implanting human blastocyst does not need a uteroglobin-like protein in the uterine cavity during the phase before invasion. If the latter is true, one may find such proteins as "tissue-bound" components in the endometrium, probably in the local vicinity of the implantation site. These thoughts underline the importance of studying the nature of the mutual interactions between the blastocyst and the uterus and the necessity to search for relevant models in available animals.

ACKNOWLEDGEMENTS

Cordial thanks are due to my wife, Dr.med. Karin Beier-Hellwig, who always cooperated in my research on Reproductive Biology and never failed to keep in mind the clinical relevance of comparative or non-human reproductive physiology research.

The investigations were supported by the Deutsche Forschungsgemeinschaft (Grant Be 524/6) in the Special Research Programme "Biologie und Klinik der Reproduktion".

Excellent technical assistance by Ms. Maria Petuelli, Ms. Barbara Bonn, Ms. Gaby Bock and Ms. Ria Becht is gratefully acknowledged.

REFERENCES

Adams, C.E. (1974) Asynchronous egg transfer in the rabbit. J. Reprod. Fert. *35*, 613–614.

Aitken, R.J. (1974) Delayed implantation in roe deer (Capreolus capreolus). J. Reprod. Fert. *39*, 225–233.

Aitken, R.J. (1977) Embryonic Diapause. In: Development in Mammals, Vol. 1 (M.H. Johnson, ed.) pp. 307–359, North-Holland Publ. Comp., Amsterdam-New York-Oxford 1977.

Aitken, R.J. (1977) The protein content of mouse uterine flushings during pseudopregnancy. J. Reprod. Fert. *50*, 191–192.

Aitken, R.J. (1979) Tubal and uterine secretions; the possibilities for contraceptive attack. J. Reprod. Fert. *55*, 247–254.

Arthur, A.T., Cowan, B.D. and Daniel, J.C., Jr. (1972) Steroid binding to blastokinin. Fert. Steril. *23*, 85–92.

Arthur, A.T. and Daniel, J.C., Jr. (1972) Progesterone regulation of blastokinin production and maintenance of rabbit blastocysts transferred into uteri of castrate recipients. Fert. Steril. *23*, 115–122.

Baer, K.E. von (1827) De ovi mammalium et hominis genesi, epistolam ad Academiam Imperialem Scientiarum Petropolitanam. Lipsiae Subptibus Leopoldi Vossii (Leopold Voss), Leipzig.

Beato, M. (1977) Physico-chemical characterization of uteroglobin and its interaction with progesterone. In: Development in Mammals (Ed.: M.H. Johnson) Vol. 2, 173–198, North-Holland Publ. Comp., Amsterdam, New York, Oxford.

Beato, M. and Arnemann, J. (1975) Hormone-dependent synthesis and secretion of uteroglobin in isolated rabbit uterus. FEBS Letters *58*, 126–129.

Beato, M. and Baier, R. (1975) Binding of progesterone to the proteins of the uterine luminal fluid. Identification of uteroglobin as the binding protein. Biochim. Biophys. Acta *392*, 346–356.

Beato, M. and Beier, H.M. (1978) Binding of progesterone to the purified uteroglobin-like protein of the lung compared to uteroglobin. J. Reprod. Fert. 53, 305–314.

Beato, M. and Rungger, D. (1975) Translation of the messenger RNA for rabbit uterglobin in Xenopus oocytes. FEBS Letters 59, 305–309.

Beier, H.M. (1966) Das Proteinmilieu in Serum, Uterus and Blastocysten des Kaninchens vor der Nidation. In: Biochemie der Morphogenese, Chairman: W. Beermann, Deutsche Forschungsgemein schaft, Konstanz.

Beier, H.M. (1967) Veränderungen am Proteinmuster des Uterus bei dessen Ernährungsfunktion für die Blastocyste des Kaninchens. Verh. dt. zool. Ges. (Heidelberg 1967) 31, 139–148.

Beier, H.M. (1968a) Uteroglobin: a hormone-sensitive endometrial protein involved in blastocyst development. Biochim. Biophys. Acta 160, 289–291.

Beier, H.M. (1968b) Biochemisch-entwicklungsphysiologische Untersuchungen am Proteinmilieu für die Blastocystenentwicklung des Kaninchens (Oryctolagus cuniculus). Zool. Jb. Anat. 85, 72–190.

Beier, H.M. (1970) Hormonal stimulation of protease inhibitor activity in endometrial secretion during early pregnancy. Acta endocr. Copenh. 63, 141–149.

Beier, H.M. (1971) Die Pseudogravidität des Kaninchens nach Stimulierung mit Choriongonadotropin. Diss. Med. Fakult. Univ. Marburg/Lahn.

Beier, H.M. (1973) Die hormonelle Steuerung der Uterussekretion and frühen Embryonalentwicklung des Kaninchens. Habil.-Schrift, Med. Fakult. Univ. Kiel, pp. 1–216.

Beier, H.M. (1974) Oviductal and uterine fluids. J. Reprod. Fert. 37, 221–237.

Beier, H.M. (1976) Uteroglobin and related biochemical changes in the reproductive tract during early pregnancy in the rabbit. J. Reprod. Fertil., Suppl. 25, 53–69.

Beier, H.M. (1977) Immunologische und biochemische Analysen am Uteroglobin und dem Uteroglobin-ähnlichen Antigen der Lunge. Med. Welt 28, 788–792.

Beier, H.M. (1978) Control of implantation by interference with uteroglobin synthesis, release and utilization. In: H. Ludwig and P.F. Tauber (Eds.) Human Fertilization, 191–203, Georg Thieme Publ., Stuttgart.

Beier, H.M. and Beier-Hellwig, K. (1973) Specific secretory protein of the female genital tract. Acta endocr. Copenh. Suppl. 180, 404–425.

Beier, H.M., Bohn, H., and Müller, W. (1975) Uteroglobin-like antigen in the male genital tract secretions. Cell Tiss. Res. 165, 1–11.

Beier, H.M., Kirchner, C. and Mootz, U. (1978) Uteroglobin-like antigen in the pulmonary epithelium and secretion of the lung. Cell Tiss. Res. 190, 15–25.

Beier, H.M., Kühnel, W. and Petry, G. (1971) Uterine secretion proteins as extrinsic factors in preimplantation development. Advances Bioscien. 6, 165–189.

Beier, H.M. and Maurer, R.R. (1975) Uteroglobin and other proteins in rabbit blastocyst fluid after development *in vivo* and *in vitro*. Cell Tiss. Res. 159, 1–10.

Beier, H.M., Mootz, U., and Kühnel, W. (1972) Asynchrone Eitransplantationen während der verzögerten Uterussekretion beim Kaninchen. The 7th Int. Congr. Anim. Reprod. Artif. Insem. München, 3, 1891–1896.

Beier, H.M., Petry, G., and Kühnel, W. (1970) Endometrial secretion and early mammalian development. In: 21st Coll. Ges. Biol. Chem. Mosbach 1970, Mammalian Reproduction, pp. 264–285. Eds.: H. Gibian and E.J. Plotz. Springer, Berlin-Heidelberg-New York.

Bernstein, G.S., Aladjem, F., and Chen, S. (1971) Proteins in human endometrial washings. A preliminary report. Fert. Steril. 22, 722–726.

Bishop, D.W. (1956) Active secretion in the rabbit oviduct. Am. J. Physiol. 187, 347–352.

Bond, C.J. (1898) Preliminary note on certain undescribed features in the secretory function of the uterus and Fallopian tubes in the human subject and in some of the mammalia. J. Physiol. 22, 296.

Bond, C.J. (1899) On the experimental production of hydrosalpinx in the human subject. The Lancet 2, 200 (1899).

Bond, C.J. (1906) An inquiry into some points in uterine and ovarian physiology and pathology in rabbits. Brit. Med. J. 2, 121–127.

Bullock, D.W. and Bhatt, B.M. (1976) Studies on uteroglobin messenger RNA. ICE-Satellite Symp. "Proteins and Steroids in Early Mammalian Development", Aachen 1976, in: Reproductive

Endocrinology (Eds. H.M. Beier and P. Karlson) Springer-Verlag, Berlin-Heidelberg-New York (in press).

Bullock, D.W. and Connell, K.M. (1973) Occurrance and molecular weight of rabbit uterine "blastokinin". Biol. Reprod. 9, 125–132.

Bullock, D.W. and Willen, G.F. (1974) Regulation of a specific uterine protein by estrogen and progesterone in ovariectomized rabbits. Proc. Soc. experim. Biol. Med. 146, 294–298.

Bullock, D.W., Woo, S.L.C. and O'Malley, B.W. (1976) Uteroglobin messenger RNA. Translation in vitro. Biol. Reprod. 15, 435–443.

Bullock, D.W. (1977) Progesterone induction of messenger RNA and protein synthesis in rabbit uterus. Ann. N.Y. Acad. Scienc. 286, 260–272.

Daniel, J.C., Jr. (1968) Comparison of electrophoretic patterns of uterine fluid from rabbits and mammals having delayed implantation. Comp. Biochem. Physiol. 24, 297–299.

Daniel, J.C., Jr. (1971a) Uterine proteins and embryonic development. Adv. Biosci. 6, 191–203.

Daniel, J.C., Jr. (1971b) Growth of the preimplantation embryo of the northern fur seal and its correlation with changes in uterine protein. Devel. Biol. 26, 316–322.

Daniel, J.C., Jr. (1973) A blastokinin-like component from the human uterus. Fertil. Steril. 24, 326–328.

Daniel, J.C. Jr. (1976) Blastokinin and analogous proteins. J. Reprod. Fert. 25, 71–83.

Daniel, J.C., Jr. and Krishnan, R.S. (1969) Studies on the relationship between uterine fluid components and the diapausing state of blastocysts from mammals having delayed implantation. J. Exp. Zool. 172, 267–281.

Denker, H. W. (1977) Implantation. The role of proteinases, and blockage of implantation by proteinase inhibitors. In: Advances in Anatomy, Embryology and Cell Biology, Vol. 53, Fasc. 5, Springer-Verlag, Berlin, Heidelbert, New York.

Denker, H.-W. (1978) The role of trophoblastic factors in implantation. In: Novel Aspects of Reproductive Physiology, Ch. H. Spilman, J. W. Wilks (Eds.) Spectrum Publ., Inc., New York, London; Halsted Press, John Wiley & Sons, pp. 181–212.

Dixon, S.N. and Gibbons, R.A. (1979) Proteins in the uterine secretions of the cow. J. Reprod. Fert. 56, 119–127.

Feigelson, M., Noske, I.G., Goswami, A.K., and Kay, E. (1977). Reproductive tract fluid proteins and their hormonal control. Ann. N.Y. Acad. Sci. 286, 273–286.

Fishel, S.B. (1979) Analysis of mouse uterine proteins at pro-oestrus, during early pregnancy and after administration of exogenous steroids. J. Reprod. Fert. 56, 91–100.

Gerlinger, H. (1922) The existence of a secretory cycle in the horns of the uterus of mammals during the heat period. Compt. Rend. Soc. Biol. 87, 582.

Haller, A. von (1757, 1766) Elementa physiologiae corporis humani. Lausanne, zit. nach Bodemer, C.W.: History of the mammalian Oviduct; In: E.S.E. Hafez and R.J. Blandau (Eds.): The mammalian oviduct, the University of Chicago Press, Chicago and London, 1969.

Ham, J. and Leeuwenhoek, A. van (1677), zit. nach: Bargmann, W., Histologie und mikroskopische Anatomie des Menschen, G. Thieme-Verlag, Stuttgart 6. Aufl. 1967.

Hamana, K. and Hafez, E.S.E. (1970) Disc electrophoretic patterns of uteroglobin and serum proteins in rabbit blastocoelic fluid. J. Reprod. Fert. 21, 557–560.

Harpel, P.C., Homburger, F. and Tregier, A. (1968) Mouse uterine fluid plasminogen activator, acid phosphatase, and contraceptive hormones. Am. J. Physiol. 215, 928–931 .

Hartman, C.G. (1923) The oestrus cycle in the opossum. Am. J. Anat. 32, 353.

Hombruger, F., Grossman, M.S. and Tregier, A. (1955) Experimental hydrouteri (hydrometra) in rodents and some factors determining their formation. Proc. Soc. exp. Biol. Med. 90, 719.

Homburger, F., Tregier, A. (1957) Endocrine factors determining the rate of accumulation of endometrial secretions in experimental hydrometra of mice. Endocrinology 61, 634–639.

Johnson, M.H. (1972) The protein composition of secretions from pregnant and pseudopregnant rabbit uteri with and without a copper intrauterine device. Fertil. Steril. 23, 123–130.

Johnson, M.H. (1974) Studies using antibodies to the macromolecular secretions of the early pregnant uterus. In: Immunology in Obstetrics and Gynecology. Proc. 1st Intern. Congr. Padua 1973. pp. 123–133. Eds. A. Centaro and N. Carretti. Excerpta Medica, Amsterdam.

Joshi, S.G. (1974) Regulation of protein synthesis in baboon endometrium by endogenous estrogens and progestins. J. Steroid. Biochem. 5, 340.

Junge, J.M., Blandau, R.J. (1958) Studies on the electrophoretic properties of the cornual fluids of rats in heat. Fertil. Steril. 9, 353–367.

Kendle, K.E. and Telford, J.M. (1970) Investigations into the mechanism of the antifertility action of minimal doses of megestrol acetate in the rabbit. Brit. J. Pharmacol. 40, 759–774.

Kirchner, C. (1969) Untersuchungen an uterusspezifischen Glycoproteinen während der frühen Gravidität des Kaninchens (Oryctolagus cuniculus). Wilhelm Roux Archiv. Entw. Mech. Org. 164, 97–133.

Kirchner, C. (1972) Immune histologic studies on the synthesis of a uterine-specific protein in the rabbit and its passage through the blastocyst coverings. Fertil. Steril. 23, 131–136.

Kirchner, C. (1976) Uteroglobin in the rabbit: I. Intracellular localization in the oviduct, uterus, and the preimplantation blastocyst. Cell Tiss. Res. 170, 415–424.

Krishnan, R.S. and Daniel, J.C., Jr. (1967) "Blastokinin": Inducer and regulator of blastocyst development in the rabbit uterus. Science 158, 490–492.

Krishnan, R.S. and Daniel, J.C., Jr. (1968) Composition of "blastokinin" from rabbit uterus. Biochim. Biophys. Acta (Amst.) 168, 579–582.

Kulangara, A.C. and Crutchfield, F.L. (1973) Passage of bovine serum albumin from the mother to rabbit blastocysts. II. Passage from uterine lumen to blastocyst fluid. J. Embry. exp. Morphol. 30, 471–482.

Kunitake, G.M., Nakamura, R.M., Wells, B.G. and Moyer, D.L. (1965) Studies on uterine fluid. I. Disc electrophoretic and disc-gel Ouchterlony analysis of rat uterine fluid. Fert. Steril. 16, 120–124.

Laster, D.B. (1977) A pregnancy-specific protein in the bovine uterus. Biol. Reprod. 16, 682–690.

Lutwak-Mann, C. (1960) O naturze i skladzie chemicznym plyn w blastocystach królika. Acta biochimica Plonica 7, 331–339.

Lutwak-Mann, C. (1962) Some properties of uterine and cervical fluid in the rabbit. Biochim. biphys. Acta 58, 637–639.

Lutwak-Mann, C., Boursnell, J.C. and Bennett, J.P. (1960) Blastocyst-uterine relationships: uptake of radioactive ions by the early rabbit embryo and its environment. J. Reprod. Fert. 1, 169–185.

Maathuis, J.B. and Aitken, R.J. (1978) Protein patterns of human uterine flushings collected at various stages of the menstrual cycle. J. Reprod. Fert. 53, 343–348.

Malsky, M.L., Bullock, D.W., Willard, J.J. and Ward, D.N. (1979) Progesterone-induced secretory protein. NH_2-terminal sequence of pre-uteroglobin. J. Biol. Chem. 254, 1580–1585.

Masson, P.L. and Hermans, J.F. (1967) Studies on lactoferrin, the iron-binding protein of secretions. Protides biol. Fluids Proc. Colloq. Bruges, 14, 115–124.

Masson, P.L., Heremans, J.F. and Ferin, J. (1968) Presence of an iron-binding protein (lactoferrin) in the genital tract of the human female. I. Its immunohistochemical changes in the female gential tract. Int. J. Fertil. 14, 1–7.

Mastroianni, L., Urzua, M., Avalos, M. and Stambaugh, R. (1969) Some observations on Fallopian tube fluid in the monkey. Am. J. Obstet. Gynec. 103, 703–709.

Mastroianni, L., Urzua, M., and Stambaugh, R. (1970) Protein patterns in monkey oviductal fluid before and after ovulation. Fertil. Steril. 21, 817–820.

McCarthy, S.M., Foote, R.H. and Maurer, R.R. (1977) Embryo mortality and altered uterine luminal proteins in progesterone-treated rabbits. Fertil. Steril. 28, 101–107.

McGaughey, R.W. and Murray, F.A. (1972) Properties of blastokinin: amino acid composition, evidence for subunits, and estimation of isoelectric point. Fertil. Steril. 23, 399–404.

Maurer, R.R. and Beier, H.M. (1976) Uterine proteins and development *in vitro* of rabbit preimplantation embryos. J. Reprod. Fert. 48, 33–41.

Mintz, B. (1971) Control of embryo implantation and survival. Adv. Biosci. 6, 317–342.

Moghissi, K.S. (1970) Human fallopian tube fluid. I. Protein composition. Fertil. Steril. 21, 821–829.

Murray, F.A., McGaughey, R.W. and Yarus, M.J. (1972) Blastokinin: Its size and shape, and an indication of the existence of subunits. Fertil. Steril. *23*, 69–77.

Noske, I.G., Daniel, J.C., Jr. (1974) Changes in uterine and oviductal fluid proteins during early pregnancy in the golden hamster, J. Reprod. Fert. *38*, 173–176.

Noske, I.G., Feigelson, M. (1976) Immunological evidence of uteroglobin (blastokinin) in the male reproductive tract and in non-reproductive ductal tissues and their secretions. Biol. Reprod. *15*, 704–713.

Peplow, V., Breed, W.G., Jones, C.M.J. and Eckstein, P. (1973) Studies on uterine flushings in the baboon. Am. J. Obstet. Gynec. *116*, 771–779.

Petzoldt, U. (1974) Micro-disc electrophoresis of soluble proteins in rabbit blastocysts. J. Embryol. exp. Morphol. *31*, 479–487.

Ponstingle, H., Nieto, A. and Beato, M. (1978) Amino acid sequence of progesterone-induced rabbit uteroglobin. Biochem. *17*, 3908–3912.

Popp, R.A., Foresman, K.R., Wise, L.D. and Daniel, J.C., Jr. (1978) Amino acid sequence of a progesterone-binding protein. Proc. Natl. Acad. Sci. USA *75*, 5516–5519.

Rahman, S.S.U., Velayo, N., Domres, P. and Billiar, R.B. (1975) Evaluation of progesterone binding to uteroglobin. Fertil. Steril. *26*, 991–995.

Renfree, M.B. (1973) Proteins in the uterine secretions of the marsupial, Macropus eugenii. Devl. Biol. *32*, 41–49.

Renfree, M.B. (1975) Uterine proteins in the marsupial, Didelphis marsupialis virginiana, during gestation. J. Reprod. Fert. *42*, 163–166.

Roberts, G.P., Parker, J.M. (1974) Macromolecular components of the luminal fluid from the bovine uterus. J. Reprod. Fert. *40*, 291–303.

Roberts, G.P., Parker, J.M. and Symonds, H.W. (1976) Macromolecular components of genital tract fluids from the sheep. J. Reprod. Fert. *48*, 99–107.

Schade, A.L. (1966) Non-heme metalloproteins: their distribution, biological functions, and chemical characteristics. Protides biol. Fluids Proc. Colloq. Bruges, *14*, 13–23.

Schlafke, S., Enders, A.C. (1973) Protein uptake by rat preimplantation stages. Anat. Rec. *175*, 539–560.

Schwick, H.G. (1963) Untersuchungen über die Zusammensetzung der Uterus- und Blastocystenflüssigkeit des Kaninchens (Oryctolagus cuniculus). Inaug. Diss., Phil. Fak. Univ. Marburg, Marburg/L.

Schwick, H.G. (1965) Chemisch-entwicklungsphysiologische Beziehungen von Uterus zu Blastocyste des Kaninchens (Oryctolagus cuniculus). Wilhelm Roux Arch. Entw.Mech. Org. *156*, 283–343.

Shapiro, A.A., Jentsch, J.P. and Yard, A.S. (1971) Protein composition of rabbit oviductal fluid. J. Reprod. Fert. *24*, 403–408.

Shirai, E., Iizuka, R. and Notake, Y. (1972) Analysis of human uterine fluid protein. Fertil. Steril. *23*, 522–528.

Squire, G.D., Bazer, F.W. and Murray, F.A. (1972) Electrophoretic patterns of porcine uterine protein secretions during the estrous cycle. Biol. Reprod. *7*, 321–325.

Surani, M.A.H. (1976) Uterine luminal proteins at the time of implantation in rats. J. Reprod. Fert. *48*, 141–145.

Surani, M.A.H. (1977) Cellular and molecular approaches to blastocyst uterine interactions at implantation. In: Development in Mammals, Vol. 1, pp. 245–305. Ed. M.H. Johnson. North-Holland, Amsterdam.

Urzua, M.A., Stambaugh, R., Flickinger, G. and Mastroianni, I. (1970) Uterine and oviduct fluid protein patterns in the rabbit before and after ovulation. Fert. Steril. *21*, 860–865.

de Visser, J. (1976) Degeneration of rabbit ova by prefertilization progesterone treatment: effect on endometrium and uteroglobin secretion. ICE-Satellite Symp. "Proteins and Steroids in Early Mammalian Development". Aachen 1976, in: Reproductive Endocrinology (Eds.: H.M. Beier and P. Karlson) Springer-Verlag, Berlin-Heidelberg-New York (in press).

Voss, H.J. and Beato, M. (1977) Human uterine fluid proteins: gel Electrophoretic pattern and progesterone-binding properties. Fert. Steril. *28*, 972–980.

Wolf, D.P. and Mastroianni, L. (1975) Protein composition of human uterine fluid. Fert. Steril. *26*, 240–247.

Wyatt, C., Heap, R.B. and Perry, J.S. (1976) Protein synthesis in co-cultures of blastocyst and endometrium explants during blastocyst steroidogenesis in the pig. Proc. 5th Int. Congr. Endocr. Hamburg 266A.

Copyright 1979 by Elsevier North Holland, Inc.
F.K. Beller and G.F.B. Schumacher, eds.
The Biology of the Fluids of the Female Genital Tract

APPROACHES TO THE ANALYSIS OF HUMAN ENDOMETRIAL SECRETIONS

G.F.B. Schumacher, J.A. Holt, and F. Reale

SUMMARY

Although important knowledge about endometrial secretions has been accumulated from investigations on laboratory and farm animals, observations on human endometrial fluid are rather scarce especially quantitative data as they are related to the action of estrogen and progesterone. The *in vivo* collection of native undiluted and uncontaminated material under near physiological condition in humans is very difficult.

Two avenues have been explored to obtain information from surgical specimens immediately after hysterectomy:

1. Tissue cylinders of 5–10 mg size were removed, transferred to wells in standard agar-gel diffusion plates and sealed with melted agar to establish contact between the surfaces of the endometrial tissue and the agar-gel. This permits radial diffusion of substances into the agar-gel containing reagents suitable for visualization of specific components. Such reagents may be monospecific anti-sera or enzyme substrates in appropriate buffers. The sizes of the radial diffusion zones are proportional to the amount of substance freely diffusible

Departments of Obstetrics and Gynecology, Pathology and the Divisional Committee on Immunology, The University of Chicago, Pritzker School of Medicine, Chicago, Illinois

from the endometrial tissue. An estimation of these amounts was accomplished by running standard solutions in the same system. The quantity of the diffusible substance X was expressed in microgram per milligram wet weight of tissue.

Freely diffusing components may derive from the content of the glands as well as from cells and intercellular space. However, information on the local level of certain components and on the topographical distribution along the inner linings of the uterus can be obtained.

2. Preweight filter paper triangles were placed on the surface of the endometrium after cutting the uterine wall in the mid-sagittal plane avoiding carefully any contamination with blood or cervix mucus. The papers were removed after 1–2 minutes and weighed immediately to determine the amount of endometrial fluid which had been soaked up by the filter paper. Subsequently the filter paper was quantitatively extracted with saline, dialyzed against distilled water, lyophilized and reconstituted with a volume of saline solution equivalent to the weight of the endometrial fluid picked up by the paper. The amounts of fluid recovered varied among the first 10 cases between 30 and 220 mg.

This material contains all non-dialyzable compounds in concentrations close to the native secretions and can be analyzed by micro radial diffusion in gel methods or other microanalytical procedures. However, it does not contain the low molecular weight components, which pass the dialysis membrane.

Preliminary results indicate the usefulness of this approach. Advantages and limits of these methods are discussed.

General Considerations and Purpose

The biochemistry of endometrial secretions is of considerable interest because sperm migration, capacitation and transport of the blastocyst to the site of implantation takes place in this fluid which is produced by the glandular elements of the endometrium, a tissue highly sensitive to estrogen and progesterone. Pathologic events resulting in infertility as well as certain methods of fertility regulation which interfere with these local events including implantation are possibly mediated by or reflected in changes of the biochemical composition of endometrial secretions, although cellular mechanisms may be more obvious under certain conditions by morphological criteria. However, cellular and humoral factors interact and complement each other as it is known for many biological systems, for instance the specific and non-specific defense systems. The humoral and cellular mechanisms involved in sperm migration, capacitation and implantation and their disruption by certain contraceptive measures are not entirely clear. This applies also to the side effects of the latter, such as increased uterine bleedings after insertion of IUD's.

Although important knowledge about endometrial secretions has been accumulated from investigations on laboratory and farm animals, observations on human endometrial fluid are rather scarce especially quantitative data as they are related to the action of estrogen and progesterone. Animal experiments, although important for the elucidation of certain principles, can not always be conclusive for the understanding of phenomena in human reproduction. The same applies to certain side effects of contraceptive measures in humans for which animal models are not available. Thus, the intensive study of human and primate endometrial secretions is important. The problem is that the *in vivo* collection of native, undiluted and uncontaminated material under near physiological condition in humans is very difficult—if not impossible—in contrast to the collection of cervical secretions which are readily accessible and well investigated (Blandau and Moghissi, 1973; Elstein, Moghissi and Borth, 1973; Insler and Bettendorf, 1977; Prins, Zaneveld and Schumacher, 1979). The amount of fluid present in the endometrial cavity is very small, although the exchange of water molecules appears to be considerable (Shaw et al., 1975). Attempts to aspirate this material by introducing small cannulas or catheters results often in traumatization by introducing the instrument and applying a vacuum which is followed by local disruption of the soft endometrial tissue resulting in contamination with blood. These problems may be reduced by using uterine flushing techniques (Maathuis and Aitken, 1978). However, this approach results in dilution of the native secretions to an unknown extent. Although flushing permits a qualitative analysis and comparison with other secretions and serum it does not permit quantitative assessments of components in these secretions. Since it is known that concentrations of secretory components in other compartments of the uterus change dramatically under the influence of estrogens and progesterone or progestational agents (Schumacher 1977, Schumacher et al., 1977, Stambaugh, Seitz and Mastroianni, 1974) one may suspect that this is also the case in endometrial secretions. Histochemical findings (Wynn 1977) and animal observations (Beier 1974) indicate such changes. Although certain constituents may be found to be present or absent in qualitative test systems the *concentration* is most likely the determining factor for their biological effectiveness within the chain of events involved in the reproductive process or its disruption and for pathophysiological events associated with infertility or contraceptive side effects.

The use of diffusion chambers as described by Edwards et al. (1968) also has problems. The introduction into the human uterus is somewhat traumatic, resulting in frequent contamination with blood. It may also induce inflammatory responses during the hours (up to 14) of presence in the uterine cavity. This time is sufficient for the accumulation of factors involved in an acute local inflammatory response. The composition of the collected fluid is most likely not physiological anymore and results of studies on spermatozoa suspended in such a chamber have to be interpreted with caution.

It is certainly difficult to find a way out of this dilemma. Moreover, these methods are more or less invasive and present therefore ethical problems. The use of surgical specimens overcomes some difficulties and adds others. Besides the fact that cases have to be selected for near normal conditions of the endometrium, the justifiable question may be raised whether or not secretions taken from surgical specimens (within an hour or less, kept on ice) represent the physiological situation *in vivo*. Although the tissues are anoxic after clamping and cutting of the blood vessels, venous congestion which could lead to increased capillary permeability does, most probably, not occur since veins and arteries are usually clamped and/or ligated simultaneously. There is also little time for the same reason for the development of inflammatory responses in the uterine tissues during the surgical procedure of hysterectomy *if traumatization of the uterus is carefully* avoided during surgery. The method of obtaining material from surgical specimens has also the advantage of obtaining information on the presence of ovarian follicles or corpora lutea and of the histological evaluation of the endometrium.

Two avenues have been explored to obtain information from surgical specimens immediately after hysterectomy:

1. The assessment of free diffusible constituents of small (5–10 mg) tissue cylinders taken from different areas of the inner surface of the uterus by means of micro radial diffusion in gel methods;
2. Blotting of the endometrial fluid by filter paper and quantitative extraction, lyophilization and reconstitution to the original weight/volume.

Both methods will be described in the following sections including some results which show their usefulness and a discussion of their limitations.

The Tissue Cylinder Method

The surgical specimens were transported on ice immediately after hysterectomy to the laboratory. Figure 1 shows the method of procedure (Schumacher and Pearl 1969). Wedges were taken from the posterior and/or anterior wall from the fundus to the cervix and a superficial tissue layer of 1–2 mm thickness was prepared. Tissue cylinders were punched from this preparation with stainless steel well cutters used for punching wells in agar-gel plates for immunodiffusion experiments. The weight was quickly determined on a torsion balance and the tissue cylinders were placed in wells of agar-gel plates containing the appropriate reagents and sealed with melted agar to establish contact between tissue and gel for free radial diffusion of soluble and diffusible components into the agar gel. The agar gel may contain monospecific antisera or enzyme substrates in appropriate buffers. The diffusion zones become visible by antigen-antibody precipitation or by enzymatic action on substrates which is either visible by itself, or is made visible by staining substrates or reaction products. The immunological method is well known as radial immunodiffusion technique (Mancini, Carbonara and Heremans 1965). Monospecific antisera against numerous human proteins of serum and other body fluids are commercially available. Micro radial diffusion methods for the assessments of enzymes have been described for lysozyme, several proteases, DNA'se, RNA'se, Amylase, plasminogen activator, phosphatase, hyaluronidase* and others (Schumacher and Wied 1966, Schill and Schumacher 1973, Schill and Schumacher 1972, Schumacher and Schill 1972, *Schumacher, unpublished). The sizes of the radial diffusion zones are proportional to the amount of substance freely diffusible from the endometrial tissue. An estimation of these amounts was accomplished by running standard solutions in the same system. The quantity of the diffusible substance X was expressed in microgram per milligram wet weight of tissue.

Freely diffusing components may derive from the content of the glands as well as from cells and intercellular space. Therefore, the diffusion process is most likely somewhat slower than the diffusion of fluid samples from the wells into the gel. In order to estimate the time necessary for completion of the diffusion process, samples and standard solutions were read and evaluated in certain time intervals over a period of several days. Figure 2 shows the result of such an experi-

PREPARATION OF TISSUE CYLINDERS FROM THE INNER SURFACE OF THE UTERUS FOR RADIAL DIFFUSION TESTS IN GEL

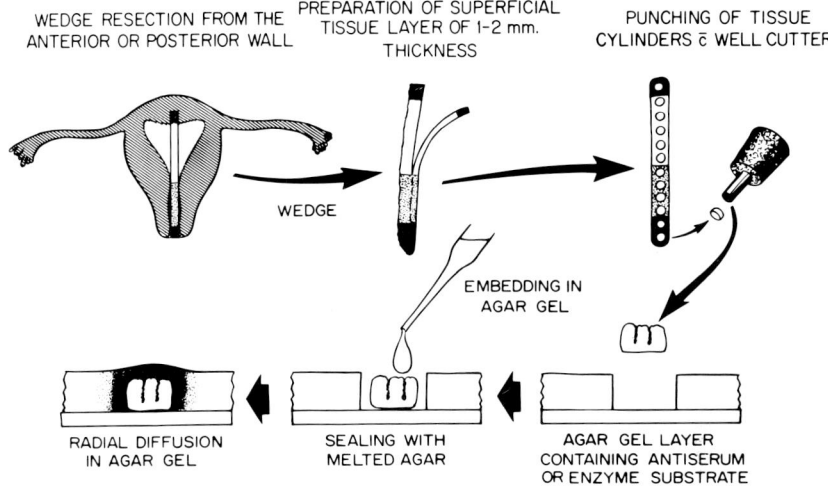

FIGURE 1. Preparation of tissue cylinders from the inner surface of the uterus immediately after hysterectomy. The size of the cylinders is approximately that of the wells, their weight is between 5 and 10 mg. A drop of melted agar establishes good contact with the surrounding agar gel which contains monospecific antisera or enzyme substrate in the appropriate buffers. Diffusible components of the tissue sample begins immediately to diffuse radially into the agar (Schumacher and Pearl 1969).

ment. In this case the protease inhibitor $alpha_1$-antitrypsin was determined. The curves show that the diffusion process especially from the tissues with a higher $alpha_1$-antitrypsin content comes virtually to an end after 2–3 days of diffusion. This experiment shows also that the highest amount of diffusible $alpha_1$-antitrypsin occurs in the lower segment of the endocervix. Similar patterns were found in Albumin, Ceruloplasmin, Immunoglobulin G and the locally produced lysozyme (Schumacher 1974). The tissue cylinder method has been used in extensive studies by Tauber (see Chapter 9) to determine proteinase inhibitors, proteinases, plasminogen activator, lysozyme, lactoferrin, immunoglobulins and complement, and the topographical distribution of these proteins in the different areas of the inner surface of the uterus at the different stages of the menstrual cycle.

The Blotting Method

The surgical specimens were transported on ice immediately after hysterectomy to the laboratory. Figure 3 illustrates the different steps. Filter paper triangles of the appropriate size were weighed in small weighing dishes with lids, labelled and their weight recorded. The filter paper triangles were placed on the surface of the endometrium after cutting the uterine wall in the mid-sagittal plane avoiding carefully any contamination with blood or cervix mucus. The papers were removed after 1 minute, transferred back to the weighing dish to avoid water

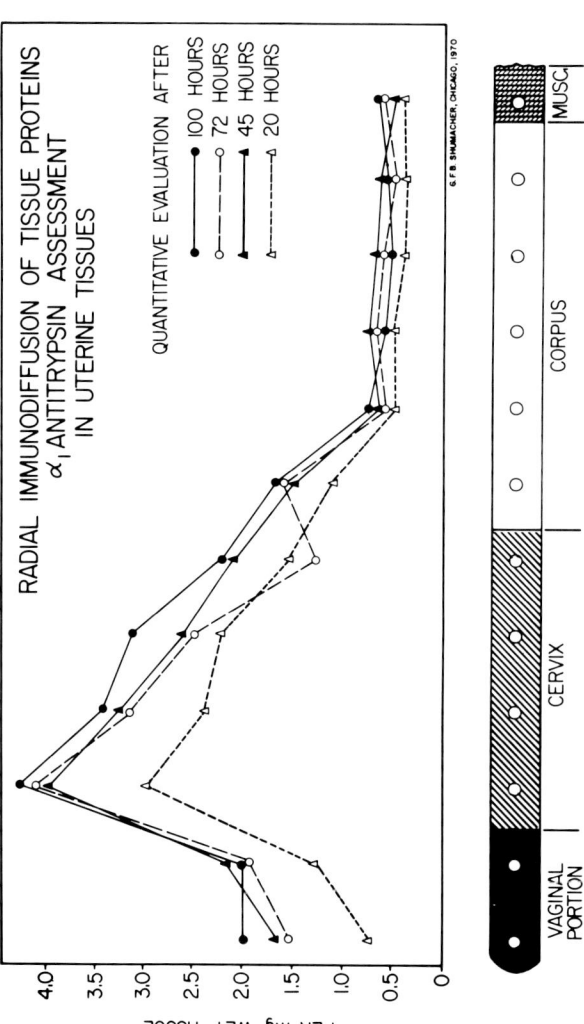

FIGURE 2. Evaluation of diffusible α_1-antitrypsin from the tissues of the inner surface of the uterus against dilutions of a reference standard solution in different time intervals over a period of 100 hours. The antigen standard solutions diffuse faster into the agar than the corresponding antigen (α_1-antitrypsin) from the tissue samples. Therefore, the readings after 20 hours show clearly lower levels than the readings after 45, 72 and 100 hours, especially in the area of higher concentration. It is interesting to note that significantly higher amounts of α_1-antitrypsin diffuse from the cervical tissue as compared to the endometrium or the uterine muscle. The order of magnitude is that of serum in the cervical tissues in contrast to cervical mucus itself where significantly lower levels have been demonstrated (Schumacher et al., 1977). On the other hand the endometrial tissues of the corpus area release α_1-antitrypsin in amounts comparable to the endometrial fluid levels listed in Table III. (see also Tauber, Chapter 9). The case characteristics of this hysterectomy specimen indicate that the 32 year old patient was on her 26th day of the cycle after administration of combined oral contraceptives.

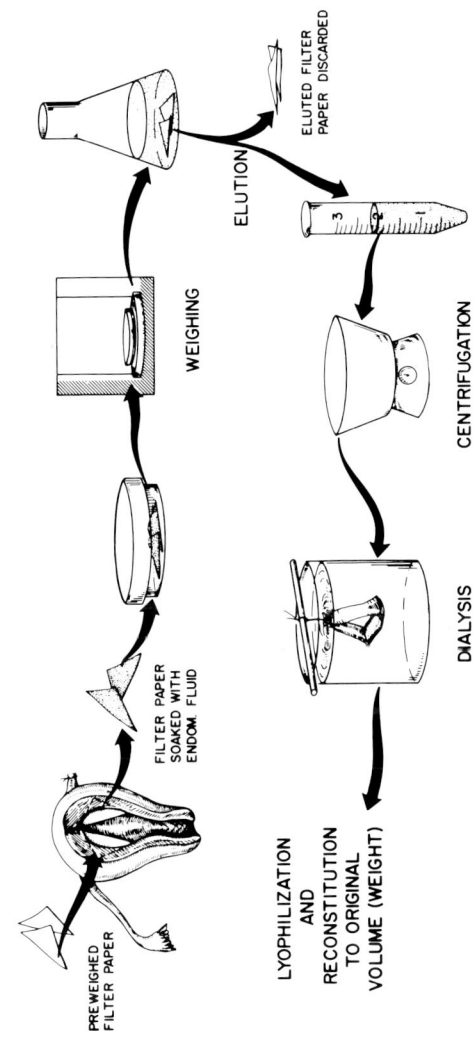

FIGURE 3. Blotting of endometrial fluid immediately after hysterectomy with filter paper triangles (Whatman No. 1) and quantitative extraction procedure (see text for details). After reconstitution to the original weight/volume the non-dialyzable constituents of the endometrial fluid may be analyzed by micro radial diffusion in gel techniques and other micro methods.

evaporation and weighed immediately to determine the amount of endometrial fluid which had been soaked up by the filter paper. Subsequently the triangles were transferred to a small flask, the weighing dish rinsed with approximately 2 ml of saline, which were then transferred to the flask for extraction of the paper. After a few seconds of mixing on a Vortex mixer the flask was kept overnight in the refrigerator. After 16–20 hours, the fluid was removed and the paper rinsed with approximately 0.5–1 ml of saline. The two fluids were combined and centrifuged in a refrigerated centrifuge at 3000 g for 15 minutes to remove cells and filter paper particles. The supernate was transferred into a small dialysis bag and dialyzed at 4°C against 1000 ml of distilled water for 18–28 hours after which it was transferred to a small vial and lyophilized. The freeze-dried material was then reconstituted with a volume of saline solution equivalent to the weight of the endometrial fluid picked up by the paper. The amounts of fluid recovered varied among the first 10 cases between 30 and 220 mg.

This material can be analyzed for non-dialyzable components, i.e. substances with a molecular weight of higher than 12,000—15,000. In case constituents of lower molecular weight would be of interest to analyze, different extraction and ultrafiltration procedures should be used. However, a variety of proteins, enzymes and enzyme inhibitors can be quantitatively assessed using micro radial diffusion in gel methods (Schill and Schumacher 1972, Schumacher and Schill 1972, Schill and Schumacher 1973) and other techniques requiring only small amounts of material such as micro-immunoelectrophoresis and polyacrylamide gel electrophoresis can be applied for further characterization and analysis. For the application of micro radial diffusion in gel methods to determine the level of some proteins present in higher concentration half of the material was quantitatively diluted (1/4) using volumetric micropipettes. In some instances tests had to be repeated with the undiluted material in case of very low levels or to establish the absence of certain constitutents.

Preliminary Results of the Blotting Method

Preliminary results of several cases investigated are being presented in the following section for three reasons:

1. to show that a considerable number of parameters can be determined with such small amounts of material available;
2. to show in parallel determinations of paired serum samples that the results are close to the expected normal serum values indicating reliability of the methods;
3. to provide information on the possible range in concentration of a variety of constituents of the human uterine fluid as a basis for further investigations, especially with respect to cyclic variations and pathological changes.

The characteristics of 8 cases investigated so far is given in Table I. Abdominal hysterectomy was performed in all instances. The histology of the endometrium did not show abnormalities except in one case with a Cu-7-IUD in situ and the histological dating is in good agreement with the hormonal values (RIA) in the peripheral blood sampled before surgery. The total amount of endometrial fluid recovered shows considerable variations. However the size of the uterus, i.e. of the

TABLE I. Case Characteristics (Total Abdominal Hysterectomy)

Case #	Age	Diagnosis	Endometrium Histol. Dating	E_1 pg/ml	E_2 pg/ml	P ng/ml	Cycle-Day (History)	Fluid Recovery mg
3346	45	Ca-in situ, Cx.	Postmenstrual	44	21	1.7	6	92
3301	47	Leiomyomata	Late Prolifer.	74	71	4.9	13	80
3344	42	Leiomyomata	Day 2/3 Post-Ovulatory	101	58	5.3	18	223
3090	32	Leiomyomata	Day 4/5 Post-Ovulatory	85	134	9.0	15	36
3331	28	Leiomyomata	Day 10/11 Post-Ovulatory	—	—	—	22	78
3277	45	Leiomyomata	Day 13/14 Post-Ovulatory	197	102	7.8	27	134
3063	33	Chron. Salpgts., adhesions	Day 13/14 Pcst-Ovulatory	—	—	—	35	35
3349	42	Stress-incont., Chronic Salpingitis	Proliferative; Endometritis Cu-7 IUD	55	70	1.1	22	218

inner surface of the uterus varied from one case to another. No blood was observed in the endometrial cavity of these cases.

Table II shows the concentrations of Immunoglobulins IgG, IgA, IgM and IgD, the presence or absence of secretory piece (TR = trace, + = approx. 10% of the concentration present in a breast milk pool) and the levels for the complement components C'1q, C'3, C'3-activator and C'4. Since no reference standard was available for C'1q, dilutions of a normal serum pool were used and the readings expressed as % of the normal serum pool. All values of the paired serum specimens show values in the expected range of normal sera. The values of most components of the endometrial fluid range between 20% and 50% of the corresponding serum values with the exception of IgD and C'1q. IgD is in 4 of 5 instances more than 2 fold higher than in serum. No explanation is available at the moment for this observation. But if it holds true in further investigations one may suspect a local production. C'1q is very low, virtually absent in 3 of 6 instances. This may be the explanation for the observation by Tauber (See Chapter 9) that only traces of hemolytic complement (C') can be detected in endometrial tissue. However other complement components are also considerably lower than in serum. The virtual absence of complement in endometrium is in agreement with our observations that hemolytic complement can not be demonstrated in human cervical mucus and rhesus monkey oviductal fluid by radial diffusion in gel methods (Schumacher and Yang, unpublished results).

Table III shows five different proteinase inhibitors in endometrial fluid and serum. The highest concentrations have been found for α_1-antitrypsin, which inhibits trypsin, chymotrypsin, plasmin, kallikrein, elastase, collagenase, cathepsin D and sperm-acrosin. Most of these enzymes are also inhibited by α_2-macroglobulin. Other inhibitors such as inter-α-trypsin inhibitor, α_1-antichymotrypsin and antithrombin III can also be detected, although in lower concentrations.

Table IV shows factors related to fibrinolysis. Plasminogen was present, in all samples, however in concentrations lower than in serum. Plasminogen activator was absent in all specimen except in case #3446 which was histologically dated as postmenstrual (sensitivity approximately 0.5–1 ploug unit/ml). Neutral proteinase activity was not detectable in all specimens using C^{++} containing buffer pH 8.0 and gelatin as substrate (sensitivity approximately $1\mu g$/ml trypsin), (Tauber et al., 1976). The immunological tests with antiserum against fibrinogen showed large rings in the radial immunodiffusion experiments which were suspicious of degradation products. Immunoelectrophoretic experiments revealed in 3 instances material of different electrophoretic mobility than fibrinogen reacting with antiserum against fibrinogen and fibrinogen split product D but not with antiserum against fibrinogen split product E. This pattern was also found in menstrual blood serum with plasminogen activator activity present.

Table V shows Albumin, Transferrin, the acute phase proteins C-reactive protein, Haptoglobin and Ceruloplasmin, the locally produced and/or from white blood cells released proteins lactoferrin and lysozyme, and α-Amylase. The Albumin concentration in endometrial fluid ranges from 980 to 3180 and represents 1/4—1/2 or more of the serum concentrations. The same applies to Transferrin; the EF/S-ratios are higher for IgM, IgD, Inter-α-trypsin Inhibitor and Antithrombin III. The EF/S ratios of the other constituents investigated are generally lower. C-reactive protein does not appear in endometrial secretions. Surprisingly it is not detectable in the endometrial fluid of the uterus with the IUD in situ, although it is weakly positive in the respective serum. The lysozyme values

TABLE II. Immunoglobulins and Complement Components in Endometrial Fluid and Serum

Case #	Phase	Immglob.G mg/dl		Immglob.A mg/dl		Immglob.M mg/dl		Immglob.D		Secr.Piece		C'1q in % of N-Ser.Pool		C'3c mg/dl		C'3 Actvr. mg/dl		C'4 mg/dl	
		EF	S	EF	S	EF	S	EF	S	EF	S	EF	S	EF	S	EF	S	EF	S
3346	Postmenstr.	388	1100	176	890	18	89	47	18	Tr	0	1	50	28	94	6	27	11	27
3301	Late Prolif.	435	1320	110	340	–	36	–	18	–	0	–	–	28	84	–	–	2	27
3344	Day +2/3	600	1280	76	130	71	142	47	10	Tr	0	25	125	28	70	11	22	4	27
3090	Day +4/5	324	1370	20	200	–	–	–	–	–	–	10	125	16	102	–	–	1	27
3331	Day +10/11	278	1460	60	365	18	149	43	10	+	0	1	125	18	70	–	24	4	27
3277	Day +13/14	336	1020	60	220	71	19	Tr	18	Tr	0	25	5	16	84	11	33	4	16
3063	Day +13/14	844	1410	–	–	–	–	–	–	–	–	–	–	–	84	–	–	11	16
3349	Proliferative, Cu-7 IUD, Endometritis	388	840	70	170	18	94	56	20	Tr	0	0	50	28	45	5	15	4	27

TABLE III. Proteinase Inhibitors in Endometrial Fluid and Serum

Case #	Phase	α_1-Antitry. mg/dl		Inter α TI mg/dl		α_1-Ant i-Chy. mg/dl		Anti Thr. III mg/dl		α_2-Macrogl. mg/dl	
		EF	S	EF	S	EF	S	EF	S	EF	S
3346	Postmenstr.	72	320	12	26	8	69	9	23	12	190
3301	Late prolif.	171	320	–	–	–	–	–	–	8	140
3344	Day +2/3	240	320	22	32	32	56	19	22	131	322
3090	Day +4/5	12	345	2	36	4	64	–	–	8	215
3331	Day +10/11	80	345	16	32	8	69	–	23	8	215
3277	Day +13/14	138	430	28	43	10	69	11	32	59	248
3063	Day +13/14	–	320	–	–	–	–	–	–	12	140
3349	Proliferative, Cu-7 IUD, Endometritis	100	295	20	29	10	73	13	23	41	156

should be looked at with reservations, since the molecular weight of approximately 15,000 is near the cut off point of the dialysis membrane. However, all samples were dialyzed and the relative values, expressed in percent of the sera show high readings for the post menstrual sample and the one deriving from the uterus with the IUD in situ. It is interesting to note that lactoferrin shows a similar pattern. In fact it was not detectable in endometrial fluid in 3 instances but present in considerable amounts in the same two cases. This iron-binding protein of body secretions does not appear in serum. Both lysozyme and lactoferrin may be locally produced and/or they derive from polymorphonuclear granulocytes (Ossermann et al., 1974, Masson et al., 1969) which are physiologically present in the endometrium during menstruation and as a result of the foreign body reaction towards intrauterine devices. The α-amylase activity measured only in 3 instances seems to be similar to the one in serum, although it may have different molecular characteristics if locally produced.

In conclusion: The amount of endometrial fluid present in human uteri appears to be very small. It can be recovered from surgical specimens by the blotting method, quantitatively extracted with saline solution, dialyzed, lyophilized and reconstituted to the original weight/volume. Depending on the amount recovered, the application of micro radial diffusion in gel allows the determination of 10–25 parameters or more. Preliminary results show that parallel determinations in paired serum samples yield meaningful results. Although the cases investigated so far are well characterized by histopathological means and hormonal data, the number is too small to draw any conclusions with respect to cyclic patterns. The range of serum proteins in endometrial fluid shows considerable variation from one protein to another. The same applies to local proteins. Immunoglobulins and proteinase inhibitors are present in considerable amounts, (for instance, IgM) which can not be demonstrated under physiological conditions in cervical mucus (Schumacher et al., 1977). Even more interesting is the fact that IgD was found in higher concentration than in serum. The results indicate further that certain proteins such as lactoferrin, lysozyme or plasminogen-activator may be present or significantly increased under certain conditions.

TABLE IV. Plasminogen, Activator, Neutral Proteinase and Fibrinogen-Related Antigens in Endometrial Fluid and Serum

Case #	Phase	Plasminogen mg/dl		Activator Ploug U/ml		Neutral Proteinase		Anti-F' gen Reactive	Anti Split D Reactive	Anti Split E Reactive
		EF	S	EF	S	EF	S	EF	EF	EF
3346	Postmenstr.	4	20	12	0	0	0	+++	–	–
3301	Late prolif.	–	11	0	0	0	0	–	–	–
3344	Day +2/3	3	15	0	0	0	0	+++	+++	0
3090	Day +4/5	5	20	0	0	0	0	+	–	–
3331	Day +10/11	1	15	0	0	0	0	++	–	0
3277	Day +13/14	4	15	0	0	0	0	++	++	0
3063	Day +13/14	5	11	0	0	0	0	–	–	–
3349	Proliferative, Cu-7 IUD, Endometritis	3	20	0	0	0	0	+++	+++	0

TABLE V. Albumin, Haptoglobin, Ceruloplasmin, CRP, Transferrin, Lactoferrin, Lysozyme and α-Amylase in Endometrial Fluid and Serum

Case #	Phase	Albumin mg/dl		Haptoglobin mg/dl		Cerulopl. mg/dl		CRP mg/dl		Transferrin mg/dl		Lactoferrin mg/dl		Lysozyme % Serum		α-Amylase μg/dl HPA-Equiv.	
		EF	S	EF	S	EF	S	EF	S	EF	S	EF	S	EF	S	EF	S
3346	Postmenstr.	1380	4250	78	293	10	36	0	0.6	80	225	39	0	562	100	–	–
3301	Late prolif.	1980	4150	53	145	–	–	–	0	110	280	–	–	–	–	–	–
3344	Day +2/3	2200	3740	60	190	16	24	0	0	184	280	0	0	37	100	220	170
3090	Day +4/5	980	3650	25	163	–	–	–	0	56	200	–	–	–	–	–	–
3331	Day +10/11	1268	4070	38	185	5	37	0	0	92	310	0	0	57	100	–	–
3277	Day +13/14	1560	3600	34	225	–	–	0	0	180	4	10	0	55	100	130	170
3063	Day +13/14	3180	4270	–	160	–	–	–	–	–	300	–	–	–	–	–	–
3349	Proliferative, Cu-7 IUD, Endometritis	1800	4070	41	155	10	33	0	1.0	68	145	14	0	100	100	130	130

Comments

Both approaches to the analysis of human endometrial secretions can provide useful information. The tissue cylinder method has the advantage that the topographical distribution of certain components in the tissues of the inner surface of the uterus can be investigated. For instance, the distribution pattern for immunoglobulins, proteinase inhibitors and plasminogen activator appears to be different between the cervix and the fundus area. (see Tauber, Chapter 9). The disadvantage is that the results of this approach provide data on secretions as well as on tissue constituents. The advantage of the blotting method described here is that *endometrial fluid only* is made available for analysis from nearly the entire inner surface of the corpus uteri. Topographical distribution studies on single components can also be done by using small pieces of paper placed in different areas as described by Parr and Shirley (1976) for the study of β-galactosidase. The disadvantage of the blotting method is that the material must be extracted with suitable electrolyte solutions which require dialysis before lyophilization in order to avoid excess electrolytes in the sample reconstituted with a physiological saline solution to the original weight/volume. The quantitative extraction procedure requires careful and accurate handling of very small amounts of material. It has to be taken into consideration, that a small percentage of the constituents may be lost during manipulations. Low molecular weight constituents are lost during the dialysis procedure. However, other procedures could be developed for low molecular weight constituents which may or may not affect the composition and molecular properties of high molecular weight constituents of endometrial secretions.

ACKNOWLEDGEMENTS
The skillful technical assistance of Mrs. Margaret Crawford is gratefully acknowledged. We thank Mrs. Evelyn Jackson for preparing the manuscript.
The work was supported in part by NIH Grant HD2682, Ford Foundation #690-0108A and the Mother's Aid Research Fund of the Chicago Lying-in Hospital.

REFERENCES

Beier, H.M.: Oviductal and uterine fluids. J. Reprod. Fert. 37 (1974) 221–237.

Blandau, R.J., Moghissi, K. (Eds.): The Biology of the Cervix. University of Chicago Press, Chicago and London, 1973.

Edwards, R.G., Talbert, L., Israelstam, D., Nino, H.V., Johnson, M.H.: Diffusion chamber for exposing spermatozoa to human uterine secretions. Am. J. Obstet. Gynec. 102 (1968) 388–396.

Elstein, M., Moghissi, K.S., Borth, R.: Cervical Mucus in Human Reproduction. Scriptor, Copenhagen, 1973.

Insler, V., Bettendorf, G. (Eds): The Uterine Cervix in Reproduction. G. Thieme Publ., Stuttgart, 1977.

Maathuis, J.B., Aitken, R.J.: Cyclic variation in concentrations of protein and hexose in human uterine flushings collected by an improved technique. J. Reprod. Fertil. 52 (1978) 289–295.

Maathius, J.B., Aitken, R.J.: Protein patterns of human uterine flushings collected at various stages of the menstrual cycle. J. Reprod. Fertil. 53 (1978) 343–348.

Mancini, G., Carbonara, A.O., Heremans, J.F.: Immunochemical quantitation of antigens by single radial immunodiffusion. Immunochemistry 2 (1965) 235–241.

Masson, P.L., Heremans, J.F., Schonne, E.: Lactoferrin, an iron-binding protein in neutrophilic leucocytes. J. Exp. Med. 130 (1969) 643–658.

Osserman, E.F., Canfield, R.E., Beychok, S. (Eds.): Lysozyme. Academic Press, New York and London, 1974.

Parr, E.L., Shirley, R.L.: Embryotoxicity of leucocyte extracts and its relationship to intrauterine contraception in humans. Fertil. Steril 27 (1976) 1067–1077.

Prins, G., Zaneveld, L.J.D., Schumacher, G.F.B.: Functional biochemistry of cervical mucus. In: Human Ovulation. Ed.: E.S.E. Hafez. Elsevier/North-Holland Biomedical Press, New York, 1979, pp. 313–325.

Schill, W.-B., Schumacher, G.F.B.: Micro radial diffusion in gel methods for the quantitative assessment of soluble proteins in genital secretions. In: The Biology of the Cervix. Eds.: R.J. Blandau and K. Moghissi. University of Chicago Press, Chicago and London, 1973, pp. 173–200.

Schill, W.-B., Schumacher, G.F.B.: Radial diffusion in gel for micro determination of enzymes. I. Muramidase, alpha-amylase, DNase I, RNase A, acid phosphatase, and alkaline phosphatase. Analyt. Biochem. 46 (1972) 502–533.

Schumacher, G.F.B., Kim, M.H., Hosseinian, A.H., Dupon, C.: Immunoglobulins, proteinase inhibitors, albumin, and lysozyme in human cervical mucus. I. Hormonal profiles and cervical mucus changes during presumably ovulatory cycles—methods and results. Am. J. Obstet. & Gynecol. 129 (1977) 629–636.

Schumacher, G.F.B.: Cervical secretions—a product of a target organ for estrogens and gestagens. In: The Uterine Cervix in Reproduction. Eds.: V. Insler, G. Bettendorf. G. Thieme Publishers, Stuttgart, 1977, pp. 101–108.

Schumacher, G.F.B., Wied, G.L.: Semiquantitative microanalysis of proteins in cervical mucus. Proc. Vth World Congr. Fertil. Steril. Stockholm 1966. Intern. Congr. Ser. No. 133, Excerpta Medica Foundation, Amsterdam—New York, 1967, pp. 713–722.

Schumacher, G.F.B., Pearl, M.J.: Muramidase (Lysozyme) in cervical secretions. In: Protides of the Biological Fluids, Vol. 16, Ed.: J. Peeters. Pergamon Press, Oxford—New York, 1969, pp. 525–534.

Schumacher, G.F.B., Schill, W.-B.: Radial diffusion in gel for micro determination of enzymes. II. Plasminogen activator, elastase and non-specific proteases. Analyt. Biochem. 48 (1972) 9–26.

Schumacher, G.F.B.: Lysozyme in human genital secretions. In: Lysozyme. Eds.: E.F. Osserman, R.E. Canfield, S. Beychok. Academic Press, New York and London, 1974, pp. 427–447.

Shaw, S.T. Jr., Azar, E., Moyer, D.L.: ^3H_2O volume and exchange in uterine cavity of monkeys. Am. J. Physiol. 229 (1975) 1465–1470.

Stambaugh, R., Seitz, H.M., Mastroianni, L., Jr.: Acrosomal proteinase inhibitors in rhesus monkey (Macaca Mulatta) oviduct fluid. Fertil. Steril. 25 (1974) 352–357.

Tauber, P.F., Zaneveld, L.J.D., Propping, D., Schumacher, G.F.B.: Components of human split ejaculates. II. Enzymes and proteinase inhibitors. J. Reprod. Fertil. 46 (1976) 165–171.

Wynn, R.M. (Ed.): Biology of the Uterus. Plenum Press, New York and London, 1977.

Copyright 1979 by Elsevier North Holland, Inc.
F.K. Beller and G.F.B. Schumacher, eds.
The Biology of the Fluids of the Female Genital Tract

BIOCHEMICAL COMPONENTS OF THE HUMAN ENDOMETRIUM

P. F. Tauber

SUMMARY

The mucosal layer of the human uterus contains considerable amounts of protein constituents which are related to the humoral defense system. Such components include the immunoglobulins G and A, the proteinase inhibitors α_1-antitrypsin and α_1-antichymotrypsin, lysozyme, plasminogen activator and to a lower extent the complement component C3. Only traces of hemolytic complement were detected. With regard to the topographic distribution of these components, highest values were found in the cervical mucosa, with the exception of plasminogen activator which was found to be low in the cervix and high in the mucosa of the fundus uteri. Cyclic changes of most of these constituents are characterized by increased values in the periovulatory phase.

INTRODUCTION

Information on quantitative aspects of biochemical and immunological protein components in tissues and secretions of the inner surface of the uterus is rather scanty. To assess freely diffusible constituents from hysterectomy specimens, two principal methods are being discussed in detail in this volume by Schumacher (see Chapter 8). Using the tissue cylinder approach according to

Frauenklinik und Poliklinik, Universitätsklinikum der Gesamthochschule, Essen, FRG

Schumacher with minor modifications the focus of our work on the various constituents of uterine epithelium has been directed to answer the following questions:

1. Which freely diffusible protein components possibly relevant to the uterine defense system are present in the mucosal layer of the human uterus and what concentrations per mg wet weight tissue can be found?
2. What distribution patterns of these constituents and their concentrations do exist at various topographic localizations in the uterus?
3. How do the concentrations and the topographic variations change with different phases of the ovarian cycle, i.e. under the influence of estrogens and progesterone?

Based upon the results of such a study one may be able to discuss the relative biological significance of the constituents with regard to physiological and/or pathophysiological phenomena occurring in the uterus under various clinical conditions, e.g. intrauterine contraception, effects of exogenously administered sex steroids during reproductive life or after menopause, and at the occasion of uterine infections and malignancies.

MATERIALS AND METHODS

Hysterectomy specimens from 36 women between 20 and 49 years of age (mean 38.8 ± 6.7) were investigated. Thirty women were multiparous, 6 women were nulliparous. The last delivery was between 8 months and 20 years prior to hysterectomy. Until this operation, all patients had a regular menstrual history with a 28.7 ± 2 days (range 26 to 32) bleeding pattern of normal intensity and an average duration of 4.8 ± 2 days (range 3 to 5 days). Hysterectomies were done for descended uteri (with or without urinary incontinence) in 23 cases, dysmenorrhoic complaints (5 cases) and sterilization (5 cases). In three women, hysterectomies were performed at the occasion of castration (bilateral oophorectomy) due to metastatic breast cancer. None of the women had received exogenous hormones within the last three months prior to the operation. Gross examinations of the hysterectomy specimens did not reveal any major uterine pathology. To determine the phase of the cycle, menstrual history and histology of the endometrium were used. Only such hysterectomy specimens were selected, which were not traumatized during surgery. Traumatization has to be considered a major factor in obtaining erroneous results.

Following removal of the uterus, the specimens were kept at +4C and within one hour or less worked up for the determinations according to the method of Schumacher and Pearl (1969) with minor modifications. Tissue cylinders of approximately 1.5 to 2.0 mm diameter and well diameters of 1.5 mm were used.

In contrast to the original method, plasminogen activator concentrations were determined at 37°C. Monospecific antisera to human IgG, IgA, α_1-antitrypsin, α_1-antichymotrypsin, complement component C3 and the bovine fibrinogen preparation for the plasminogen activator determination were obtained from Behringwerke, Marburg, West Germany, antiserum to human lactoferrin from Nordic Laboratories, Tilburg, The Netherlands. Lysozyme standard and Micrococcus luteus substrate were purchased from Boehringer, Mannheim, West Germany and urokinase from Serono, Freiburg, West Germany. The lactoferrin standard was obtained through the generosity of Dr. P. Masson, University of

Louvain, Belgium. Standard plasma or serum was provided by the Behringwerke, Marburg, West Germany. After diffusion, the tissue cylinders were removed from the agar(ose) gel layer and were quickly weighed with a precision balance. The precipitation or lysis zone diameters were measured under dark field illumination with a calibrating viewer (Transidyne Corporation, Ann Arbor, Michigan). Since the sizes of the precipitation or lysis zones are proportional to the amount of substance freely diffusible from the tissue cylinders, the amounts were determined from standard solutions applied to the same system and expressed in μg or Units (plasminogen activator, complement activity) per mg wet weight tissue.

For the determination of the total complement activity in the uterine mucosa, commercially available agar gel plates containing sensitized sheep erythrocytes (Biotest Serum Institute, Frankfurt, West Germany) were used. As standard served a guinea pig serum preparation.

Hysterectomy specimens from days 4 to 10 of the cycle were considered as proliferative phase preparations, those from days 11 to 16 as periovulatory and from days 17 to 32 as secretory phase uteri. Studied were only tissue cylinders from the posterior wall of the uterus. The dissection areas and their topographic localization are demonstrated in Figure 7. Three tissue samples were taken from the uterine cervix (external os, cervical canal, internal os), 3 from the center of the corpus, 2 from the fundus and one from each tubal corner. The results obtained from both sides were averaged for further evaluation. A more detailed description of the exact performance of the investigations including the statistical analysis procedure were published elsewhere (Tauber 1979).

RESULTS

Qualitative Pilot Studies

In order to obtain preliminary information about the presence or absence of various diffusible components in the uterine mucosa, a pilot study was done using 4 hysterectomy specimens from different stages of the menstrual cycle. The results are listed in Table I: Of the components present in both uterine cervix and corpus, higher amounts were found in the cervical mucosa (IgG, IgA, α_1-antitrypsin, α_1-antichymotrypsin, complement component C 3 and lysozyme), with the exception of the plasminogen activator that revealed much higher activities in the corpus mucosa, and albumin which showed similarly high amounts in both areas. Secretory piece to IgA, lactoferrin and the complement component C1q were detectable only in traces in the cervical mucosa, but were virtually absent in the endometrium. Total complement activity was very low in the cervix and corpus, while the complement component C1r was not detectable. Neutral proteinase activity was not found in the mucosa samples.

Quantitative Determinations: Cyclic Variations

Both immunoglobulins (Figures 1 and 2) and proteinase inhibitors (Figures 3 and 4) show highest concentrations in the periovulatory phase of the cycle. With the exception of α_1 =antichymotrypsin the changes from low values during the proliferative phase to high concentrations during the midcycle period are statistically significant (p< 0.0001). All values obtained during the secretory phase show

TABLE I. Diffusible Protein Components in Mucosal Tissues of the Human Uterus—Pilot Study Results*

Component	Presence in uterine mucosa	
	Cervix	Corpus
IgG	++	+
IgA	+	(+)
T-piece	((+))	∅
α_1AT	++	+
α_1ACT	+	(+)
Albumin	++	++
Lactoferrin	((+))	∅
C1q	((+))	∅
C1r	∅	∅
C3	+	(+)
C4	(+)	((+))
TCA	(+)	(+)
Lysozyme	++	+
P1-Activator	(+)/∅	+
Neutral Protease	∅	∅

* from 4 human uteri at different phases of cycle
∅ = *not present*/ ((+)) = *traces*/ (+) = *small amounts*/ + = *measurable amounts present*/ ++ = *large amounts*

lower levels but do not reach the postmenstrual concentrations. In contrast to the immunoglobulins and the proteinase inhibitors, lysozyme shows its highest concentrations during the proliferative phase (Figure 5) of the cycle. Plasminogen Activator exhibits a concentration pattern similar to the immunoglobulins and the proteinase inhibitors during the cycle (Figure 6). There was not enough material available to study samples from the different phases of the cycle with respect to complement and the C3 component of the complement system.

Quantitative Determinations: Topographic Variations

Figures 1 to 6 show clearly that the endocervical tissue contains higher amounts of these diffusible components as compared to the endometrium, with the exception of the plasminogen activator which exhibits a completely reversed pattern of distribution throughout all phases of the cycle. The distribution pattern of α_1-antichymotrypsin, however, shows less pronounced differences between the cervix and the corpus uteri.

Quantitative Determinations: IgG/IgA Ratio in Uterine Mucosa

IgG/IgA ratios were presented in Figure 7 with regard to their topographic localization in the uterus. During the proliferative and the secretory phase, the ratio values are rather high (approximately 20:1) in the cervical and the fundal areas. The ratio decreases to about 10:1 around midcycle indicating a relative increase of diffusible IgA.

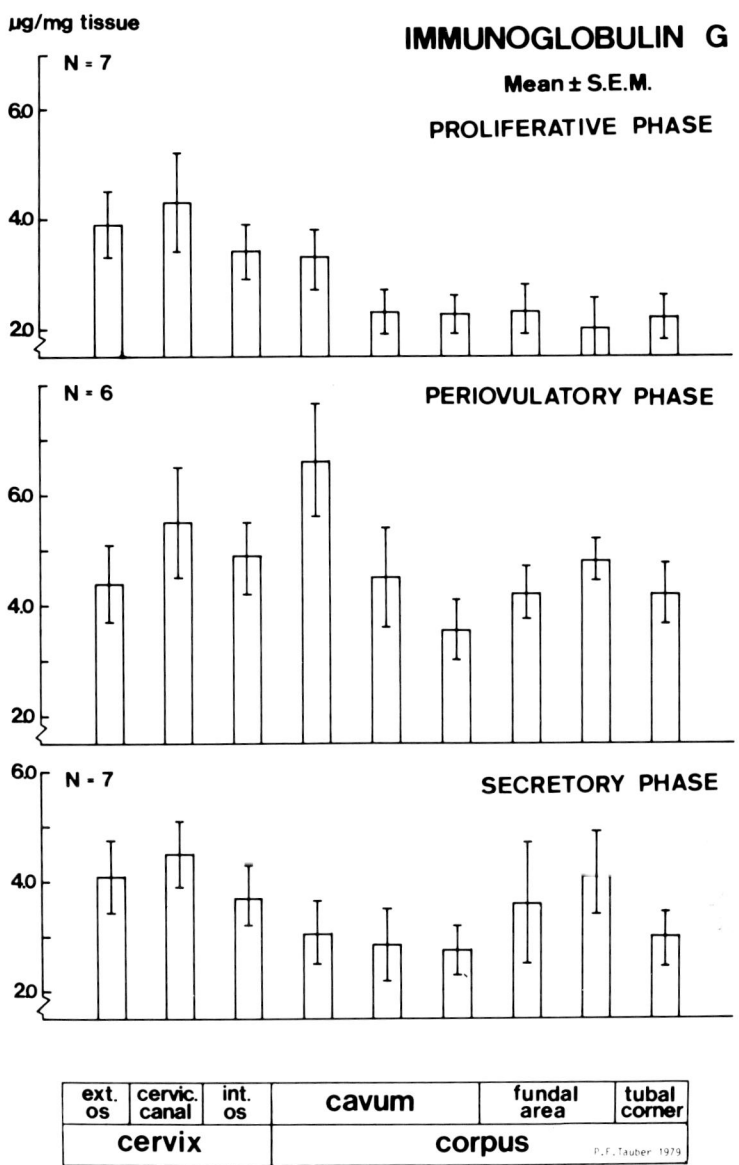

FIGURE 1. Cyclic and topographic variations of Immunoglobulin G concentrations (μg/mg wet weight tissue) at the inner epithelial layer of the human uterus. Considerably higher concentrations are found in the periovulatory phase (days 11 to 16). The increase in concentrations vs. the proliferative phase is statistically significant ($p < 0.0001$). In specimens from the secretory phase, IgG concentrations are lowered again, but not to the values during the proliferation. Note the remarkably high IgG concentration at tissue localization 4 in periovulatory specimens. It appears that this functionally important localization is particularly well guarded by the available immunoglobulin in the epithelium.

Values are means ± S.E.M.; N represents number of investigated hysterectomy specimens.

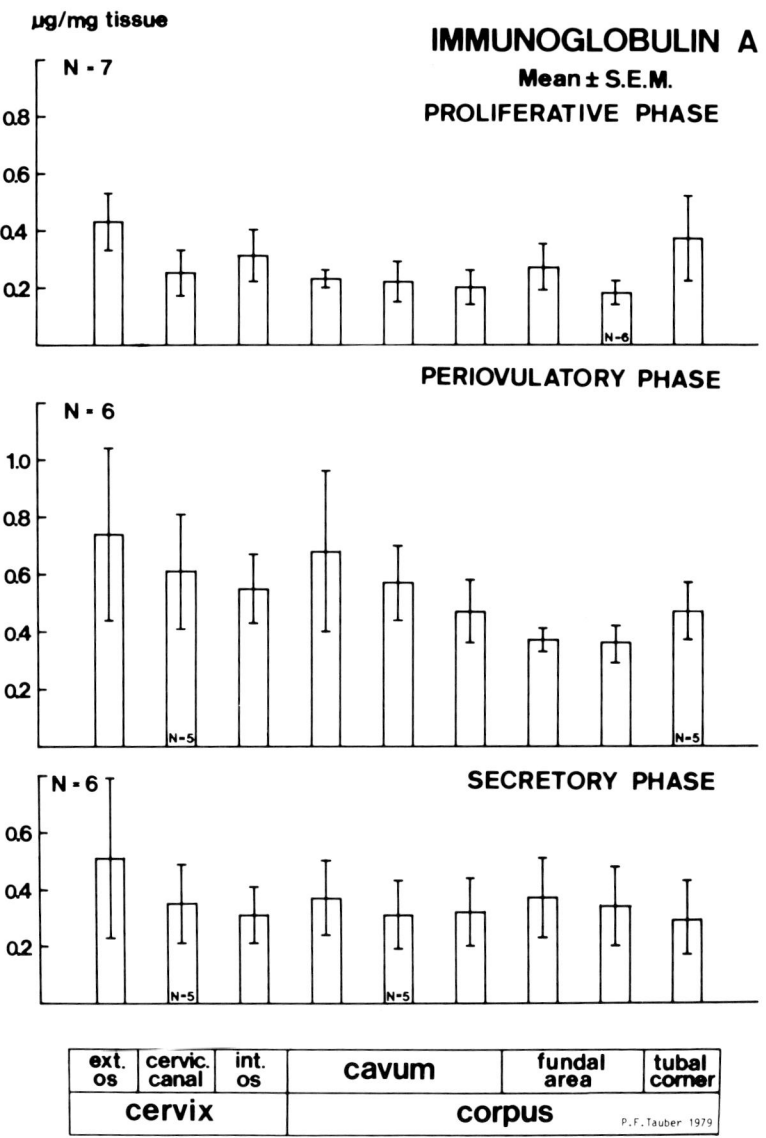

FIGURE 2. Cyclic and topographic variations of Immunoglobulin A concentrations (μg/mg wet weight tissue) at the inner epithelial layer of the human uterus. Similarly to IgG, Immunoglobulin A exhibits highest concentrations in the periovulatory specimens. The values are statistically significant ($p < 0.0001$) vs. the proliferative phase. Again, the localization 4 shows some prominence in IgA concentration during periovulation.

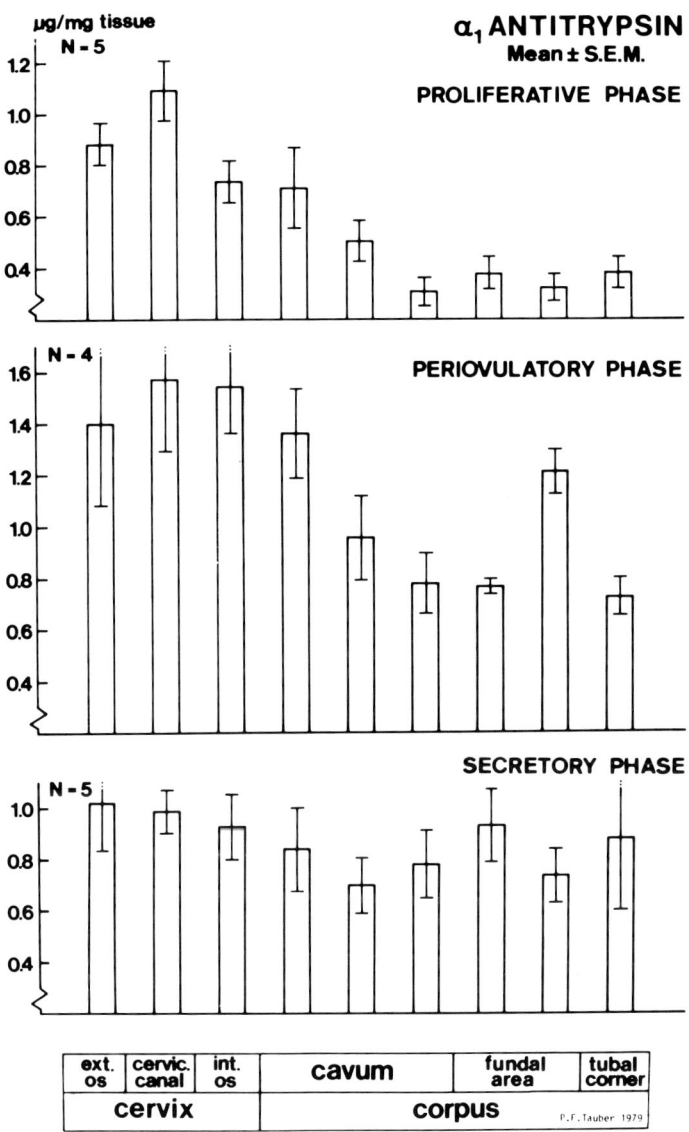

FIGURE 3. Cyclic and topographic variations of α_1-Antitrypsin concentrations (μg/mg wet weight tissue) in the mucosal layer of the human uterus. The values obtained from periovulatory specimens are remarkably higher than those in the proliferation phase ($p < 0.0001$), but return to lower concentrations in the secretory phase. Note the prominent inhibitor concentrations in the cervical mucosa during the periovulation.

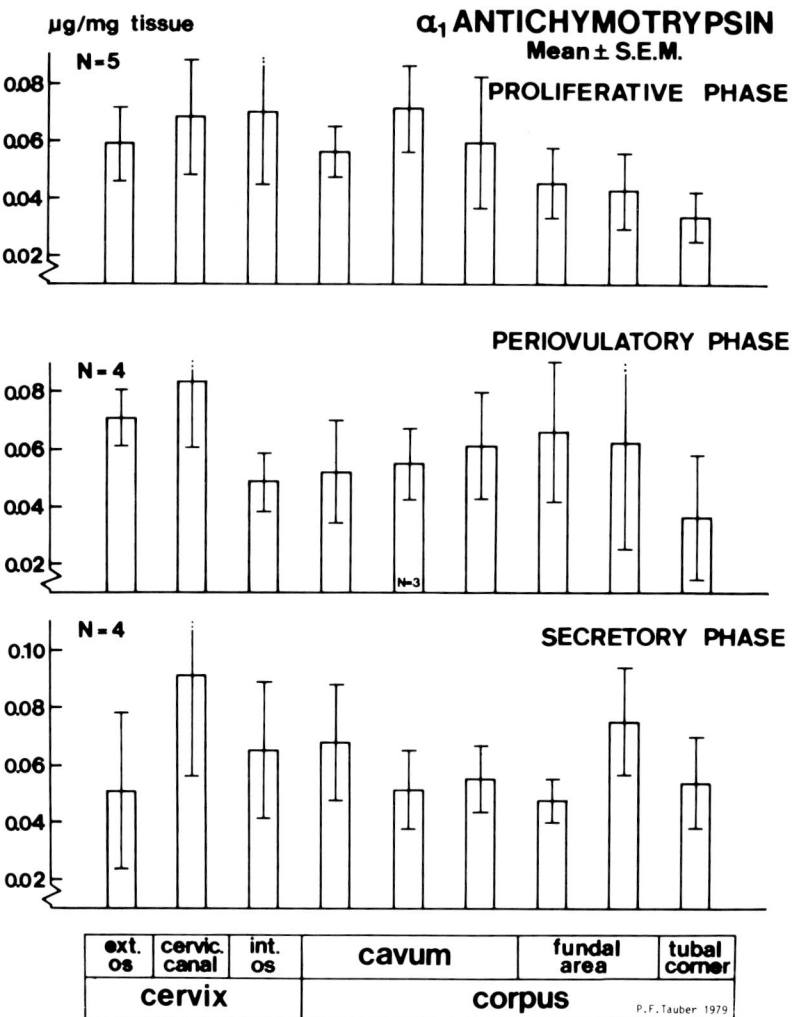

FIGURE 4. Cyclic and topographic variations of α_1-Antichymotrypsin concentrations (μg/mg wet weight tissue) in mucosal tissue cylinders from human uteri. Values are approximately 1/10 as compared to α_1-Antitrypsin and do not exhibit major changes during the different phases of the menstrual cycle. Compared to the distribution pattern in Figure 4, the preference of the cervix is not as pronounced.

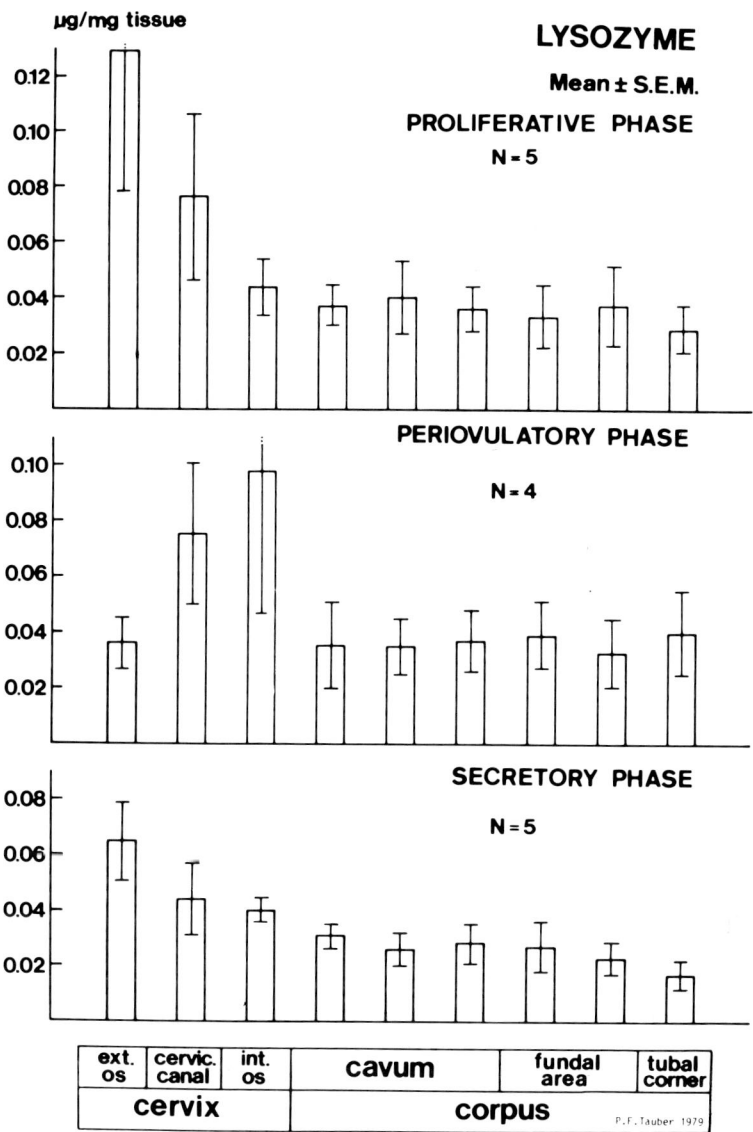

FIGURE 5. Cyclic and topographic variations of concentrations (μg/mg wet weight tissue) of diffusible Lysozyme in the mucosal layer of human uteri. Smooth distribution patterns are found in the corpus and fundus area without major variations during the menstrual cycle. The cervix mucosa contains much higher concentrations and exhibits a reversed pattern in the periovulatory phase as compared to the proliferative phase. The high values in the cervix are statistically significant vs. the low values in the corpus.

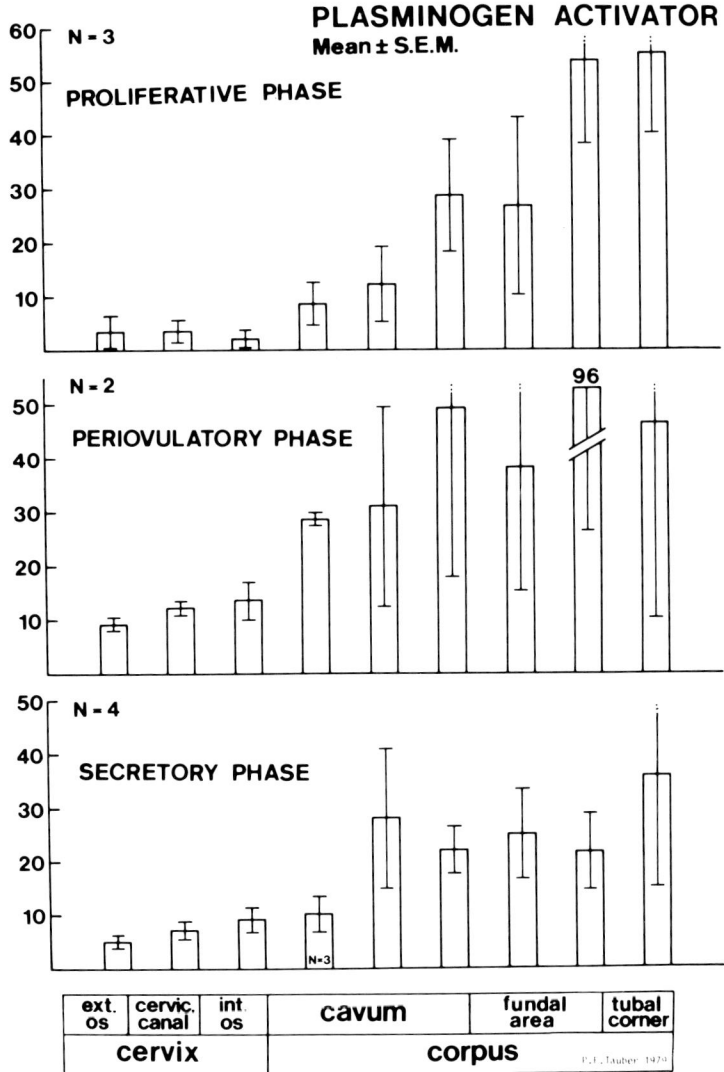

FIGURE 6. Plasminogen activator concentrations (International Units/mg wet weight issue) in the mucosa of human uteri. Extremely high concentrations are found in the fundal area which also shows peak concentrations in the periovulatory phase. Concentrations in the cervix are consistently low through all phases.

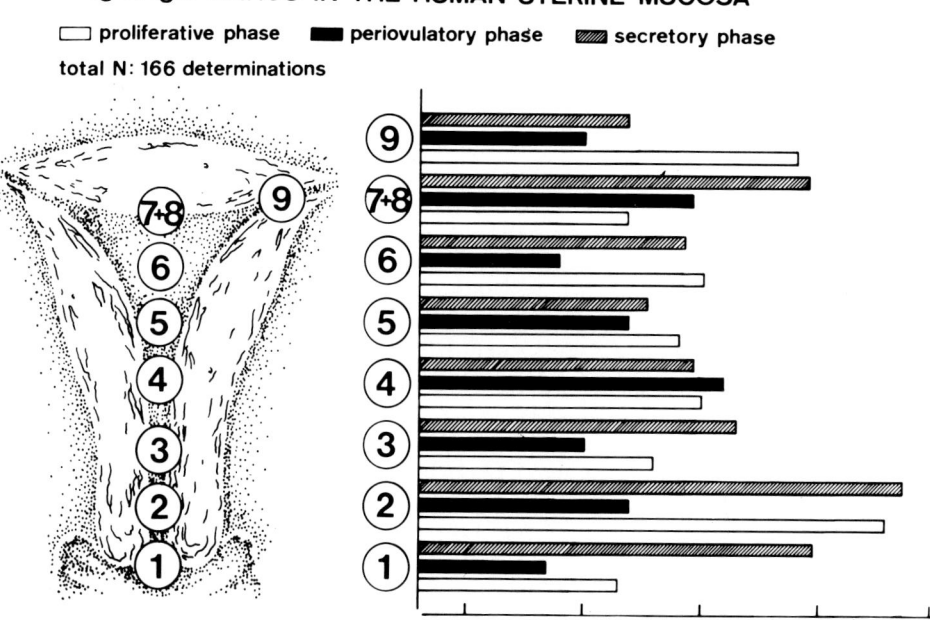

FIGURE 7. IgG/IgA ratios in the inner epithelial layer of human uteri (right panel). Corresponding topographic localizations for tissue dissections are demonstrated in the left panel. At midcycle values are generally lower than in the other phases, possibly indicating a relative increase of IgA concentrations. Proliferative phase and secretory phase patterns of localizations #1 (external os) and #9 (tubal corner) exhibit reversed patterns which suggests a functionally synergistic, but topographically antagonistic principle of immune defense during the cycle.

Overall Concentrations in the Uterine Mucosa

Figures 8 and 9 demonstrate the overall distribution of the diffusible components at different levels of the inner surface of the uterus (summary of all cases studied). The graphs emphasize again the preference for higher concentrations of some diffusible constituents in the cervical mucosa (immunoglobulins, proteinase inhibitors, lysozyme and complement component C3), and the reversed pattern of distribution for the plasminogen activator.

COMMENTS AND DISCUSSION

Methodological Considerations

Assessment of concentrations of soluble protein components in female genital tract secretions is associated with numerous problems mostly due to the limited access and to sampling methods. The data presented here indicate, however, that the tissue cylinder method offers the possibility to study components which diffuse freely from the tissues of the inner linings of the uterus, with sufficient accuracy, reproducibility and comparability. When hysterectomy specimens are used, traumatization of the tissues during operation should be carefully avoided in order to prevent contamination with blood constituents. The contamination with blood still present in blood vessels of non-traumatized specimen seems to be rather limited since complement activity is missing or negligible. In addition, the significantly higher values found in the cervical mucosa as compared to the corpus uteri speak also for themselves in favor of minor blood contamination, if one considers the fact that the blood flow in the uterus is much lower in the cervix than in the uterine corpus (Prill 1963). Thus, it can be concluded that the values obtained by the tissue cylinder method provide data on the presence of diffusible components in these tissues and their distribution on the inner surface of the uterus which give at least some indication whether or not one should expect higher or lower concentrations (or absence) of these components in the secretions of the respective compartments of the uterus.

The Defense System in the Uterus

The presence of the immunoglobulins G and A, the proteinase inhibitors α_1-antitrypsin and α_1-antichymotrypsin, and lysozyme in considerable amounts at the innermost epithelial layer of the uterus underlines the importance of the non-specific defense mechanisms in the female genital tract which are directed against microbial invaders. These proteins may play a biological role as specific or nonspecific immune factors against bacteria (immunoglobulins), and neutralizers of numerous proteolytic enzymes involved in tissue inflammation (proteinase inhibitors) or reproductive processes. Since the uterine cervix carries the major part of this biochemical-immunological defense system, both principles, anatomical and humoral barrier, work hand in hand with each other in order to protect the anatomically unique open connection between the outside environment and the peritoneal cavity.

While a considerable amount of information exists on the presence of these proteins and their concentrations in cervical secretions (Schumacher et al., 1977), reports from the uterine mucosal tissues are rather rare. Cyclic concentration changes in cervical mucus show lowest values during midcycle and it is interesting to note from the data presented here that the concentration in the *tissues* exhibit a completely reversed pattern (Table II). So far, no other explanation for this phenomenon can be found than the possibility that the female genital tract mucosa owns a more or less selective storage mechanism for these and possibly other pro-

---

FIGURE 8. Overall concentrations of diffusible IgG, IgA, α_1-Antitrypsin and α_1-Antichymotrypsin according to various localizations in the mucosal layer of human uteri (material of all phases of the cycle). *IgG*: Markedly lower concentrations in the corpus mucosa vs. the cervix ($p < 0.0001$). *IgA*: Concentrations in the corpus are not as pronounced low vs. the cervix as compared to IgG, but are statistically significantly different ($p < 0.0001$). α_1-*Antitrypsin*: Highest values in the cervical mucosa. Differences to corpus are statistically significant ($p < 0.0001$). α_1-*Antichymotrypsin*: Highest concentration in the cervical canal. Remarkably low value at the tubal corner. Difference between cervix and corpus not significant.

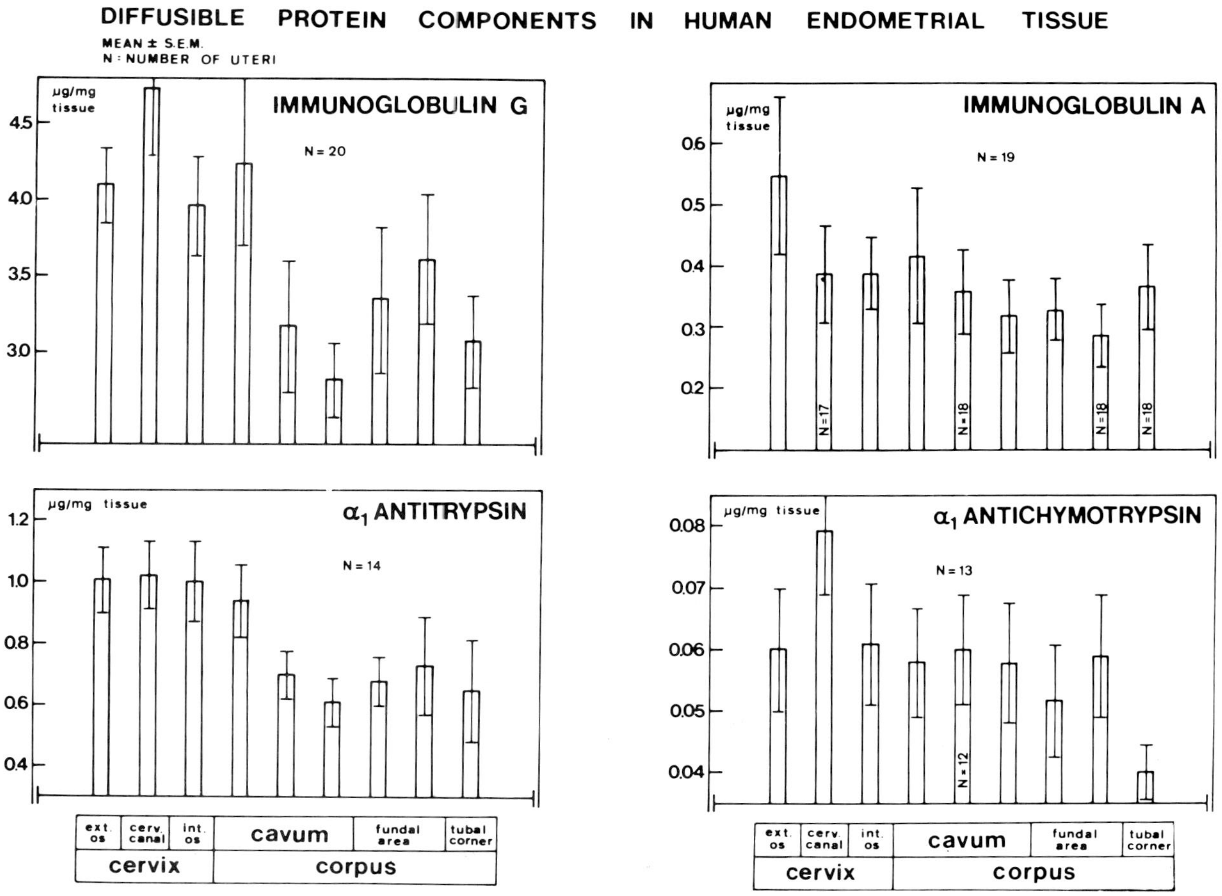
DIFFUSIBLE PROTEIN COMPONENTS IN HUMAN ENDOMETRIAL TISSUE
MEAN ± S.E.M.
N : NUMBER OF UTERI
IMMUNOGLOBULIN G
N = 20
µg/mg tissue
4.5
4.0
3.5
3.0
IMMUNOGLOBULIN A
N = 19
0.6
0.5
0.4
0.3
0.2
N = 17
N = 18
N = 18
N = 18
α1 ANTITRYPSIN
N = 14
1.2
1.0
0.8
0.6
0.4
α1 ANTICHYMOTRYPSIN
N = 13
0.08
0.07
0.06
0.05
0.04
N = 12
ext. os
cerv. canal
int. os
cavum
fundal area
tubal corner
cervix
corpus

FIG. 8

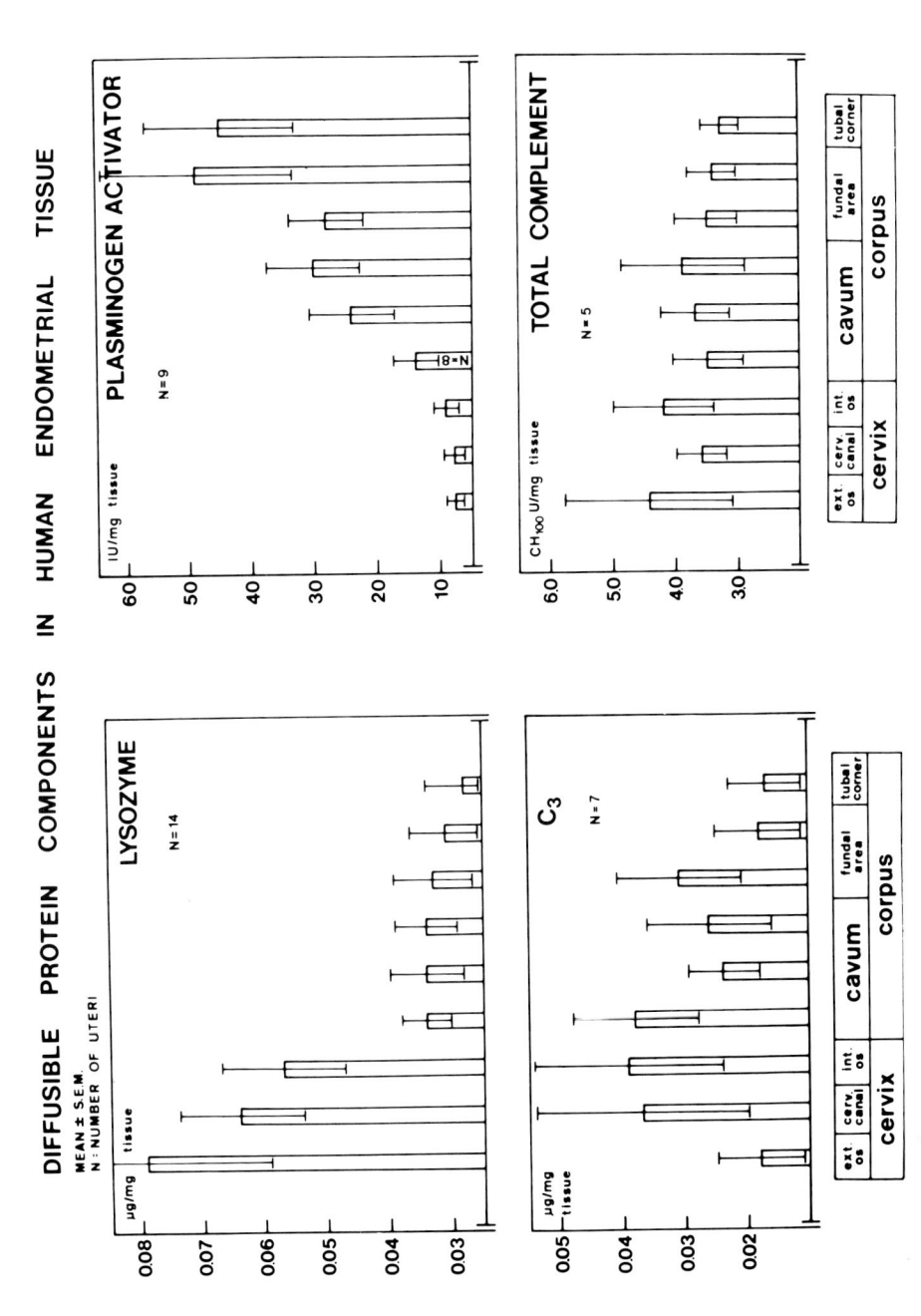

TABLE II. Diffusible Protein Components in the Human Uterine Mucosa

Component	Overall Concentration Differences—Cyclic and Topographic Variations				
	Pre	Peri*	Post	Cervix*	Corpus
Immunoglobulin G	−40%	4.80	−25%	4.26	−20%
Immunoglobulin A	−47%	0.53	−43%	0.42	−20%
α_1 Antitrypsin	−50%	1.14	−25%	1.10	−20%
α_1 Antichymotrypsin	− 5%	0.06	+ 5%	0.07	−20%
Lysozyme	+ 8%	0.05	−30%	0.07	−50%
PlG Activator	−40%	36**	−50%	<10**	+300%
C 3	—	—	—	0.03	−12%
TCA	—	—	—	4.0^+	−10%

*Concentrations in ug/mg wet weight tissue; **in International Units/mg tissue; + in CH 100 Units/mg tissue.

FTCA = Total Complement Activity

teins during the various phases of the cycle. It is obvious that the control over the release from the tissues to the secretions is strictly hormone dependent.

Immunoglobulins

As in our results, the hormonal influence upon the presence of immunoglobulins in the uterine mucosa has been suggested also by other authors. (Lippes et al., 1970; Tourville et al., 1970; Schiller and Donat, 1975; Hurlimann et al., 1978; Kelly and Fox, 1977). There is considerable disagreement in the literature, however, as to what extent sex steroids, estrogen and progesterone, trigger changes in immunoglobulin concentrations. Estrogens increase RNA and protein biosynthesis in the uterus and in other organs (Segal et al., 1977) and participation of immunoglobulins in this increase is possible (Schiller and Donat, 1975). The estrogenic, i.e. proliferative phase of the cycle may indeed stimulate the presence of higher amounts of immunoglobulins in the uterine epithelium. However, there have also been observations ascribing a stimulating effect for the presence of components related to the local immune system in the endometrium to progesterone (Hirsch et al., 1976; Kelly and Fox, 1977). So far, the question as to whether estrogens or progesterone or a combination of both are responsible for higher and lower concentrations of diffusible immunoglobulins in the uterine mucosa remains still to be solved.

There is also conflicting evidence on the presence of a local immune system in uterine tissues. A sparse population of immunocytes in the endometrium was observed by Tourville et al., (1970) and Vaerman and Ferin (1975), but was not

FIGURE 9. Overall concentrations of diffusible Lysozyme, Plasminogen Activator, Complement component C3 and Total Complement Activity at various localizations in the mucosal layer of human uteri (material of all phases of the cycle). *Lysozyme*: Extremely high concentrations in the cervix vs. corpus ($p < 0.0001$). *Plasminogen Activator*: Very low values in the cervix which increase consistently to reach extremely high values in the fundus. Differences cervix vs. corpus are statistically significant ($p < 0.0001$). International units equate to CTA units. *C3*: Cervical concentrations somewhat higher than in corpus, but statistically not significant. *Total complement activity*: Consistently low values at all localizations with weak preference of the cervical area. Hemolytic complement was detectable in only 5 out of 9 human uteri. The activity found represents less than 5% of normal human serum.

found by others (Hurliman et al., 1978; Kelly and Fox, 1979). Similarly contradictory results have been obtained in studies on cervical tissue (Chipperfield and Evans, 1972; Rebello et al., 1975). Sen and Fox (1967) reported on the presence of lymphoid tissue aggregations in endometrial tissues from premenopausal women, but found only sparse indications in women with endometrial cancer. This might explain the observation from our laboratory of extremely low concentrations of immunoglobulins in edometrial cancer tissues (Tauber, unpublished). The results presented in this paper on immunoglobulin concentrations in the uterine mucosa leave it open, however, whether or not a local synthesizing or a storage system, or both, are involved in the immune defense system of the uterus.

The concentrations of immunoglobulin G in the uterine epithelium are approximately 5 to 8 times in excess of the IgA. It must be considered, however, that the IgA values were determined by using a serum standard containing 7 S IgA as reference. IgA may therefore be underestimated in concentrations if secretory (11S) IgA is predominant as it has been described for other secretions (Greenberg et al., 1978). The presence of relatively high amounts of immunoglobulins in the endometrium may also be a major factor in immunological sterility in the female.

Proteinase Inhibitors

Similar to the immunoglobulins, the concentrations of diffusible proteinase inhibitors in the uterine mucosa are also hormone dependent. Exogenous application of certain oral contraceptives increase these concentrations in the case of α_1-antitrypsin (Schumacher, 1971). Whether or not high α_1-antitrypsin levels in the endometrium can interfere with proteolytic processes associated with implantation (Denker, 1976) is not yet known. It is, however, conceivable that these inhibitors do interact with a number of physiological and/or pathophysiological events which occur in the uterine cavity and known to be proteolytic in nature, e.g. menstruation, uterine woundhealing post partum, inflammation and microbial invasion.

The regulating influence of an "antitryptic activity" during the process of menstruation has been assumed already by Huggins et al. (1943), although by that time α_1-antitrypsin had not been discovered as yet. The hormone dependent increase of inhibitors could also explain biochemically why women under oral contraceptive medication do usually bleed with lower intensity and duration. The presence of high concentrations of α_1-antitrypsin in post partum fluid (Tauber, 1979) is particularly interesting since this inhibitor inhibits the activation of utcrine collagenase, an enzyme shown to be involved in uterine involution post partum in the human (Woessner, 1975). Proteinase inhibitors protect epithelial surfaces against proteolytic influences during inflammatory processes which are usually associated with the migration of large numbers of white blood cells. Elastase from neutrophil granulocytes is strongly inhibited by α_1-antitrypsin (Ohlsson et al., 1976). Heavy inflammatory reactions lead to a complete or partial consumption of locally available inhibitors, as in the case of cervicitis (Wallner and Fritz, 1974) or in IUD-wearing women with heavy menstrual periods (Tauber et al., 1977). The latter observation, in combination with an increase in local fibrinolysis (Larsson et al., 1974), has led to the therapeutic concept of local treatment with suitable proteinase inhibitors in IUD-wearers with increased uterine bleeding (Tauber and Wolf, 1975; Tauber et al., 1977).

Complement Components and Total Complement Activity

The fact that total complement, i.e. hemolytic activity, has been found in traces only in some hysterectomy specimens, sheds an interesting light on the concept of immunological sterility associated with the presence of circulating spermatozoa immobilizing antibodies. The immobilizing activity of such antibodies are strictly dependent on the presence of an intact complement system (Menge et al., 1977). From our preliminary results and from observations of others (see Schumacher et al., p. 115 this volume, Schumacher et al., 1977) it might be concluded that an intact hemolytic complement system is virtually absent in the uterine secretion. This applies also to uterine fluid post partum and from IUD-wearing women (Tauber, 1979). However, one has to consider that under certain pathophysiological circumstances activation of the complement system could occur through the alternate pathway, i.e. through the presence of proteolytic enzymes such as plasmin, trypsin, or elastase and collagenase from lysosomes (Johnson et al., 1976) and other components (complexes). Further investigations into the presence or absence of complement components other than C3 or C4 or C1q/C1r in uterine mucosal tissues and secretions are therefore needed in order to define the biological role of this important system in the female genital tract.

Lysozyme

The results in this paper confirm the previous observations by Schumacher and Pearl (1969) and Schumacher (1974) concerning the cyclic and topographic variations of this enzyme in the uterine mucosa. The bacteriolytic action of lysozyme has been known for a long time (Fleming, 1922). From this and later observations (Adinolfi et al., 1966; Nakazawa et al., 1966; Grossgebauer and Langmaack, 1968) it appears that this enzyme which is ubiquitously distributed in the mammalian and other organisms (Jollès, 1969) plays a major role in humoral defense reactions against microbial invaders. The bacteriolytic effect of lysozyme has also been demonstrated in human cervical tissues (Schumacher, 1974) which indicates that this enzyme participates in the non-specific humoral defense system of the uterus to protect the upper female genital tract.

High lysozyme concentrations are also found in uterine fluid specimens from women shortly after insertion of an intrauterine device (Tauber, 1979). Approximately 6 months postinsertion, the values return to normal. This suggests that the short time increase of the enzyme is mainly due to the large number of white blood cells, particularly neutrophils, in the uterine environment as a response to the foreign body. (Moyer et al., 1978) Neutrophil granulocytes contain large amounts of lysozyme (Baggiolini et al., 1970). It has also been suggested from animal experiments that lysozyme may exert lytic effects towards blastocysts (Parr et al., 1967). Whether this holds true for the human, remains to be established.

Plasminogen Activator

The presence of plasminogen activator in the endometrium is particularly important because of its biochemical association with the process of menstruation. The intensity of the menstrual blood flow appears to be dependent on the amount of plasminogen activator in the endometrial layer (Rybo, 1966; Nilsson, 1975). Plasminogen activator activity was demonstrated in high quantities in cervical mucus (Beller and Weiss, 1966; Weiss and Beller, 1969) but it appears to be absent in endometrial secretions (Schumacher this volume; see Chapter 8). The distribution pattern in the uterine secretions is reversed to the one found in tissue specimens of the uterine epithelia where highest concentrations were demonstrated in the fundus of the uterus and lowest in the cervix. It appears obvious therefore that the plasminogen activator in the uterine mucosa is bound to the tissues as it also was shown earlier by others (Schmidt-Matthiessen, 1967). From our results it can also be concluded that the plasminogen activator concentrations in the uterine mucosa vary with the different stages of the cycle. Highest concentrations were found during the periovulatory phase which is different from the observations by Rybo (1966) who found a maximum 1 to 2 days before the onset of menstruation, and by Schmidt-Matthiessen (1967) who demonstrated the highest values in midsecretory phase, i.e. around day 20 of the cycle. An explanation for this discrepancy is possibly the small number of uteri investigated in our studies where no specimen from the immediate premenstrual phase was available and also through the pooling of data for the three major phases of the cycle. The localization of plasminogen activator in the uterine epithelium may also be of biological significance for various pathophysiological processes in the uterus. The high concentrations in the fundus could be related to the onset of menstruation as it was reported as early as in 1929 by von Mikulicz-Radecki and later by Schroeder in 1934. This "mechanical" concept of menstruation as it can be developed from hysteroscopic techniques has again recently been reported by Lindemann (see page 225), but has been doubted by others (Ludwig and Metzger, 1976; Wagner see page 187) from morphological and ultramorphological observations of the inner surface of the uterus during menstruation. Intensive uterine bleeding from IUD-wearing women might also be related to this plasminogen-activator distribution in the endometrium particularly when the IUD has transversal arms covering the fundal mucosa which contains highest plasminogen-activator concentrations. It is however possible that heavy uterine bleeding in IUD-wearers is also initiated by other proteolytic enzymes provoked by the IUD-induced inflammatory reaction occurring in the endometrium. Plasminogen-activator concentrations in the uterine fluid from IUD-wearing women do at least not exhibit significantly increased values (Tauber 1979).

ACKNOWLEDGEMENTS
Thanks are due to Ms. Bettina Winkemann for excellent technical assistance and to Mr. Franz Warnking for preparation of the graphs. Part of this research presented here was supported by a grant from the Department of Science and Research, The State of North-Rhine Westfalia, West Germany.

REFERENCES

Adinolfi, M., Glynn, A.A., Lindsay, M., Milne, C.M.: Serological properties of γ-A antibodies to Escherichia coli present in human colostrum. Immunology 10: 517–526, 1966.
Baggiolini, M., De Duve, C., Masson, L., Heremans, J.F.: Association of lactoferrin with specific granules in rabbit heterophil leukocytes. J. Exp. Med. 131: 559–570, 1970.
Beller, F.K., Weiss, G.: The fibrinolytic enzyme system in cervical mucus. Fertil. Steril. 17: 654–662, 1966.

Chipperfield, E.J., Evans, B.A.: The influence of local infection on immunoglobulin formation in the human endocervix. Clin. Exp. Immunol. 11: 219–223, 1972.

Denker, H.-W.: Interaction of Proteinase Inhibitors with Blastocyst Proteinases involved in Implantation. In: Protides of the Biological Fluids, Vol. XXIII. H. Peeters (ed.) Pergamon Press, Oxford-New York, 1976, pp. 63–67.

Fleming, A.: On an remarkable bacteriolytic element found in tissues and secretions. Proc. Roy, Soc. London 93: 306–317, 1922.

Greenberg, St.B., Rossen, R.D., Six, H.R., Baxter, B.D., Couch, R.B.: Determination of Immunoglobulin A concentrations in nasal secretions with a serum immunoglobulin A standard. J. Clin. Microbiol. 8: 465–467, 1978.

Grossgebauer, K., Langmaack, H.: Lysozyme, Ergebnisse und Probleme. Klin. W.schr. 46: 1121–1127, 1968.

Haspels, A.A.: The "morning-after pill"—a preliminary report. I.P.P.F. Med. Bull. 3: 6, 1969.

Hirsch, P.J., Fergusson, I.L.C., King, R.J.B.: Protein composition of human endometrium and its secretions at different stages of the menstrual cycle. Ann. N.Y. Acad. Sci. 233–245, 1976.

Huggins, C., Vail, C.V., Davis, E.M.: Fluidity of menstrual blood: proteolytic effect. Am. J. Obstet. Gynecol. 46: 78–84, 1943.

Hurlimann, J., Dayal, R., Gloor, E.: Immunoglobulins and secretory component in endometrium and cervix: influence of inflammation and carcinoma. Virchows Arch. A. Path. Anat. Histol. 377: 211–223, 1978.

Johnson, U., Ohlsson, K., Olsson, I.: Effects of granulocyte neutral protease on complement components. Scand. J. Immunol. 5: 421–426, 1976.

Jollès, P.: Lysozymes: A chapter of molecular biology. Angew. Chem. Int. Ed. Engl. 8: 227–239, 1969.

Kelly, J.K., Fox, H.: The local immunological defense system of the human endometrium. J. Reprod. Immunol. 1: 39–45, 1979.

Larsson, B., Liedholm, P., Sjöberg, N.O., Astedt, B.: Increased fibrinolytic activity in the endometrium of patients using copper-IUD. Contraception 9: 531–537, 1974.

Lindemann, H.J.: Hysteroscopic data during menstruation. In: The Biology of the Fluids of the Female Genital Tract. Beller, F.K. and Schumacher, G.F.B. (eds) Elsevier North Holland, Inc., New York, 1979, pp. 225.

Lippes, J., Ogra, S.S., Tomasi, T.B. Jr., Tourville, D.R.: Immunohistological localization of γG, γA, γM, secretory piece and lactoferrin in the human genital tract. Contraception 1: 163–168, 1970.

Ludwig, H., Metzger, H.: The Human Female Reproductive Tract. A Scanning Electron Microscopic Atlas. Springer Verlag, Berlin-Heidelberg-New York, 1976.

Menge, A.C., Schwanz, M.L., Riolo, R.L., Greenberg, V.N., Neda, T.: The role of the cervix and cervical secretions in immunologic infertility. In: The Uterine Cervix in Reproduction. Insler, V., Bettendorf, G. (eds.) Georg Thieme Publishers, Stuttgart, 1977, pp. 221–230.

Mikulicz-Radecki, F. von: Weitere Erfahrungen mit der Hysteroskopie insbesondere beim Studium des Endometriums. Zbl. Gynäkol. 53: 258–269, 1929.

Moyer, D.L., Shaw, S.T., Fu, J., Hohmann, R., Thompson, R.S.: Preclinical Intrauterine Contraception. In: Human Fertilization. Ludwig, H., Tauber, P.F. (eds.) Georg Thieme Publishers, Stuttgart, 1978, pp. 226–236.

Nakazawa, S., Itagaki, M., Yokota, T., Otani, Y., Miwa, M., Onitake, J., Nakayama, T., Fusaoka, N.: Fundamental studies on the antibiotic action of lysozyme. Jap. J. Antibiot. Ser. B. 19: 34–47, 1966.

Nilsson, I.M.: Local Fibrinolysis as a Mechanism for Haemorrhage. Thrombos. Diathes. haemorrh. (Stuttgart) 34: 623–631, 1975.

Ogra, P.L., Ogra, S.S.: Local antibody response to poliovaccine in the human female genital tract. J. Immunol. 110: 1307–1311, 1973.

Ohlsson, K., Olsson, I., Delshammar, M., Schiessler, H.: Elastases from Human and Canine granulocytes. I. Some proteolytic and esterolytic properties. Hoppe-Seyler's Z. Physiol. Chem. 357:

1245–1250, 1976.

Parr, E.L., Schaedler, R.W., Hirsch, J.G.: A possible role for granulocytes in the action of intrauterine contraceptive devices. Trans. Assoc. Am. Phys. 80: 123–132, 1967.

Prill, H.J.: Durchblutung. In: Das normale menschliche Endometrium. Schmidt-Matthiesen, H. (Hrsg.) Thieme Verlag, Stuttgart, 1963, pp. 245–267.

Rebello, R., Green, F.H.Y., Fox, H.: A study of the secretory immune system of the female genital tract. Brit. J. Obstet. Gynecol. 82: 812–816, 1975.

Rybo, G.: Plasminogen activators in the endometrium. II. Clinical Aspects. Acta Obstet. Gynaecol. Scand. 45: 429–450, 1966.

Schiller, S., Donat, H.: Immunglobulinkonzentrationen der Zervixschleimhaut. Zbl. Gynäkol. 97: 1502–1506, 1975.

Schmidt-Matthiesen, H.: Die fibrinolytische Aktivität von Endometrium und Myometrium, Dezidua und Plazenta, Kollum- und Korpus-karzinomen. Physiologie, Pathophysiologie und klinisch-therapeutische Konsequenzen. Fortschr. Geburtseh. Gynäkol. 31: 1–117, 1967.

Schroeder, C.: Über den Ausbau und die Leistungen der Hysteroskopie. Arch. Gynäkol. 156: 407–449, 1934.

Schumacher, G.F.B., Pearl, M.J.: Cyclic changes of muramidase (lysozyme) in cervical mucus. J. Reprod. Med. 3: 171–178, 1969.

Schumacher, G.F.B.: Alpha$_1$antitrypsin in Uterine secretions. In: Proceedings of the International Research Conference on Proteinase Inhibitors. Munich, 1970. H. Fritz, H. Tschesche (eds.) De Gruyter, Berlin, 1971, pp. 253–256.

Schumacher, G.F.B.: Lysozyme in human genital secretions. In: Lysozyme. Osserman, E.F., Canfield, R.E., Beychock, Sh. (eds.) Academic Press Inc. New York-London, 1974, pp. 427–447.

Schumacher, G.F.B., Kim, M.H., Hosseinian, A.H., DuPont, C.: Immunoglobulins, proteinase inhibitors, albumin, and lysozyme in hyman cervical mucus. I. Hormone profiles and cervical mucus changes during presumably ovulatory cycles—methods and results. Amer. J. Obstet. Gynecol. 129: 629–636, 1977.

Schumacher, G.F.B., Holt, J.A., Reale, F.: Approaches to the analysis of human endometrial secretions. This volume. pp. 000–000.

Segal, Sh.J., Scher, W., Koide, S.S.: Estrogens, Nucleic Acids, and Protein Synthesis in Uterine Metalbolism. In: The Biology of the Uterus. Wynn, R.M. (ed.) Plenum Press, New York-London, 1977, pp. 139–201.

Sen, D.K., Fox, H.: The lymphoid tissue of the endometrium. Gynaecologia 163: 371–378, 1967.

Tauber, P.F.: Biochemische und immunologische Untersuchungen über Proteine im menschlichen Endometrium und in uterinen Sekreten unter verschiednen klinischen Bedingungen. Habilitationsschrift an der Med. Fakultät der Universität Essen, West Germany 1979.

Tauber, P.F., Wolf, A.S.: Beeinflussung unerwünschter IUD-Neben-wirkungen durch lokale Antifibrinolyse. Oberrh. Ges. Gebh. Gynäkol., Ulm, 2.–3.5. 1975.

Tauber, P.F., Wolf, A.S., Herting, W., Zaneveld, L.J.D.: Hemorrhage induced by intrauterine devices: control by local proteinase inhibition. Fertil. Steril. 28: 1375–1377, 1977c.

Tourville, D.R., Ogra, S.S., Lippes, J., Tomasi, T.B.: The human female reproductive tract: Immunhistological localization of γA, γM secretory piece and lactoferrin. Am. J. Obstet. Gynceol. 108: 1102–1108, 1970.

Vaerman, J.P., Ferin, J.: Local immunological response in the vagina, cervix and endometrium. Acta endocrin. (Kbh.) 78: Sppl. 194, 281–305, 1975.

Wagner, H.: Vaginal transudation. In: The Biology of the Fluids of the Female Genital Tract. Beller, F.K. and Schumacher, G.F.B. (eds.) Elsevier North Holland, Inc., New York, 1979, pp. 187.

Wallner, O., Fritz, H.: Characterization of an acid-stable proteinase inhibitor in human cervical mucus. Hoppe-Seyler's Z. physiol. Chem. 355: 705–715, 1974.

Weiss, G., Beller, F.K.: Tissue activator of the fibrinolytic enzyme in the female reproductive system. Obstet. Gynecol. 34: 809–819, 1969.

Woessner, J.F.jr.: Regulation of collagenase activity. Scand. J. Rheum. 4 (Suppl. 8), 15–30, 1975.

Copyright 1979 by Elsevier North Holland, Inc.
F.K. Beller and G.F.B. Schumacher, eds.
The Biology of the Fluids of the Female Genital Tract

INHIBITORS OF TROPHOBLAST PROTEINASES

H.-W. Denker

Why with the time do I not glance aside
To new-found methods, and to compounds strange?
(Shakespeare, Sonnet 76)

SUMMARY

Certain proteinases of the trophoblast and of uterine secretions play an important role in the initiation of embryo implantation as suggested by investigations done in the rabbit and mouse. Blastolemmase, a trophoblast-dependent endopeptidase studied in detail in the rabbit, appears to be a major factor in the disintegration of the blastocyst coverings during the initiation phase of implantation. Regulation of this proteinase activity may involve the action of proteinase inhibitors present in the endometrium and the uterine secretion, of the human as well as in some animal models although nothing is known about proteinases of early implantation stage human trophoblast. A first attempt at studying a model system was made by investigating the interaction between rabbit blastocyst proteinase (blastolemmase) and plasma inhibitors present in human endometrium and uterine secretion. Examples of other proteinase inhibitors from animal tissues were also included for comparison. Recently developed biochemical tests based on the hydrolysis of synthetic tripeptide p-nitroanilide substrates were used in order to obtain quantitative data on enzyme-inhibitor interactions, and the results were com-

Abteilung Anatomie, Rheinisch-Wesfaelische Technische Hochschule, Aachen, FRG

pared with those obtained with gelatin substrate film tests. Biochemical and physiological aspects of the relationship between blastolemmase and other proteinases of the trypsin family present in implantation stage trophoblast are discussed.

INTRODUCTION

Proteinase activity associated with implantation, in particular with its first phase, i.e. attachment of the trophoblast to the uterine epithelium, has recently received increased interest (for review see Denker 1977, 1978). There is good evidence that certain enzymes of the trypsin family, which are found in the trophoblast and the uterine secretion and which have been studied in detail in the rabbit, play a significant role in initiation of implantation since it was shown that inhibition of these enzymes by administration of specific proteinase inhibitors *in vivo* results in blockage of implantation (Denker 1977, 1978).

As far as other species are concerned, only few data on implantation associated proteinases are available, most of them for the mouse. A specific role in dissolution of the zona pellucida and in implantation initiation has been suggested for a uterine secretion proteinase in this species ("implantation initiating factor", Mintz 1971, Pinsker et al., 1974). On the other hand, trypsin-like and chymotrypsin-like enzymes were shown to be present in late preimplantation stage mouse blastocysts (Dabich and Andary, 1976). Intrauterine administration of proteinase inhibitors caused embryonic loss also in this species (Dabich and Andary, 1974), although it has not been shown that this treatment interferes in fact with the process of implantation as in the rabbit. Cathepsin-like enzymes as demonstrated in the guinea pig (Owers and Blandau, 1971) and the cat (Denker et al., 1978) can be assumed primarily to play a role in intracellular protein degradation rather than in implantation initiation. Little is known about trypsin-like enzymes which may also be present in these species.

PROTEINASES

The most detailed data available so far have been presented for *blastolemmase*, a trophoblast-dependent enzyme which seems to play an important role in the process of dissolution of the extracellular blastocyst coverings (which is the prerequisite for attachment of the trophoblast to the uterine epithelium) in the rabbit. Blastolemmase shows enzymatic properties which are in many respects closely related to those of trypsin. However, it shows different electrophoretic mobility (Denker 1977, Denker and Petzoldt, 1977) and has more restricted substrate specificity: while there is a general specificity for arginyl bonds as in the case of trypsin, blastolemmase seems to be more selective with respect to the conformation and nature of the protein/peptide to be split: hydrolysis rates as measured in rabbit blastocyst extracts are strongly influenced by the type of amino acid present in subsite position P_2 and P_3 preceding the residue (P_1) which fits to the specificity pocket of the enzyme (Denker and Fritz 1979). Only little general proteolytic activity can be measured with conventional protein substrates like casein. It has been suggested, therefore, that the physiological function of this enzyme does not involve complete digestion of the blastocyst coverings but may lie more in hydrolyzing a limited number of peptide bonds. This may result in a change of the physicochemical properties of the blastocyst coverings at the abembryonic pole of the blastocyst, i.e. the region of maximal blastolemmase activity. These changes may have physiological significance in the following processes: 1. Increased stickiness of the blastocyst coverings at the abembryonic pole has been suggested to provide the mechanism for ensuring the correct orientation of the blastocyst with its abembryonic pole facing the antimesometrial endometrium (Böving, 1963) (for a hypothesis concerning the possible mechanism, taking into account the alkaline pH optimum of blastolemmase and higher alkalinity of the antimesometrial as compared to the mesometrial endometrial surface, see Denker 1978). 2. Softening of the blastocyst coverings, resulting from limited hydrolysis of certain peptide bonds by blastolemmase, may be sufficient to allow the trophoblastic knobs to penetrate them, with the vis a tergo provided by the continuing expansion of the blastocyst. 3. The so altered glycoproteins of the coverings may become more susceptible to the action of other enzymes present (like glycosidases, see Denker, 1970b, 1971a, 1977). 4. Limited proteolysis might also change properties of cell surface-bound receptors possibly involved in the attachment of the trophoblast to the uterine epithelium, although experimental support for this hypothesis is lacking so far.

The presence, in the implanting trophoblast of the rabbit, of additional proteinases has been deduced from experiments with various substrates and inhibitors (Denker and Fritz, 1979) and has been shown electrophoretically (Denker and Petzoldt, in preparation). In particular, a possibly kallikrein-like enzyme and a plasminogen activator have been demonstrated in the non-gelatinolytical fractions. More detailed studies of these enzymes are in progress.

Proteinase Inhibitors

The presence of various *proteinase inhibitors in the endometrium and in the uterine secretion* is well known. It seems reasonable to assume that such inhibitors act as physiological regulators of the described proteinase activities. In fact, this concept had already been developed around the turn of the century when it was found that human decidua had antitryptic activity able to counteract the proteolytic activity of the trophoblast (Gräfenberg, 1909, 1910; Halban and Frankl, 1910) This was confirmed and extended by Schmidt-Matthiesen (1967). More recently, numerous investigations have identified various proteinase inhibitors in the endometrium and the uterine secretion in the human as well as in laboratory animals (Schumacher, 1970, Beier, 1970, Somerville and Dabich, 1974). Two fractions have been demonstrated by agar gel and starch gel electrophoresis, in rabbit uterine fluid, particularly after treatment of the animals with large doses of estradiol-17β and/or with progesterone (Beier 1970). Purified preparations of uteroglobin, the predominant protein in rabbit uterine secretion in the preimplantation phase, were recently shown to possess trypsin-inhibiting activity (Beier 1977). It is still not completely sure, however, whether uteroglobin can be identified on this basis as a proteinase inhibitor, and further investigations are certainly needed in order to clarify this. Interestingly, the uteroglobin-like protein from lung tissue does not show trypsin inhibition in the same assay (fibrin agar gel electrophoresis). Uteroglobin binds more or less strongly a number of different compounds like progesterone (Beato 1977) so that it is not completely excluded so far that it may perhaps also carry a low molecular weight proteinase inhibitor. Since the quantities of uteroglobin applied in published trypsin inhibition tests (using the fibrin agar gel electrophoresis technique) appear relatively high, it remains to be determined whether the kinetic constants for trypsin binding by this protein are in the range typical for true proteinase inhibitors.

As far as the *human* endometrium and uterine fluid are concerned, the presence of various plasma proteinase inhibitors (α_1-antitrypsin, α_1-antichymotrypsin, α_2-macroglobulin) has been described by several authors using semiquantitative radial diffusion tests (Schumacher, 1970, Tauber, 1979 and this volume) and qualitative immunological tests (Beier and Beier-Hellwig, 1973). The concentration of α_1-antitrypsin found in the uterine mucosa from the corpus was, however, much lower than in the cervix, and only minor cyclical variations have been shown in the corpus (Schumacher, 1970, Tauber 1979 and this volume).

Unfortunately, detailed biochemical data on the counterpart, i.e. on individual proteinases of the trophoblast and of the uterine secretion which might play a role in initiation of implantation are totally missing for the *human*. Recently, biochemical investigations of various proteinases found in mature human placentae have been performed (Unger and Struck, 1977, 1978); however, it is questionable whether they are at all related to those postulated enzymes which might have a physiological function in the phase of implantation initiation.

In this situation, it may appear justified to take a somewhat speculative look at the problem, discussing the interaction of: 1. Trophoblast-dependent proteinase (blastolemmase) available so far only from the rabbit, and 2. inhibitors known to be present in the endometrium and uterine secretion in the human as discussed above.

RESULTS AND DISCUSSION

Experiments of this type will be described below. Naturally, they cannot give any information on the proteinase: proteinase inhibitor system present *in vivo* in the two species, but they may help to develop some ideas and concepts useful for further investigations. These experiments are based primarily on quantitative photometric assays developed since synthetic chromogenic tripeptide p-nitroanilide substrates became available (Denker and Fritz, 1979). This technology will improve the investigation of blastocyst proteinases (previously based primarily on qualitative (or, at the best, semi-quantitative) gelatin substrate film tests (Denker, 1971, 1972, 1974, 1976). As long as purification of trophoblast proteinase(s) has not been achieved, non-purified extracts of late preimplantation rabbit blastocysts are used (for the methodological details, see Denker and Fritz, 1979). This material contains, in addition to blastolemmase, two other enzymes electrophoretically distinguishable enzymes (see above) which are able to split arginyl and lysyl bonds and which can, therefore, contribute to the photometer readings obtained with the tripeptide p-nitroanilide substrates used. Therefore, interpretation of the photometric tests has to be done cautiously if interest is focused on blastolemmase alone. On the other hand, the relative homogeneity of results of kinetic investigations (Denker and Fritz, 1979) and experiments with highly specific inhibitors (like BSTI-II, see below) suggest that one enzyme seems to dominate in the hydrolysis rate, if the substrate N-tosyl-glycyl-L-prolyl-L-arginine-p-nitroanilide *(TosGlyProArgPNA)* is used. Since the accompanying proteases can be easily distinguished from blastolemmase due to the fact that they do not digest gelatin membranes (Denker and Petzoldt, in preparation) we are not basing our investigations only on tests with the synthetic substrates but are also including qualitative tests with the gelatin substrate film method.

The results obtained with various proteinase inhibitors from human plasma are summarized in Table I. Notice that the inhibitor concentrations indicated can

TABLE I. Inhibitors of Rabbit Blastocyst Proteinase

	Lowest effective concentration[1]	
	Biochemical test system[2] (substrate: TosGlyProArgPNA)	Histochemical test system[3] (substrate: gelatin)
Inhibitor		
Human plasma inhibitors:		
α_1-antitrypsin	$3 \cdot 10^{-6}$ M[4]	$1 \cdot 10^{-5}$ M
α_1-antichymotrypsin [5]	$3 \cdot 10^{-5}$ M	$1 \cdot 10^{-4}$ M
inter-α-trypsin inhibitor	($>1 \cdot 10^{-7}$ M) [6]	$1 \cdot 10^{-6}$ M
α_2-macroglobulin	($>1 \cdot 10^{-7}$ M) [6]	($>1 \cdot 10^{-5}$ M)
Other inhibitors: (selected examples)		
boar seminal plasma trypsin-acrosin inhibitor (BSTI-II)	$7 \cdot 10^{-8}$ M	$5 \cdot 10^{-6}$ M
aprotinin (basic trypsin-kallikrein inhibitor from bovine organs, Trasylol)	$1 \cdot 10^{-10}$ M	$1 \cdot 10^{-6}$ M

1) In the range of ~50% inhibition
2) Test performed as described by Denker and Fritz (1979). Preincubation of enzyme with inhibitor: 5 min. at 37° C if not indicated otherwise.
3) For details of the test see Denker (1974,1976). This basically qualitative test gives no information on kinetic constants. Inhibitor concentrations indicated are as present in the solution used for soaking the gelatin, not identical with actual concentration during the test.
4) Progressive inhibition; preincubation 2 hours.
5) Contains 1-2% α_1-antitrypsin.
6) At higher concentrations, TosGlyProArgPNA-splitting activity present as an impurity in the inhibitor preparation influenced photometer readings.

    Human plasma inhibitors were obtained from Behringwerke Marburg; purity given as determined by immunological test; α_1-antitrypsin: ca. 98% pure; no contamination by other proteinase inhibitors; α_1-antichymotrypsin: ca. 98% pure, contains 1-2% α_1-antitrypsin; inter-α-trypsin inhibitor: ca. 98% pure, no contamination by other proteinase inhibitors; α_2-macroglobulin: purity ca. 90% (values corrected accordingly), main contaminant IgA but no other proteinase inhibitors, 1/3 of dry matter glycin added. Other chemicals used were as indicated by Denker and Fritz (1979).

allow to draw conclusions on the kinetics of the interaction only in the case of the biochemical test system (substrate: TosGlyProArgPNA) and not in the case of the histochemical gelatin film test. The latter shows clearly that blastolemmase is inhibited by the inhibitors of trypsin-like enzymes, *inter-α-trypsin inhibitor*, *α_1-antitrypsin*, and, from the group of other inhibitors from animal tissues included for comparison, by *boar seminal plasma trypsin-acrosin inhibitor (BSTI-II)* and by *aprotinin* (basic trypsin-kallikrein inhibitor from bovine organs, Trasylol[R]). No inhibition was obtained, in the range tested, with α_2-macroglobulin (concerning the specificity of the plasma inhibitors, see Heimburger, 1975; for BSTI see Fritz et al., 1975, 1976; for further references see Denker, 1976, 1977).

The results obtained in the biochemical test system show that the plasma inhibitors are less effective than the inhibitors from animal sources. This is particularly obvious when they are compared to aprotinin, the most effective inhibitor of blastolemmase known so far (K_i estimated below 10 pM, Denker and Fritz, 1979). The interaction with inter-α-trypsin inhibitor and α_2-macroglobulin could not be studied in the biochemical test system because the sensitivity of this system is so high that traces of proteinases present in the inhibitor preparations influenced the photometer readings at concentrations higher than $1 \cdot 10^{-7}$ M. The histochemical gelatin substrate film test, however, shows that the inter-α-trypsin inhibitor does inhibit blastolemmase efficiently.

The inhibitory effect seen with α_1-*antichymotrypsin* is somewhat surprising because this inhibitor is rather specific for chymotrypsin (Heimburger, 1975) while the blastocyst proteinases discussed here are trypsin-like enzymes. This phenomenon had already been observed (Denker, 1976) at a time when only the gelatin substrate film test was available. At that time it appeared possible that a chymotrypsin-like enzyme, perhaps present at the same sites as blastolemmase, would contribute to the results of the test and its inhibition could account for the effect seen with α_1-antichymotrypsin. It seems interesting, therefore, that inhibition is now also seen in the biochemical test system using TosGlyProArgPNA, a substrate which is being hydrolyzed quite specifically by trypsin-like enzymes. The preparation of α_1-antichymotrypsin used contains 1–2% α_1-antitrypsin. However, according to the inhibitor concentrations found effective (see Table), the presence of these impurities does not explain the observed effect satisfactorily. Further investigations are needed in order to prove whether α_1-antichymotrypsin is in fact able to interact with blastolemmase.

α_1-*antitrypsin* was found to inhibit rabbit blastocyst proteinase activity in a progressive manner (Figure 1). This has been shown likewise for the interaction of this inhibitor with acrosin (Fritz et al., 1972), kallikrein and plasmin.

Boar seminal plasma trypsin-acrosin inhibitor (BSTI-II) has been included in the study for comparison (Table, Figure 2) although this inhibitor is not a constituent of the implantation phase uterine milieu. As the biochemical test shows, a relatively strong inhibition is obtained with this compound. BSTI is known to inhibit trypsin and acrosin but not the related enzymes with very restricted substrate specificity, i.e. plasminogen activator and kallikreins. It inhibits blastolemmase strongly as seen in the gelatin substrate film test. Incomplete inhibition is seen, on the other hand, in the biochemical test system using TosGlyProArgPNA as a substrate, in the indicated range of inhibitor concentrations (Figure 2). The residual activity is, however, only low. This indicates that blastolemmase probably accounts for most of the activity measured with this substrate, and the other proteinases present in this material and mentioned above seem to influence the test only to a minor degree.

The described investigations show that proteinase inhibitors, known to be present in the plasma and in the endometrium and uterine lumen in the human, modulate trophoblast proteinase activity, as demonstrated using the rabbit as a model, *in vitro*. Since blastolemmase has previously been shown to play a major role in implantation initiation in the rabbit, we may hypothesize that uterine pro-

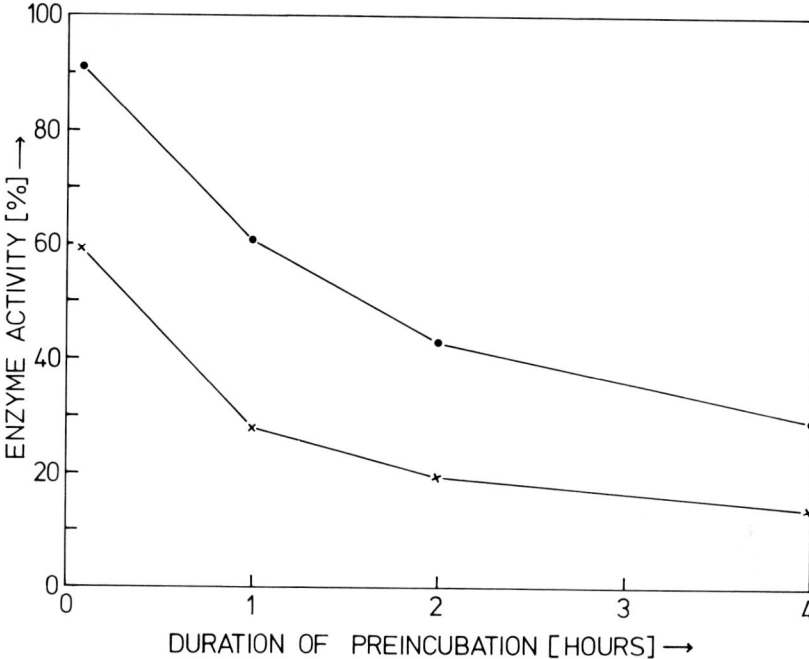

FIGURE 1. Progressive inhibition of rabbit blastocyst proteinase by α_1-antitrypsin. Biochemical test system as indicated in the Table. The inhibition concentration was maintained during preincubation as well as during the test: ● ——— ● $3.3 \cdot 10^{-6}$ M; x ——— x $1 \cdot 10^{-5}$ M.

teinase inhibitors are one of the factors which *regulate implantation events from the maternal side in vivo*. Regulation by proteinase inhibitors is well documented for other systems in which proteinases are being produced, activated, and play a biological role (like digestive enzymes in salivary glands and the intestinal tract, the blood clotting and fibrinolytic system, etc.). It can be regarded as a rule that, *in vivo*, proteinases are always controlled by a well-developed and often complicated system of activators and inhibitors.

Experimental evidence indicates that the uterine milieu is not particularly favorable for implantation but rather contains, at least in certain stages, implantation inhibiting factors (Weitlauf, 1978; Finn, 1974; McLaren, 1973; Psychoyos and Bitton-Casimiri, 1969). Implantation-like events, in particular invasive growth of the trophoblast, starts readily in ectopic sites, independent of the hormonal status of the host (Kirby, 1970). In rodents, the implantation-initiating effect of the estrogen surge is possibly based on depression of uterine inhibitor. After experimental delay of implantation, implantation can be induced by administration of actinomycin D, which is again thought to result from blockage of inhibitor synthesis (Finn, 1974). Although this view of the *uterus as an organ that regulates implantation* is not very new (for discussion and references see Denker, 1977), these recent experiments seem to accentuate this aspect. Identification of inhibitory factors of the uterus as proteinase inhibitors is speculative, at present. In a general sense, the following physiological functions of uterine proteinase inhibitors may

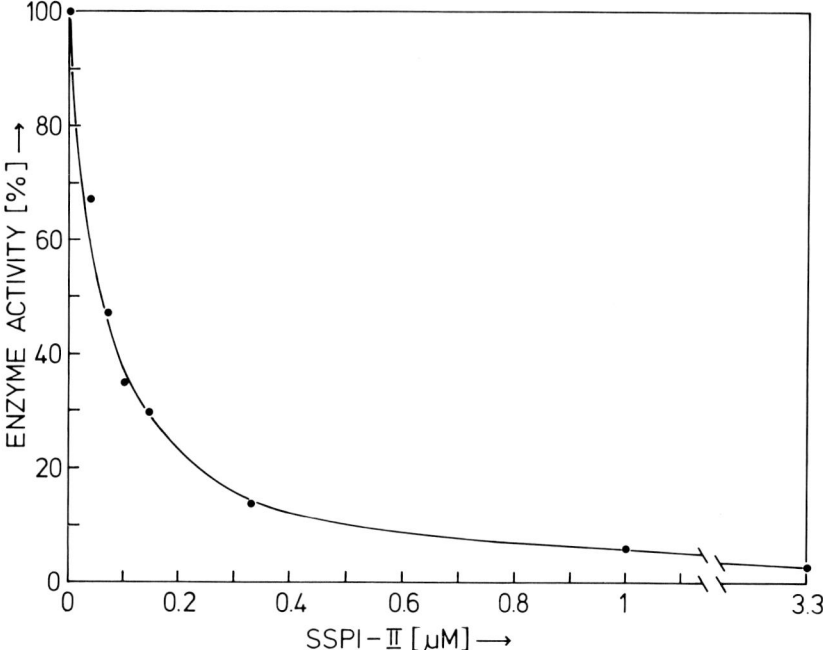

FIGURE 2. Titration of rabbit blastocyst proteinase with various concentrations of boar seminal plasma trypsin-acrosin inhibitor (BSTI-II). Biochemical Test system as indicated in the Table.

be envisaged: 1) a general protective role, i.e. prohibiting spreading of proteinase activity and localizing it in space and time where it is needed for implantation; 2) a more specific regulatory function in the initiation of implantation by influencing the equilibrium between trophoblastic (and uterine) protease on the one hand and uterine inhibitors on the other.

As mentioned above, in addition to blastolemmase, a number of different proteinases are present in the blastocyst and the uterine secretion—even the trypsin family is represented by a number of individual members for which different physiological functions must be envisaged. Such functions include partial dissolution of the blastocyst coverings (as an element of the implantation initiation process) by blastolemmase; digestion of remnants of the blastocyst coverings by trypsin-like (and a chymotrypsin-like ?) proteinase(s) of the uterine secretion; fibrinolysis (and promotion of invasion ?) by the plasminogen activator—plasmin system; liberation of biologically active peptides by kallikrein-like enzymes, etc. Far too little is known about the presumed differential effects of the present inhibitors on these different proteinases and proteinase systems, and we therefore feel that this field merits further investigations.

Finally, one aspect of practical relevance may be mentioned. At present, animal experiments as well as clinical trials with intrauterine administration of proteinase inhibitors into the uterine lumen are being performed in several institutions to prevent increased menstrual blood loss associated with IUD use (Tauber et al.,

1977, WHO 1978). In the light of the cited *in vivo* studies performed in the rabbit, it must be considered that one "side"-effect of such treatment is interaction with those proteinases (of the trophoblast and the uterine secretion) which are involved in implantation initiation. In fact, exactly those inhibitors used in the IUD studies, i.e. aprotinin (Trasylol ^{R}) (Tauber et al., 1977) and aromatic diamidines (WHO 1978) are effective in blocking the dissolution of the blastocyst coverings and implantation initiation in the rabbit experiments (Denker, 1977 and unpublished data). Therefore, more detailed investigation of proteinase systems involved in implantation and/or in various functions of the uterus seems desirable.

ACKNOWLEDGEMENTS
The author expresses his gratitude to Prof. Dr. H.G. Schwick and Dr. N. Heimburger, Behringwerke Marburg, for providing samples of α_1-antitrypsin, α_1-antichymotrypsin, inter- α -trypsin inhibitor and $\alpha_2$macroglobulin, to Prof. Dr. H. Fritz, München, for a sample of BSTI-II and for valuable discussions and suggestions, and to Dr. E. Truscheit, Bayer AG Wuppertal-Elberfeld, for gifts of Trasylol ^{R}. Sincere thanks are due to Mrs. Gerda Bohr and Edith Höricht for excellent technical assistance, to Mrs. Ursula Grässler for typing the manuscript, and to Mr. W. Graulich for drawing the diagrams. These investigations were supported by Deutsche Forschungsgemeinschaft grant De 181/8 (Schwerpunktprogramm "Biologie und Klinik der Reproduktion").

REFERENCES

Beato, M.: Physico-chemical characterization of uteroglobin and its interaction with progesterone. In: Development in Mammals. Vol. 2. Ed.: M.H. Johnson, North-Holland Publishing Comp., Amsterdam-New York-Oxford 1977, pp. 173–198.

Beier, H.M.: Hormonal stimulation of protease inhibitor activity in endometrial secretion during early pregnancy. Acta endocr. (Kbh.) 63: 141–149, 1970.

Beier, H.M.: Immunologische und biochemische Analysen am Uteroglobin und dem Uteroglobinähnlichen Antigen der Lunge. Med. Welt 28: 788–792, 1977.

Beier, H.M., Beier-Hellwig, K.: Specific secretory protein of the female genital tract. Acta endocr. (Kbh.) Suppl. 180: 404–425, 1973.

Böving, B.G.: Implantation mechanisms. In: Conference on Physiological Mechanisms Concerned with Conception. Ed.: C.G. Hartman, Pergamon Press, Oxford etc. 1963, pp. 321–396.

Dabich, D., Andary, T.J.: Prevention of blastocyst implantation in mice with proteinase inhibitors. Fertil. Steril. 25: 954–957, 1974.

Dabich, D., Andary, T.J.: Tryptic- and chymotryptic-like proteinases in early and late preimplantation mouse blastocysts. Biochim. Biophys. Acta 444: 147–153, 1976.

Denker, H.-W.: Topochemie hochmolekularer Kohlenhydratsubstanzen in Frühentwicklung und Implantation des Kaninchens. I. Allgemeine Lokalisierung und Charakterisierung hochmolekularer Kohlenhydratsubstanzen in frühen Embryonalstadien. Zool. Jahrb. Abt. Allgem. Zool. u. Physiol. 75: 141–245, 1970a.

Denker, H.-W.: Topochemie hochmolekularer Kohlenhydratsubstanzen in Frühentwicklung und Implantation des Kanichens. II. Beiträge zu entwicklungsphysiologischen Fragestellungen. Zool. Jahrb. Abt. Allg. Zool. u. Physiol. 75: 246–308, 1970b.

Denker, H.-W.: Enzym-Topochemie von Frühentwicklung und Implantation des Kaninchens. II. Glykosidasen. Histochemie 25: 268–285, 1971a.

Denker, H.-W.: Enzym-Topochemie von Frühentwicklung und Implantation des Kaninchens. III. Proteasen. Histochemie 25: 344–360, 1971b.

Denker, H.-W.: Blastocyst protease and implantation: effect of ovariecctomy and progesterone substitution in the rabbit. Acta endocr. (Kbh). 70: 591–602, 1972.

Denker, H.-W.: Protease substrate film test. Histochemistry 38: 331–338, 1974 and 39: 193, 1974.

Denker, H.-W.: Interaction of proteinase inhibitors with blastocyst proteinases involved in implantation. In: Protides of the Biological Fluids; Proceedings of the 23rd Colloquium. Ed.: H. Peeters, Pergamon Press, Oxford and New York 1976, pp. 63–68.

Denker, H.-W.: Implantation: The Role of Proteinases, and Blockage of Implantation by Proteinase Inhibitors. Springer-Verlag, Berlin-Heidelberg-New York 1977 (= Adv. Anat. Embryol. Cell Biol. Vol. 53 Fasc. 5).

Denker, H-W.: The role of trophoblastic factors in implantation. In: Novel Aspects of Reproductive Physiology. Eds.: Ch. H. Spilman and J.W. Wilks, Spectrum Publications, New York and London 1978, pp. 181–212.

Denker, H-W., L.A. Eng. C.E. Hamner: Studies on the early development and implantation in the cat. II. Implantation: proteinases. Anat. Embryol. 154: 39–54, 1978.

Denker, H-W., Fritz, H.: Enzymic characterization of rabbit blastocyst proteinase with synthetic substrates of trypsin-like enzymes. Hoppe-Seyler's Z. Physiol. Chem. 360: 107–113, 1979.

Denker, H-W., Petzoldt, U.: Proteinases involved in implantation initiation in the rabbit: microdisc electrophroetic studies. Cytobiologic (Europ. J. Cell Biol.) 15:363–371, 1977.

Denker, H-W., Petzoldt, U.: Microdisc electrophoretic separation of blastolemmase and other implantation-associated proteinases in the rabbit. (In preparation).

Finn, C.A.: The induction of implantation in mice by actinomycin D. J. Endocr. 60: 199–200, 1974.

Fritz, H., Heimburger, N., Meier, M., Arnhold, M., Zaneveld, L.J.D., Schumacher, G.F.B.: Humanakrosin: Zur Kinetik der Hemmung durch Human-Seruminhibitoren. Hoppe-Seyler's Z. Physiol. Chem. 353: 1953–1956, 1972.

Fritz, H., Schiessler, H., Schill, W.-B, Tschesche, H., Heimburger, H., Wallner, O.: Low molecular weight proteinase (acrosin) inhibitors from human and boar seminal plasma and spermatoza and human cervical mucus—Isolation, properties and biological aspects. In: Proteases and Biological Control. Eds.: E. Reich, D.B. Rifkin and E. Shaw (= Cold Spring Harbor Conferences on Cell Proliferation, Vol. 2) Cold Spring Harbor Laboratories, Cold Spring Harbor 1975, pp. 737–766.

Fritz, H., Tschesche, H., Fink, H.: Proteinase inhibitors from boar seminal plasma. In: Methods in Enzymology (Eds.: S.P. Colowick and N.O. Kaplan) Vol. XLV: Proteolytic Enzymes, Part B. Vol. Ed.: L. Lorand. Academic Press, New York, 1976, pp. 834–847.

Gräfenberg, E.: Der Antitrypsingehalt des mütterlichen Blutserums während der Schwangerschaft. Münch. med. Wschr. 56: 702–704, 1909.

Gräfenberg, E.: Beiträge zur Physiologie der Eieinbettung. Z. Geburtsh. Gyn. 65 1–35 1910.

Halban, J., Frankl, O.: Zur Biochemie der Uterusmukosa. Gynäk. Rundschau (Wien) 4: 471–484, 1910.

Heimburger, N.: Proteinase inhibitors of human plasma—Their properties and control functions. In: Proteases and Biological Control. Eds.: E. Reich, D.B. Rifkin and E. Shaw (Cold Spring Harbor Conferences on Cell Proliferation, Vol. 2) Cold Spring Harbor Laboratories, Cold Spring Harbor 1975, pp. 367–386.

Kirby, D.R.S.: The extra-uterine mouse egg as an experimental model. In: Schering Symposium on Mechanisms Involved in Conception (= Adv. Biosciences 4). Ed.: G. Raspé, Pergamon Press/Vieweg, Oxford, 1970, pp. 255–273.

McLaren, A.: Blastocyst activation. In: The Regulation of Mammalian Reproduction. Eds.: S.J. Segal, R. Crozier, P.A. Corfman and P.G. Condliffe, Charles C. Thomas, Springfield (Illinois) 1973, pp. 321–328.

Mintz, B.: Control of embryo implantation and survival. In: Schering Symposium on Intrinsic and Extrinsic Factors in Early Mammalian Development (= Adv. Biosciences 6). Ed.: G. Raspé, Pergamon Press/Vieweg, Oxford, Braunschweig 1971, pp. 317–342.

Owers, N.O., Blandau, R.J.: Proteolytic activity of the rat and guinea pig blastocyst *in vitro*. In: The Biology of the Blastocyst. Ed.: R.J. Blandau, The University of Chicago Press, Chicago and London 1971, pp. 207–223.

Pinsker, M.C., Sacco, A.G., Mintz, B.: Implantation-associated proteinase in mouse uterine fluid. Develop. Biol. 38: 285–290, 1974.

Psychoyos, A., Bitton-Casimiri, V.: Captation *in vitro* d'un précurseur d'acide ribonucléique

(ARN) (uridine-5-³H) par le blastocyste du rat: différences entre blastocystes normaux et blastocystes en diapause. C.R. hebd. Séances Acad. Sci. (Paris) 268: 188–190, 1968.

Schmidt-Matthiesen, H.: Die fibrinolytische Aktivität von Endometrium und Myometrium, Decidua und Plazenta, Kollum- und Korpuskarzinomen. Physiologie, Pathologie und klinischtherapeutische Konsequenzen. Fortschr. Geburtsh. Gyn. 31. S. Karger, Basel/New York 1967.

Schumacher, G.F.B.: Alpha$_1$-antitrypsin in uterine secretions. In: Inter. Res. Conf. on Proteinase Inhibitors, Munich 1970. Eds.: H. Fritz and H. Tschesche, Walter de Gruyter, Berlin/New York 1970, pp. 253–256.

Somerville M., Dabich, D.: Changes in trypsin-like inhibitors in mouse uteri during early gestation. Fed. Proc. 33: 282a, 1974.

Tauber, P.F.: Biochemische und immunologische Untersuchungen über Proteine im menschlichen Endometrium und in uterinen Sekreten unter verschiedenen klinischen Bedingungen. Habilitationsschrift, Essen 1979.

Tauber, P.F., Wolf, A.S., Herting, W., Zaneveld, L.J.D.: Hemorrhage induced by intrauterine devices: control by local proteinase inhibition. Fert. Steril. 28: 1375–1377, 1977.

Unger, Th., Struck, H.: Aminosäure-p-Nitroanilide spaltende Enzymakitivitoäten der reifen menschlichen Plazenta. I. Arch. Gynäk. 222: 311–318, 1977.

Weitlauf, H.M.: Factors in mouse uterine fluid that inhibit the incorporation of ³H uridine by blastocysts *in vitro*. J. Reprod. Fert. 52: 321–325, 1978.

WHO—Special Programme of Research, Development and Research Training in Human Reproduction. Seventh Annual Report, 1978.

MENSTRUATION: ENDOCRINE ASPECTS

H. D. Taubert and H. Kuhl

SUMMARY

Menstruation is the end point of regressive changes which are initiated in the endometrium of the human female and in certain non-human primates when fertilization fails to take place, and the production of progesterone in the corpus luteum declines.

The cyclic changes in the plasma level of estradiol and progesterone are reflected in similar changes in the endometrium. Both sex steroids are bound to the endometrial cell by specific cytosol receptor proteins. Estradiol induces the synthesis of its own receptor and that of the progesterone receptor. Progesterone has the opposite effect.

Although menstruation is caused by progesterone withdrawal, endometrial shedding of similar nature can also occur from a proliferative endometrium in cases of anovulation.

INTRODUCTION

Menstruation, defined as regularly occurring uterine bleeding due to endometrial desquamation, is causally an endocrinological phenomenon inasmuch as menstrual bleeding commences in normally cyclic women within a few days after

Abteilung für gynäkologische Endokrinologie, Zentrum der Frauenheilkunde und Geburtshilfe, Johann Wolfgang Goethe Universität, Frankfurt am Main / FRG

plasma progesterone falls to the low levels of the preovulatory phase. The temporal relationship between a decline in plasma progesterone and the onset of menstrual bleeding indicates that it is not caused by an abrupt breakdown of the endometrium with subsequent shedding, but should rather be considered as the final phase of a complex process of regression which is initiated at the moment conception failed, and the function of the corpus luteum was not maintained beyond its normal life span of approximately 12 days by the action of chorionic gonadotropin. As a regular, normal menstrual flow has been considered throughout the ages and in nearly any type of culture as a token of normal reproductive function and womanhood, *"menstrual cycle"* has generally been accepted as a descriptive term for what should more properly be called the "ovarian cycle".

The menstrual cycle is a variant of the estrus cycle which made its appearance at a relatively late stage of evolution. Even though there is some uterine bleeding during proestrus and estrus in some species such as the domestic dog or *Tupaia javanica*, genuine endometrial shedding with external, i.e. vaginal bleeding of varying degrees is only found in catarrhine monkeys, the anthropoid apes, and in the human female, while some endometrial desquamation with slight intrauterine bleeding is also seen in some platyrrhine monkeys (*review*: Marshall).

There is no uterine bleeding at the end of an ovulatory cycle in other mammals comparable to menstruation, even though some species such as the guinea pig have a corpus luteum-phase of comparable length. The ability of the endometrium to shed its functional layer seems in some ways to be related to the presence of a highly specialized and unique vascular apparatus, the *spiral* or *coiled arteries*, which react readily to changes in the blood level of ovarian steroid hormones. It should, however, be pointed out that this special feature is missing in the endometrium of certain menstruating new world monkeys (Kaiser, 1947).

Disturbances of menstrual function do not only encompass a wide spectrum of *deviations from the normal bleeding pattern* ranging from amenorrhea to poly- and hypermenorrhea, but are often accompanied by pain, discomfort, anemia, the inability to conceive, and they interfere generally with normal activity. Irregular and abnormal uterine bleeding and menstruation-linked symptoms such as dysmenorrhea or premenstrual spotting motivate in all likelihood more women to seek medical advice than any other cause of gynecologic illness. As a consequence, the investigation of the causes of normal and deranged uterine bleeding is of utmost clinical concern, particularly with respect to a more physiological approach to therapy with sex steroids than the prevailing one which is more or less based on the simplified concept that an *estrogen-dominated proliferative phase* of the cycle is followed by a *secretory phase* governed by *progesterone*. It should be mentioned in this context that there are as yet no preparations available which would bring about fluctuations in the blood level of the synthetic steroid hormones approximating that of an ovulatory cycle.

Even before the introduction of radioimmunochemical techniques into the field of reproductive physiology, the cyclic pattern of the secretion of ovarian sex steroids had been well established (Brown et al., 1958; Hammerstein, 1962; Ross et al., 1970), and it could reasonably well be linked to morphological changes that the endometrium undergoes throughout the menstrual cycle (Schröder, 1928). As considerable progress has been made in recent years in elucidating the complex interactions between the cyclic changes in plasma steroids, the amount of specific receptors located in the target organs, and the metabolism and elimination of hormones at the tissue level, we are in the initial stages of understanding in which manner sex steroids exert their effects on the endometrium and eventually bring on menstruation.

Cyclic Changes of Sex Steroids in Plasma

The plasma level of estradiol and of progesterone undergoes great changes during the ovarian cycle (Figure 1). In the early follicular phase, estradiol is low and the mean level approximates 50 pg/ml. There is a marked increase in the mid-follicular phase which culminates in the mid-cyclic surge of estradiol reaching peak levels of 200 to 300 pg/ml (Abraham et al., 1972; Holmdahl et al., 1972;

FIGURE 1. Cyclic changes of serum estradiol and progesterone in eumenorrhoic women. The values represent means ± SD. The day of the LH peak depicted as "Day 0".

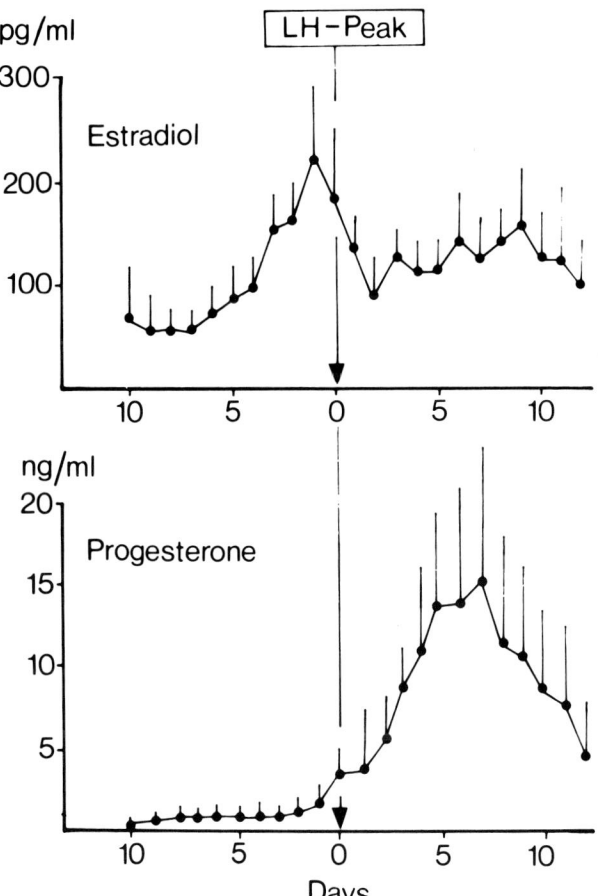

Moghissi et al., 1972). After ovulation, there is a decline, and this is followed in women, and in the female chimpanzee (Graham et al., 1972), by another peak of 80 to 100 pg/ml in the former during the height of the luteal phase. The main difference compared to the cyclic pattern of estradiol secretion in other non-human primates is the second rise in estradiol during the corpus luteum-phase which is probably caused by estrogen secretion from the largest non-atretic follicle (Baird and Scaramuzzi, 1976).

During the proliferative phase, plasma progesterone levels range from 0.5 to 1.0 ng/ml both in women and in non-human primates. This is followed by a small albeit clearly demonstrable rise of progesterone at the time of the preovulatory LH peak. Three to 4 days after ovulation, the plasma level of progesterone reaches its maximum (10 to 25 ng/ml in women, [Abraham et al., 1972; Holmdahl et al., 1972; Moghissi et al., 1972], 3 to 7 ng/ml in non-human primates [Graham et al., 1972; Bosu et al., 1973]), and remains at this level until the demise of the corpus luteum becomes apparent by the declining progesterone levels during the three days preceding menstruation. 20α-Hydroxyprogesterone is secreted in a pattern similar to that of progesterone, and the cyclic changes of 17α-Hydroxyprogesterone resemble those of estradiol (Abraham et al., 1972; Holmdahl et al., 1972).

Protein Binding of Sex Steroids

The concentration of sex steroids in plasma depends to a large degree upon the presence of proteins which bind these hormones. As a consequence of protein binding, only one to three per cent of the total circulating steroids occur in the blood stream as "free" or "unbound" hormones which represent the biologically available form (*review*: Träger, 1977). Protein binding protects steroid hormones from metabolic inactivation, and the protein-bound form represents a protected reserve (Träger, 1977).

There are two steroid-binding proteins with *high affinity* and *low capacity*, SHBG and CBG. Their synthesis is stimulated by estradiol in the liver. SHBG binds estradiol and, with even higher affinity, testosterone. Progesterone is bound with high affinity by CBG (Table I). The synthesis of a third steroid-binding protein, albumin, is not regulated by steroid hormones. Albumin binds sex steroids with a much lower affinity than SHBG and CBG (Träger, 1977), but has an enormous capacity (Haskins and Taubert, 1963), and it buffers the effect of steroid metabolites and conjugates upon the high-affinity binding proteins. Contrary to steriods bound to SHBG or CBG, albumin-bound steroid hormones are easily eliminated during liver passage. Although it has clearly been shown that estrogens

TABLE 1. Protein-binding of Sex Steroids in Plasma

Type	Concentration	Synthesis stimulated by	Binding affinity to		
			Estradiol	Testosteron	Progesteron
CBG	40 mg/l	Estrogen	−	−	+ +
SHBG	3 mg/l	Estrogen	+ +	+ + +	(+)
Albumin	38 g/l	?	+	+	+

stimulate the production of SHBG in the liver resulting in increased binding of estradiol, there is little information available on the level and cyclic changes of free estradiol and progesterone, respectively.

Binding of Sex Steroids to Target Tissue

Although sex steroids act also upon other organs such as the hypothalamus, the liver, or the mammary gland, the uterus has to be considered as a main target organ for estradiol and particularly for progesterone. It is shown in Figure 2 that R 5020, a synthetic and highly specific progestogen is bound by the cytosol prepared from immature rabbit uteri 10 to 20 times more as compared to other tissues (Philibert et al., 1977).

The presently available evidence suggests that the regulation of endometrial function by sex steroids is mediated by specific receptor proteins for estradiol and progesterone in accordance with the concept developed by Jensen et al. (1968). Receptor proteins do not only serve as vehicles for the transport of steroids into the nucleus, and for storage. They also protect the minute amounts of steroids contained in the cytoplasm against enzymatic degradation and loss due to unspecific binding to plasma proteins. It has recently been shown that the actual biologic code does not appear to be an inherent property of the steroid hormones but rather of their receptors, and is in fact merely optimized when binding occurs. Therefore, steroids do not seem to initiate biological processes but rather regulate rates (Jungblut et al., 1976).

The human endometrium contains specific binding proteins, the *cytosol receptors* for *estradiol* and *progesterone*, and possibly *uteroglobin*. The latter is a protein having a molecular weight of approximately 14 000 to 15 000 which binds progesterone in endometrial secretions of the rabbit (Beato and Beier, 1975). It's function is in some way comparable to that of androgen-binding globulin (Hansson et al., 1974) in the testis in that it mediates the biologic effect of progesterone for the maintenance of the blastocyst.

Every clinician in the field of gynecology is aware of the fact that progesterone is not capable of eliciting any specific effect in the female genital tract unless the tissue has been primed by the action of estradiol. An example for such a priming effect is given in Figure 3 which shows that the number of cytosol binding sites for progesterone in uterine tissue of immature rabbits is markedly elevated after pretreating the animals with estradiol. The clinical observation showing that progesterone cannot induce secretory transformation of the glandular epithelium unless the endometrium has been preexposed to the growth-stimulating effect of estradiol, is supported by the results of recent investigations showing that estradiol not only stimulates the synthesis of its own receptor but also that of progesterone (*review*: Brenner and West, 1975). An increase in the number of binding sites for ^{3}H-estradiol has been correlated with estrus in the rat (Gorski et al., 1971; Hsueh et al., 1975; Mester et al., 1974) and the mouse, the guinea pig (Freifeld et al., 1974; Milgrom et al., 1972; Thi et al., 1975), and in the cow (Kimball and Hansel, 1974; Senior, 1975). Similarly changes in cytosol receptor content have been demonstrated in endometrial tissue obtained from normally cycling women (Evans et al., 1973, 1974, 1975; Flickinger et al., 1977; Gabb and Stone, 1974; Schmidt-Gollwitzer, 1978; Tseng and Gurpide, 1972).

It was found by most investigators that the concentration of the estradiol re-

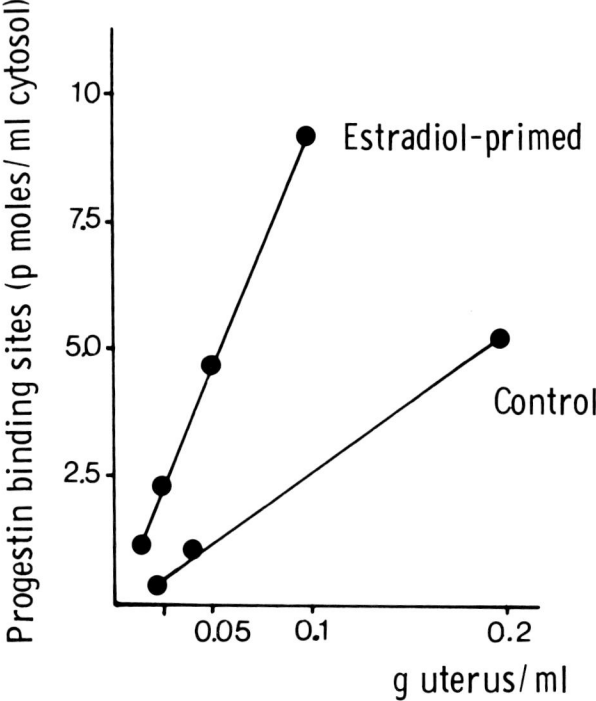

FIGURE 2. Linearity of binding measurement with respect to cytosol concentration. The cytosol was obtained from estradial-primed or control immature rabbits. Bound radioactivity was measured by DCC absorption following incubation of aliquots for 2h at OC with 50 nM (^{3}H) R 5020 in the presence or absence of 5000 nM radioinert R 5020 (from: Philibert et al., Endocrinology 101:1850 (1977).

ceptor in endometrium was high during the midproliferative phase of the cycle, i.e. between day 8 to 11, which represents the phase of highest mitotic activity (Figure 4). Robertson et al. (1971) and Crocker et al. (1974) observed maximal values in the periovulatory phase. In the mid-proliferative phase, the estradiol concentration in endometrial tissue just begins to increase. The highest estradiol content is found in mid-cycle concomitantly with that of plasma estradiol. In contrast to the latter, there is no increase in endometrial tissue during the luteal phase.

As a result of estrogenic stimulation, the number of cytosol binding sites for progesterone rises steeply in mid-cycle. This increase parallels that of estradiol in plasma during the preovulatory peak (Milgrom et al., 1973; Toft and O'Malley, 1972). The enhanced synthesis of the progesterone receptor, and the rising level of progesterone in plasma result in an approximately five-fold increase in the concentration of progesterone in the endometrium (Porias et al., 1978; Schmidt-Gollwitzer, 1978). The decline in the number of binding sites for estradiol during the late proliferative phase is followed by a fairly rapid decrease in progesterone

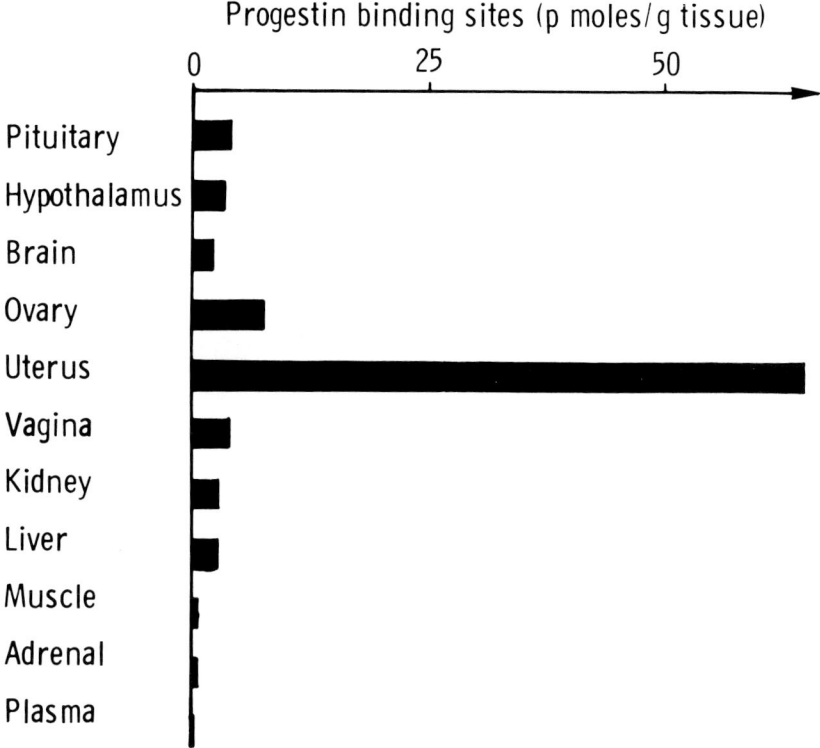

FIGURE 3. Progestin binding sites in the cytosol of various tissues of the estradiol-primed immature female rabbit. (From: Philibert et al., Endocrinology 101:1850 (1977).

receptor content which remains at a low level comparable to that of the early follicular phase for the remainder of the cycle.

A simplified diagram depicting possible pathways for the interaction between sex steroids and their receptors is given in Figure 5. After a binding of estradiol to the cytosol receptor, the hormone-receptor complex is translocated into the nucleus where it induces the chain of events resulting in increased synthesis of receptors for both estradiol and progesterone. After progesterone has bound to the progesterone receptor, the hormone-receptor complex exerts a negative effect upon the formation of the estradiol and progesterone receptor. This antagonistic effect of progesterone upon the estradiol cytosol receptor is in all probability mediated by a progesterone-specific enzyme, estradiol dehydrogenase (17β-Hydroxysteroid-Dehydrogenase). This enzyme, whose activity rises in mid-cycle by a factor of 10 (Pollow et al., 1977; Tseng and Gurpide, 1974), converts estradiol to estrone. The latter is eliminated from the cell without entering the nucleus, possibly due to a high K_d of the estrone-receptor complex. This results in a decreased supply of estradiol and a decrease in the synthesis of the estradiol receptor (Gurpide et al., 1977).

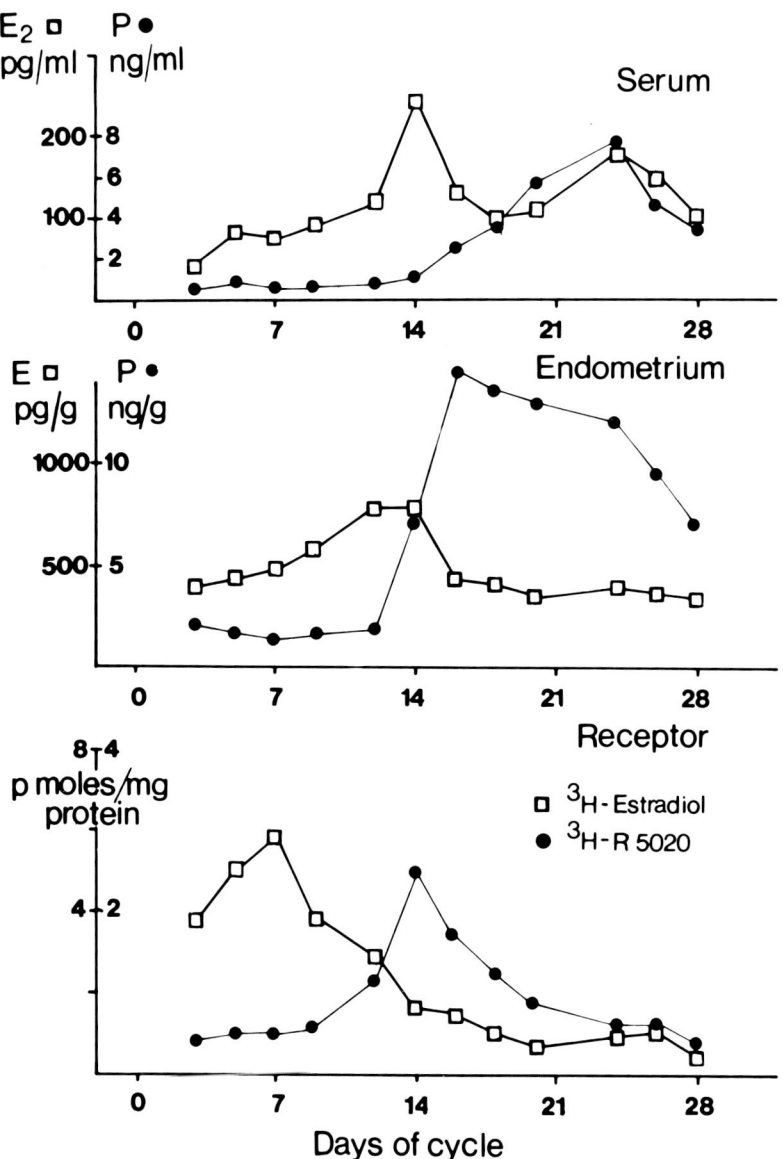

FIGURE 4. Comparison of the cyclic profile of estradiol and progesterone concentration in serum (upper frame) and endometrium (middle frame) of normally cyclic women to that of the cytosol receptor for estradiol and progesterone (lower frame). Adapted from: Schmidt-Gollwitzer, 1978).

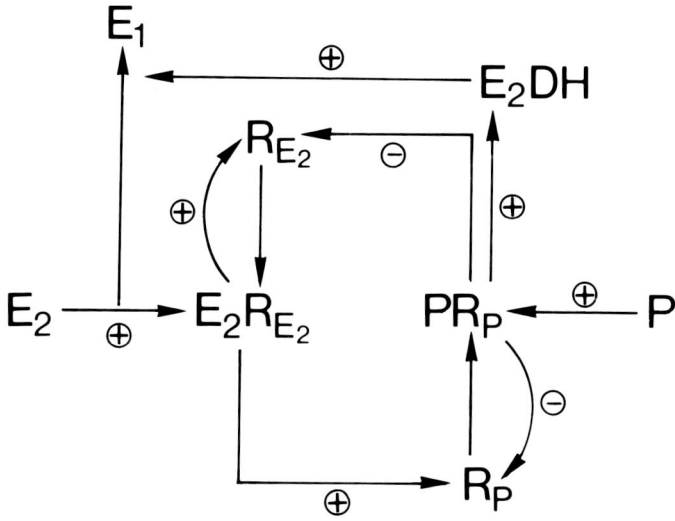

FIGURE 5. Schematic presentation of the interactions of estradiol and progesterone with their respective receptors in the endometrium. E_1 = estrone, E_2 = estradiol, P = progesterone, R_{E2} = estradiol-receptor, P_{RP} = Progesteron-receptor, E_2R_{E2} = estradiol/estradiol-receptor complex, PR_P = Progesterone/progesterone-receptor-complex, E_2DH = estradiol dehydrogenase.

Events after Receptor-Binding of Steroids

When free estradiol enters the cytoplasm of the endometrial cell, its binding to the cytosol receptor induces a conformational change which results in the formation of an active dimeric complex or of even higher aggregates (Jungblut et al., 1976). In the case of estradiol the receptor is dimerized from a MW of 75 000 to 150 000, and in the case of progesterone aggregation from a MW of 80 000 to 320 000 is observed. This is followed by the synthesis of specific mRNA which is transferred to ribosomes where it stimulates the synthesis of enzymes and other proteins, e.g. the estradiol and progesterone receptors (*review*: Gorski and Gannon, 1976). There is as yet little information concerning the pathways for the degradation of steroid-receptor complexes in the nucleus (Figure 6).

Regression and Menstruation

When a menstrual cycle approaches its end, and fertilization and nidation fail to occur, the interaction of estradiol and of progesterone has produced the following situation:

1. The glandular epithelium is in a state of secretory exhaustion. This is plausible, as the optimal time for implantation has long passed, and there is no longer any need for the glands to provide nutrient and to maintain a milieu for the yet unattached blastocyst. It was shown by Ferenczy et al. (1979) that DNA activity reaches its absolute zero point in the days preceding menstruation. This is

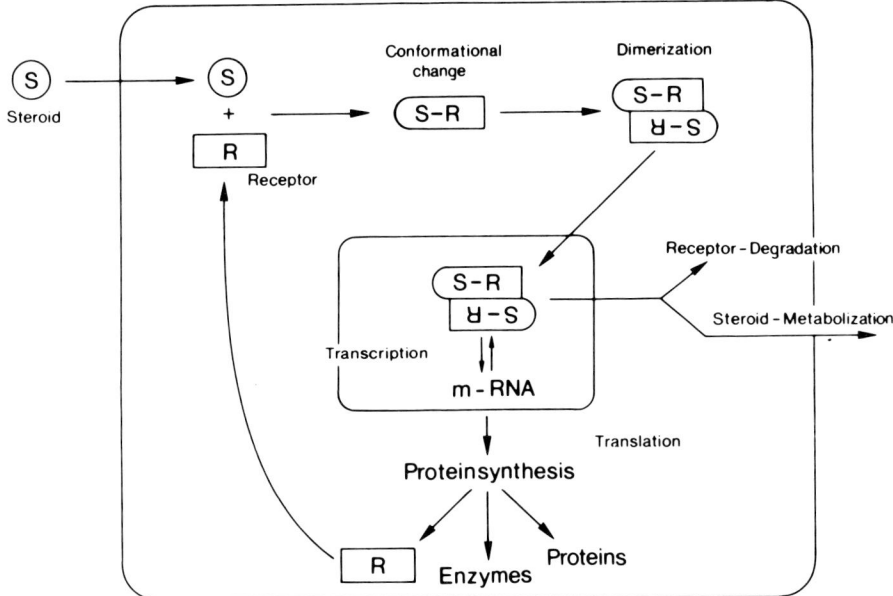

FIGURE 6. Hormone-receptor interactions at the target cell.

accompanied by irreversible cell injury which should be considered as a prelethal state, as the secretory differentiation is apparently inconsistent with further proliferation (Epinova, 1971).
2. In the endometrial stroma, progesterone has stimulated the growth of the coiled arteries and, in synergism with estradiol, the transition of stromal fibroblasts into glycogen-rich predecidual cells as a matrix for the nidus.

When the level of progesterone begins to decline both in plasma and in endometrial tissue, regressive changes are elicited in a cascade-like fashion. One to 5 days prior to the onset of menstruation, the microcirculation within the functional layer becomes progressively slower. As regression advances, the endometrium becomes thinner, and the coiling of the spiral arteries increases. Within 24 hours before the beginning of bleeding constriction of the basal portions of the spiral arteries occurs. This vasoconstriction persists throughout menstruation except during bleeding of individual arteries. This is followed by anoxemia, derangement of metabolism, and an activation of proteolytic enzymes resulting in histiolysis. It is very likely that prostaglandins play a role in bringing on menstruation, as both PGE_1 and $PGF_{2\alpha}$ are found in human endometrium. The highest concentration is reached just prior to the onset of menstruation, and at least in the guinea pig their binding to uterine tissue can be stimulated by treatment with progesterone (Wakeling and Wyngarden, 1974).

The endocrine parameters of the menstrual cycle and menstruation itself are consistent with the well-known clinical observation that the normal menses is a progesterone-withdrawal bleeding which can be delayed almost indefinitely by progestogens. As approximately 10% of eumenorrhoic cycles are in fact anovulatory, menstruation is quite obviously frequently induced by a mechanism other than progesterone-withdrawal. It had been recognized by Allen and others (cited by Riley) that menstruation-like bleeding ("pseudomenstruation") can be caused by the deprivation of estrogen. Based on the observation that 1) bleeding will occur following oophorectomy even in the absence of a corpus luteum, and after the discontinuation of a course of treatment with a synthetic estrogen, and 2) bleeding episodes can be observed at unpredictable intervals in anovulatory women, the concept of *estrogen-withdrawal-bleeding* and *estrogen-breakthrough-bleeding* was formulated. Withdrawal bleeding will occur according to Markee (cited by Riley) when the circulating level of estrogen is decreased by approximately 50%. This is seen in anovulatory women showing some evidence of follicular maturation. Contrary to that, breakthrough bleeding was believed to occur in the presence of a rather stabile estrogen level, when the growing demands of the endometrium cannot be met any longer. It was very recently shown by Wu and Mikhail (1979) that this type of bleeding does not only occur in anovulatory women with high plasma estradiol but with a normal or low one, too. Moreover, in contradiction to previously held tenets stating that the bleeding pattern in anovulatory oligomenorrhea is usually a breakthrough bleeding, their data showed it quite often to be a withdrawal bleeding. Although Gorski et al. (1977) demonstrated that prolonged application of estradiol impedes rather than enhances nucleic acid synthesis, and Karnary (1948) observed actual atrophy of the endometrium during long-term application of stilbestrol by a step-up scheme in cases of endometriosis, the causes of bleeding from a non-secretory endometrium need further elucidation, even though Markee contended that bleeding from a secretory or proliferative endometrium is caused by the same fundamental mechanisms.

REFERENCES

Abraham, G.E., Odell, W.D., Swerdloff, R.S. and Hopper, K.: Simultaneous radioimmunoassay of plasma FSH, Lh, progesterone, 17-hydroxyprogesterone, and estradiol 17-β during the menstrual cycle. J. Clin. Endocrin. Metab. 34:312, 1972.

Baird, D.T., Scaramuzzi, R.J.: The source of ovarian oestradiol and androstendione in the sheep during the luteal phase. Acta endocr. (Kbh.) 83:402, 1976.

Beato, M., Beier, R.: Binding of progesterone to the proteins of the uterine luminal fluid. Identification of uteroglobin as the binding protein. Biochem. biophys. Acta 392:346, 1975.

Bosu, W.T., Johansson, E.D.B. and Gemzell, C.: Peripheral plasma levels of oestrone, oestradiol-17β and progesterone during the ovulatory menstrual cycle in the rhesus monkey with special reference to the onset of menstruation. Acta endocr. (Kbh.) 74:732, 1973.

Brenner, R.M., West, N.B.: Hormonal regulation of the reproductive tract in female mammals. Ann. Review Physiol. (Eds.: J.H. Comroe, Jr., R.R. Sonnenschein and I.S. Edelmann), 37:273, 1975.

Brown, J.B., Klopper, A. and Lorraine, J.A.: The urinary excretion of oestrogens, pregnanediol and gonadotropins during the menstrual cycle. J. Clin. Endocrin. Metab. 17:401, 1958.

Crocker, S.G., Milton, P.J.D. and King, R.J.B.: Uptake of (6,7-^{3}H)-oestradiol-17β by normal and abnormal human endometrium. J. Endocr. 62:145, 1974.

Epinova, O.I.: Effects of hormones on the cell cycle, *in* Barerga, R. (Editor): The cell cycle and cancer. New York, 1971, Marcel Dekker Inc., pp. 145–190.

Evans, L.H., Haehnel, R.: Distribution of oestrogen receptors in cell fractions of human uterine tissue. J. Endocr. 56:503, 1973.

Evans, L.H., Martin, J.D. and Haehnel, R.: Estradiol receptor concentration in human uterine tissues. Studies on empty and filled sites. Proc. Endocr. Soc. Aust. 18:5, 1975.

Evans, L.H., Martin, J.D. and Haehnel, R.: Estradiol concentration in normal and pathologic human uterine tissues. J. Clin. Endocrin. Metab. 38:23, 1974.

Evans, L.H., Gardiner, M. and Haehnel, R.: Estradiol receptors in human uterine tissues. Studies on empty and filled sites. Proc. Endocr. Soc. Aust. 18:5, 1975.

Ferenczy, A., Bertrand, G. and Gelfand, M.M.: Proliferation kinetics of human endometrium during the normal menstrual cycle. Amer. J. Obstet. Gynec. 133:859, 1979.

Flickinger, G.L., Elsner, C., Illingsworth, D.V., Muechler, E.K. and Mikhail, G.: Estradiol and progesterone receptors in the female tract of humans and monkeys. Ann. N.Y. Acad. Sci. 286:180, 1977.

Freifeld, M.L., Feil, P.D. and Bardin, C.W.: The *in vivo* regulation of progesterone "receptor" in guinea pig uterus. Dependence on estrogen and steroids. Steroids 23:93, 1974.

Gabb, R.G., Stone, G.M.: Uptake and metabolism of tritiated estradiol and estrone by human endometrial and myometrial tissue. J. Endocr. 62:109, 1974.

Gorski, J., Sarff, M., and Clerk, J.H.: The regulation of uterine concentration of estrogen binding protein. Adv. Biosc. 7:5, 1971.

Gorski, J., Gannon, F.: Current models of steroid hormone action: A Critique. Ann. Review Physiol. 38:425, 1976.

Gorski, J., Stormshak, F., Harris, J. and Wertz, N.: Hormone regulation by growth: Stimulatory and inhibitory influences of estrogens on DNA synthesis. J. Toxicol. Environ. Health 3:271, 1977.

Graham, C.E., Collins, D.C., Robinson, H. and Preedy, J.R.K.: Urinary levels of estrogen and plasma levels of progesterone during the menstrual cycle of the chimpanzee: relationship to sexual swelling. Endocr. 99:12, 1972.

Gurpide, E., Tseng, L., and Gusberg, S.G.: Estrogen metabolism in normal and neoplastic endometrium. Am. J. Obstet. Gynecol. 129:809, 1977.

Hammerstein, J.: Hormonanalytische Untersuchungen zur Frage der endokrinen Korrelationen im biphasischen Menstruationszyklus der Frau. Arch. Gynäk. 196:504, 1962.

Hansson, V., Ritzen, E.M. and French, F.S.: Androgen transport mechanism in the testis and epididymis. Acta endocrin. (Kbh.) 77, Suppl. 191:191, 1974.

Haskins, A.L., Jr., Taubert, H.-D.: Progesterone transportation in blood. Obstet. Gynec. 21:395, 1963.

Holmdahl, T.H., Johansson, E.D.B.: Peripheral plasma levels of 17α-Hydroxyprogesterone, progesterone, and oestradiol during the normal menstrual cycle in women. Acta endocrin. (Kbh.) 71:743, 1972.

Hsueh, A.J.W., Peck, E.J. and Clark, J.H.: Progesterone antagonism of oestrogen receptor and oestrogen-induced uterine growth. Nature 254:337, 1975.

Jensen, E.V., Suzuki, T., Kawashami, T., Stumpf, W.E., Jungblut, P.W. and DeSombre, R.: A two-step mechanism for the interaction of estradiol with rat uterus. Proc. Natl. Acad. Sci. 59:632, 1968.

Jungblut, P.W., Gauers, J., Hughes, A. et al.: Activation of transciption regulating proteins by steroids. J. Steroid Biochem. 7:1109, 1976.

Kaiser, I.H.: Absence of coiled arterioles in the endometrium of menstruating new world monkeys. Anat. Rec. 99:353, 1947.

Karnary, K.J.: The use of stilbestrol for endometriosis; preliminary report. South. Med. J. 41:1109, 1948.

Kimball, F.A., Hansel, W.: Estrogen cytosol binding protein in bovine endometrium and corpus luteum. Biol. of Reprod. 11:566, 1974.

Marshall's Physiology of Reproduction (Ed. A.S. Parkes) Vol. I, Part One, Longman's, 1965.

Mester, I., Martel, D., Psychoyos, A. and Baulieu, E.-E.: Hormonal control of estrogen receptors in uterus and receptivity for ovoimplantation in the rat. Nature 250:776, 1974.

Milgrom, E., Thi, L., Atger, M. and Baulieu, E.-E.: Progesterone in uterus and plasma. An assay of the progesterone cytosol receptor of the guinea pig. Endocrinology 90:1064, 1972.

Milgram, E., Thi, L., Atger, M. and Baulieu, E.-E.: Mechanism regulating the concentration and confirmation of progesterone receptor(s) in the uterus. J. Biol. Chem. 248:6366, 1973.

Moghissi, K.S., Syner, F.N. and Evans, T.N.: A composite picture of the menstrual cycle. Amer. J. Obstet. Gynec. 114:405, 1972.

Philibert, D., Ojasoo, T. and Raynaud, J.P.: Properties of the cytoplasmic progestin-binding protein in the rabbit uterus. Endocrinology 101:1850, 1977.

Pollow, K., Schmidt-Gollwitzer, M., Boquoi, E. and Pollow, B.: Estrogen receptor in normal human myometrium and leiomyoma. J. Mol. Med. 2:61, 1977.

Porias, H., Sojo, I., Carranco, A., Gonzalez-Martinez, R. and Cortes-Gallegos, V.: A simultaneous assay to quantitate plasma and endometrial hormone concentrations. Fertil. Steril. 30:66, 1978.

Robertson, D.M., Mester, J., Beilby, J., Steely, S.J. and Kellie, A.E.: The measurement of high affinity estradiol receptor in human endometrium and myometrium. Acta endocrin. (Kbh.) 68:534, 1971.

Riley, G.M.: Gynecologic Endocrinology, Hoeber-Harper, 1960.

Ross, G.T., Cargille, C.M., Lipsett, M.B., Rayford, P.L., Marshall, J.R., Strott, C.A. and Rodbard, D.: Pituitary and gonadal hormones in women during spontaneous and induced ovulatory cycles. Rec. Prog. Horm. Res. 26:1, 1970.

Schmidt-Gollwitzer, M.: Korrelation zwischen den Sexualsteroiden im Serum und im Endometrium, den östradiol- und progesteron-bindenden Rezeptorproteinen und der Aktivität der 17β-HSD während des mensuellen Zyklus. Habilitationsschrift, Berlin, 1978.

Schröder, R.: Der mensuelle Genitalzyklus des Weibes und seine Störungen, in: Hdb. der Gynäkologie (Ed. W. Stöckel), Bd.I/2, W.F.J. Bergmann, München, 1978.

Senior, B.E.: Cytoplasmic oestrogen-binding sites and their relationship to oestrogen content in the endometrium of the cattle. J. Reprod. Fertil. 44:501, 1975.

Thi, L., Baulieu, E.-E. and Milgrom, E.: Comparison of the characteristics and of the hormonal control of the endometrial and myometrial progesterone receptors. J. Endocr. 66:349, 1975.

Toft, D.O., O'Malley, B.W.: Target tissue receptors for progesterone. The influence of estrogen treatment. Endocrinology 91:738, 1972.

Träger, L.: Steroidhormone, Springer, Berlin/Heidelberg, 1977.

Tseng, L., Gurpide, E.: Nuclear concentration of estradiol in superfused slices of human endometrium. Amer. J. Obstet. Gynec. 114:995, 1972.

Tseng, L., Gurpide, E.: Estradiol and 20αdihydroprogesterone activity in human endometrium during the menstrual cycle. Endocrinology 94:419, 1974.

Wakeling, A.F., Wyngarden, L.J.: Prostaglandin receptors in the human, monkey and hamster uterus. Endocrinology 95:55, 1974.

Wu, Ch. H., Mikhail, G.: Plasma hormone profile in anovulation. Fertil. Steril 31:258, 1979.

Copyright 1979 by Elsevier North Holland, Inc.
F.K. Beller and G.F.B. Schumacher, eds.
The Biology of the Fluids of the Female Genital Tract

THE HISTOLOGY AND PROLIFERATION KINETICS OF MENSTRUAL ENDOMETRIUM

A. Ferenczy and M. S. Guralnick

SUMMARY

During normal menstruation, physiologic loss of the functionalis layer of the endometrium is followed by mucosal healing which involves both the migration and replication of surface epithelial cells. These originate from the gland stumps of the residual basalis and the persistent surface epithelium peripheral to the denuded basalis of the endometrial cavity. Endometrial degeneration and regeneration are completed within four days and occur independent of hormonal influence.

INTRODUCTION

According to Blakiston's New Gould Medical Dictionary the term menstruation refers to a "periodic discharge of sanguineous fluid from the uterus occurring during the period of a woman's sexual activity, from puberty to the menopause". In our opinion, the term menstruation should further imply that bleeding is the result of the breakdown of a postovulatory secretory phase endometrium.

The morphologic phenomena involved in endometrial remodelling during the normal menstrual period have been studied by several investigators (Schröder 1915; Bohnen, 1927; Sturgis and Meigs, 1936; Bartelemez, 1957; McLennan et al., 1965; Baggish et al., 1967; Dallenbach-Hellweg, 1971; Ferenczy, 1976 a, b;

Departments of Pathology and Obstetrics and Gynecology, Jewish General Hospital and McGill University.

Ludwig et al., 1976; Flowers and Wilborn, 1978; Nogales-Ortiz et al., 1978; and Ferenczy et al., 1979) without reaching uniform conclusions and understanding. Issues of controversy are related to the extent of endometrial mucosal shedding and to the cellular origin and mechanisms of renewal of post-desquamation regenerative endometrium. There are three schools of thought: One favors the concept of total loss of the functionalis layer of the endometrium followed by a reepithelialization of the denuded basalis. The regenerative epithelium originates from the stumps of the residual basal glands and surface epithelium of the persistent endometrium adjacent to denudation (Bohnen, 1927; Sturgis and Meigs, 1936; Schröder, 1945; Dallenbach-Hellweg, 1971; Ferenczy, 1976 a, b; Ludwig et al., 1976; and Ferenczy et al., 1979). Others believe that desquamation involves only the upper ⅓-½ of the functionalis and regeneration takes place de novo from the residual spongiosa. The latter undergoes rapid metamorphosis, i.e., conversion from secretory to proliferative tissue (Bartelemez, 1957; McLennan et al., 1965; Flowers and Wilborn, 1978; Nogales-Ortiz et al., 1978). Still other workers are of the opinion that following variable loss of the functionalis layer, the regenerative epithelium derives from the residual stromal fibroblasts through metaplastic transformation (Baggish et al., 1967). The discrepancies in observations and conclusions are largely due to different interpretations of cellular changes occurring during the premenstrual and menstrual periods as well as to different techniques used for sampling and studying uterine specimens.

In the following discussion we will review the histological sequences of events that we have observed over the years in both routine and experimental human specimens (Ferenczy, 1976 a, b). The findings will be correlated with results derived from *in vitro* proliferation kinetic studies (Ferenczy, 1977; Ferenczy et al., 1979) and steroid receptor measurements of menstrual endometrium as well as radioimmunoassays of cyclic plasma sex-steroids and serum gonadotropins.

RESULTS AND DISCUSSION

The endometrium in between cycle days 28 and 1 is thick, red and gelatinous. There may be superficial ulcerations and foci of bleeding. These rapidly become generalized so that the surface becomes rough, friable and hemorrhagic. When seen in cross section on a large block of tissue, the "functionalis" of endometrium occupies the upper two thirds of the entire thickness, the lower third, the basalis changing very little during the endometrial cycle (Figure 1a). On cycle day 2 the functionalis becomes disorganized, containing predecidual stromal cells admixed with epithelial glandular cells. Both cellular systems undergo severe degenerative changes. There is present a heavy polymorphonuclear exudate as well as many red blood cells providing for a bloody, purulent state of dead and dying tissue which flows from the uterine cavity (Figure 1b). During cycle days 1 and 2, synthesis of nuclear DNA is near zero levels in the secretory functionalis layer of the endometrium as determined by *in vitro* short term incubation historadioautography (Ferenczy et al., 1979). The findings are consistent with with previous ultrastructural observations which have indicated that the cellular components of the functionalis layer undergo irreversible cell injury prior to expulsion during periods of menstruation (Ferenczy, 1976 b). The observations also agree with those of Epifanova (1971) according to whom secretory differentiation implies an arrest in cell growth on the one hand and a prelethal state on the other.

On cycle days 2-3, the functionalis layer becomes gradually cleaved off

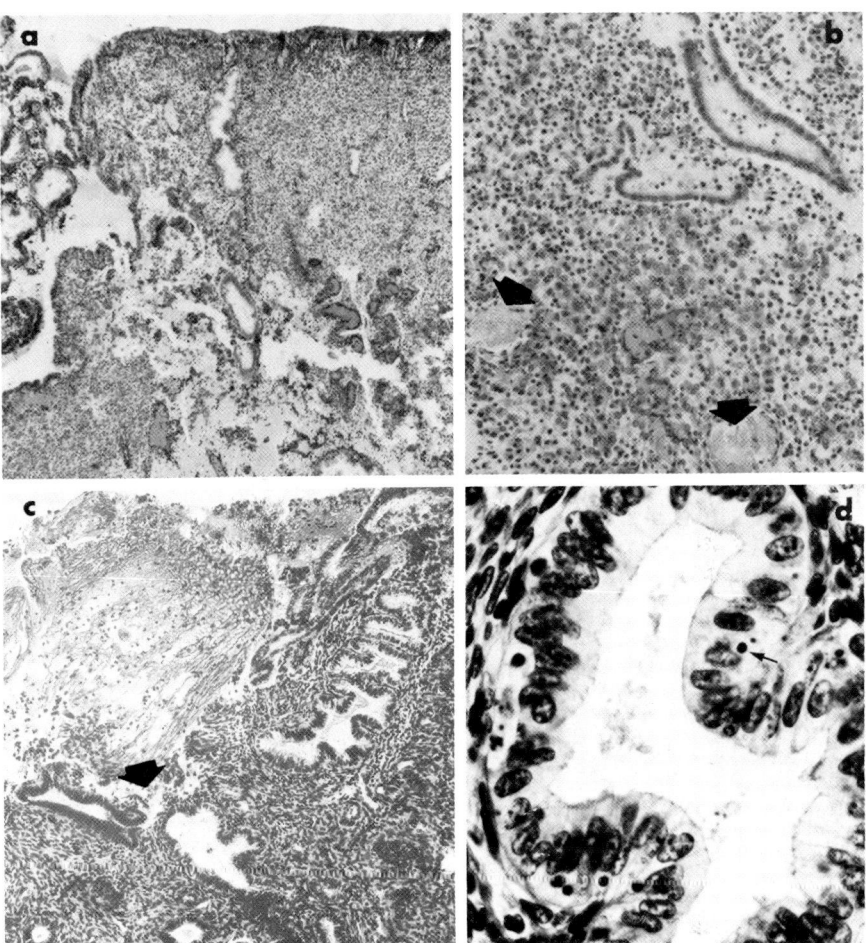

FIGURE 1. *Menstrual endometrium.* a) Cycle day 1. Partly collapsed functionalis (on the left) in the process of cleavage from the underlying basalis. Note edema, broken tissue at cleavage site (x 60). b) Detailed view of degenerated functionalis with broken glands, collapsed stroma, inflammatory exudate and thrombosed vessels (arrows) (x 100). c) Cycle days 2–3. Endometrial shedding extends to the basalis layer (arrow) (x 100). d) "Poly dust" or nuclear debris of inflammatory origin (arrow) in residual basal gland cells characteristic feature of recent uterine bleeding and tissue necrosis (x 400).

from the underlying basalis. As a result, the latter demonstrates a thin, denuded layer with open residual basal gland stumps (Figure 1c). During the menstrual period, nuclear fragments of inflammatory exudate origin, the so-called "poly dust" are found within the intercellular spaces of basal gland cells as well as within the cytoplasmic substance of basal cells (Ferenczy, 1976 b)—another sequence of recent tissue dehiscence and necrotic phase of the menstrual cycle (Figure 1d).

During the 2nd day and especially the following two days, proliferation of the basal gland epithelium begins in areas of denudation. The surface of the endo-

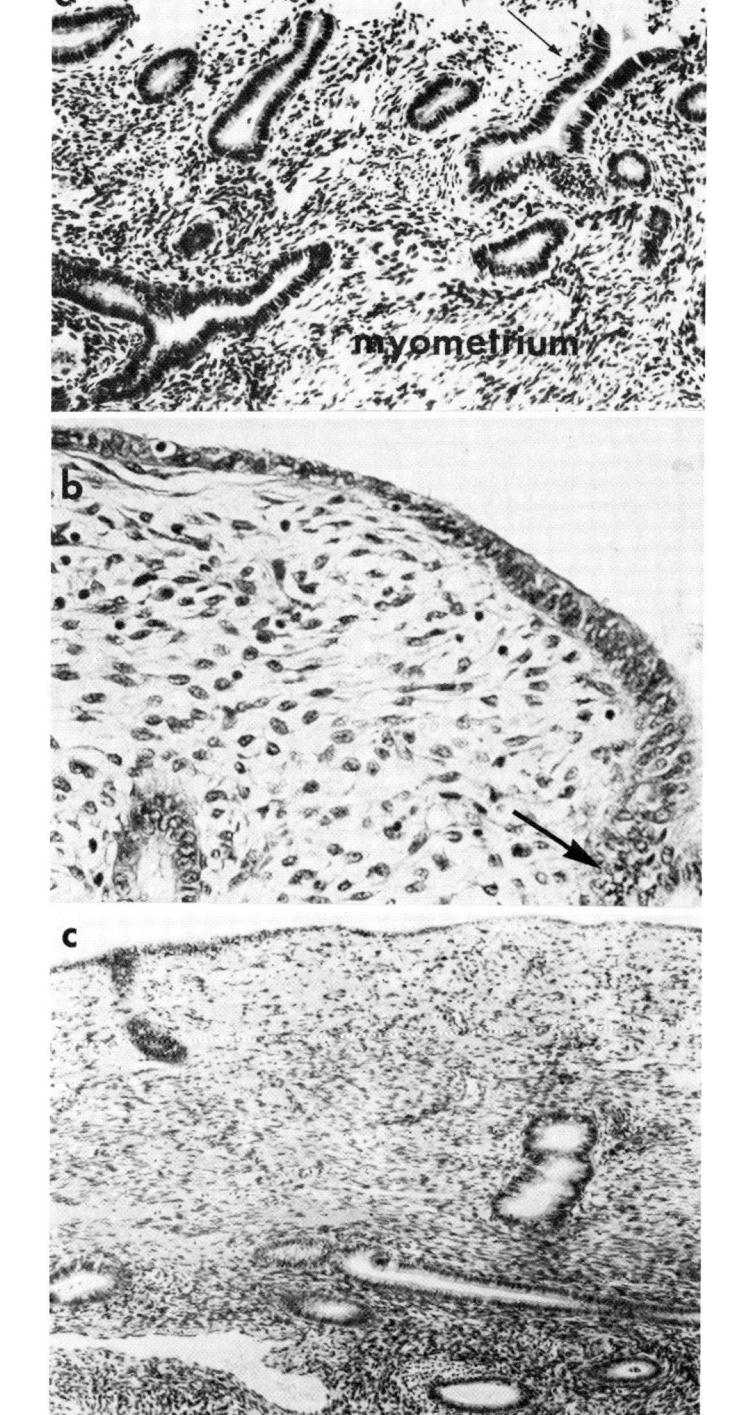

metrium is reepithelialized by a spreading of the residual glandular epithelium over the denuded surface (Figure 2a & b). Another source of resurfacing epithelium is the surface epithelium of peripheral regions of the endometrial cavity such as the lower uterine segment and peritubal-ostium which remain intact during the menstrual period (Ferenczy, 1976 a,b). The subsequent development of interanastomoses between converging epithelial proliferations lead ultimately to complete reconstruction of a new surface epithelium by cycle day 5 (Figure 2c). Complete reepithelialization of the surface coincides with the cessation of bleeding.

According to radiothymidine tracing studies (Ferenczy et al., 1979), DNA synthesis is confined to the basalis of the body-fundus of the uterus as well as the isthmic and peritubal-ostial endometrial mucosa all of which remain intact during menstruation (Figure 3a-c). Significant increase in Labelling Index (LI) in these regions occur only following complete denudation of the zona basalis by cycle day 3 (Figure 4). The significant rise in labelling intensity of the glandular epithelium (but not of stromal fibroblasts) followed by the appearance of resurfacing epithelial cells concur with the concept that the newly formed surface lining derives principally from the persistent glandular epithelium of the basalis layer. A similar labelling pattern observed in the isthmic and peritubal-ostial mucosae adjacent to the denuded endometrial cavity indicates their contribution to the peripheral repair of lost tissue. These observations are in agreement with previous experimental studies in the rabbit (Ferenczy, 1977). Indeed, partial removal of the entire thickness of the endometrial mucosa including the basalis is reconstructed by the peripheral ingrowth of surface epithelial cells originating in the endometrium adjacent to mechanical denudation.

Postmenstrual endometrial repair involves cellular migration and replication of surface epithelial cells (Ferenczy, 1976 a, b; Ferenczy et al., 1979). During the first 6–12 hours of the regenerative period starting from about day 3, spreading and migration unassociated with a significant DNA-synthesis and mitotic activity are the principal means to rapidly initiate endometrial reconstruction. The resurfacing cells are flattened, spindle-shaped and, in the rabbit endometrial regeneration model have intracellular microfillamentous-microtubular systems and pseudopodial projections (Ferenczy, 1977). These features are consistent with ameboid contraction-expansion mediated motility. For the period thereafter, cell division and migration operate simultaneously until a confluent surface layer has been regenerated on cycle day 5. Following the initial amitotic epithelial spread, the sudden increase in LI associated with very short DNA-synthesis phase and accelerated tissue turnover time explains the spectacularly rapid wound healing capability of the human endometrium (Table I).

The mechanism of induction of endometrial proliferation during menstruation does not seem to be influenced by estradiol-17β. Indeed, during cycle days 3–4, despite increased DNA activity (limited to the regenerative epithelial and endothelial cellular systems) plasma estrogens, serum gonadotropins and progester-

---

FIGURE 2. *Menstrual endometrium.* a) Cycle days 2–3. Denuded basalis with residual gland stumps (arrow) (myometrium) (x 150). b) Cycle days 3–4. New surface epithelial cells originate from the residual basal glands (arrow) and spread over the denuded surface (x 150). c) Cycle days 4–5. Endometrial resurfacing is complete; there is stromal edema scattered with a few glands and postmenstrual, residual inflammatory exudate (x 100).

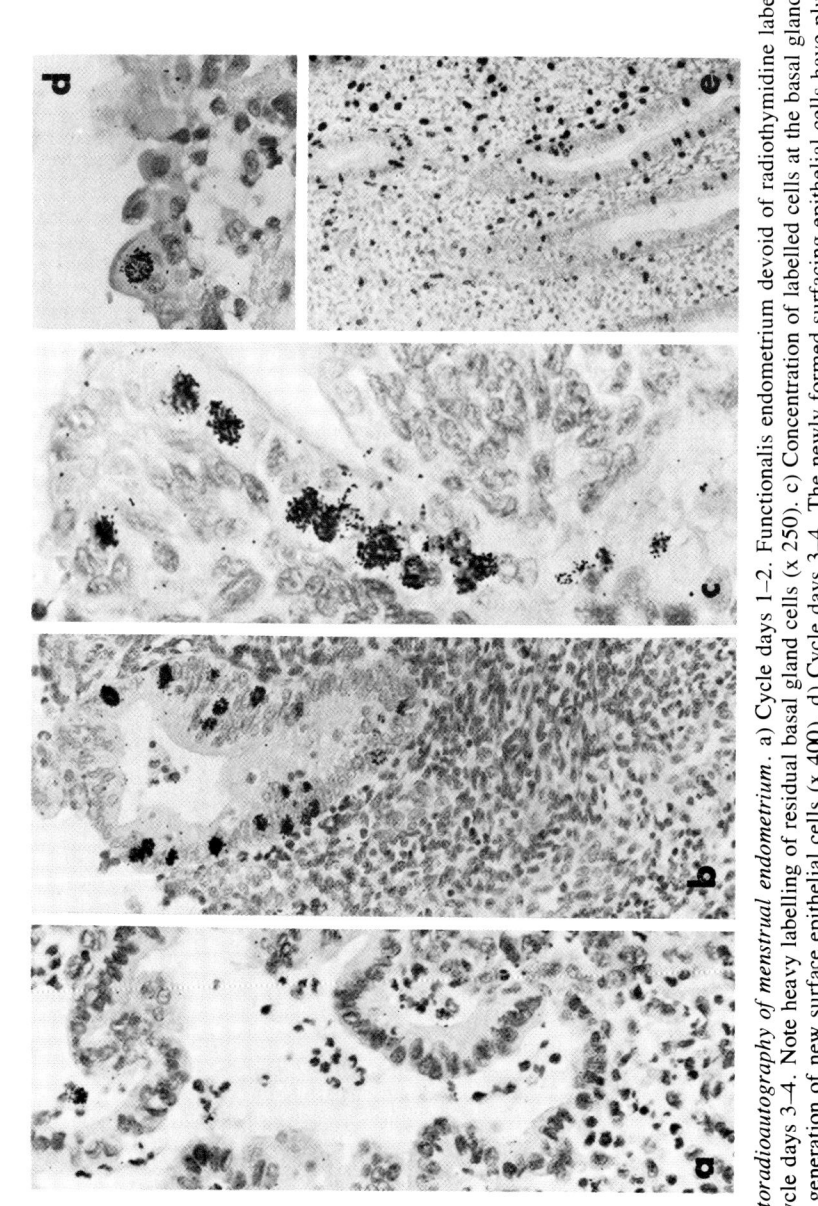

Figure 3. *Historadioautography of menstrual endometrium*. a) Cycle days 1–2. Functionalis endometrium devoid of radiothymidine labelled cells (x 250). b) Cycle days 3–4. Note heavy labelling of residual basal gland cells (x 250). c) Concentration of labelled cells at the basal gland neck region precedes generation of new surface epithelial cells (x 400). d) Cycle days 3–4. The newly formed surfacing epithelial cells have plump cytoplasmic substance and a few labelled nuclei (x 320). e) Cycle day 10. Note heavy nuclear labelling of glandular and stromal endometrial cells (x 80). (From: Ferenezy, A., G. Bertrand, M.M. Gelfand: Studies on the cytodynamics of human endometrial regeneration. III. *In vitro* short-term historadioautography. Amer. J. Obstet. Gynecol. 134, 1979, pp. 297-304.)

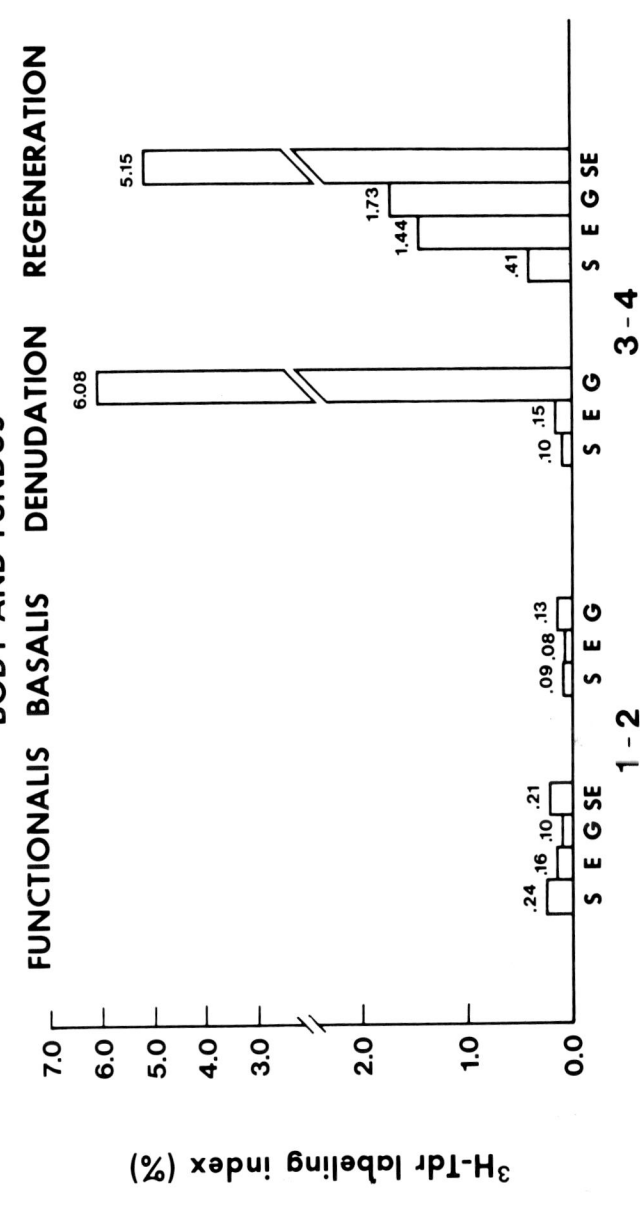

FIGURE 4. *Zonal and cellular distribution of mean ³H-thymidine labelling intensity of endometrial mucosa during epriods of menstrual breakdown and regeneration.* Note negligible LI on cycle days 1–2 and sharp increase in the residual basalis glands and newly formed surface epithelium on cycle days 3 and 4. S, stromal fibroblasts; E, capillary endothelium; G, glandular epithelium; SE, surface epithelium. (From Ferenczy, A., Bertrand, G., Gelfand, M.M.: Studies on the cytodynamics of human endometrial regeneration. III. *In vitro* short-term historadioautography. Amer. J. Obstet. Gynecol. 134, 1979, pp. 297-304.)

TABLE 1. Mean Endometrial Proliferation Kinetics, Receptor Content, Blood Estrogens and Gonadotropins by Cycle Days

Cycle Days	No. Patients	Age (yr)	Kinetics			Receptors	Steroids	Gonadotropins	
			LI %	DNA-S-Phase (hr)	TpD (hr)	PR (fmoles/mg protein)	E_1-E_2 (ng/100 ml)	FSH (mIU/ml)	LH (mIU/ml)
1–2	4	36 ± 2	0.2 ± 0.1	NM	NM	231 ± 19	3.4 ± 1.2	11.5 ± 2.8	9.7 ± 1.8
3–4	4	39 ± 3	7.3 ± 2.4	3.5 ± 0.1	54 ± 15	216 ± 34	4.6 ± 1.5	14.3 ± 8.0	8.2 ± 1.1
7–12	7	40 ± 3	7.5 ± 3.5	7.4 ± 3.1	91 ± 35	1131 ± 206	33.1 ± 6.3	10.8 ± 2.0	6.7 ± 8.5
25–28	7	32 ± 4	0.3 ± 0.1	NM	NM	254 ± 95	3.4 ± 0.9	10.0 ± 3.1	11.2 ± 3.3

± mean standard errors; TpD: potential doubling time; PR: progesterone receptors, fmoles: femtomoles; E_1: estrone; E_2: estradiol; ng: nanogram; NM: not measurable; LI: labelling index.

one receptors are low and unchanged from the premenstrual values (Table I). Also in experimental endometrial regeneration in the rabbit, proliferation kinetics and morphologic alterations of the regenerative but estrogen-deprived atrophic endometrium associated with ovariectomy are similar to animals with intact ovaries (Ferenczy, 1977).

On the other hand, on cycle days 7–12 there is a sudden increase in both nuclear DNA synthesis (Figure 3d) and mitosis in the stomal, vascular and gland cell components of regenerated human endometrium. This is accompanied by an increase in progesterone receptor concentrations and plasma estrogens and a decrease in serum pituitary hormones (Table I). These alterations are consistent with target cell sensitivity and response to preovulatory estradiol-17β.

ACKNOWLEDGEMENTS

Supported in part by Grant MA 5137 from the Medical Research Council of Canada. The authors are indebted to Miss Rosemary De Marco for typing the manuscript.

REFERENCES

Baggish, M.S., Pauerstein, C.J., Woodruff, J.D.: Role of stroma in regeneration of endometrial epithelium. Amer. J. Obstet. Gynecol. 99, 1967, p. 453

Bartelemez, G.W.: The phases of the menstrual cycle and their interpretation in terms of the pregnancy cycle. Amer. J. Obstet. Gynecol. 74, 1957, p. 931

Bohnen, P.: Wie weit wird das Endometrium bei der Menstruation abgestossen. Arch. Gynaekol. 104, 1927, p. 459

Dallenbach-Hellweg, G.: Histopathology of the endometrium. Springer-Verlag, New York, 1971, pp. 62–70

Epifanova, O.I.: Effects of hormones on the cell cycle. In: The Cell Cycle and Cancer, by ed. R. Baserga, M. Dekker, Inc., New York, 1971, pp. 145–190

Ferenczy, A.: Studies on the cytodynamics of human endometrial regeneration. I. Scanning Electron Microscopy. Amer. J. Obstet. Gynecol. 124, 1976 a, p.64.

Ferenczy, A.: Studies on the cytodynamics of human endometrial regeneration. II. Transmission Electron Microscopy and Histochemistry. Amer. J. Obstet. Gynecol. 124, 1976 b, p. 582.

Ferenczy, A.: Studies on the cytodynamics of experimental endometrial regeneration in the rabbit. Historadioautography and ultrastructure. Amer. J. Obstet. Gynecol. 128, 1977, p. 536.

Ferenczy, A., Bertrand, G., Gelfand, M.M.: Studies on the cytodynamics of human endometrial regeneration. III. *In vitro* short-term historadioautography. Amer. J. Obstet. Gynecol., 1979, in press.

Flowers, C.E. Jr., Wilborn, W.H.: New observations on the physiology of menstruation. Obstet. Gynecol. 51, 1978, p. 16

Ludwig, H., Metzger, H.: The reepithelialization of endometrium after menstrual desquamation. Arch. Gynak. 221, 1976, p. 51

McLennan, C.E., Rydell, A.H.: Extent of endometrial shedding during normal menstruation. Obstet. Gynecol. 26, 1965, p. 605.

Nogales-Ortiz, F., Puerta, J. and Nogales, F.F., Jr.: The normal menstrual cycle. Chronology and mechanism of endometrial desquamation. Obstet. Gynecol. 51, 1978, p. 259.

Schröder, R.: Anatomische Studien zur normalen und pathologischen Physiologie des menstrual Zyklus. Arch. Gynaekol. 104, 1915, p. 27.

Sturgis, S.H., Meigs, J.V.: Endometrial cycle and mechanism of normal menstruation. Amer. J. Surg. 33, 1936, p. 369.

ULTRASTRUCTURAL ASPECTS OF HUMAN ENDOMETRIUM DURING MENSTRUATION

H. Wagner and F.K. Beller

SUMMARY

The menstruating endometrium was studied in 16 hysterectomy specimens of normal women with biphasic cycles by electron microscopy and scanning electron microscopy. There seems to be agreement that the repair mechanism of the early menstruating endometrium is a unique feature of the organism and not a function of rising estrogen levels. Impressive is the interrelation between desquamation and repair which is shown by a semiquantitative technique. These are present and functioning in regard to the endometrium only on day 6 or later. The regeneration starts from the glands and the surface epithelium adjacent to denuded areas. However, there is no evidence that stromal cells can transform into surface epithelial cells. There is evidence that not only glandular stumps but also compact remaining glands can contribute to regeneration. The problem of the amount of shedding seems to be more a matter of semantics than anything else.

INTRODUCTION

The endometrium has a very high rate of regeneration. The cyclical nature of its morphological kinetics is well known (Themann and Schuenke, 1963; Wynn, 1977; Ludwig and Metzger, 1976). Little information is available regard-

Frauenklinik, Abteilung Geburtshilfe und Gynäkologie, Westfälische Wilhelms-Universität Münster/Westf

TABLE I. Distribution of Patients in Our Study (DC = Day of Cycle)

No	Name	Age (Years)	D.C.
1	W.F.	32	1
2	F.E.	42	1
3	H.D.	44	2
4	K.H.	4o	2
5	B.B.	39	2
6	R.E.	32	2
7	S.C.	47	2
8	F.E.	42	3
9	V.D.	39	3
lo	M.H.	46	4
11	K.I.	45	4
12	H.H.	27	5
13	V.G.	36	5
14	H.E.	4o	6
15	V.M.	38	6
16	K.U.	48	6

ing the morphological changes occurring during menstruation and dysfunctional bleeding. Extensive electron and scanning electron microscopic data are available on menstrual changes in the endometrium (Ferenczy, 1976). SEM-studies elucidating ciliogenesis during menstruation were reported by Ludwig (1976). The observations of Ferenczy agree with the older ones of Schröder (1947) obtained by light microscopy. Rockenschaub (1960), however, did not believe that there was a general shedding of the endometrium during menstruation.

MATERIALS AND METHODS

Hysterectomy specimens were investigated from patients with biphasic cycles. The indication was vaginal prolaps and stress incontinence. The distribution is indicated in Table I. Patients had not taken any medication including hormones. Basal-body temperature curves were available from a few patients to indicate ovulation. Serum concentrations of estrogen and progestrone (Radio immune assay) were obtained to indicate the phase of the cycle. There were 16 uteri investigated.

Immediately following hysterectomy the uterus was opened along the left lateral border. The surface of the endometrium was carefully washed either with saline or with glutaraldehyde 3%. The surface was then fixed in glutaraldehyde 3% for 30 minutes. Pieces of tissue of 0.5 to 1 cm² were removed from identical areas of the uterus (Figure 1). For transmission electron microscopy (TEM) four slices were taken from the edges of these pieces. The tissue was fixed in glutaraldehyde 3%, washed with saline and fixed again with OsO_4 1, 33% for 2 hours. Dehydration of the sample was achieved by subjecting the tissue to an increasing alcohol concentration followed by directional embedding in Epon. For scanning electron microscopy (SEM) the preparation was transferred to Freon,

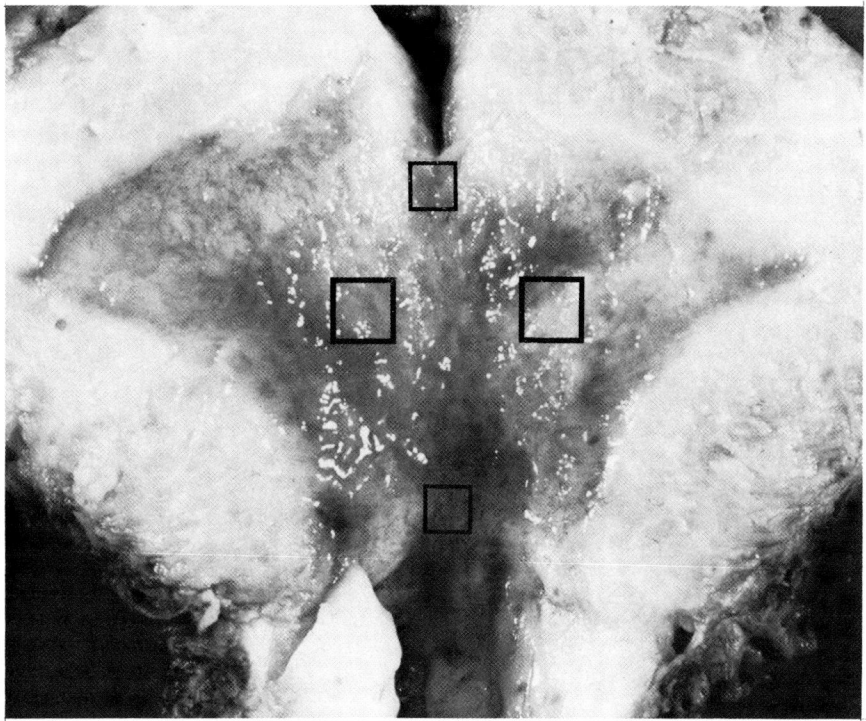

FIGURE 1. Uterus opened at the left margin. Black squares mark the area from where the specimen was taken.

dried at critical point and spattered with gold. The thick and very thin sections were prepared with an ultramicrotome Porter Blum MT 1 B. The sections were taken up on foil, and again contrasted with uranyl-acetate in a wet chamber. Microscopic examination was performed with a Phillips EM 301 and a Cambridge Stereoscan 150, working with voltages of 60 and 20 KV respectively.

RESULTS

On the first day of the cycle there was a generalized edema of the stroma, which had begun in the late luteal phase. Partial epitheliolysis with desquamation of the target epithelium resulted or was due to the presence of focal bleeding (Figure 2a). Diapedesis of the stromal blood vessels was striking during this phase. Also deposits of blood cells were observed close to ruptured endothelial walls (Figure 2c). The focal subepithelial bleeding was frequently located next to the gland mouths where the epithelial tissue showed early indications of break up (2b). As a result epithelial defects were seen (2d). SEM pictures confirmed these observations in the tissue around the gland openings. The intercellular junctions broke up with subsequent defects (Figure 3a). This in turn resulted in desquamation of epithelium between the glandular lumina (3b). Extreme prominent glandu-

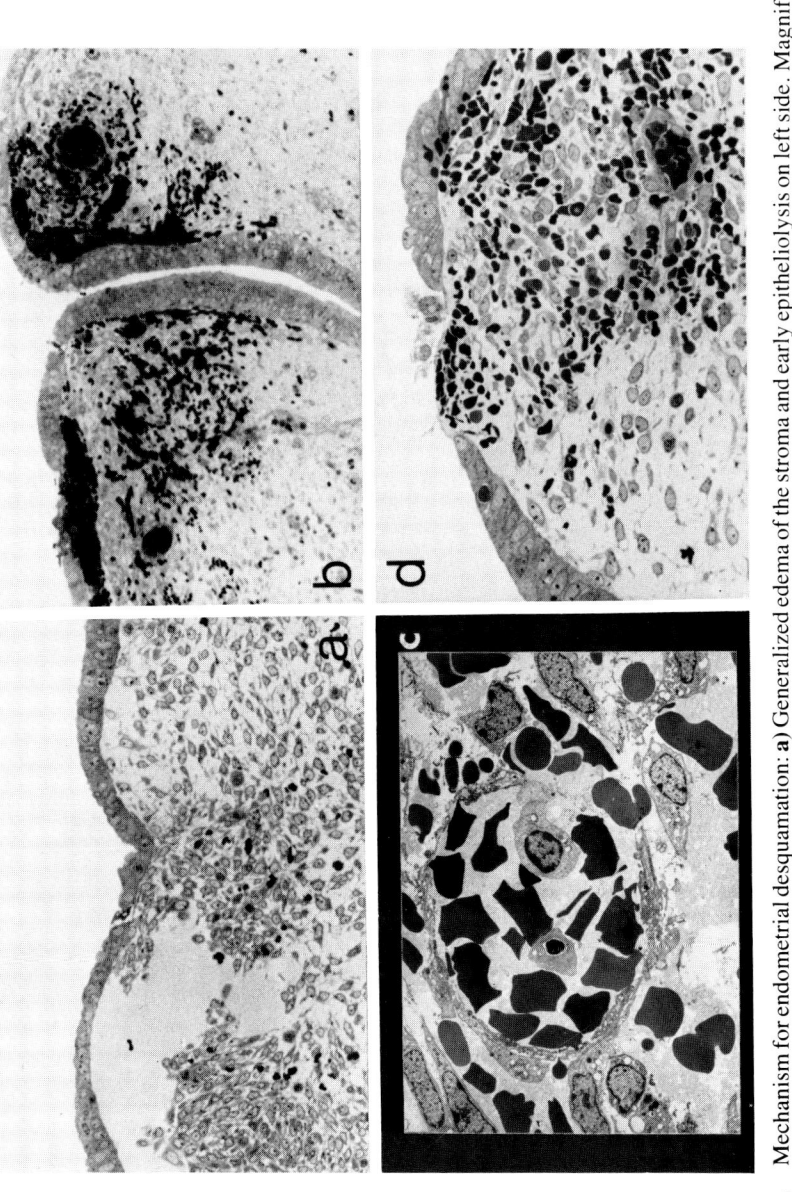

FIGURE 2. Mechanism for endometrial desquamation: **a)** Generalized edema of the stroma and early epitheliolysis on left side. Magnification: 780:1; LM (light microscopic photograph). **b)** Focal subepithelial bleeding with engorged blood vessels are seen frequently next to glands' openings. Magnification: 500:1; LM. **c)** Blood capillary of the stroma. Ruptured endothelium with passing blood elements. Diapedesis is also apparent. Magnification: 2.500:1; TEM (Transmission electron microscopic photograph). **d)** Focal subepithelial bleeding and epithelium break. Magnification: 1200:1; LM.

lar openings were left in the middle of such degenerated areas. The edges of these stumps projected upwards and then rolled outwards. We believe that they are of significance for regeneration of the epithelium (Figure 4). The denuded areas were covered with blood cells, cell debris, fibrin, and predominantly microphages. Adjacent to these areas of desquamation luteal phase endometrium was identified distant to the cornual and isthmic regions. As a characteristic feature of the luteal phase endometrium, apical secretion was seen (Figure 5b), together with cilia and microvilli on the surface of the cells (Figure 5c). The endometrium covering the focal points of bleeding, revealed cellular organelles with signs of degeneration. The lipid granules lost their content and formed predominantly small vesicles which then ran together to form vacuoles. The intercellular junctions became enlarged and the cell membranes showed projections and involutions indicating cell degeneration. Pyknosis was also observed (Figure 5d).

The largest extension of destructed areas is reached on day 3 of the new menstrual cycle. Besides mitotic activity we found migration processes of white blood cells and microphages (Figure 6). This is considered to be the multicentric beginning of epitheliol reparation. Beginning with glandular stumps, the cornua of the fallopian tube, the area around the internal os and rarely from islands of endometrium in the midst of the uterus tissue, tongs are seen which grow together and epithelialize the interglandular areas (Figure 7). Cell form and size varies in the regenerating epithelium. There are however predominantly cuboidal cells (Fig. 8). The surface is smooth, microvilli can be seen on day 5 of the cycle with now predominant regenerated epithelium. Defects are small and scanty (Figure 8b). On electron microscopy we were impressed by the dense plasma of the cells, which explained the dark appearance. The cell type was at that time cuboidal with round nuclei and well developed nucleoli.

On day 6 we found cilia also in the middle part of the endometrium. They may be considered as the early result of estrogenic activity (Figure 9).

Considerable variation on the various days of the cycle was seen relating denuded and intact epithelium of the endometrium. Therefore we tried to establish some semiquantitative data. Since we took a piece of tissue of 1 cm^2 from the anterior and posterior wall of the uterus, we used areas of similar size of the region of the cornua of the fallopian tube and the internal os as a control. The entire surface of the cavum uteri was examined by reflected light microscope, planimetered and set in relation to the 4 cm^2 of the tissue seen by SEM, using small magnification. The normal and defect areas per square centimeter were measured and related to the total surface area, which was considered to be 100%. The relation between destructed and repaired endometrium was expressed at the various days of the cycle as a deviation of 100% (Figure 10). In our material the largest destruction was seen on day 3 of the cycle. However, there were already regenerated areas present. On day 6 approximately 20% of the total area of the endometrium was completely re-epithelialized. We had no controls of days 7 and 8 of the cycle, but on day 9 the endothelium surface was completely repaired.

DISCUSSION

There is room for ample discussion regarding the basic phenomenon of repair. We are in agreement with Ferenczy that ultrastructure fails to provide evidence for the assumption that regeneration is due to stromal cell transformation

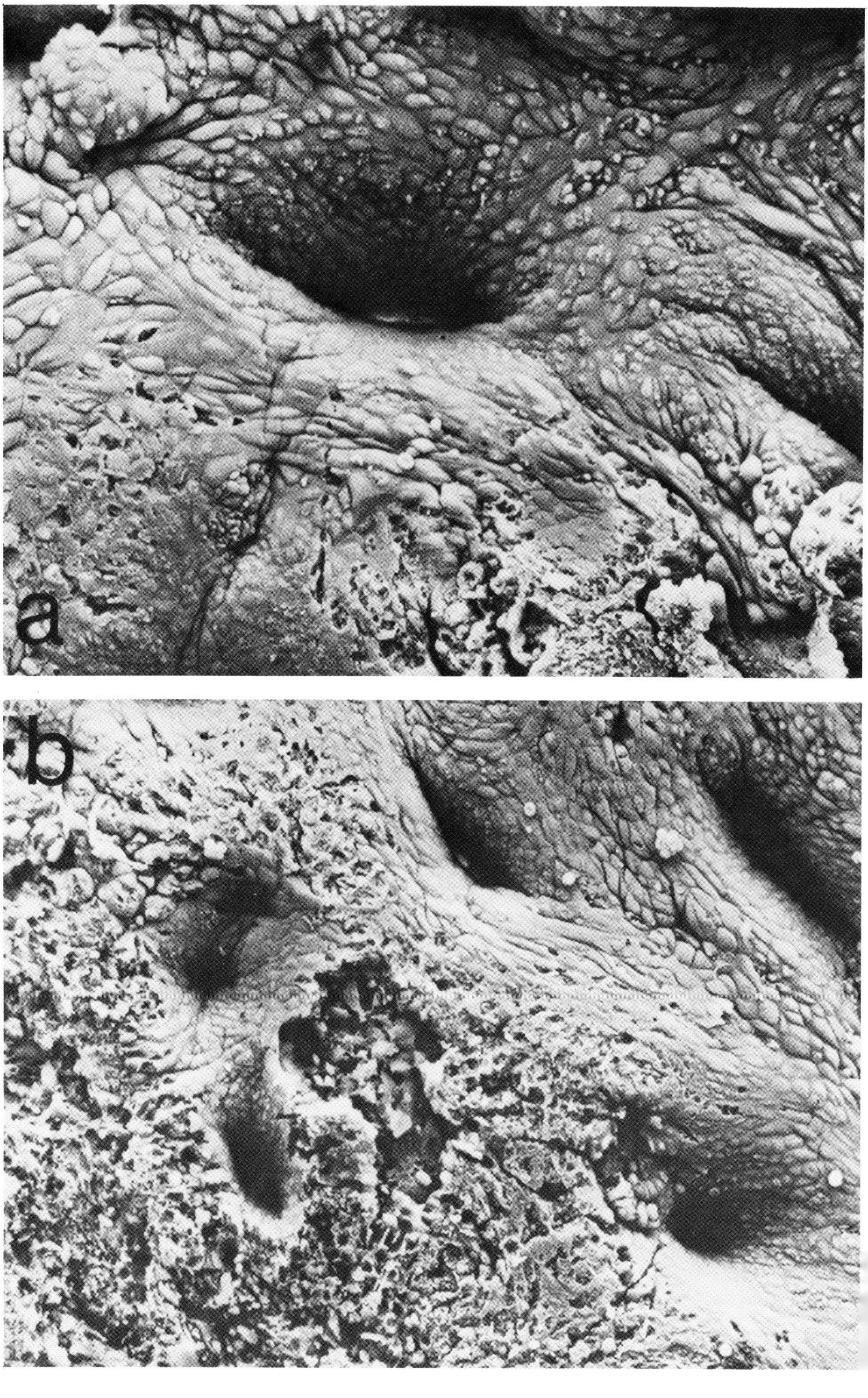

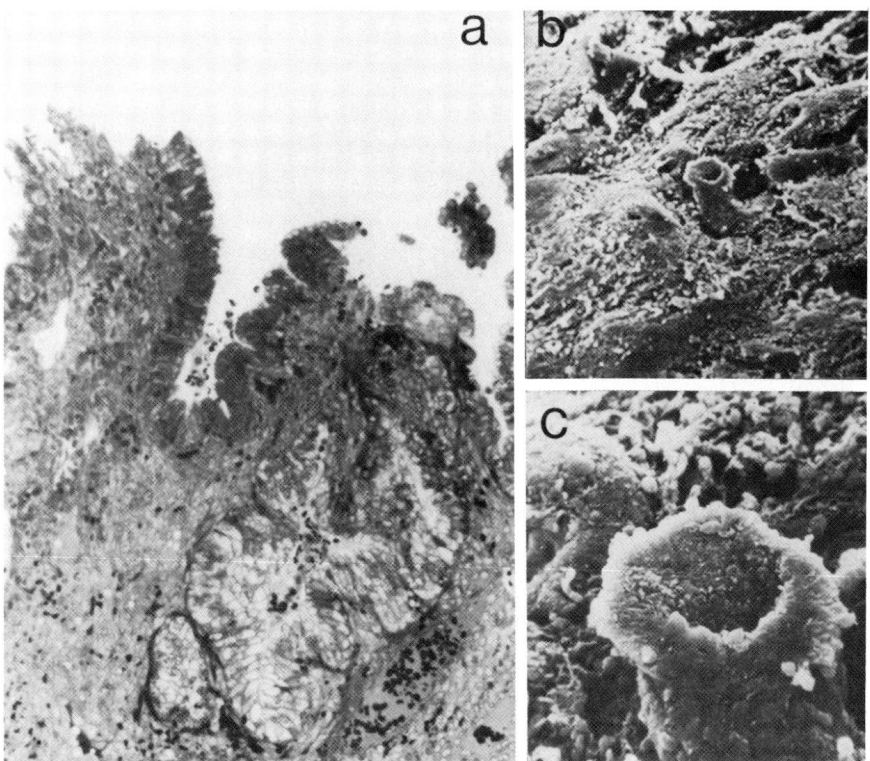

FIG. 4

FIGURE 4. Destroyed endometrial areas on the third day of the cycle. a) A solitary endometrial gland surrounded by denuded stroma. Some glandular structure exhibit already secretory function. Magnification: 500:1; LM. b) In the destroyed areas glandular stumps protrude the surface Magnification: 50:1; SEM. c) Other glandular stumps form collars which roll outwards. Re-epithelization starts from this area. Magnification: 250:1; SEM.

FIGURE 3. Scanning electron microscopic picture (SEM) showing the menstruating endometrial surface on the first day of the cycle. a) Gland opening with circularly splitting of the epithelium. Magnification: 200:1. b) Interglandular areas reveal partial desquamation of the surface epithelium. The remaining glandular openings show tendency to protuse. The denuded areas are covered with blood cells, fibrin, collagen fibrils and cellular debris. Magnification: 100:1.

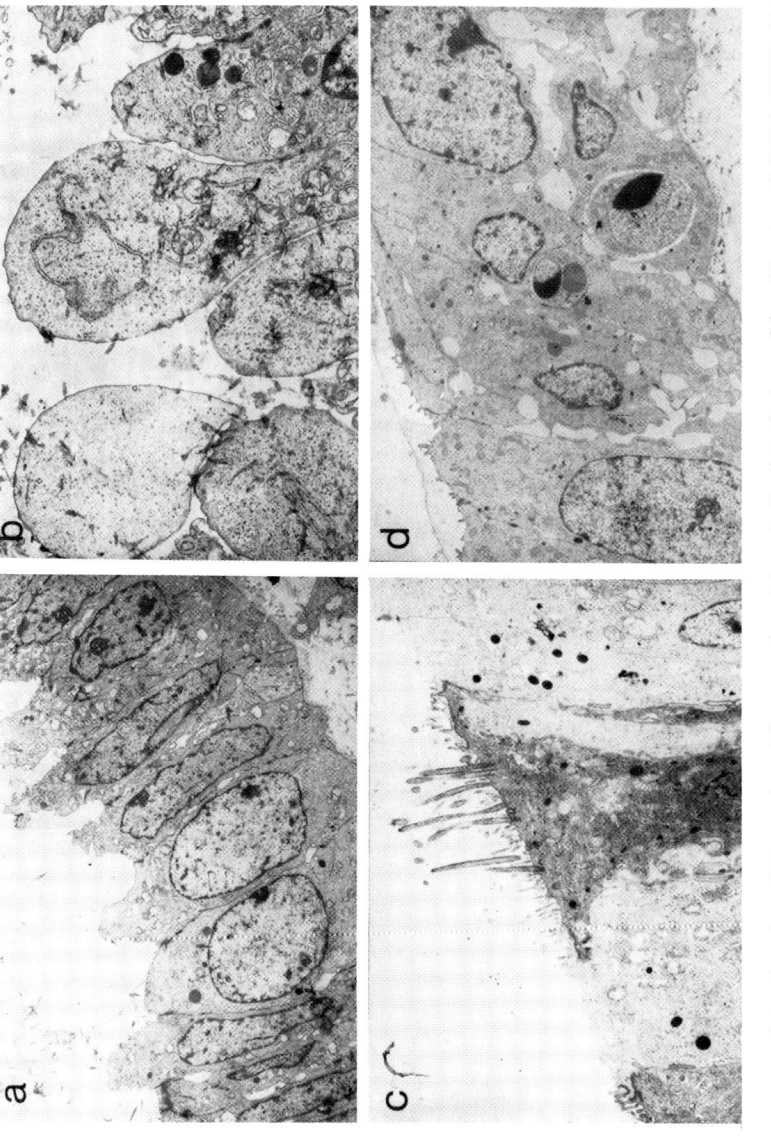

FIGURE 5. Observation of the first day of the cycle. **a)** Intact endometrium in the luteal phase. Magnification: 2.500:1; TEM. **b)** Partial apical secretion of the epithelial cells. Magnification: 3.400:1; TEM. **c)** Cilia, microvilli and intracellular lipid granules are found in the mid endometrial area. Magnification: 4.500:1; TEM. **d)** The endometrial epithelium of other areas revealed variation of destruction. The cell structures were indistinct, nucleoli disappeared and the lipid granules dissolved. The cells changed in form and size and showed signs of epitheliolysis Magnification: 3.400:1; TEM.

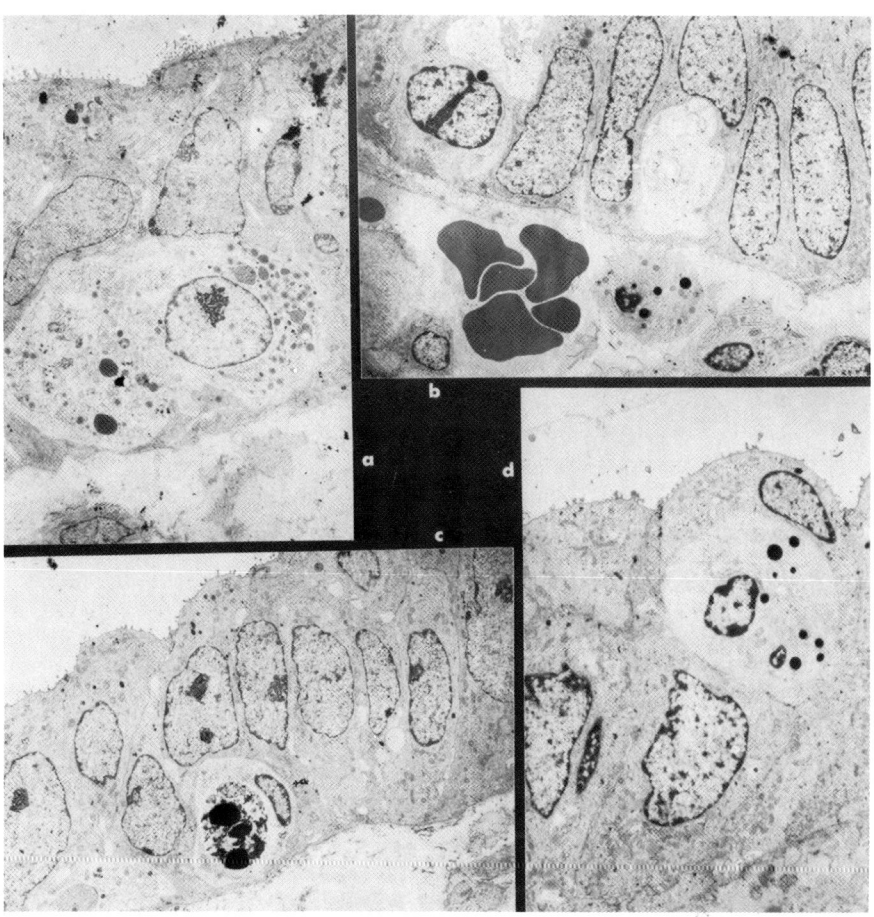

FIGURE 6. Mechanism of cell migration through the endometrial surface epithelium on the 3rd day of the cycle. **a)** Part of a microphage in the endometrial epithelium. **b)** Erythrocytes and Lymphocytes directly subepithelial. On the upper left side is early mitosis seen. **c)** Microphage with phagozyted lipid granules. **d)** Interepithelial migration of a lymphocyte. Magnification: 3.400:1; TEM.

---

into surface epithelial cells as suggested by light microscopy studies (Hitschmann and Adler, 1908; McLennan and Rydell, 1965; Baggish et al., 1967). Predominantly regeneration is related to the exposed glandular stumps and the surface epithelium of isthmic and cornual regions as indicated by Ferenczy (1976). However, we have observed in two uteri, islands of intact endometrium which remained intact. Both were on day 4 of the cycle. From the border areas tongue like reparation seemed to occur. We are therefore suggesting that denudation of the overlying spongiosa is not necessary in all instances but that remaining islands of glands have the potential of regenerating the endometrium from their border lines.

Further discussion applies to the time sequence of regeneration. Our data do not support the assumption that complete denudation of the interglandular surface has occurred on day 2 of the cycle. By using our semiquantitative technique we found that on day 2 only 70% of the entire midarea of the endometrium was destroyed. Desquamation was greatest on day 3 with 80% of the total area. On the other hand we observed on day 3 20% regenerating epithelium which then increased on the following days. On day 6 of the cycle 20% of the total area failed to be regenerated. In our study regeneration was completed on day 9 of the cycle. Regeneration can be completed in 48 hours but it is very difficult at present to make statements in regard to the normality of this time sequence. The clinical scholar of menstruation is well aware of the variation of duration of menstrual bleeding, as indicated in another paper (see above). It is our assumption that hemostasis is more related to regeneration processes than to clotting (Beller, 1971).

We expect large individual variation in regard to the onset of estrogen production. We do not regard the reported difference in time sequences of ciliogenesis as disagreement. In our material we have observed cilia on day six of the cycle as it was seen by Ludwig and Metzger, 1976).

The problem of "shedding" of the epithelial surface of the endometrium or partial shedding in a certain time sequence remains speculative. The distinction between a basal layer and a layer of functional spongiosa came from light microscopy studies of the endometrium. Certainly scanning electron microscopy is not a very good tool for delineating the two layers.

There are schemes in the literature based on the older experiments of Markee (1940) that the endometrium would regress 48 hours before the onset of bleeding. This does not agree with our observation. Bleeding starts when the endometrium is high and edematous. Desquamation is not a general phenomenon but develops in between glandular structures. Stromal edema is regressing when bleeding has started and desquamation of interglandular tissue has begun. This can be demonstrated by the greater cellularity seen in stromal tissue and as a result the glandular stumps protrude. Taken together it is very difficult to decide how and if these mechanisms occur together since layers of basalis and functionalis are difficult to distinct during menstruation.

However, it should be stressed in agreement with Ferenczy that the repair process of menstruation is not a result of early rising estrogen levels but a regeneration process of unique feature in the organism which may require much more work for complete understanding.

FIGURE 7. Endometrial re-epithelization on the fourth day of the cycle. a) Tongue-like epithelial growth covering the denuded stroma. b) Union of two epithelial growing sites, covering the stroma surface. Magnification: 1.200:1; LM.

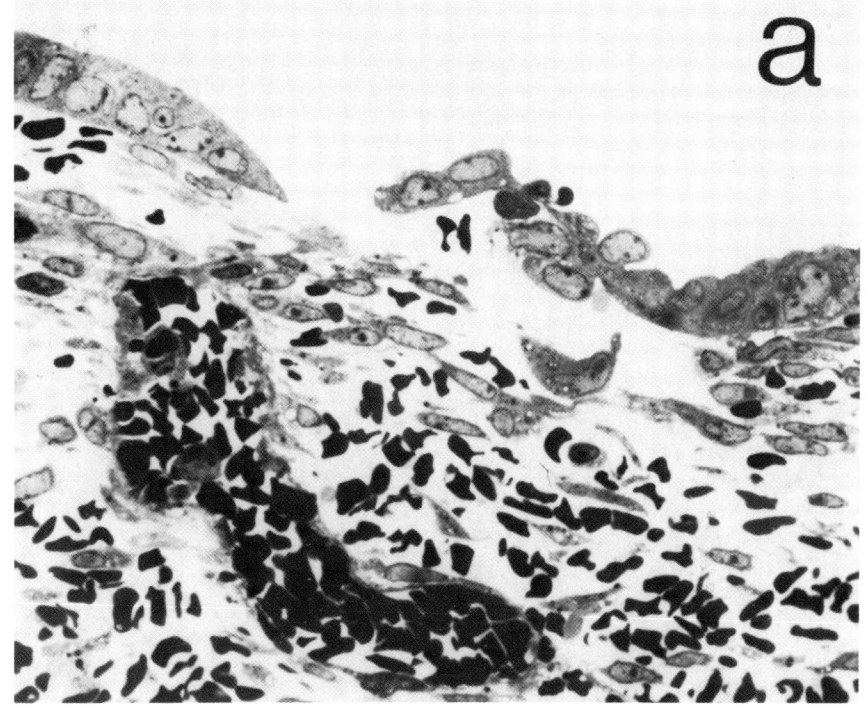
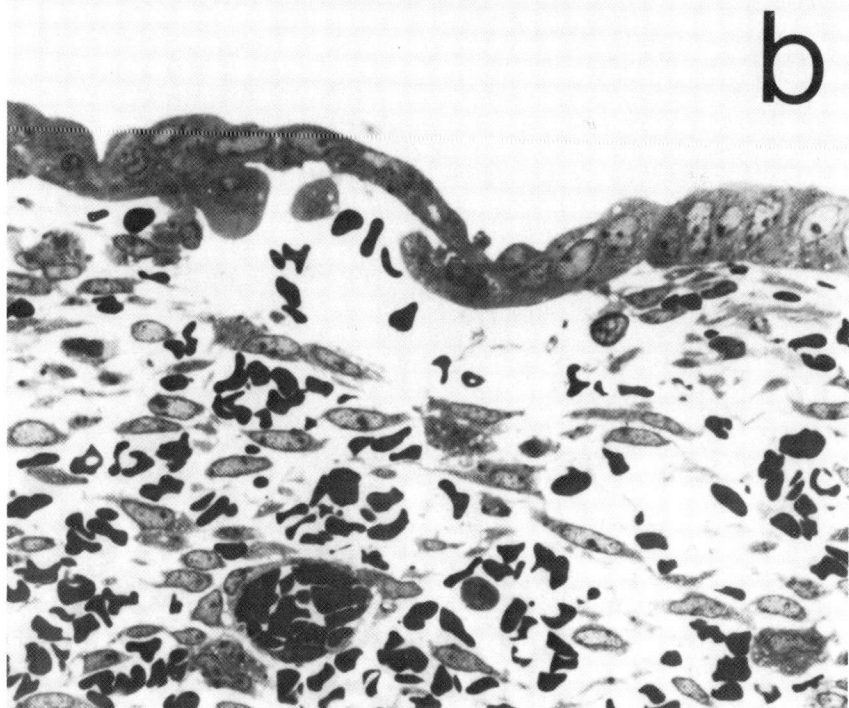

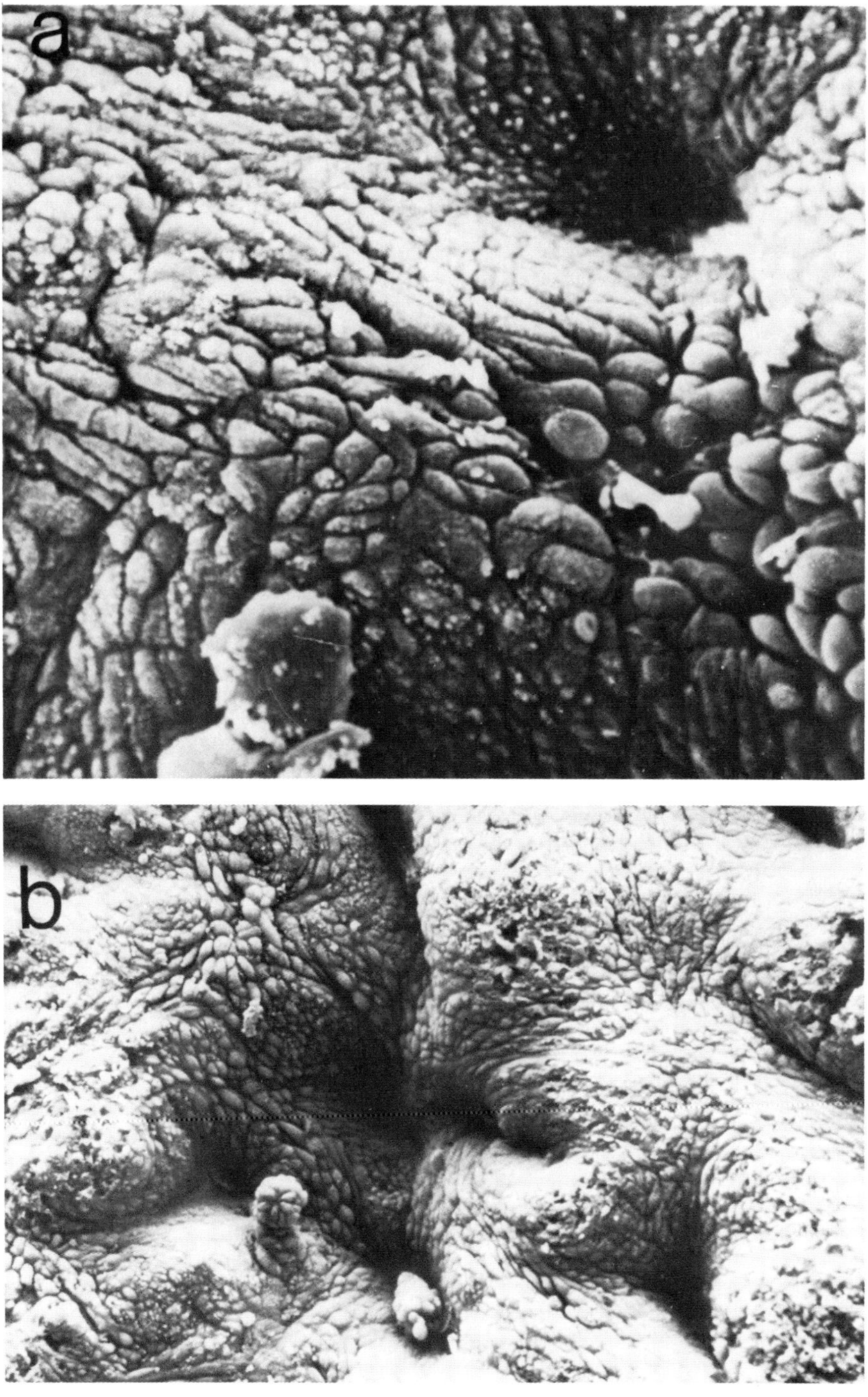

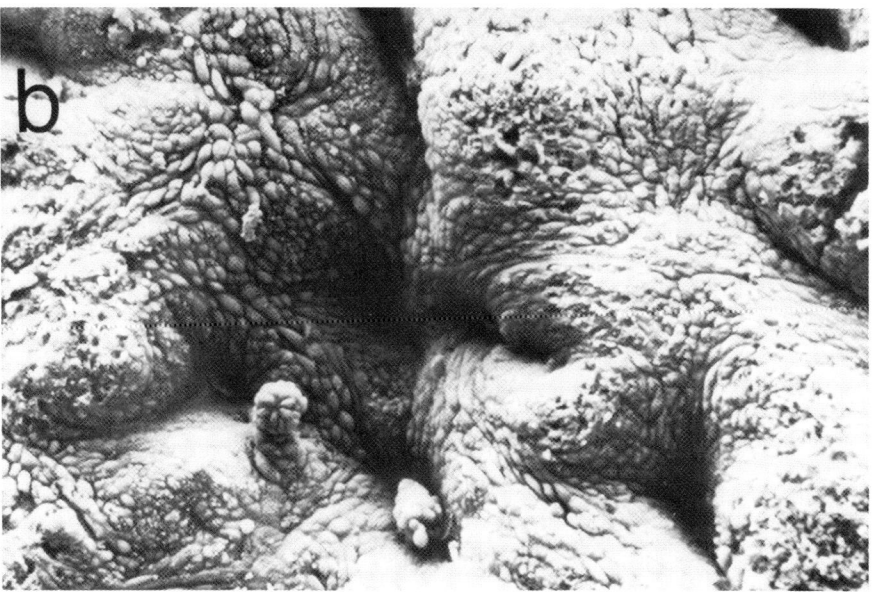

FIG. 8

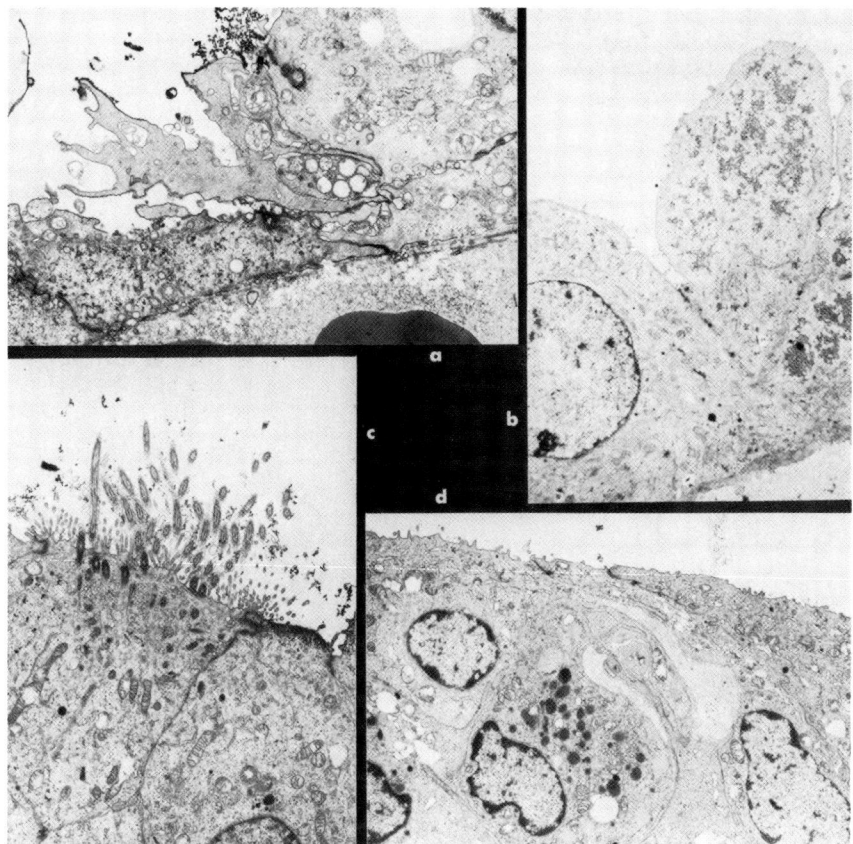

FIG. 9

FIGURE 9. Regenerated epithelium on the sixth day of the cycle. **a)** Regenerating epithelium with a bizarre dark cytoplasmic cell. Magnification: 7.100:1; TEM. **b)** Beginning of glycogenosis in a cuboidal endometrial cell with round nucleus. Magnification: 3.400:1; TEM. **c)** Beginning of cilogenesis at the same time. Magnification: 5.700:1; TEM. **d)** Re-epithelized area with cuboidal cells, round nuclei, dark cytoplasma and distinct lipid granules. Magnification: 4.500:1; TEM.

FIGURE 8. Mechanism of endometrial repair. **a)** Re-epithelized area surrounding a gland opening. The predominant cuboidal epithelial cells reveal a lack of microvilli and cilia. At the lower glandular border a small epithelial defect is preserved. Magnification: 400:1; SEM. **b)** Nearly complete repaired interglandular areas. Polygonal cells are characteristic for this regenerated area. Small epithelial defects were preserved at the borderline. Magnification: 100:1; SEM.

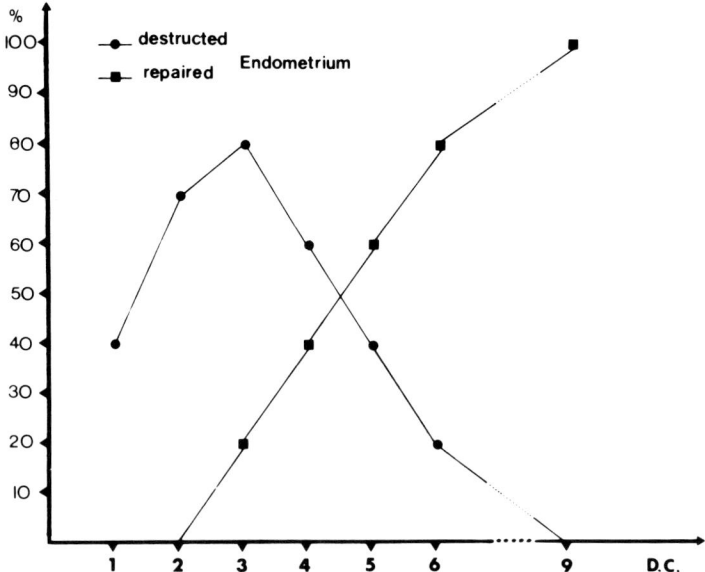

FIGURE 10. Relationship between destroyed and repaired endometrial areas correlated to the days of cycle.

ACKNOWLEDGEMENT

Supported by a Grant of Deutsche Forschungsgemeinschaft (Contract Nr. 648/5)

REFERENCES

Baggish, M.S., Pauerstein, C.J., Woodruff, J.D.: Role of stroma in regeneration of endometrial epithelium. Am. J. Obstet. Gynecol. 99:453, 1967.

Beller, F.K.: Observations on the clotting of menstrual blood and clot formation. Am. J. Obstet. Gynecol. 111:535, 1971.

Ferenczy, A.: Studies on the cytodynamics of human endometrial regeneration. I. Scanning electron microscopy. Am. J. Obstet. Gynecol. 124:64, 1976.

Ferenczy, A.: Studies on the cytodynamics of human endometrial regeneration. II. Transmission electron microscopy and histochemistry. Am. J. Obstet. Gynecol. 124:582, 1976.

Hitschmann, F., Adler, L.: Der Bau der Uterusschleimhaut des geschlechtsreifen Weibes mit besonderer Berücksichtigung der Menstruation. Mschr. Geburtsh. Gynäk. 27:1, 1908.

Ludwig, H., Metzger, H.: Human Female Reproductive Tract. A scanning electron microscopy atlas. Springer (1976) Berlin-Heidelberg-New York.

Ludwig, H., Metzger, H.: The Re-Epithelization of the Endometrium after menstrual desquamation. In: Scanning Electron Microscopy (Part IV). Proceedings of the Workshop on SEM in reproductive Biology. JIT Research Institute (1976) Chicago.

Markee, J.E.: Menstruation in intraocular endometrial transplants in the Rhesus monkey. Contr. Embryol. Carneg. Instn. 28:219, 1940.

McLennan, C.E., Rydell, A.H.: Extent of endometrial shedding during normal menstruation. Obstet. Gynecol. 26:605, 1965.

Rockenschaub, A.: Wie wird das Endometrium abgebaut? Gynaecologia 149:176, 1960.
Schröder, R.: Gynäkologie. Springer Verlag Berlin (1947).
Themann, H., Schünke, W.: Die Feinstruktur der Drüsenepithelien des menschlichen Endometriums. Elektronenoptische Morphologie. In: H. Schmidt-Mattiesen. Das normale menschliche Endometrium. Georg Thieme (1963) Stuttgart.
Wynn, R.M.: Biology of the uterus. Plenum Press (1977) New York.

HISTOENZYMOLOGY OF THE HUMAN ENDOMETRIUM DURING MENSTRUATION (II)

C. E. Flowers and W. H. Wilborn

SUMMARY

Menstruation represents a failure in the important biologic process of reproduction. The endometrium immediately attempts to prepare itself for a successful reproductive cycle by rapidly healing injured areas and remodeling its structure. This is accomplished by regressing and eliminating waste products. Cellular debris is phagocytized and expelled into the gland lumen. The manufacture of glycoprotein is discontinued and expelled directly from its cell; lipid is phagocytized. Lysosomes aid in the internal digestion of cellular wastes and the digestion of dead cells. Mucins within the endometrium protect its undamaged cells from the lytic effect of lysosomal enzymes.

INTRODUCTION

Menstruation is a remarkable biological process which is peculiar to primates. It has captured the interest of clinicians and researchers for many years and still poses many interesting and unanswered questions.

One question of continued interest concerns the extent to which the endometrium is shed during menstruation. The traditional belief is that the compact and

Department of Obstetrics and Gynecology, The University of Alabama in Birmingham, Birmingham, Alabama and Department of Anatomy, University of South Alabama, Mobile, Alabama

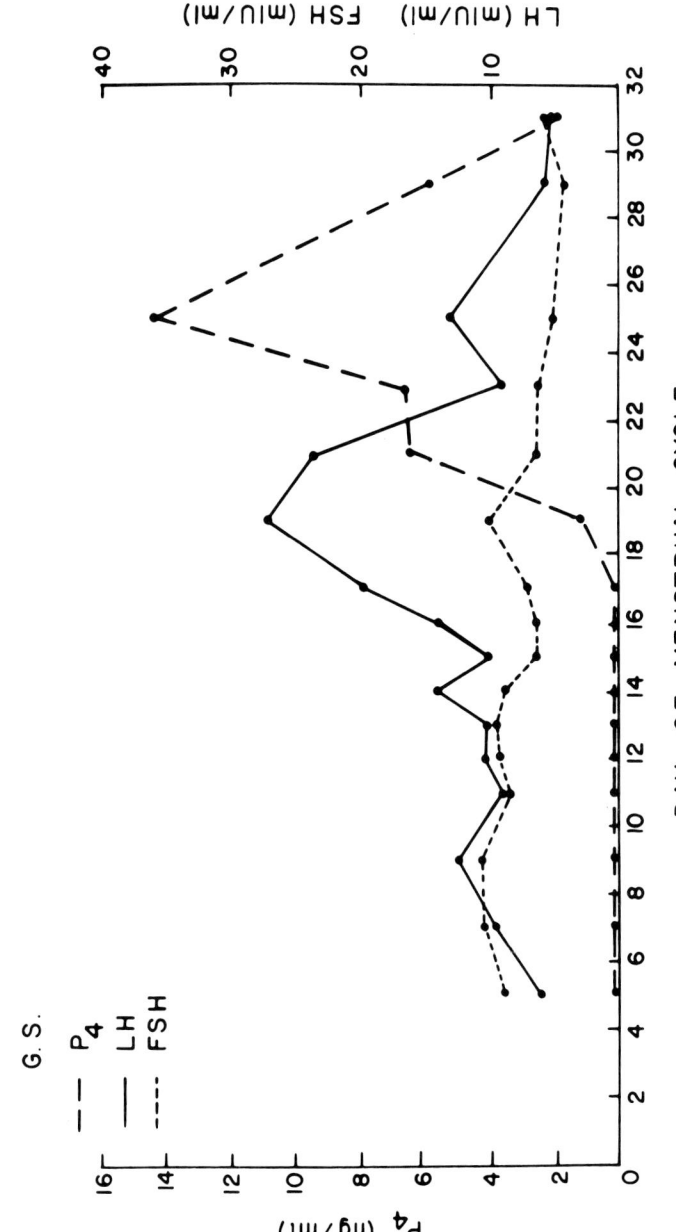

FIGURE 1. Follicle stimulating hormone (FSH), luteinizing hormone (LH), and progesterone (P_4) levels in one patient (GS).

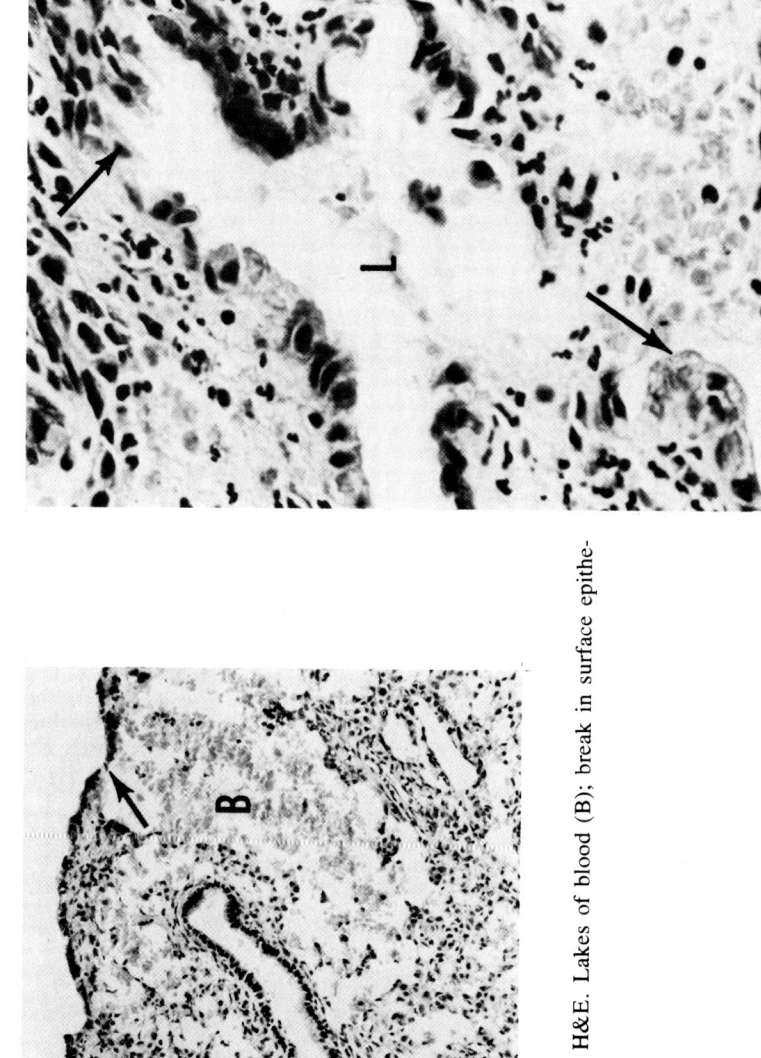

FIGURE 2. Day 1, Paraffin section, H&E. Lakes of blood (B); break in surface epithelium (arrow). X120

FIGURE 3. Day 2, Paraffin section, H&E. Degenerating segment of gland showing stromal elements in lumen (L), gland cells that have been retained, and basement membrane (arrows). X480

spongy zones are lost and regeneration takes place at the basal layer (Bohnen, 1927). This idea is propagated in certain textbooks of histolology (Greep, 1973), pathology (Robbins, 1974), and gynecology (Taylor, 1962). The recent studies of Ferenczy (1976a, 1976b) also support the traditional view. Contrarily, others believe that the compact layer may undergo total or partial desquamation but part or all of the spongy layer remains and participates in the regeneration process (Bartelmez, 1931; Bartelmez and Culbertson, 1933; Rockenschaub, 1960a, 1960b; McLennan and Rydell, 1965; Flowers and Wilborn, 1978).

This study was designed to contribute additional information on the histoenzymological and morphological processes involved in endometrial shedding. We take this opportunity to present some of our work in a unified form and to present our own opinions and interpretations in an effort to unravel the fascinating process involved in menstruation.

MATERIALS AND METHODS

These studies were performed on the endometria of three normal ovulating patients (23, 27, and 28 years in age). The adequacy of the luteal phase was established by the criteria of Noyes et al. (1950) on sections stained with hematoxylin and eosin (H&E). The occurrence of ovulation and the adequacy of progesterone were determined through follicle stimulating hormone (FSH), luteinizing hormones (LH), and progesterone (P_4) radioimmunoassay studies.

Human LH and FSH levels were determined in serum according to standard radioimmunoassay procedures. A total of 60 biopsies were obtained over nine menstrual cycles from the three patients. The women had regular cycles and the approximate time bleeding would begin was highly predictable. Biopsies were adequate and carefully made two days prior to bleeding, on each day of menses, and on days 6–9 following cessation of menstrual flow. The curette was maneuvered with sufficient pressure to include the basalis. At least three generous biopsies were obtained from different areas of one-half of the endometrial cavity. When two biopsies were taken during one month, the second series were obtained from the previously unbiopsied sites. Biopsies were taken only every third month in order that complete regeneration of the endometrium could occur.

Each biopsy was cut into smaller portions to be used for histology, histochemistry, transmission electron microscopy, and scanning electron microscopy. These procedures and their importance to the study have been described in previous publications (Flowers et al., 1974; Flowers and Wilborn, 1978; Wilborn and Flowers, 1979) and in a preceding paper of this symposium. Histochemical procedures employed to evaluate the endometrium during menses included periodic acid-Schiff, alcian blue (pH 2.5 and pH 0.5), alkaline phosphatase, acid phosphatase, and succinate dehydrogenase. In addition to these methods, sudan black B and oil red O were used according to standard techniques to demonstrate lipids in 10 μm frozen sections fixed in 10% calcium formol. Lipids were also studied in tissues fixed in osmium tetroxide.

RESULTS

Our findings deal with the main endometrial components: the surface epithelium, glands, stroma, and blood vessels. It should be noted that our results concern elements in the spongy and compact zones of the functionalis, and not those in the basalis. Furthermore, it should be indicated for clarity that cells closely associated with glands, surface epithelium, and blood vessels are referred to as predecidual cells while other cells of the stroma are termed stromal cells.

A graph illustrating levels of FSH, LH, and P_4 in one patient is shown in Figure 1. These data were obtained for each patient to document normal ovulation and the adequacy of progesterone.

Alkaline phosphatase activity was consistently weak during menstruation. Succinate dehydrogenase activity varied from weak to moderate. Sections stained with alcian blue likewise require little comment because of the variations in staining intensities encountered during menstruation. The most important observation was the presence of a cell coat of alcian blue-positive material which remained throughout menstruation. The coat contained both sialomucins and sulfomucins and, as shown later, was vividly demonstrated by the ruthenium red techniques and transmission electron microscopy.

Although it would be convenient and helpful to stereotype certain events of menstruation as occurring on day 1, others on day 2, etc., it was found early in our studies that this simply could not be done. Some cells, for example, manifested the features on day 1 that other cells showed on day 3. We have chosen, therefore, to emphasize the events of menstruation since the cells involved did not all respond identically or at the same time.

Hematoxylin and Eosin

The histology of menstruating endometrium closely approximated that described in the elegant works of Rockenschaub (1960a, 1960b) and McLennan and Rydell (1965).

Examination of histological sections from biopsies taken on days 27–28 of the cycle before the onset of clinical bleeding showed that the endometrium had regressed to approximately one half its height in the secretory phase. Significant amounts of extravascular blood in the stroma indicated that bleeding actually began at least two days before blood appeared in the vagina. Within the spongiosa, some glands were more tortuous than others. They were relatively straight in the compacta. Some cell apices were frayed and entered the lumina as secretory products. Small breaks were present in the gland wall which permitted stromal cells, leukocytes, and erythrocytes to reach the gland lumina for passage to the uterine cavity. Predecidual cells showed varying degrees of hypertrophy and were most abundant in the compact layer beneath the surface epithelium.

On day 1 of menstruation, the surface epithelium was intact except at a few sites (Figure 2). Large lakes of blood were present in the spongiosa and occasionally extended into the narrow compact zone beneath the surface epithelium. Extravascular blood in the compacta escaped through breaks in the surface epithelium into the lumen of the uterine cavity. There was insufficient pressure from the pools of blood to evaginate the surface epithelium. It appeared, therefore, that epithelial detachment and the concomitant release of blood resulted from the lytic action of blood and/or stromal enzymes.

At no time during menstruation was there complete denudation of the surface epithelium. Reepithelialization of broken areas began immediately after the majority of blood in the lake had escaped into the uterine cavity. Areas of healing were numerous by the second day of menstruation and were easily recognized by the presence of surface epithelial cells with pale cytoplasm. These cells resembled

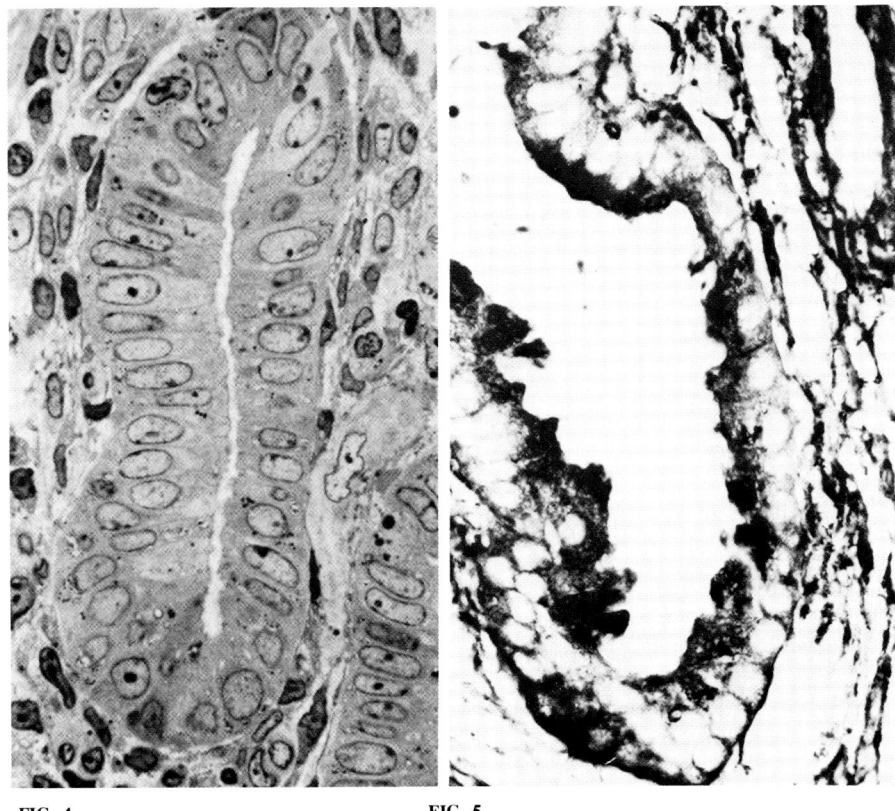

FIG. 4 FIG. 5

FIGURE 4. Day 2, Plastic section, toluidine blue. Unaltered gland. X480

FIGURE 5. Day 2, Paraffin section, PAS. Gland with PAS-positive material concentrated in cell apices. Stromal and predecidual cells are also PAS-positive. Nuclei are unstained. X480

the "clear cells" described by others (Feyrter, 1949, 1952; Fuchs, 1959) as representing newly formed cells.

Glands on the first day of menstruation contained foci of dead or degenerating cells separated by areas of viable cells. Large intercellular spaces were present between many cells. There were breaks in the gland wall through which stromal elements passed into the gland lumen which resulted in the accumulation of erythrocytes, all types of leukocytes, and stromal cells within the lumen. Predecidual cells were closely applied to the basement membrane at most sites along the gland base. It was interesting that breaks in the gland wall were not seen where layers of predecidual cells were contiguous with the gland base. Thus, even at the light microscopic level, predecidual cells seemed to support the glands, maintain their intactness, prevent their invasion by stromal elements, and provide nourishment for the epithelial cells and blood vessels.

As menstruation continued through the third day, larger breaks appeared in the walls of some glands, more cells degenerated, and the glands became smaller. By careful study of serial sections, however, it was obvious that only portions of some glands were lost (Figure 3). The basement membrane was retained at such sites. The cells which remained underwent mitoses and began repopulation and repair of the gland. Clear cells in regenerating glands resembled those of the surface epithelium. The basement membrane acted as a sleeve along which newly formed epithelial cells moved in reepithelialization of the defective area.

One Micron Epoxy Sections Stained with Toluidine Blue

Thin plastic sections stained with toluidine blue provided better cytological detail than conventional paraffin sections and clearly showed that many glands did not undergo significant alterations during menstruation (Figure 4). Unaltered segments occurred throughout the functionalis. Predecidual cells were abundant about viable glands.

Viable cells in glands had moderately dense cytoplasm and were not associated with the large intercellular spaces which were often adjacent to dead or degenerating cells. Nuclei were somewhat pale and contained nucleoli.

Glands in menstruating endometrium sometimes contained degenerating cells on one side of the lumen and viable cells on the opposite side. Degenerating cells possessed dark cytoplasm, a hallmark which readily distinguished them from viable cells with ligher cytoplasm. They demonstrated the classical characteristics of impending cell death, including pyknotic nuclei, karyorrhexis, numerous cytoplasmic vacuoles, and fragmentation. Predecidual cells seldom bordered the basement membrane and in their absence stromal elements readily migrated into the gland lumina.

Periodic Acid-Schiff

The PAS technique showed much PAS-positive material in the surface epithelium, glands, and stroma on days 27–28 and during the first three days of menstruation (Figure 5). Most of the PAS-positive had been expelled by the cessation of menstrual flow. Incubation of sections in diastase greatly reduced the staining and indicated that glycogen was a main component of the PAS-positive material.

The PAS-positive material was concentrated in the apices and lumina of glands. In contrast, it was present in both the basal and apical region of surface epithelial cells. Stromal cells, laden with glycogen, and small extracellular particles of PAS-positive material migrated through the basement membrane to reach the grand lumina.

The conclusion was reached from the accumulation of material in gland lumina that the glands and stroma were expelling their secretory products during the process of menstruation. Since the surface epithelium was intact at most sites, the gland lumina provided avenues for the elimination of the discharged secretory products.

Large sacculated glands contained more PAS-positive material and were more infiltrated with stromal cells than smaller glands. Cells of such glands appeared degenerative. In contrast, cells with little or no PAS-positive material or with PAS-positive material only in their apices were viable. Cells with glycogen and other PAS-positive material were seen throughout menstruation. They had obviously survived menstruation since glycogen and glycoproteins are not normally synthesized during menses.

Acid Phosphatase

Activity of this lysosomal enzyme was high in most cells of the surface epithelium, glands, and stroma on days 27–28 and during the first three days of menstruation. The Sigma technique for acid phosphatase demonstrated lysosomes as small, distinct granules (Figure 6). With the Gomori method, the reaction was more intense and individual lysosomes were distinguishable only in areas of weak to moderate enzyme activity (Figure 7). Both methods showed that activity was highest on day 1 and gradually subsided on subsequent days.

The majority of glands demonstrated intense activity; a few showed moderate to weak activity. Some glands contained cells with varying degrees of activity (Figure 7). The fact that cells with the least activity were associated with degenerative areas suggested that a high level of enzyme activity was necessary for cell survival.

Many stromal cells with varying degrees of enzyme activity migrated through patent zones in the gland wall and accumulated in the lumen along with other menstrual debris. Decrease in luminal material after day 2 suggested that most of the debris was digested during early menses. The fact that enzyme activity remained high in the gland cells after day 3 indicated continued intracellular digestion of secretory products and effete organelles.

Lipid

Sudan black or oil red O demonstrated numerous lipid droplets in cells of the surface epithelium, glands, and stroma. The number of lipid droplets seemed to increase from the time regression began to the onset of menstruation. Most droplets were located at the base of gland and surface epithelial cells; a few were present in cell apices and lumina. They were randomly distributed in stromal cells and some were in the interstices. One micron plastic section of tissues fixed in osmium tetroxide also showed the small lipid droplets (Figure 8). Such sections confirmed results obtained with the classical lipid dyes and offered the additional advantage of permitting electron microscopic examination of the droplets in thinner sections of the same piece of tissue.

Transmission Electron Microscopy

Cells of the surface epithelium, glands, and stroma exhibited remarkable heterogeneity during menses. Some cells were dying, others were recovering from insult, and many appeared unaffected by menstruation.

The amount of lipid in the epithelial and predecidual cells was particularly striking in transmission electron micrographs (Figure 9). The rise in lipid content before the onset of menstruation was interpreted as due to the shutdown of

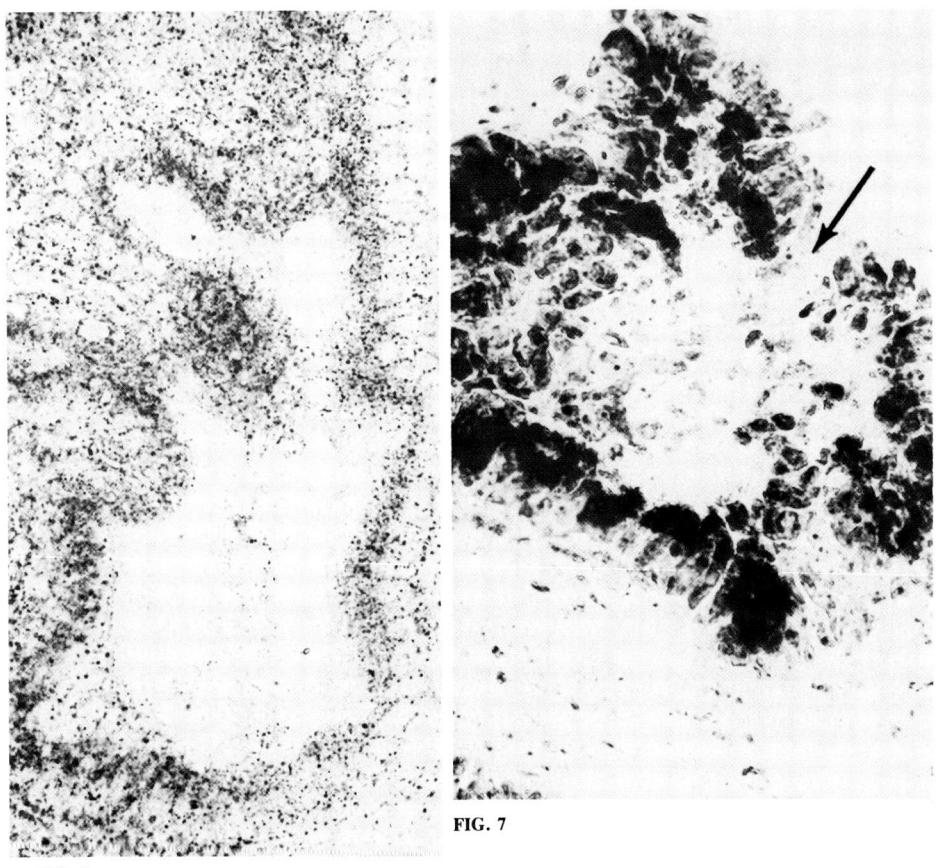

FIG. 7

FIG. 6

FIGURE 6. Day 28, Frozen section, Acid Phosphatase (Sigma). Small granules represent individual lysosomes and sites of enzyme activity in the large gland and surrounding stroma. X480

FIGURE 7. Day 1, Frozen section, Acid Phosphatase (Gomori). Gland cells with least activity are degenerating and associated with broken area (arrow) in gland wall. X480

cytological and enzymatic pathways previously used for the manufacture of secretory products. This, in turn, resulted in the conversion to lipid of the raw materials previously used for the formation of secretory products. Schmidt-Matthiesen (1963) held a similar view regarding the accumulation of lipid during menses.

Mitochondria in some cells contained aggregates of electron dense granules in their matrices. These granules (Figure 9) may have resulted from hemorrhagic shock. This idea correlates with the fact that similar granules have been observed in mitochondria of the liver and kidney of the rat following hemorrhagic shock by

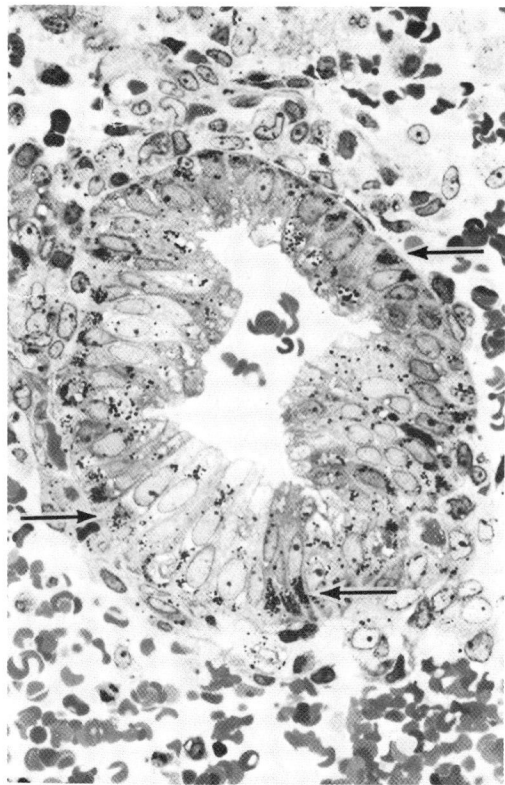

FIGURE 8. Day 1, Plastic section, Osmium tetroxide. Numerous lipid droplets (arrows) in gland cells. X480

lethal hemorrhage (White et al., 1973; Mela, 1974). It would seem that a similar condition in menstruating endometrium could result from necrosis of blood vessels. Mitochondria with electron dense granules in the rat have been found to have reduced respiratory activity (Mela, 1974). This finding corresponds with the reduced succinate dehydrogenase activity in menstruating endometrium.

Cells of the glands and surface epithelium of menstruating endometrium manifested a remarkable capacity to phagocytose vesicles, cell fragments, and basement membrane-like material. Short processes, not unlike pseudopodia, sometimes extended from the cell base and entrapped these stromal elements. As the vesicles and vacuoles of phagocytosed materials migrated from the basal to the apical cytoplasm, they focused with similar structures and many became large and pleomorphic (Figure 10). They were expelled by reverse pinocytosis into the gland lumen or into the lumen of the uterine cavity.

Cell bodies or processes of predecidual cells were closely apposed to the basal lamina at many sites during days 1–3 of menstruation. Vesicles of secretory material passed from the cell bodies or their processes into the gland or surface ep-

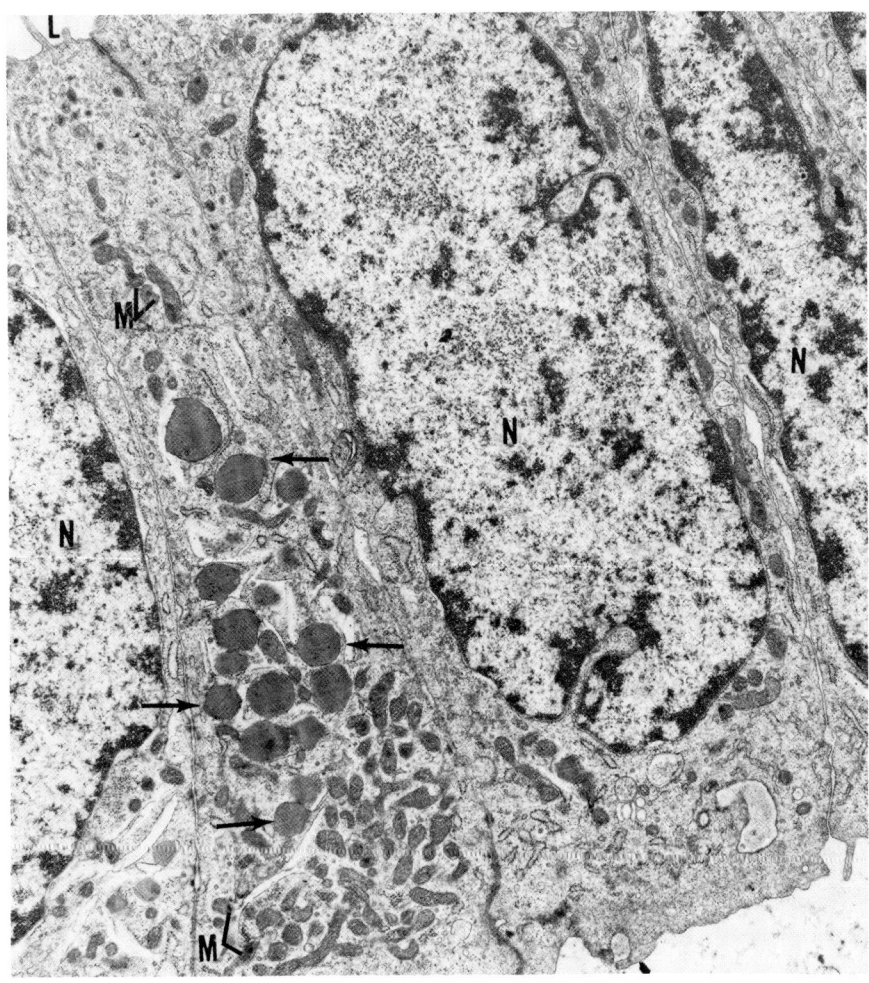

FIGURE 9. Day 1, TEM, base, apex, and lumen of gland. Droplets of lipid (arrows), nucleus (N), and mitochondria (M). X11,250

ithelial cells. The close apposition greatly reduced the distance that materials traversed in passing from predecidual cells into gland or surface epithelial cells.

As shown in photomicrographs, acid phosphatase activity was greater in viable cells of glands, surface epithelium, and stroma than in degenerating cells. Since acid phosphatase is a lysosomal enzyme, this finding correlates with the electron micrographs which also showed far greater numbers of lysosomes in viable cells than in degenerating cells. Lysosomes were membrane-bound electron dense bodies which ranged in size from about 0.2 μm to 5 or 6 μm (Figure 11). Use of the acid phosphatase technique at the electron microscopic level validated

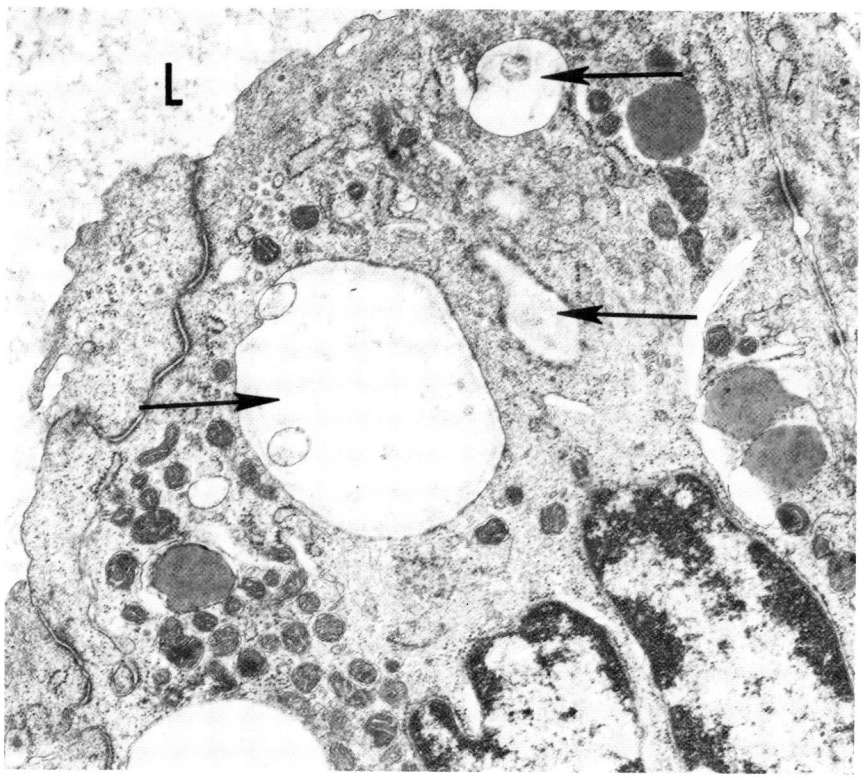

FIGURE 10. Day 2, TEM, gland apex. Large vacuoles of pleomorphic masses of material (arrows) in apical cytoplasm prior to passage into gland lumen (L). X22,000

that these bodies were lysosomes. Their membranes often coalesced with autophagic vacuoles which contained entrapped effete organelles and cytoplasmic inclusions. It was apparent that the lysosomes were essential in clearing the cytoplasm of secretory products and aged organelles. This view is in agreement with their function in other tissues (Aronson and DeDuve, 1968).

Cells of glands and surface epithelium in the process of dying had similar characteristics. They contained autophagic vacuoles of various sizes and much glycogen (Figure 12). Some lysosomes were present and they tended to fuse with the autophagic vacuoles. Intercellular spaces were prominent and contained flocculent material, cell fragments, or cells that had migrated from the stroma. Nuclei were irregular and often indented. Lipid droplets were particularly abundant at the cell base.

Macrophages, laden with lysosomes and vesicles, were present in menstruating endometrium (Figure 13). There was evidence that the macrophages developed from extravascular monocytes since all morphological variations were seen between them and typical monocytes. Some of the material which macrophages by heterophagocytosis had an electron dense core (Figure 13). Macro-

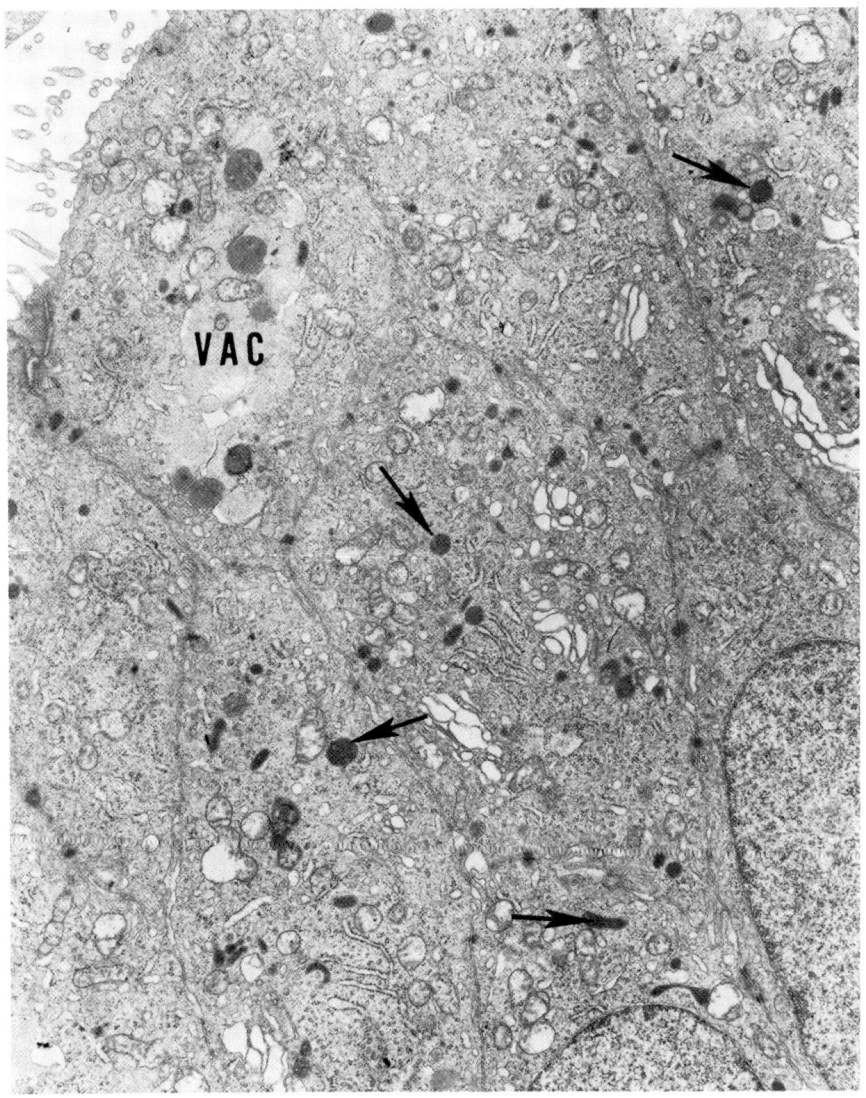

FIGURE 11. Day 4, TEM, gland apex. Numerous lysosomes (arrows) of various sizes are present. Several are associated with an autophagic vacuole (VAC). X8,100

phages or their processes which contained this material were easily identified as they migrated between cells of glands and surface epithelium to reach the lumina. It was interesting that dead or degenerating cells attached more macrophages than viable cells. This finding indicates that cells in the process of degeneration are releasing a macrophage attractant.

A few ciliated cells were present among the secretory cells of the glands and

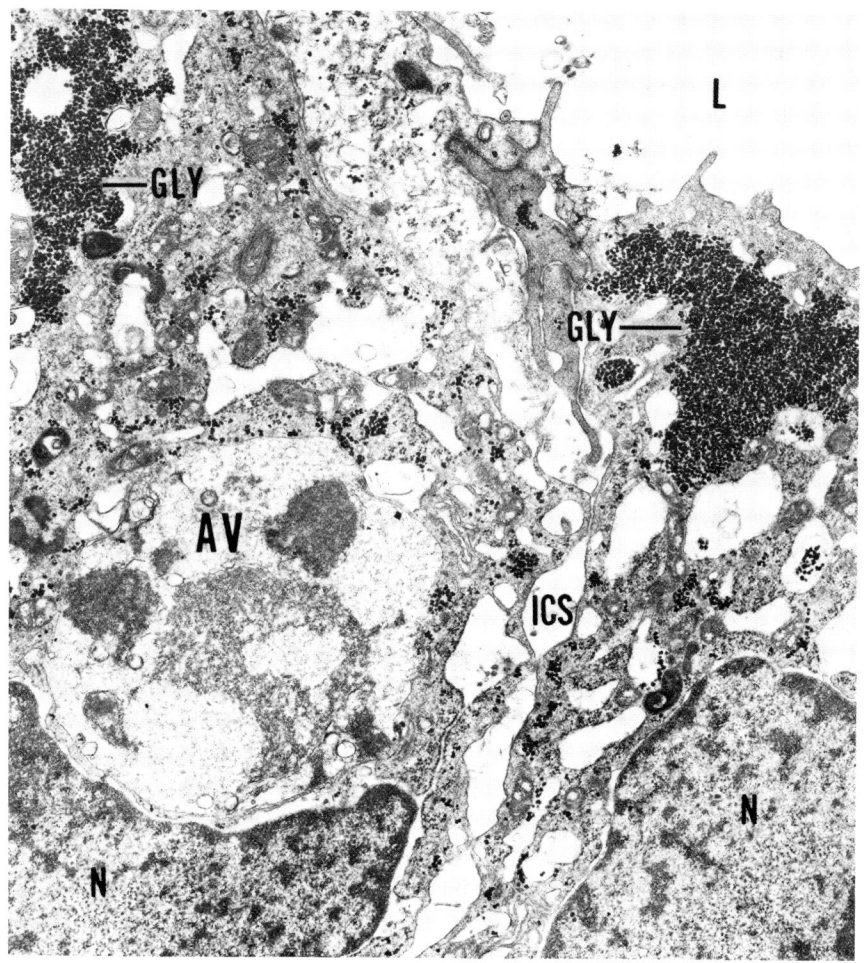

FIGURE 12. Day 1, TEM, gland apex, degenerating cells. Lumen (L), large autophagic vacuole (AV), glycogen (GLY), intercellular space (ICS), and nucleus (N). X22,000

surface epithelium. They had a somewhat electron lucent cytoplasm and in this respect resembled the pale, newly formed cells observed in histological sections. Ciliated cells were more numerous about the openings of glands and were important in expediting the flow of menstrual debris.

Reticular fibers of the stroma were also affected by menstruation. Lysosomes which escaped from disintegrating cells were present in certain areas of the stroma. Undoubtedly, the fibers in such areas were bathed in enzymes which had passed through defective or ruptured lysosomal membranes. The first sign of fiber destruction was loss of periodicity. This was followed by aggregation of the fibers into amorphous masses (Figure 14).

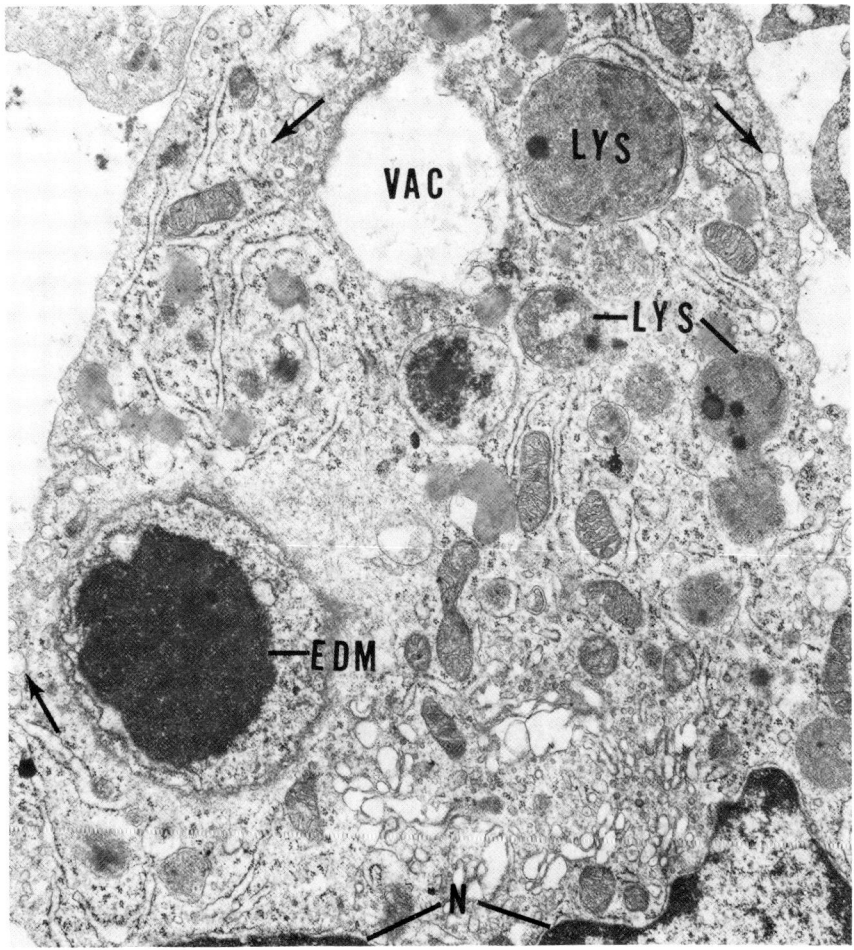

FIGURE 13. Day 2, TEM, macrophage in stroma. Lysosomes (LYS), vesicles (arrows), electron dense material (EDM), vacuole (VAC), and nucleus (N). X18,200

Many fibroblast-like stromal cells were present at some sites and new fiber formation took place concomitantly with fiber destruction. It was interesting that these cells were capable not only of synthesizing tropocollagen molecules for the formation of reticular fibers, but they were also capable of phagocytosing and degrading reticular fibers (Figure 15). This ability of the fibroblast-like stromal cells to degrade their own product provided the cellular basis for much of the remodeling and turnover of the stromal connective tissue.

Blood vessels of menstruating endometrium differed markedly in appearance. Most were perfectly normal but a few were dead or dying. Endothelial cells of viable vessels contained clearly defined organelles and numerous pinocytotic

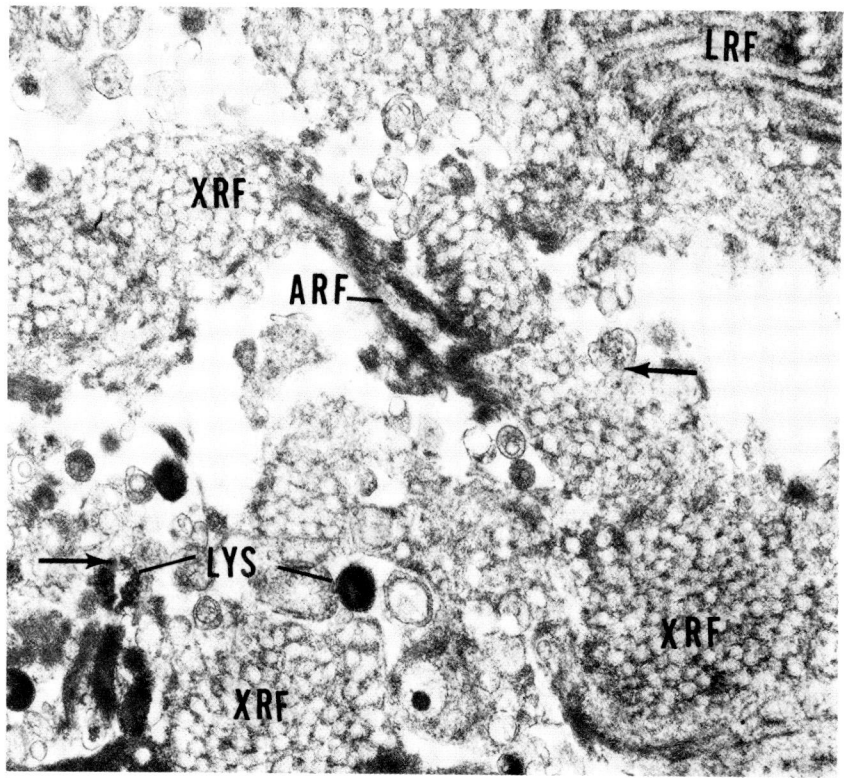

FIGURE 14. Day 1, TEM, reticular fibers of stroma. Reticular fibers in longitudinal section (LRF) showing cross striations. Reticular fibers in cross section (XRF). Amorphous masses of reticular fibers (ARF). Lysosomes (LYS). X27,500

vesicles. The vesicles indicated that waste products and nutrients were passing between blood and stroma. Predecidual cells occupied the periphery of these vessels.

Endothelial cells of dead or degenerating vessels contained ill-defined, greatly altered organelles, numerous vacuoles, and few pinocytotic vesicles. Nuclei were pyknotic and each was surrounded by a dilated perinuclear cisterna. Disrupted and vacuolated predecidual cells surrounded these vessels and their mitochondria often contained large granules. The reason some vessels degenerated was uncertain, but it was apparent that viable vessels were necessary for the survival of the surrounding tissue.

The extensiveness of cell death was estimated with the ruthenium red technique which stained the cytoplasm of dead or damaged cells, but did not stain viable cells with intact cell membranes. By counting the number of cells stained with ruthenium red on each day of menses, it was found that not more than 5% of the cells were dead or degenerating on any one day. This finding indicates that the vast majority of cells survive menstruation.

Ruthenium red demonstrated intracellular lipid droplets (including those in

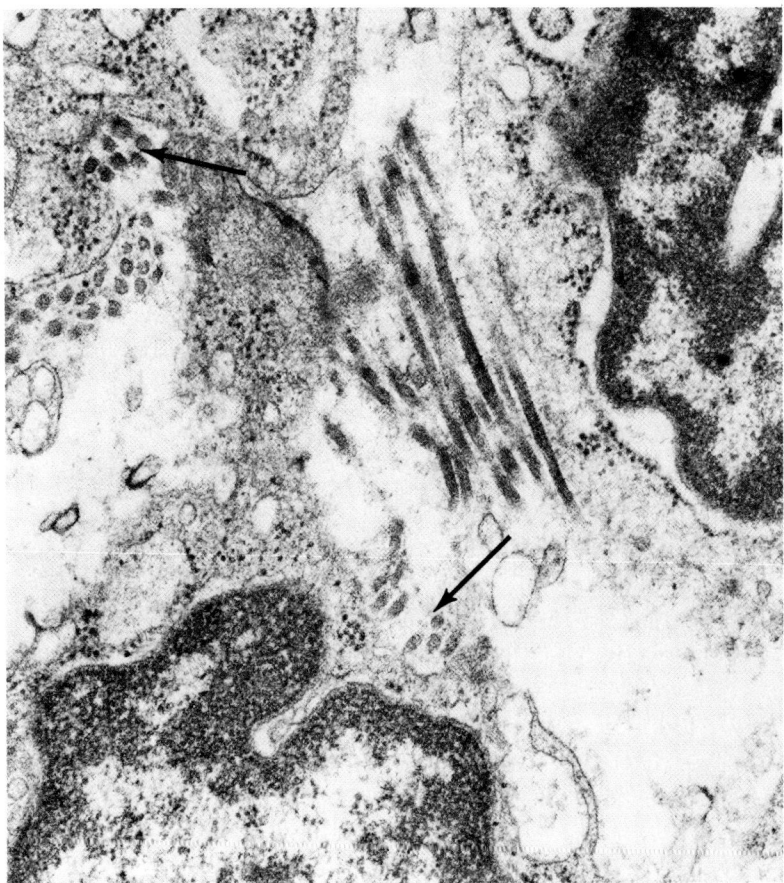

FIGURE 15. Day 4, TEM, fibroblast-like stromal cells and reticular fibers. Some of the reticular fibers (arrows) are in the process of being phagocytosed by the stromal cells. X45,000

certain types of lysosomes and autophagic vacuoles), intercellular spaces, the basement membrane, and the cell coat of carbohydrate at the apices of gland and surface epithelial cells. Widening of the intercellular spaces which occurred during menstruation allowed debris and macrophages a more direct passage to the lumina of the glands and uterine cavity. The cell coat was thickest on days 1–3 of menses.

Large amounts of ruthenium red-positive extracellular carbohydrates were present in the stroma. This material appeared to arise from the stromal and predecidual cells and to form their cell coat. Since ruthenium red stains acid carbohydrates, such as the mucins which protect the stomach from being digested by its own enzymes, it is tempting to speculate that the extracellular carbohydrates of the endometrium perform a similar function during menses (Figure 16).

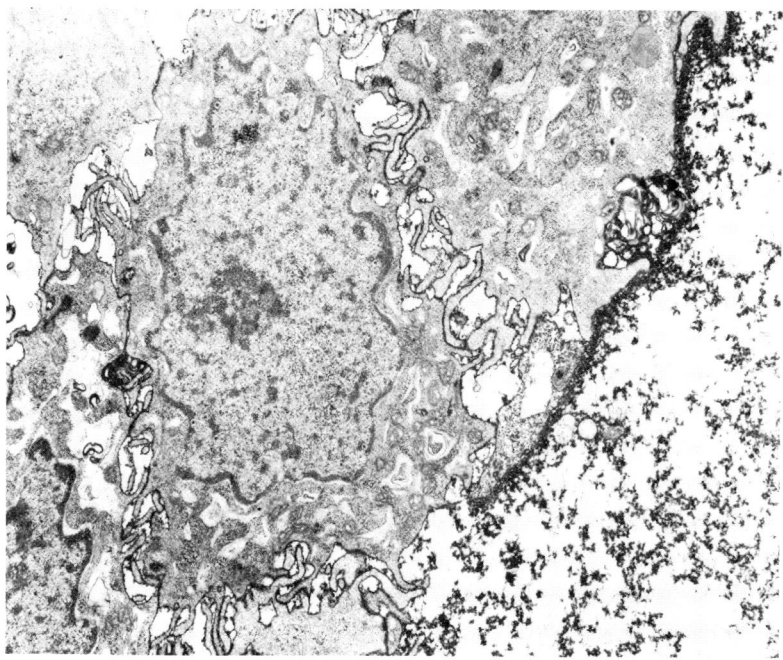

FIGURE 16. Day 6, TEM, stromal cells with interdigitating processes. Ruthenium red-positive material covers the surfaces of the processes as the cell coat and occupies much of the area outside the stromal cells. X13,650

An intriguing feature of the stromal and predecidual cells was their many interdigitating processes which were covered with ruthenium red-positive material. Furthermore, there were junctions between the cells and the membranes of adjacent cells appeared to fuse at some sites. We have previously proposed that the interlocking cell processes encrusted with secretory products constitute a conservatory force which helps to maintain the intactness of the functionalis during menses (Wilborn and Flowers, 1979).

Scanning Electron Microscopy

A tridimensional study of the endometrium during menses by scanning electron microscopy (SEM) provided new information and confirmed findings made by other techniques. The conclusion was reached with the PAS-technique that the cells were expelling secretory products during menses. This finding was vividly shown by SEM. Although most secretory products were expelled in the middle secretory phase, a second wave of expulsion began shortly before the onset of menstruation. This resulted in a thick population of small secretory droplets on the microvilli and cilia. The expelled secretion corresponded to the ruthenium red-positive material observed by TEM. Its role in protecting the endometrium from destruction during menses has already been proposed.

SEM supported the view that most of the surface epithelium remained during menstruation. It occasionally contained small breaks and in some areas it was hidden from view by a layer of fibrin and blood cells mixed with stromal elements. Cell apices flattened as the cells expelled their secretory products. Some areas showed more regression than others. Openings of glands extended above the surface epithelium in areas of greatest regression.

DISCUSSION

The most remarkable feature of menstruating endometrium was its valiant attempt to survive. This was manifested by lysosomal activity, expulsion and digestion of secretory materials, uptake of material from the stroma for passage to the uterine cavity, and macrophage activity. These events are set into motion only when conception does not occur and they are designed to save as much of the endometrium as possible and to prepare it for another attempt at reproduction.

Ruthenium red as a marker for dead cells illustrated that the vast majority of cells are viable at all times during menstruation. This impression was first gained while observing menstruating endometrium through a dissecting microscope. It resembled a burned over forest with stumps of varying heights and some areas which seemingly were unaffected. Further observations in a day or two showed the "greening of the forest" with healing of the scars. It was, however, only by the study of serial sections and the combined techniques of histochemistry and electron microscopy that the cellular events of menstruation could be appreciated.

Electron micrographs showed that the cells were in different phases of functional activity and in various stages of biological aging. Perhaps one of the adaptations of human endometrium is to have cells which age at various times. This would insure the availability of a sufficient number of cells for rapid regeneration and would, therefore, permit more frequent pregnancies.

Our results show that the chief event of menstruation is regression, rather than cell death. Regression occurs in a manner quite similar to the involution of the mammary gland following lactation (Helminen and Ericsson, 1968a, b, c; Helminen et al., 1968). Both endometrial regression and mammary gland involution are characterized by the physiological remodeling of cells, connective tissue, and certain types of degenerative processes. They involve autophagocytosis, heterophagocytosis, and the release of enzymes from leaky or damaged lysosomes. Autophagocytosis in the endometrium is attributable to lysosomes which digest portions of the cell's own cytoplasm, either by direct uptake of cytoplasmic constituents or by fusion with vacuoles which contain such constituents. Heterophagocytosis involves the phagocytosis of materials by macrophages. Digestion of reticular fibers results from the release of enzymes by extracellular lysosomes and by the phagocytosis of reticular fibers by fibroblast-like stromal cells. Individually and collectively, all of these processes contribute to the great regression that the endometrium undergoes during menstruation. Just as the slowing of these processes can be produced in the mammary gland by the administration of hormones (Helminen and Ericsson, 1968c), it is likely that cessation of endometrial regression is dependent on estrogen reaching a biologically effective level.

Identical findings for endometrial regression have been reported in lower animals, such as the rat and in a primitive mammal, the opossum (Padykula and

Taylor, 1976; Padykula and Campbell, 1976). The same events of endometrial regression also occur in epithelial and stromal cells of the nonpregnant bitch (Barrau et al., 1975).

The pinocytotic activity observed at the basal surface of cells of glands and surface epithelium is another mechanism for endometrial regression. It differs from the others which are largely concerned with the elimination of solid wastes. We have studied the microvillous-like processes at the cell base by means of ruthenium red staining and have found that they, like the microvilli of the intestine, are coated with acid carbohydrates. Thus, they are equipped chemically to attract and bind many types of molecules to their surfaces for eventual uptake by the cell. Basal pinocytosis seems to be the major mechanism for discharge of fluid wastes from the stroma during menstruation.

The basis for the disparity in views concerning the events of menstruation may be related to the frequent use of hysterectomy specimens. We found considerable microscopic hemorrhage within the endometrium when the hysterectomy was performed in the premenstrual phase, but this was particularly dramatic when the hysterectomy was done during the first day or two of menstruation. There was trauma to the endometrium during the operation, and more importantly, the hypoxia secondary to clamping the vessels apparently causes rupture of lysosomal membranes and, therefore, endometrial destruction. Further confusion may result from the use of hysterectomy specimens from patients with inadequate estrogen and progesterone levels. For these reasons, we avoided the use of hysterectomy specimens and chose instead to study endometrial biopsies from normal ovulating young women who had normal estrogen and progesterone values by radioimmunoassays.

REFERENCES

Aronson, N.N., Jr., and DeDuve, C.: Digestive activity of lysosomes. II. The digestion of macromolecular carbohydrates by extracts of rat liver lysosomes. J. Biol. Chem. 243:4564–4573, 1968.

Barrau, M.D., Abel, J.H., Jr., Uerhage, G., and Tietz, W.J., Jr.: Development of the endometrium during the estrous cycle of the bitch. Am. J. Anat. 142:47–66, 1975.

Bartelmez, G.W.: The human uterine mucous membrane during menstruation. Amer. J. Obstet. Gynecol. 21:623–625, 1931.

Bartelmez, G.W., and Culbertson, C.: Histological studies on the menstruating mucous membranes of the human uterus. Contrib. Embryol. 24:143–186, 1933.

Bohnen, P.: Wie weit wird das Endometrium bei der Menstruation abestossen. Arch. Gynak. 129:459–472, 1927.

Ferenczy, A.: Studies on the cytodynamics of human endometrial regeneration. I. Scanning electron microscopy. Am. J. Obstet. Gynecol. 124:64–74, 1976a.

Ferenczy, A.: Studies on the cytodynamics of human endometrial regeneration. II. Transmission electron microscopy and histochemistry. Am. J. Obstet. Gynecol. 124:582–595, 1976b.

Feyrter, F.: Uber die Vermehrung der Hellen Zellen bei der Hyperplasia glandularis endometrii cystica. Vichows Arch. path Anat. 316:435–438, 1949.

Feyrter, F.: Zur Frage der Hellen Zellen der menschlicken Gebamutterschleimhaus. Virchows Arch. path Anat. 321:134–137, 1952.

Flowers, C.E., Jr., and Wilborn, W.H.: New observations on the physiology of menstruation. Obstet. Gynecol. 51:16–24, 1978.

Flowers, C.E., Jr., Wilborn, W.H., and Enger, J.: Effects of quingestanol acetate on the histology, histochemistry, and ultrastructure of the human endometrium. Amer. J. Obstet. Gynecol. 120:589–612, 1974.

Fuchs, M.: Uber die "Hellen Zellen" im Epithel der menschlichen Uterusschleimhaut. Acta. anat. (Basel) 39:244–259, 1959.

Greep, R.O., and Weiss, L.: *Histology*. Blakiston, New York, 1973.

Helminen, H.J., and Ericsson, J.L.E.: Studies on mammary gland involution. I. On the ultrastructure of the lactating mammary gland. J. Ultrastruct. Res. 25:193–213, 1968a.

Helminen, H.J., and Ericsson, J.L.E.: Studies on mammary gland involution. II. Ultrastructural evidence for auto- and heterophagocytosis. J. Ultrastruct. Res. 25:214–227, 1968b.

Helminen, H.J., and Ericsson, J.L.E.: Studies on mammary gland involution. III. Alterations outside auto- and heterophagocytic pathways for cytoplasmic degradation. U. Ultrastruct. Res. 25:228–239, 1968c.

Helminen, H.J., Ericsson, J.L.E., and Orrenius, S.: Studies on mammary gland involution. IV. Histochemical and biochemical observations on alterations in lysosomes and lysosomal enzymes. J. Ultrastruct. Res. 25:240–252, 1968.

Markee, J.E.: Menstruation in intraocular endometrial transplants in the rhesus monkey. Contrib. Embryol. 28:219–308, 1940.

McLennan, C.E., and Rydell, A.H.: Extent of endometrial shedding during normal menstruation. Obstet. Gynecol. 26:605–621, 1965.

Mela, L.M.: *Current Concepts: Physiology and Pathology of Mitochondria*. The Upjohn Company, Kalamazoo, Michigan, pp. 1026, 1974.

Noyes, R.W., Hertig, A.T., and Rock, J.: Dating the endometrial biopsy. Fertility and Sterility. 1:3–25, 1950.

Padykula, H.A. and Campbell, A.G.: Cellular mechanisms involved in stromal renewal of the uterus. II. The albino rat. Anat. Rec. 184:27–48, 1976.

Padykula, H.A. and Taylor, J.M.: Cellular mechanisms involved in cyclic stromal renewal of the uterus. I. The opossum, *Didelphis virginiana*. Anat. Rec. 184:5–26, 1976.

Robbins, S.L.: *Textbook of Pathology*. W.B. Saunders Co., Philadelphia, 1974.

Rockenschaub, A.: Der menstruelle Zyklus. Z. Geburtsh. Gynäk. 155:105–115, 1960a.

Rockenschaub, A.: Wie wird das Endometrium abgebaut? Gymaecologia (Basel) 149:176–187, 1960b.

Schmidt-Mattiesen, H.: Histochemistry. In: The Normal Human Endometrium. Ed.: H. Schmidt-Mattiesen, Blakiston Division of McGraw-Hill Book Company, New York, 1963, pp. 135–207.

Taylor, E.S.: *Essentials of Gynecology*. Lea and Febiger, Philadelphia, 1962.

White, R.R., Mela, L., Bacalzo, L.V., Jr., Olofsson, K., and Miller, L.D.: Hepatic ultrastructure in endotoxemia, hemorrhage, and hypoxia: Emphasis on mitochondrial changes. Surg. 73:525–534, 1973.

Wilborn, W.H. and Flowers, C.E., Jr.: Mechanisms of uterine bleeding with oral contraceptives. Transactions of the American Association of Obstetritions and Gynecologists, Vol. LXXIX, for the year 1978. Published by the C.V. Mosby Company, St. Louis, 1979.

Copyright 1979 by Elsevier North Holland, Inc.
F.K. Beller and G.F.B. Schumacher, eds.
The Biology of the Fluids of the Female Genital Tract

HYSTEROSCOPIC DATA DURING MENSTRUATION

H.J. Lindemann

SUMMARY

The surface reaction during desquamation of the endometrium is described using the technique of CO_2-Hysteroscopy. The data indicate that desquamation commences generally at the fundus spreading downwards to the isthmus. In agreement with histological and ultrastructural data is the observation that signs of new proliferation co-exist with desquamation.

HYSTEROSCOPIC OBSERVATIONS

The data to be presented demonstrate the surface of the endometrium during the menstrual cycle and especially of the desquamation of the endometrium *in vivo*. The method used was CO_2 hysteroscopy. CO_2 gas in a constant rate deflates the uterine cavity. The gas is a dry medium providing a refraction index of 1.0 which like air conveys a natural non-distorted picture. Target extractions can be performed from the cavity and tubes. (Lindemann 1973, 1976, 1976)

The photographs demonstrate the course of menstruation at various stages of desquamation of the endometrium. The uterine cavity can be appreciated by turning the hysteroscope and the openings of the fallopian tube are clearly seen in

Geburtshilfliche-Gynäkologische Abteilung des Elisabeth-Krankenhauses Hamburg/FRG

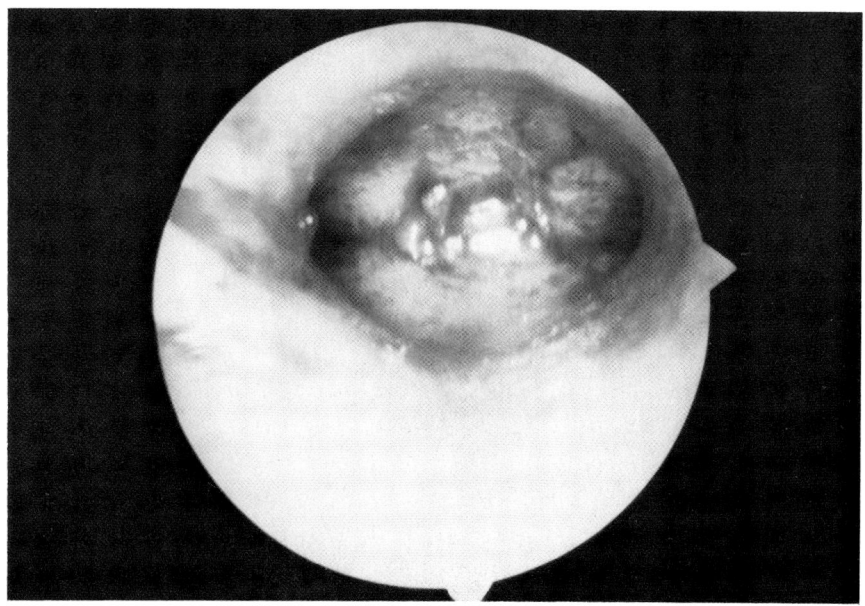

FIGURE 1. View of the uterine cavity during the early proliferate phase. The wall is lined by a thin endometrium. The mucous membrane looks like a smooth close-cropped carpet. Slight bleeding is occasionally seen at the end of the desquamation stage.

FIGURE 2. View of the cornu of the uterus with the tubal orifice in the back. The shape of the endometrium with slight bleeding between the isolated clots indicates early menstruation.

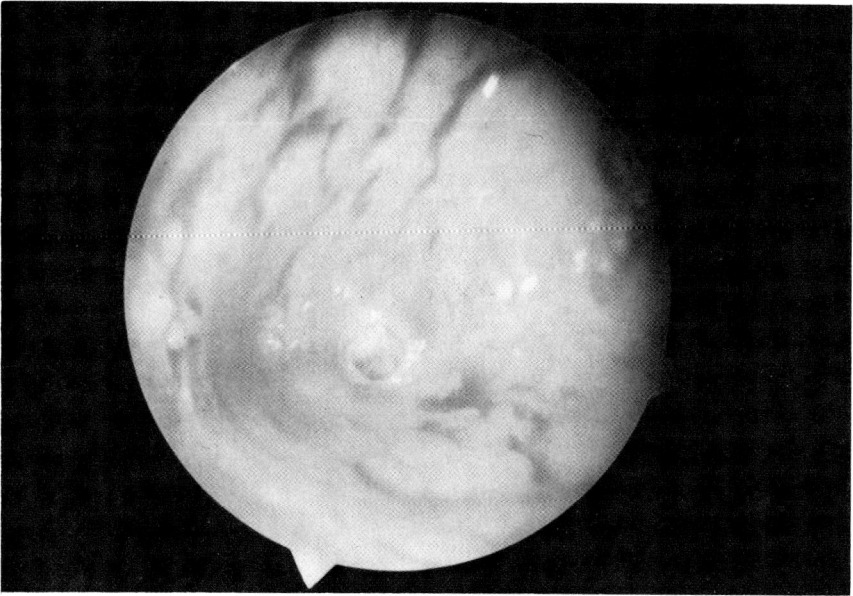

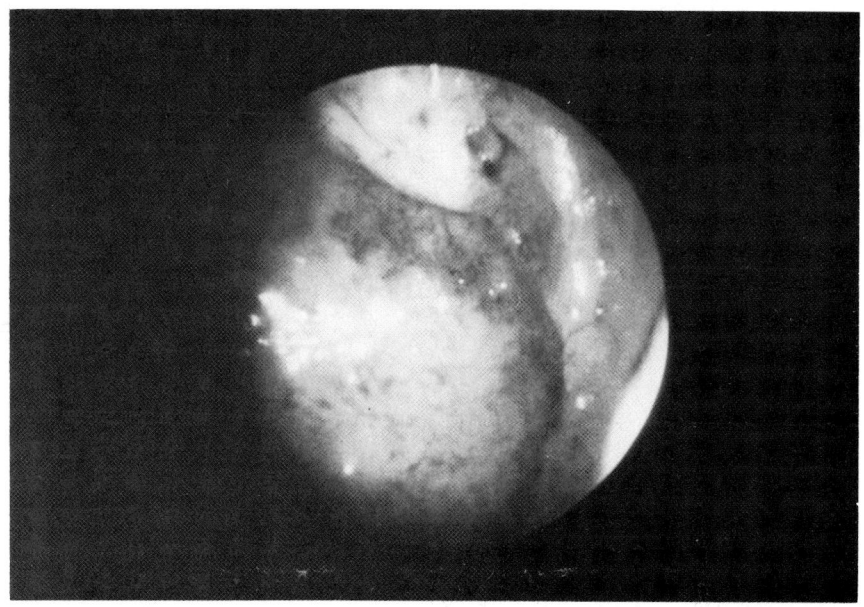

FIGURE 3. Secretory phase. The tissue is edematous and puffy and of greasy lustre.

FIGURE 4. Second day of menstruation. The endometrium is desquamating in large plaques. Between the shreds of mucous membrane is non-coagulated blood.

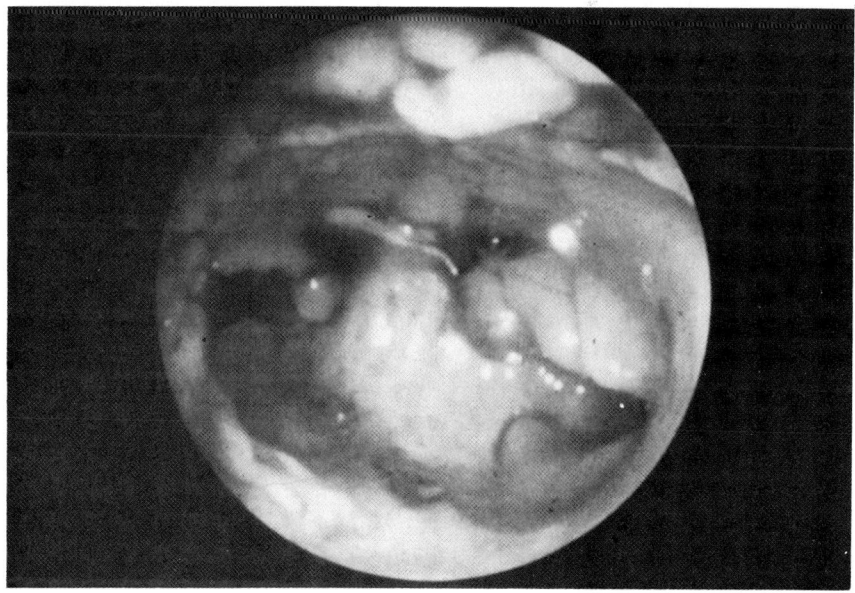

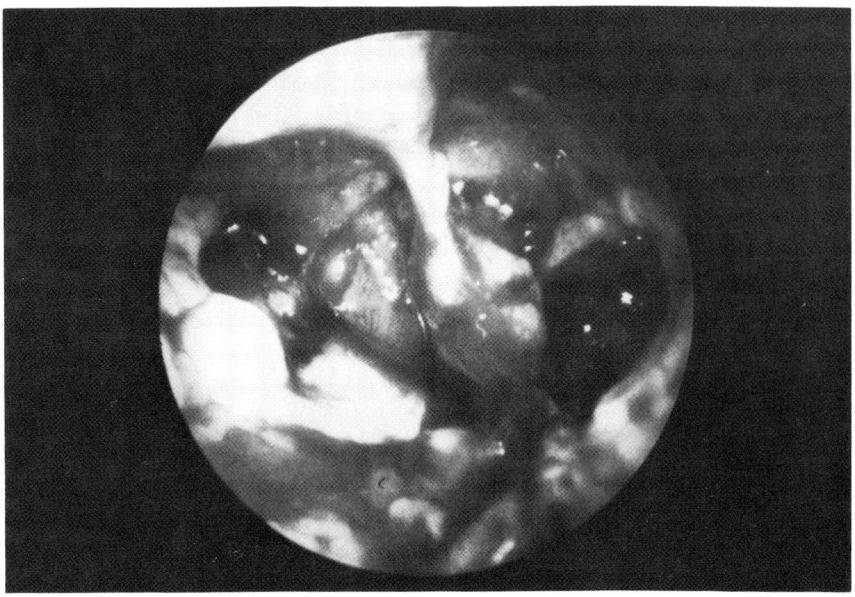

FIGURE 5. Third day of menstruation. The desquamation is starting from the fundal region spreading downwards to the isthmus. The tissue looks like rolled packages.

a round fashion. The uterine cavity of a female in the reproductive age group is lined by a mucous membrane. During the proliferative phase the endometrium is best described as a smooth close-cropped carpet of reddish-yellow coloring. At ovulation it appears somewhat fluffy and yellowish. The diffuse oozing of blood is not caused artificially but is a natural event which may be explained as an abundant rest of ovulatory bleeding. Vascularization of the mucous membrane is pronounced.

Similar to the cervix (Insler and Bettendorf, 1977), there is a watery transparent mucus in the endometrium. During the secretory phase and particularly close to menstruation the endometrium becomes puffy, polypous and very rugged. Just before onset of menstrual bleeding the epithelium turns into a reddish violet color. It is edematous and of greasy lustre, indicating pronounced hyperemia. These observations confirm the histological findings of the endometrium. (Schröder, 1948; Schmidt-Mathiessen, 1963)

Figure 3 demonstrates desquamation at an early stage. If this can be confirmed by repeated observation this would contradict the assumption first expressed by Markee, (1940, 1950), that the endometrium shrinks before menstruation. Further examinations will give more information.

At desquamation the endometrium has a gangrenous appearance. It seems to be ejected in forms of rolled up packages at its borders. The blood is oozing from the surface mostly uncoagulated. This confirms the observations by Beller (1957, 1964). However several blood clots of various shape and size are present. From our observation it seems apparent that desquamation starts from the fundal region spreading downwards to the cervix. This may be related to the pattern of uterine contractions. (Csapo and Pinto-Dantas, 1966; Knaus, 1953) At a time when desquamation passes, proliferation is in an early stage, therefore desquamation and proliferation can be seen abreast. The new proliferation look like budding sprouts with occasional slight bleeding.

REFERENCES

Beller, F.K., Graf, H.: Gerinnungsphysiologische und Plasmaeiweißuntersuchungen bei normaler und pathologischer uteriner Blutungen. Arch. Gynäk. 188, 441 (1957).

Beller, F. K., Goebelsmann, U., Douglas G.W., Johnson A.: The fibrinolytic system during the menstrual cycle. Obstet. and gynec. 23, 12 (1964).

Csapo, A. I., Pinto-Dantos, C.R.: The cyclic activity of the nonpregnant uterus. Fertil. and Steril. 17, 34 (1966).

Insler, V., Bettendorf G.: The uterine cervix in reproduction. Thieme Stuttgart, 1977.

Knaus, H.: Die Physiologie der Zeugung des Menschen; 4. Aufl. Maudrich, Wien 1953.

Lindemann, H.-J.: Pneumometra für die Hysteroskopie, Geburtsh. u. Frauenheilk. 33, 18 (1973).

Lindemann, H.-J., Mohr J., Gallinat A., Buros, M.: Der Einfluß von CO_2-Gas während der Hysteroskopie. Geburtsh. u. Frauenheilk. 36, 153 (1976).

Lindemann, H.-J., Gallinat A.: Physikalische und physiologische Grundlagen de CO_2-Hysteroskopie. Gerburtsh. u. Frauenheilk. 36, 729 (1976).

Markee, J. E.: Menstruation in intraocular endometria (Transplants in the rhesus monkey. Carnegie Inst. Wash. Publ. 518, 219 (1940).

Markee, J.E.: The relation of blood flow to endometrial growth and inception of menstruation. In: E. T. Engle: Menstruation and its disorders. Thomas, Springfield (1950).

Schmidt-Matthiesen, H.: Vaskolarisierung. In: Das normale menschliche Endometrium, hsg. von H. Schmidt-Matthiesen. Thieme, Stuttgart 1963.

Schröder, R.: Gynäkologie. Springer Verlag, Berlin, 3. und 4. Aufl. 1948.

Shettles, L. B.: Die klinische Bedeutung der zyklischen Veränderungen der Mukosa der Cervix uteri und deren Absonderungen. In: Klinische Fortschritte, Gynäkologie, hsg. T. Antoine, Urban und Schwarzenberg, Wien und Innsbruck 1954.

Copyright 1979 by Elsevier North Holland, Inc.
F.K. Beller and G.F.B. Schumacher, eds.
The Biology of the Fluids of the Female Genital Tract

REVIEW ON THE BIOLOGY OF MENSTRUAL BLOOD

F. K. Beller and K. W. Schweppe

SUMMARY

Although menstrual blood is easily obtained by the gynecologist limited information is available describing this material. The literature on blood loss is discussed together with data on cellularity and biochemistry of menstrual blood which is in essence serum.

Menstrual blood provides by virtue of a natural experiment insight about the mechanism, whereby the organism renders blood incoagulable.

Blut ist ein ganz besonderer Saft (Blood is a very special fluid) J.W. Goethe, Faust I. Teil.

INTRODUCTION

Blood was to our ancient forebears the symbol for the secret of life. The presence of menstruation was considered an indication for fertility and therefore was a sign of femininity. Many of our patients refuse hysterectomy for this reason. The presence of menstrual blood also rendered a female unclean for many

Frauenklinik, Abteilung: Geburtshilfe und Gynäkologie der Westfälischen Wilhelms Universität; Münster/Westf., FRG centuries. This is referred back to the Holy Books like the Talmud, the Bible and the Koran.

Since the earliest knowledge of human life menstruation is known. But if one tries to understand the physiological significance of menstruation, very little can be said for a good reason even if one tries to establish teleological explanations.

In 1945 Smith and Smith reported on a substance in menstrual blood which they called "Menotoxin". They injected menstrual blood into rats and found a high lethality. These experiments and their data were never confirmed and it is assumed that the lethality was due to infectious contamination or allergic reactions to foreign body protein. The observed inhibition of coagulation was not the result of heparin but rather, as will be later explained, it results from the presence of fibrin(ogen) breakdown products.

Discussion seems to be appropriate regarding terminology. Menstrual blood does not contain fibrinogen even in trace amounts. We have therefore proposed for scientific purpose the term menstrual "serum" rather than menstrual "plasma" (Beller and Graf, 1957).

Blood Loss

The continuous drainage of blood every 4 weeks devoids the female of blood constituents predominantly iron (Hytten et al., 1964; Jacobs and Butler, 1965). This is presumably the reason that more than 75% of our patients enter pregnancy with more or less depleted iron storages.

To establish a "normal" value in this regard is rather difficult. "Menorrhagia" is the term for a bleeding which lasts too long and "Hypermenorrhoea" is the term for a blood loss exceeding normal values. But what are normal values for a process which is not needed. Ober reported that women of primitive tribes experience a menstrual bleeding of half an hour and few drops (1952). The loss in the subhuman primate is scanty at best. A menstruation lasting 6 days and more is considered quite normal in New York City, but too long in Muenster. Regional differences have therefore to be considered if normal values are established.

A review of the literature on blood loss is given in Table I, which indicates the large variation found by several investigators. Table II indicates the amount of loss per day (Callard et al., 1966). The amount of blood loss in a study done by Cole (1971) is given in Figure 1.

The large variation in results is explainable by the already mentioned difference in population but also by the difference in technique used. The question to the patient: "Is the menstrual period normal?" is answered by very few women intelligently because they have no reference. It is therefore better to ask about the number of pads or tampons. A completely wet pad absorbs approximately 90 ml and a tampon approximately 40 ml of menstrual blood.

Organic and inorganic data on menstrual blood were elaborated by Büssing (1957). Table IV gives the known physical data, Table V the inorganic substances and Table VI the organic substances, as assayed by this author.

Hematological Data

The cellularity was studied by a number of investigators (Burnhill and Birnberg, 1965; McDonald and McDonald, 1977; Pohle, 1959; Rotter, 1927) and is summarized in Table VII. There is no data regarding the function of platelets or

TABLE I. Review of the Literature on Blood Loss During Menstruation

Menstrual Blood Loss

SOURCES		n (number of cycles)	MEAN (ml)	RANGE (ml)
Baldwin, R. M., Whalley, P. J. and Pritchard, J. A.	1961	54	25	10 - 55
Cole, S. K., Billewicz, W. Z.	1971	89	34, 4	± 23, 6 (S.D.)
Poon, C. H., Moyer, D. L. Forino, R V, Shaw, S T. jr.[++]	1972	271	29, 62	3 - 130 ; 18, 56 (S.D.)
Hahn, L, Rybo, G.	1975	15	30	8 - 60
Haynes, P. J., Hodgson, A. B. M., Anderson, H., Turnbull, A. C.	1977	12	28	9 - 61

[++]Combined data from Baldwin et al., 1961; Hallberg and Nilsson, 1964; Jacobs and Butler, 1965; Hytten et al., 1964; and Hallberg et al., 1966.

FIGURE 1. Menstrual blood loss in ml in a surveyed population.

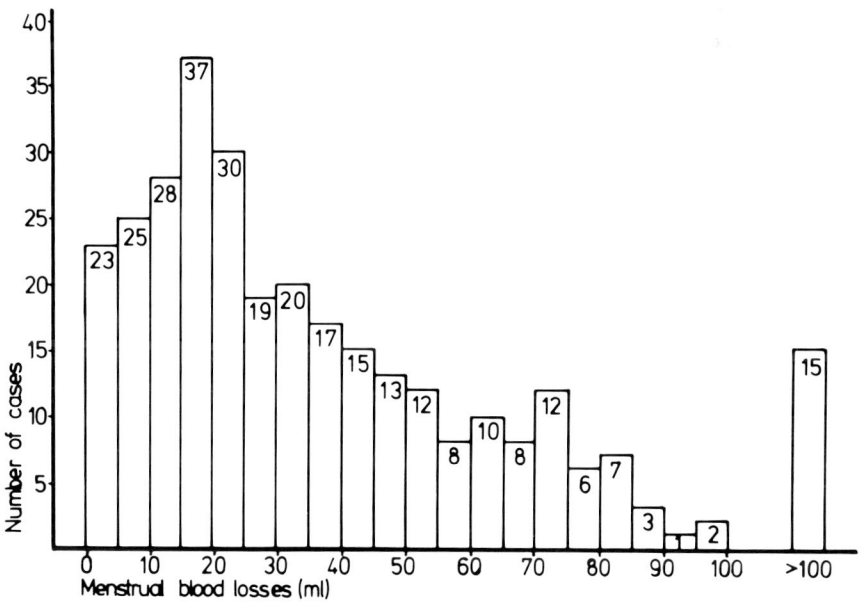

TABLE II. Amount of Menstrual Blood Loss Per Day

Day of period	Donors (No.)	Observations (No.) Cycles	Samples	Vol. (ml./hr.)	± S.E.
1	27	108	167	1,45	± 0,07
2	28	113	183	1,36	± 0,07
3	21	68	87	0,82	± 0,08 ++
4 +	13	18	21	0,36	±0,10 ++

++ P = 0,001 compared to previous day.
(Callard, G.V. Litofsky, F.S., DeMerre, L.J., 1966)

leucocytes. However, it is well known that patients with idiopathic thrombocytopenic purpura have frequent menorrhagia and excessive blood loss. Numbers are of less interest since these patients can adjust to a rather low platelet count normal for them, but pathologic for normal individuals (Quick, 1966; Vinazzer, 1966). This is indicated by the normal bleeding time seen in patients with platelet numbers below 50.000 mm^2. Quite often the number of circulating platelets falls even below this level and explains uterine bleeding. The frequent episodes of menorrhagia in patients with ITP seem to indicate the significance of platelets for hemostasis and we will focus on this mechanism later.

Plasma Protein

The only available data were reported by our group (Figures 2 and 3) some 20 years ago.

Enzymatic Activity

The few studies available concerning enzyme activity in menstrual blood are summarized in Table III (Callard and DeMerre, 1966; DeMerre and Litofsky, 1968; DeMerre et al., 1968: Fuhrmann, 1963; Goldberg and Jones, 1954; Henzl et al., 1972; Meyer, 1952; Rao, 1973; Wood, 1969).

Blood Coagulation

Attempts to explain the mechanism for incoagulability refers back to World War One. Bell assumed that menstrual blood clotted in response to the release of tissue thromboplastin in the uteri (1912). The serum as the result of coagulation would subsequently drain through the cervical canal. This concept was taken up by a variety of investigators (Elert and Nold, 1956; Glueck and Mirsky, 1941; Lozner et al., 1942).

In contrast Whitehouse presented data in a remarkable lecture before the

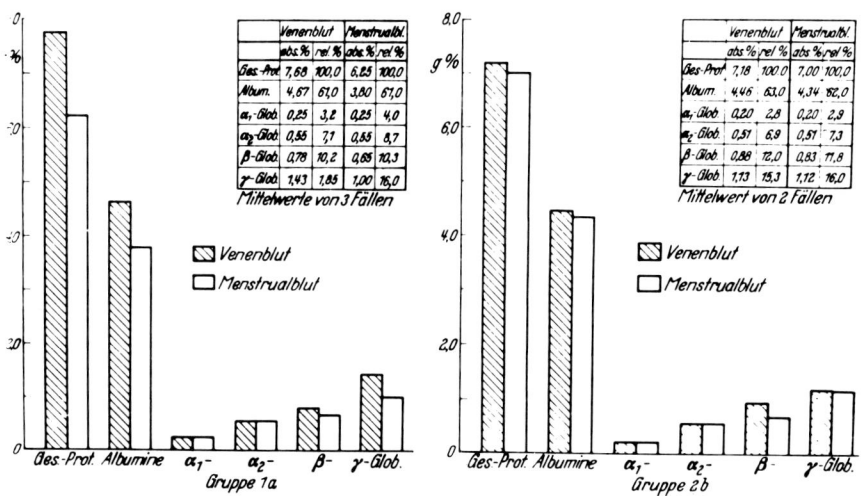

FIGURE 2. Electrophoretic pattern (Antweiler) in menstrual serum and peripheral blood. Group 1a marked differences compared to peripheral blood; 2b no differences. Menstrual blood obtained before day 3. (Beller and Graf)

FIGURE 3. Electrophoretic pattern (Antweiler) as in figure 2. Group 2a marked differences: group 1b no differences. Menstrual blood obtained after day 3. (Beller and Graf).

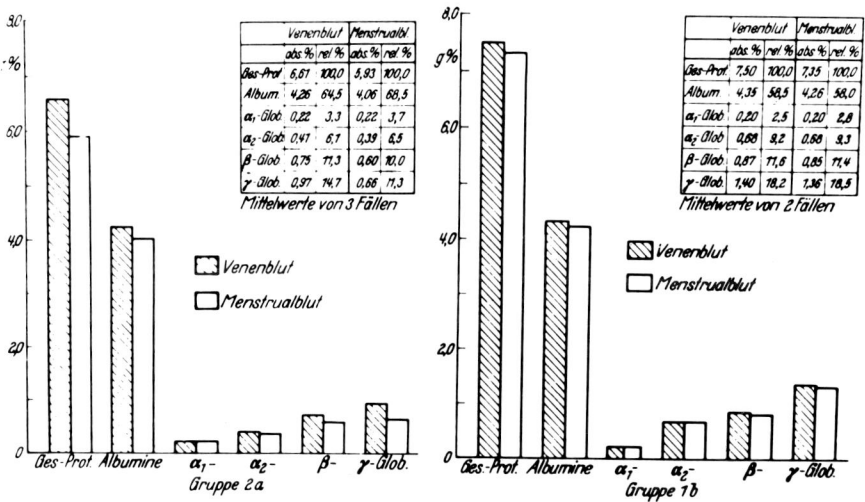

TABLE III. Enzyme Activity in Menstrual Blood

sources	enzyme	day of cycle	No. of samples	MEAN	± S.E.
Callard, G. V. and DeMerre, L. J. (1966)	beta-glucuronidase (menstr. discharge)	1 2 3+ all	45 46 33 124	3450 (U/100 ml) 3953 " 4774 " 3989 "	296 (U/100 ml) 354 " 385 " 202 "
	beta-glucuronidase (venous plasma)	2 9 - 11 21 - 22 all	23 16 14 53	418 (U/100 ml) 379,8 " 401,1 " 402,0 "	33,2 (U/100 ml) 36,8 " 27,1 " 19,3 "
DeMerre, L. J. and Litofsky, F. S. (1968)	alkaline-phosphatase (menstr. discharge)	1 2 3 all	32 37 31 100	7,20 (SigmaU/hr) 5,54 " 4,24 " 6,24 "	1,04 (Sigma U/hr.) 0,47 " 0,64 " 0,35 "
	alkaline - phosphatase (venous plasma)	all	64	1,10 (SigmaU/hr)	0,08 (Sigma U/hr.)

TABLE IV. Physical Data in Menstrual Blood*

	MEAN		RANGE
	venous blood	menstrual blood	menstrual blood
specific weight	1,055	1,040	1,033 - 1,048
viscosity	1,8	2,4	
refrective index	1,350	1,346	1,345 - 1,349
pH - value	7,4	7,0	6.9 - 7.2
depression of freezing point	0,56°	0,51°	
surface tension	0,86	0,80	
water content	80 %	88 %	

* Büssing, H.J., 1957.

TABLE V. Anorganic Substances in Menstrual Blood*

	MEAN		RANGE
	venous blood	menstrual blood	menstrual blood
Natrium	330 mg%	260 mg%	230 - 310 mg%
Calcium	10,5 mg%	10,0 mg%	9,0 - 11,0 mg%
Magnesium	3,3 mg%	3,3 mg%	2,5 - 3,6 mg%
Iron	120 gam.%	150 gam.%	
Cupper	100 gam.%	90 gam.%	
Chloride	360 mg%	350 mg%	320 - 390 mg%
Rhodanide	70 gam.%	50 gam.%	
anorg. Sulfat	1,5 mg%	1,2 mg%	
Phosphat (total)	27 mg%	37 mg%	32 - 45 mg%
Phosphat (anorg.) Serum	4,0 mg%	8,0 mg%	8,0 - 10,0 mg%
Phosphat (esterified)	0,5 mg%	2,0 mg%	
Phosphat (soluble in acid)	4,8 mg%	10,0 mg%	8,0 - 13,0 mg%

* Büssing, H.J., 1957.

Physiological Society in memory of the Physiologist Hunter in 1914. Evidence was presented for his assumption that menstrual blood is rendered incoagulable by a different mechanism namely proteolysis and digestion. We elaborated on this concept and focused attention on the mechanism of fibrinolysis, which means the enzymatic breakdown of fibrinogen rather than fibrin. (Beller and Graf, 1957; Beller, 1971).

The possibility that changes of the blood coagulation system in the circulation could be held responsible (Flähmig et al., 1965; Marx and Rovatti, 1952) were excluded by previous data from this laboratory (Beller et al., 1964) and older studies (Bayerle and Marx, 1947; Cederblad et al., 1977; Genell, 1936; Hengstmann and Klien, 1958; Kraus, 1952; Moebius and Johannes, 1956). The observation of Pepper of a rise of blood platelets to indicate ovulation is today only of historical interest. However, it may be related to the observations that oral contraceptives may stabilize the platelet number in patients with cyclic thrombocytopenia (Beller, 1971). Maki and Saito (1963) observed an increased activator concentration in the draining venous channels of the uterus at menstruation and we have confirmed this (Beller et al., 1968). However, the amount is rather small and it is unable to activate the fibrinolytic enzyme system in the circulation.

Therefore local mechanisms in the endometrium must be held responsible for the incoagulability. Halban and Fraenkel (1910) and later Caffier (1930) reported on proteolytic enzyme activity in the endometrium and menstrual blood.

In agreement with Elert and Nold (1956) we found in various days of menstrual bleeding low activities of nearly all coagulation factors except factor IX. A

TABLE VI. Organic Substances in Menstrual Blood*

	MEAN		RANGE
	venous blood	menstrual blood	menstrual blood
Protein	7,0 g%	6,5 g%	5,9 - 7,5 g%
Nitrogen	35 mg%	80 mg%	50 - 100 mg%
Urea	40 mg%	15 mg%	10 - 20 mg%
Uric acid	2,5 mg%	1,5 mg%	0,5 - 1,8 mg%
Creatinin	1,2 mg%	1,5 mg%	1,3 - 2,2 mg%
Aminoacids	10 mg%	25 mg%	16 - 35 mg%
Bloodsuggar	90 mg%	50 mg%	30 - 50 mg%
Glycogen	35 mg%	50 mg%	40 - 60 mg%
Lactidacid	11 mg%	30 mg%	24 - 37 mg%
Aceton	1,5 mg%	1,9 mg%	
Fatacids	350 mg%	300 mg%	220 - 330 mg%
Cholesterin (total)	175 mg%	150 mg%	135 - 170 mg%
Cholesterin (free)	60 mg%	50 mg%	41 - 55 mg%
Cholesterin (esterified)	115 mg%	100 mg%	90 - 110 mg%
Hemoglobin	15 g%	5 g%	3 - 10 g%
Bilirubin	0,7 mg%	0,4 mg%	0,3 - 0,7 mg%

* Büssing, H.J., 1957.

TABLE VII. Cellularity in Menstrual Blood

HEMATOLOGIC DATA OF MENSTRUAL DISCHARGE

Sources	N samples	RBC (x 10^6 cu. mm)	Hb (mg%)	WBC (per cu. mm.)	Platelets (per cu. mm.)	Eos. (%)	Bas. (%)	Neut. (%)	Lym. (%)	Mono. (%)	Day of cycle
STICKEL, M. and ZONDEK, B. (1920)	13	2,6 - 3,59	8,0 -10,2	21000 - 36400	/ / /	1 1,6 1,6	1 1 1	52,3 49,6 25,3	44,7 46,8 71,1	1 1 1	1 2 3
DEMERRE, L.J. MOSS, J.D. and PATTISON, D.S. (1967)	96	2,44 2,82 2,42	9,1 9,7 10,3	21444 9901 15492	33000 31000 32000	1 1 1	0 0 0	59,7 50,0 61,0	37,0 46,6 36,0	2,3 2,4 2,0	1 2 3

tendency for these activities to raise towards the end of menstruation was also noted (Beller and Graf, 1957) (Figure 4). Fibrinogen activity was never demonstrated in our studies nor by other investigators which seemed to be in agreement with the lack of fibrin. We have reported previously that clots in the vagina do not stain positively with any of the stains against fibrin and fibrin is rarely seen in the endometrium (Beller, 1971; Picoff and Luginbuhl, 1964; Salvatore, 1969). Only occasionally does the mechanism of incoagulability fail and in such cases fibrin strands are detectable by scanning and electron microscopy (see paper Ebert et al.).

We have discussed various sources of proteolytic enzymes (another paper at this symposium), whose activity generates large concentrations of fibrin(ogen) breakdown products in MS (Basu, 1970; Beller, 1971; Cole and Billwicz, 1971; Hahn et al., 1976; Hahn and Rybo, 1975; Marx et al., 1972). The clot inhibitory activity of FDP is an important factor in rendering blood incoagulable. The effect in older experiments was confused with heparin like activity, complicated by the evidence for a therapeutic effect of toluidine blue and protamine sulfate on intrauterine bleeding (Beller and Naegele, 1956; Elgehammer et al., 1949; Hahn, 1974). But this effect is also attributable to inhibition of FSP by these substances (Beller, 1971).

There is evidence now, that the proteolytic activity is not solely due to plasmin activated by KSCN extractable activators (Albrechtsen, 1956; Albrechtsen, 1959; Fuhrmann, 1962) or cytokinase (Lack and Ali, 1964). Indeed, our

FIGURE 4. Activity of coagulation factor in menstrual blood. (Beller)

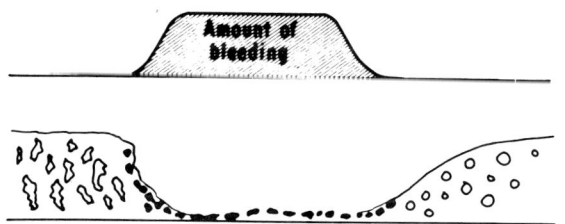

Menses	Early	Middle	End	Peripheral Plasma
1. Fibrinogen		Absent		300 mg %
2. Prothrombin	Below 5%	5 to 30%	5 to 80%	100%
3. Factor V		Below 5%		100%
4. Factor VII	Below 10%	40 to 80%	40 to 80%	100%
5. Factor VIII	Below 20%	40%	20 to 80%	80 to 150%
6. Factor IX		Normal		100%
7. Platelets		Approximately 10,000 mm^3		>200,000 mm^3

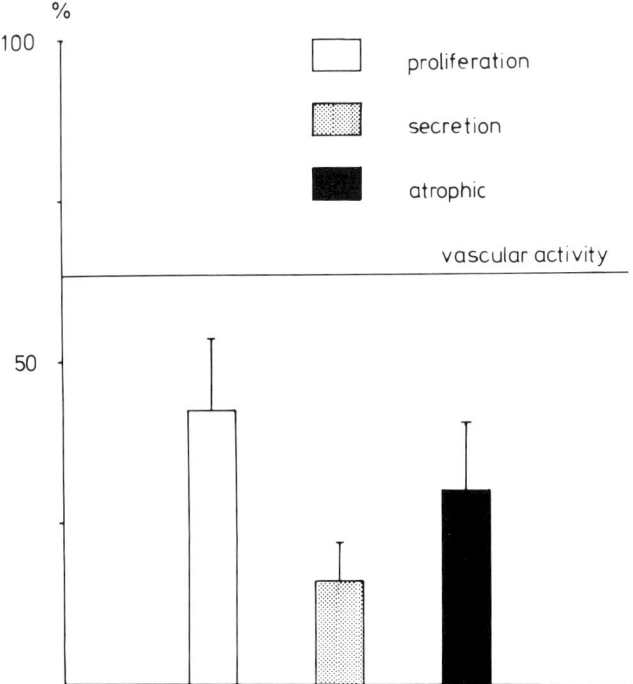

FIGURE 5. Activator activity in endometrium during various stages of the endometrium (from Schmidt et al., unpublished)

studies have revealed that the activator in MS is the same or lower in concentration in the secretory than in the proliferative phase (Figure 5). This can also be seen by the histochemical electron of activator by the technique of Todd (Figure 6) (Glas-Greenwalt, 1971; Luginbuhl, 1966). Data previously reported (Beller and Weiss, 1966; Weiss and Beller, 1969) indicate that the activator present in cervical mucus contributes to the activation of plasminogen to plasmin. This mechanism can therefore be considered as an additional line of defense in preventing clotting.

Little information is present regarding the onset and termination of menstrual bleeding. The morphology will be discussed intensively at this meeting. The pioneer experiments of Markee (1940), who implanted endometrium into the anterior chamber of the eye of Rhesus monkeys, is extremely difficult to duplicate. We were successful in transplanting endometrium in a similar fashion in baboons and the pieces menstruated. However, we were unsuccessful in observing the endometrium at a magnification of 100-fold even with very sophisticated equipment because of rapid eye movement at this magnification.

There is little doubt that the mechanism for rendering the blood incoagulable is different from a similar, but distinctly different mechanism excurring in the intraperitoneal cavity during ectopic pregnancy (Beller et al., 1968).

There is little known about the physiology of menstruation and even less in

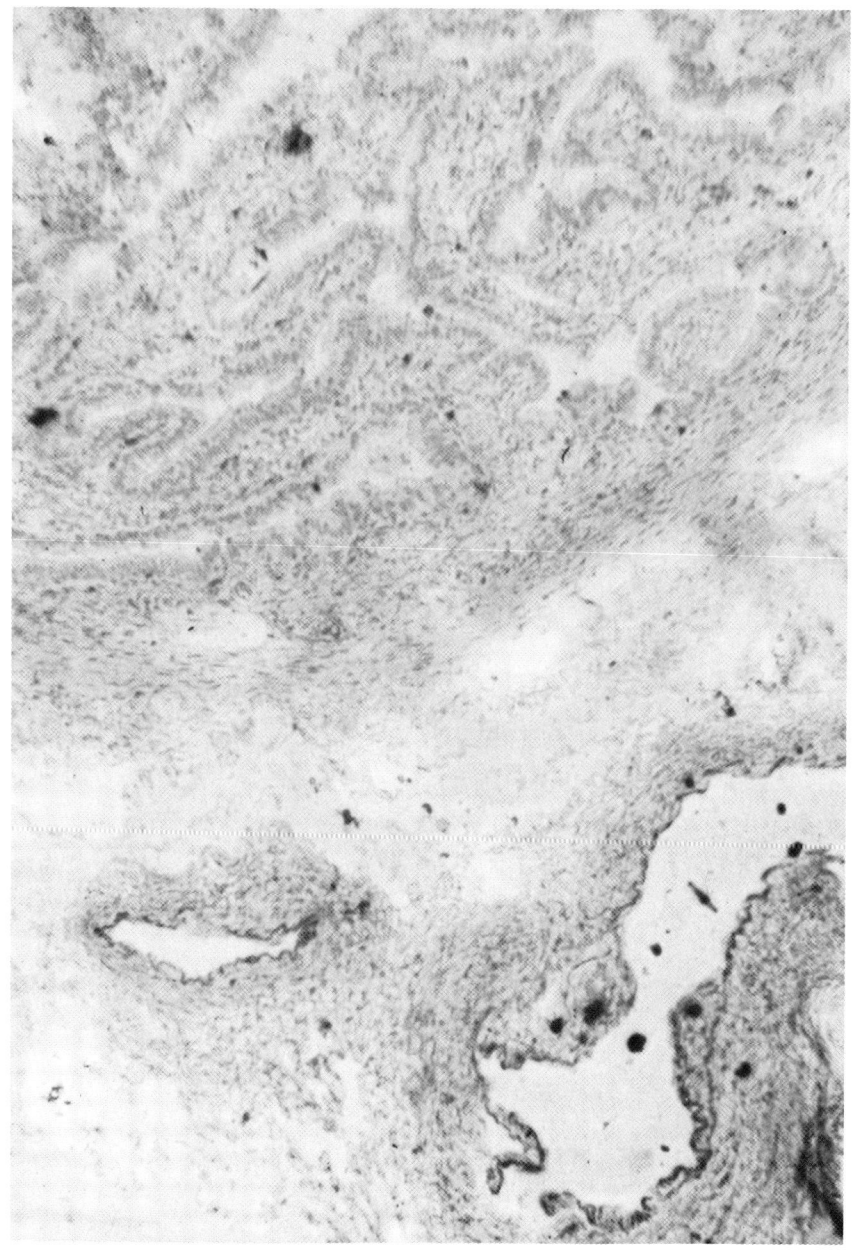

FIGURE 6. Activator activity in endometrium. Note the large activity in endometrium compared to endometrium.

regard to the mechanism for breakthrough bleeding, dysfunctional bleeding or even postmenopausal bleeding. We believe that it will be difficult to approach experimentally any such pathological entities as long as information on the physiology of menstruation is inadequate. However, this discussion will hopefully serve to stimulate more research in this area.

ACKNOWLEDGEMENT ·
Supported by a Grant of Deutsche Forschungsgemeinschaft (Contract Nr. 648/5)

REFERENCES

Albrechtsen, O.K.: The fibrinolytic activity of the human endometrium. Acta Endocrinol. (Kbh.) 23:219–226, 1956.

Albrechtsen, O.K.: The fibrinolytic activity of menstrual blood. Acta Endocrinol. (Kbh.) 23:207, 1956.

Albrechtsen, O.K.: Fibrinolytic activity in the organism. Acta Physiol. Scand. Suppl. 47:165, 1959.

Baldwin, R.M., Whalley, P.J. and Pritchard, J.A.: Measurement of menstrual blood loss. Am. J. Obstet. Gynec. 81:739–742, 1961.

Bayerle, H. and Marx, M.: Zur Frage der Abhängigkeit des Prothrombinspiegels des Blutes vom Menstruationszyklus. Geburtsh. Frauenheilk. 8:767, 1947.

Basu, H.K.: Fibrin degration products in sera of women with normal menstruation and menorrhagia. Br. Med. J. 1:74, 1970.

Bell, W.B.: Further investigations into chemical composition of menstrual fluid and the secretions of the vagina. J. Obstet. Gynecol. Brit. Cwlth. Emp. 91:209, 1912.

Beller, F.K.: Physiologie der uterinen Hämostase des nicht schwangeren Uterus. H. Hardert and H. Ludwig (ed.): Antithrombin, uterine Hämostase, Herz und Blutgerinnung. Schattauer, Stuttgart, 1971.

Beller, F.K.: Observations on the clotting of menstrual blood and clot formation. Am. J. Obstet. Gynecol. 111:535–546, 1971.

Beller, F.K., Douglas, G.W., Morris, R.H. and Johnson, A.J.: The fibrinolytic enzyme system in pregnancy. Am. J. Obstet. Gynecol. 101:587, 1968.

Beller, F.K., Goebgelsmann, U., Douglas, G.W. and Johnson, A.J.: The fibrinolytic system during menstrual cycle. Obstet. and Gynec. 23:12, 1964.

Beller, F.K., Graf, H.: Gerinnungsphysiologische und Plasmaeiweißuntersuchungen bei normalen (Menses) und patholgischen uterinen Blutungen. Arch. Gynaecol. 188:411–442, 1957.

Beller, F.K. and Maki, M. and Epstein, M.D.: Incoagulability of intraperitoneal blood. Am. J. Obstet. Gynec. 102:1121, 1968.

Beller, F.K., Naegele, M.: Untersuchungen über die Hämostase uteriner Blutungen durch Protaminsulfat und Toluidinblau. Arch. Gynäk. 188:123, 1956.

Beller, F.K., Weiss, G.: The fibrinolytic enzyme system in cervical mucus. Fertil. Steril. 17:654, 1966.

Büssing, H.J.: Zur Biochemie des Menstrualblutes. Zbl. Gynaec. 79:456, 1957.

Burnhill, M.S. and Birnberg, C.H.: Contents of menstrual fluid: An analysis of 260 samples. Am. J. Obstet. Gynec. 92:183, 1965.

Caffier, P.: Die Rolle des menschlichen Uterus als mesodermales Verdauungsorgan. Münch. med. Wschr. 77:389, 1930.

Callard, G.V., DeMerre, L.J.: Beta-Glucuronidase During Menstruation. Fertil. Steril. 17:547–555, 1966.

Callard, G.V., Litofsky, F.S. and DeMerre, L.J.: Menstruation in women with normal and artificially controlled cycles. Fertil. Steril. 17:684, 1966.

Cederblad, G., Hahn, L., Korsan-Bengtsen, K., Pehrson, N.G. and Rybo, G.: Variations in

Blood Coagulation, Fibrinolysis, Platelets Function and Various Plasma Proteins during the Menstrual Cycle. Haemostasis 6:294–302, 1977.

Cole, S.K., Billewicz, W.Z.: Sources of Variation in Menstrual Blood Loss. J. Obstet. Gynaec. Brit. Cwlth. 78:933–939, 1971.

Cole, S.K., Clarkson, A.R.: Menstrual blood loss and fibrin degration products. Br. Med. J. 1:78, 1972.

Daron, G.H.: The arterial pattern of the tunica mucosa of the uterus in macacas rhesus. Am. J. Anat. 58:349, 1936.

DeMerre, L.J., Gilbreath, E.B. and Pattison, D.S.: Cholesterol Content of Menstrual Discharge. Obstet. Gynecol. 32:645–648, 1968.

DeMerre, L.J., Litofsky, F.S.: Alkaline-Phosphatase Activity During Menstruation. Fertil. Steril. 19:593–597, 1968.

DeMerre, L.J., Moss, J.D. and Pattison, D.S.: The Hematological study of menstrual discharge. Obstet. and Gynec. 30:830, 1967.

Dausset, J., Beregerot-Blondel, Y. and Colin, M.: Fibrinolyse du sang peripherique au cours de flux menstrual physiologique. C. R. Soc. franc. Gynéc. 28:191, 1958.

Ebert, R., Nold, B.: Gerinnungsphysiologische Studien am Menstrualblut. Schweiz. Med. Wochenschr. 36:999, 1956.

Elgehammer, R.M., Grossman, B.J., Koff, A.K., Moulder, P.V. and Allen, J.J.: Observation on the clotting mechanism in menstruation and menorrhagia. Surg. Gynec. Obstet. 89:764, 1949.

Flähmig, M., Sieg, U. and Vogel, G.: Fibrinolytische Störungen im uterinen Blut. Münch. med. Woschenschr. 107:2007, 1965.

Fuhrmann, K.: Die fibrinolytische Aktivität im Endometrium. Zbl. Gynäk. 84:1457, 1962.

Fuhrmann, K.: Stoffwechsel. in: H. Schmidt-Matthiesen: Das normale menschliche Endometrium. G. Thieme, Stuttgart, S.268–293, 1963.

Glas-Greenwalt, P., Beller, F.K. and Astrup, T.: Comparative assays of tissue plasminogen activator in myometrium, cervix and fibromas of the human uterus. Am. J. Obstet. Gynec. 110:721–725, 1971.

Genell, S.: Study of variations in number of blood platelets during menstrual cycle. J. Obstet. Gynaec. Brit. Emp. 43:1124, 1936.

Glueck, H.I. and Mirsky, A.: The clotting mechanism of menstrual fluid. Am. J. Obstet. Gynec. 42:267, 1941.

Goldberg, B., Jones, II.W., Jr.: Some characteristics of the acid phosphatase of the human endometrium. Obstet. and Gynec. 4:426, 1954.

Hahn, L., Cederblad, G., Rybo, G., Pehrson, N.G. and Korsan-Bengtsen, K.: Blood coagulation, fibrinolysis and plasma proteins in women with normal and with excessive blood loss. Brit. Med. J. Obstet. Gynaec. 83:974–980, 1976.

Hahn, L., Rybo, G.: Fibrinogen-fibrin degration products in menstrual blood from women with normal and excessive menstrual blood loss. Acta Obstet. Gynec. Scand. 54:119, 1975.

Hahn, L.: On fibrinolysis and coagulation during parturition and menstruation. Acta obstetr. gynec. Scand. Suppl. 28:5–39, 1974.

Halban, J., Fraenkel, O.: Zur Biochemie der Uterus Mucosa. Gynäkol. Rundschau 4:471, 1910.

Hallberg, L., Hogdahl, A., Nilsson, L. and Rybo, G.: Menstrual blood loss: A population study. Acta Obstet. Gynec. Scand. 45:320–351, 1966.

Hallberg, L., Nilsson, L.: Determination of menstrual blood loss. Scand. J. Clin. Lab. Invest. 16:244–248, 1964.

Hallberg, L., Nilsson, L.: Constancy of individual menstrual blood loss. Acta Obstetr. Gynec. Scand. 43:352, 1964.

Hengstmann, H. and Klien, D.: Über die Abhängigkeit der Faktoren des Prothrombinkomplexes vom weiblichen Zyclus. Arch. Gynäk. 191:283, 1958.

Haynes, P.J., Hodgson, H., Anderson, A.B.M. and Turnbull, A.C.: Measurement of menstrual blood loss in patients complaining of menorrhagia. Brit. J. Obstet. Gynaec. 84:763–768, 1977.

Henzl, M.R., Smith, S.E., Boost, G. and Tyler, E.T.: Lysosomal concept of menstrual bleeding in humans. J. Clin. Endocrinol. Metab. 34:860, 1972.

Hytten, F.E., Cheyne, G.A. and Klopper, A.I.: Iron loss at menstruation. J. Obstet. Gynaec. Brit. Cwlth. 71:255–259, 1964.

Jacobs, A. and Butler, E.B.: Menstrual blood loss in Iron deficiency anemia. Lancet II:407–409, 1965.

Kraus, H.H.: Ursachen der Prothrombinspiegelschwankungen während des normalen Zyclus. Zbl. Gynäk. 24:1661, 1952.

Lack, C.H., Ali, S.Y.: Tissue activator of plasminogen. Nature 201:1030, 1964.

Lozner, El., Taylor, Z.E. and Taylor, F.H.L.: The so called defect coagulation in menstrual blood. New Engl. J. Med. 226:481, 1942.

Luginbuhl, W.H., Picoff, R.C.: The localization and characteristics of endometrial fibrinolysis. Am. J. Obstet. Gynec. 95:462, 1966.

McDonald, R.G., McDonald, H.N.: Erythrocyte 2,3-Diphosphoglycerate and associated haematological parameters during the menstrual cycle and pregnancy. Brit. J. Obstet. Gynaec. 84:427–433, 1977.

Maki, M. and Saito, H.: Pathophysiology of plasminsystem III. Contribution to the mechanism of incoagulability of menstrual and intraperitoneal blood. Tohoka J. exp. Med. 79:125, 1963.

Markee, J.E.: Menstruation in intraocular endometrial transplants in the Rhesus monkey. Contr. Embryol. Carneg. Instn. 28:219, 1940.

Marx, R., Rovatti, B.: Untersuchungen über das Verhalten der Fibrinolyse im Serum des Menstrualzyclus. Haematologica 36:685, 1952.

Marx, R., Weinzierl, W., Schwick, G. and Störiko, K.: Zum Nachweis und Vorkommen und zur Bedeutung intracorporal endstandener Fibrin(nogen)-Abbauprodukte mit besonderer Berücksichtigung des Nachweises von hochmolekularen Fibrin-Abbauprodukten im Menstrualblut. Blut 12:22, 1965.

Meyer, R.K.: Relation of beta-glucuronidase to action of gonadal hormones. in: Ciba Foundation Colloquia on Endocrinology. J. & A. Churchill, London, 1952.

Moebius, W. and Johannes, S.: Schwankungen der Zahl der Thrombocyten während des weiblichen Genitalzyklus. Zbl. Gynäk. 84:489–450, 1956.

Ober, K.G.: Die Behandlung der unzulänglichen Keimdrüsenfunktion: in: Seitz-Amreich II.S.726 ff. Urban and Schwarzenberg, Berlin, 1952.

Pepper, H.S. Lindsay: Elevation of platelets in midcycle: An indication of ovulation. Science 124:180, 1956.

Picoff, R. and Luginbuhl, W.H.: Fibrin in the endometrial stroma, in uterine bleeding. Am. J. Obstet. Gynec. 88:642, 1964.

Quick, A.J.: Menstruation in hereditary bleeding disorders. Obstet. and Gynec. 28:37, 1966.

Pohle, F.J.: The blood platelets count in relation to the menstrual cycle in normal women. Amer. J. med. Sci. 197:40, 1939.

Rao, A.R.: Viskosity, alkaline phosphatase and beta-glucuronidase in menstrual blood. Int. J. Gynaecol. Obstet. 11:247–248, 1973.

Rasmussen, J., Roberts, H.R.: Fibrinolytic activity of the normal and fibromyomatous human uterus. Surg. Gynec. Obstet. 118:1277, 1964.

Rotter, H.: Mikroskopische Untersuchung des genitalen Blutes. Zbl. Gynaek. 51:607, 1927.

Rybo, G.: Plasminogen activator in the endometrium. I. Methodological aspects. Acta Obstet. Gynec. Scand. 45:411, 1966.

Rybo, G.: Plasminogen activator in the endometrium. II. Clinical aspects. Acta Obstet. Gynec. Scand. 45:429–450, 1966.

Salvatore, C.A.: Identification of fibrin in menstrual endometrium. Am. J. Obstet. Gynec. 103:537, 1969.

Schmidt-Matthiesen, H. and Schreinert, B.: Die Bestimmung von Gewebegängigkeit und therapeutischer Dosis von e-Aminocapronsäure, AMCHA und Trasylol mittels direkter Homogenat-Eigenplasma-Thrombelastographie am Beispiel des fibrinolytisch aktiven Myomentrium. Klin. Wochenschr. 46:730–731, 1968.

Schmidt-Matthiesen, H.: Die fribrinolytische Aktivität von Endometrium und Myometrium, Dezidua und Plazenta, Kollum- und Korpuskarzinomen. Bibl. Gynaecol. 44, Karger, 1967.

Shaw, S.Z., Elsahwi, S.Y. and Moyer, D.L.: Menstrual blood quantification in the Rhesus monkey: An experimental tool for improving intrauterine contraceptive devices (IUDS). Fertil. Steril. 23:257–263, 1972.

Skipetrov, V.P.: The role of tissue factors of the endometrium in noncoagulability of the uterine blood. Akush Ginekol. 3:3, 1966, reviewed in Excerpta Med. Section 10: Obstet. Gynecol. 19:764, 1966.

Skjodt, P. and Albrechtsen, O.K.: Coagulation and fibrinolysis in uterine blood. Acta Obstet. Gynec. Scand. 44:180, 1966.

Smith, O.W., Smith, C.V.S.: A fibrinolytic enzyme in menstruation and late pregnancy toxemia. Science 102:253, 1945.

Smith, O.W.: Menstrualtoxin: experimental studies. Am. J. Obstet. Gynec. 54:221, 1947.

Stickel, M. and Zondek, B.: Das Menstruationsblut. Z. Geburtsh. u. Gynäkol. 83:1–26, 1920.

Todd, A.S.: The historical localization of fibrinolysin activator. J. Path. Bact. 78:281, 1959.

Todd, A.S.: Localization of fibrinolytic activity in tissues. Br. Med. Bull. 20:210, 1964.

Vinazzer, H.: Über Störungen der Hämostase als Ursache von Menorrhagien. Geburtsh. Frauenheilk. 26:743, 1966.

Weiss, G. and Beller, F.K.: Tissue activator of the fibrinolytic enzyme in the female reproductive system. Obstet. Gynec. 34:809, 1969.

Whitehouse, B.H.: The Physiology and Pathology of uterine Haemorrhage. Lancet I:879–951, 1914.

Wood, J.C., Williams, E.A., Barley, V.L. and Cowdell, R.H.: The activity of hydrolytic enzymes in the human endometrium during the menstrual cycle. J. Obstet. Gynaecol. Br. Commonw. 76:724, 1969.

Copyright 1979 by Elsevier North Holland, Inc.
F.K. Beller and G.F.B. Schumacher, eds.
The Biology of the Fluids of the Female Genital Tract

BIOCHEMISTRY OF MENSTRUAL BLOOD

C. Ebert, F.K. Beller, K.W. Schweppe, and H. Wagner

SUMMARY

Menstrual blood taken at various days of the menstrual cycle was studied for the presence of plasma proteins and proteolytic enzymes.

Activity towards a substrate which is cleaved by factor Xa, subtilisin, factor IXa and papain-like enzymes was missing. High activities of plasmin, trypsin-like and other proteolytic enzymes of undetermined nature were found. There was also activity present for a substrate which was cleaved by kallikrein. In agreement with previous reports, a high concentration of fibrin(ogen) degradation products was found. Inhibitors of the coagulation system like α_2 macroglobulin, α_1 trypsin inhibitor were below peripheral plasma concentrations as was the concentration of antithrombin III.

Clottable fibrinogen was absent, however, in some clots there were discrete network structures appearing in scanning and transmission electron micrographs as fibrin indicating an incomplete mechanism of rendering the blood incoagulable.

Frauenklinik, Abt. Geburtshilfe and Gynäkologie der Westfälischen Wilhelms-Universität Münster / Westf

INTRODUCTION

The mechanism by which blood is rendered incoagulable during menstruation is an unusual enzymatic process in the human organism. It is aimed to achieve a special mechanism of breakdown and repair and it is therefore not surprising that the mechanism is biochemically complicated. The end result is menstrual blood or serum.

The present status of mind is focused on the enzymatic cleavage of fibrinogen by proteases as the significant enzyme system for rendering the blood incoagulable. In previous papers one of us (Beller, 1971) has suggested that fibrinogenolysis is the principle mechanism for incoagulability. In the meantime biochemical methodology has improved and we have reinvestigated the process which we consider fascinating since it provides the opportunity to study the biological mechanisms associated with incoagulable blood by the feature of a naturally occurring experiment.

The present paper presents data employing modern enzyme technology to provide additional information of the incoagulability of menstrual blood.

MATERIALS AND METHODS

Menstrual blood was obtained from patients age 17 to 38 on various days of the menstrual cycle. The blood was taken from the vagina in some instances by a suction cannula from the external os of the cervix. The menstrual blood was centrifuged for 30 min. at 3000 xg and 5° C. The supernatent "menstrual serum" (MS) was used for study.

1. The assay included the use of the following chromogenic substrates (Kabi Laboratories: Stockholm, Schweden) S 2251 (plasmin) S 2302 (kallikrein) S 2238 (thrombin) S 2222 (Factor Xa) S 2160 (serine proteases). For each substrate 10 μl of the MS was incubated with 590 μl tris buffer pH 7.4 or 8.4 respectively. The extinction was measured at 405 nm and 37°C for 30 min. after adding the chromogenic substrate.
2. Immuno assays were performed on Partigen plates (Behring Werke, Marburg FRG) for antithrombin III, α_1 trypsin inhibitor and α_2 macroglobulin.
3. Fibrin degradation products were assayed by Laurell electrophoresis with antibodies against D and E (Behring Werke, Marburg FRG). The antibody concentration was 1% for Anti D and 2% for Anti E in 1% Agarose. Running time: 5 hours at 6V/cm in barbiturate buffer pH 8.6.
4. "Clots were taken from the vagina following insertion of a pair of specula. It was fixed immediately in 3% glutaraldehyde. The clots were broken in slices of 0.5 cm for scanning electron microscopy.

For transmission electron microscopy small pieces of about 1 x 1 x 5 mm were prepared. Contrast was obtained by exposure to OsO_4 (1.33%) and samples were dehydrated in ethanol. Inbedding was performed in Epon and specimens were incubated in Freon for SEM. The latter were dried at critical point, coated with gold and the broken surface was observed in a Cambridge stereo scan 150 at 20 KV. A Philips EM 301 operated at 60 KV was employed for TEM.

RESULTS

The pH of menstrual blood was 7 to 7.5 independent of whether it was taken from the cervical os or the vagina.

1.0 *Proteolytic activities of menstrual blood.*

1.1 Substrate S 2222 which is cleaved by factor Xa, trypsin, acrosin, subtilisin, kallikrein and papain like enzymes: there was more activity present than in peripheral plasma (Figure 1).

1.2 Substrate 2251: Plasmin which cleaves the substrate 2251 was present in high activities. The enzymatic activity was equivalent to approximately 4,0 n catalytic units plasmin/ml "menstrual serum". It is inhibited completely by the inhibitors aprotinin and EACA (Figure 2).

1.3 Substrate 2160: This substrate is cleaved by serine proteases like thrombin, trypsin, brinase and others. The enzyme activity for this substrate was very high in MS (Figure 3) and it was not inhibited by added soy bean trypsin inhibitor.

1.4 Substrate 2238: This substrate is cleaved by thrombin. The enzyme activity was very high in MS, higher than the activity measured with substrate 2160. Hirudin as a thrombin inhibitor and soy bean trypsin inhibitor did not change the activity. Aprotinin produced only a small decrease of enzyme activity (Figure 4).

FIGURE 1. Cleavage kinetics of two menstrual sera (representative for 20 samples). Cleavage of substrate S 2222 (substrate for F Xa, trypsin ect.) in comparison to normal plasma.

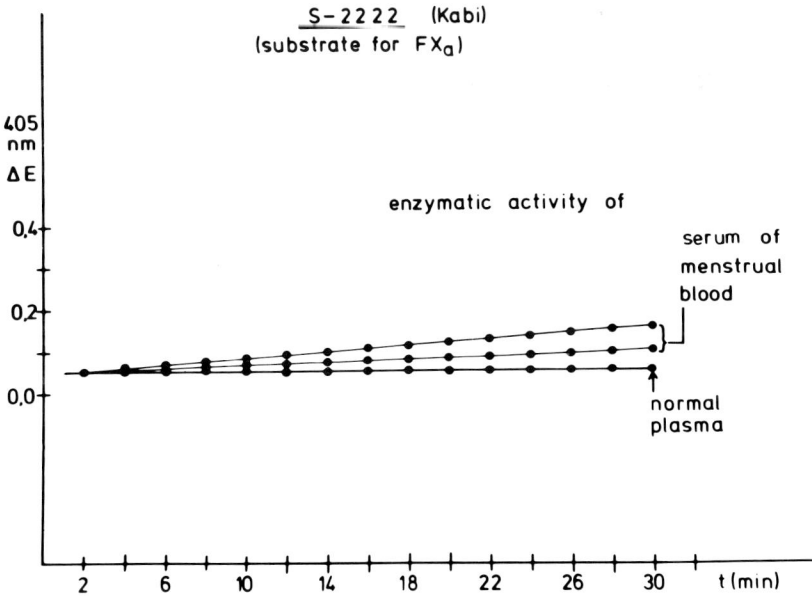

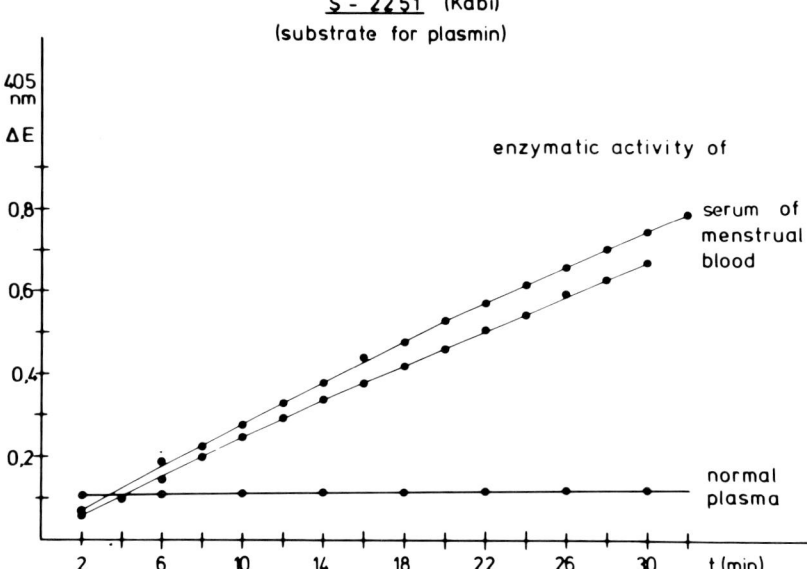

FIGURE 2. Cleavage kinetics of two menstrual sera (representative for 18 samples). Substrate S 2251 (substrate for plasmin) in comparison to normal plasma.

FIGURE 3. Cleavage kinetics of two menstrual sera (representative for 20 samples). Cleavage of substrate S 2160 (substrate for serin proteases) in comparison to normal plasma.

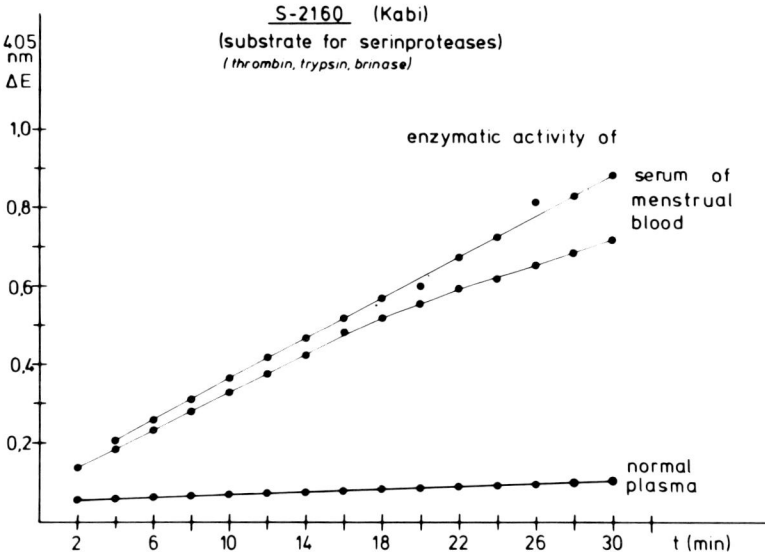

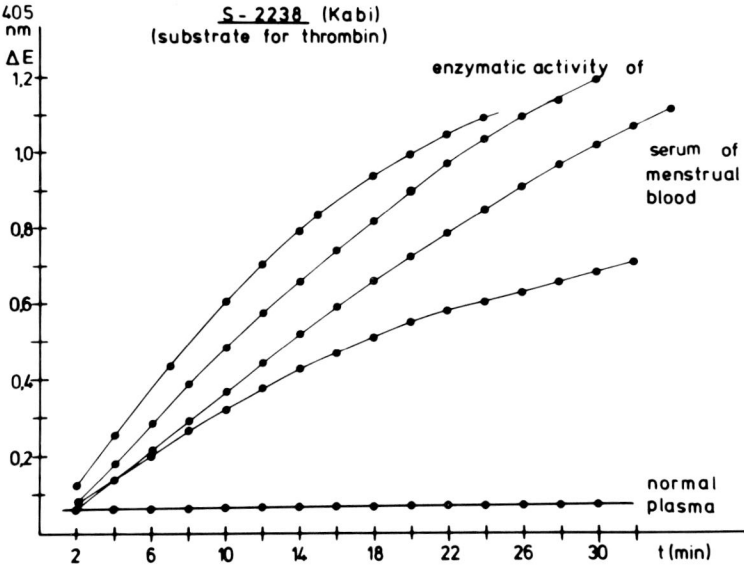

FIGURE 4. Cleavage kinetics of four menstrual sera (representative for 18 samples) for the cleavage of substrate S 2238 (substrate for thrombin) in comparison to normal plasma.

FIGURE 5. Cleavage kinetics of two menstrual sera (representative for 18 samples) for the cleavage of substrate S 2302 (substrate for kallikrein) in comparison to normal plasma.

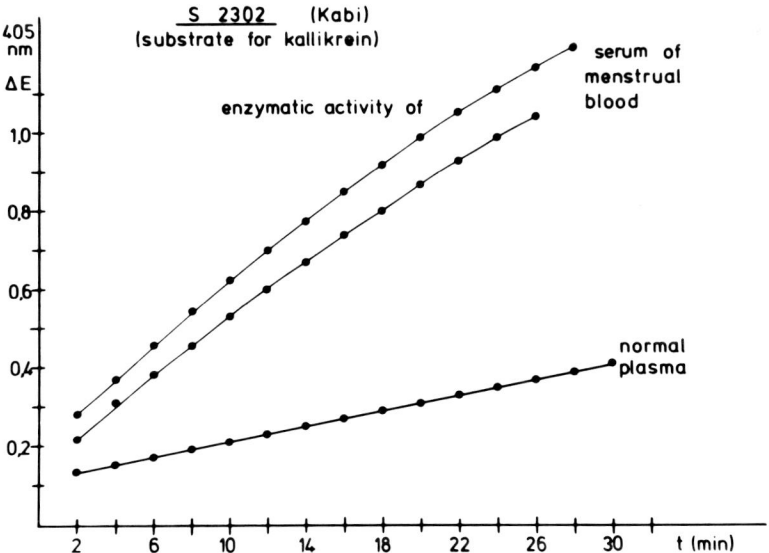

1.5 Substrate 2302 which is cleaved by kallikrein: There was enzyme activity present which was not inhibited by hirudin (Figure 5).

The enzymatic activities as measured with the substrates mentioned here are equivalent to 50 units thrombin/ml MS.

2.0 *Fibrin degradation products:*

The concentration for FDP E is in the range of 10 to 300 μg/ml ($\overline{M}$ 108 μg/ml) and for FDP D 30-2000 μg/ml ($\overline{M}$ 528 μg/ml. Considering the amount in peripheral blood (0.5–1.0 μg/ml), this concentration is (Figure 6) very high.

3.0 *Inhibitors:*

The values of α_2 MG and α_1 AT were 190 mg / 100 ml and 170 mg / 100 ml respectively below the concentration in peripheral plasma. The activity of antithrombin III was equivalent to peripheral plasma. Noteworthy is the small variation in the concentration of this inhibitor (Figure 7).

4.0 *Fibrinogen:*
Clottable Fibrinogen was not detectable in any sample.

FIGURE 6. Distribution of FDP (E) in menstrual plasma.

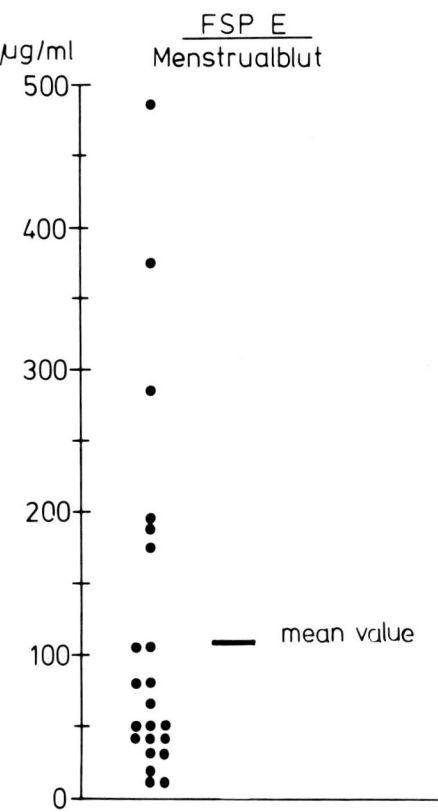

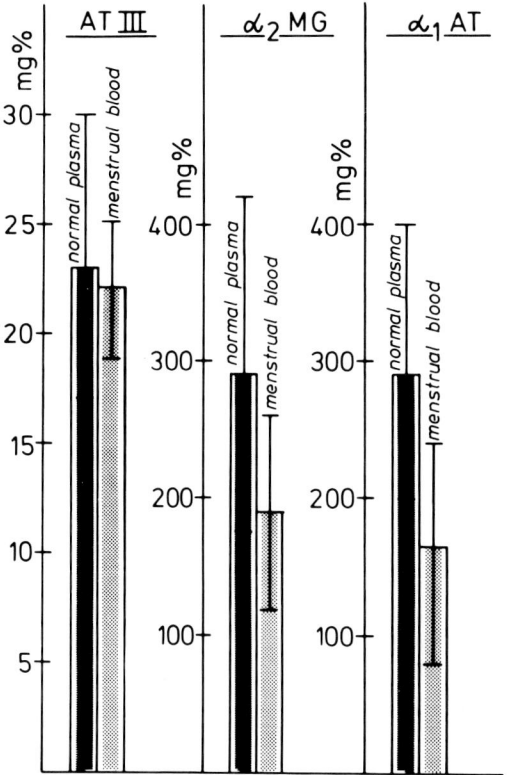

FIGURE 7. Concentration of AT III, α_2 MG and α_1 AT in menstrual sera (mean values and standard deviation) compared with peripheral plasma.

5.0 *Fibrin:*

In several menstrual clots we found discrete strands of a network (Figure 8) with a periodicity of 180 Å revealed by scanning and transmission electron microscopic examination. It is therefore likely that these strands are composed of fibrin-like material.

COMMENTS

The proteolytic activity demonstrated against various chromogenic substrates needs further discussion. Substrate S 2222 which is cleaved by factor Xa is not cleaved by menstrual serum consistent with the absence of activity for this substrate in peripheral plasma.

Substrates 2160, 2238 and 2302 are cleaved preferentially by thrombin but at different rates. Although the activity in MS is high, it cannot be equated with thrombin since hirudin a potent thrombin inhibitor does not inhibit this activity. It is therefore assumed that we are dealing with some as yet undetermined proteolytic activity other than thrombin or plasmin.

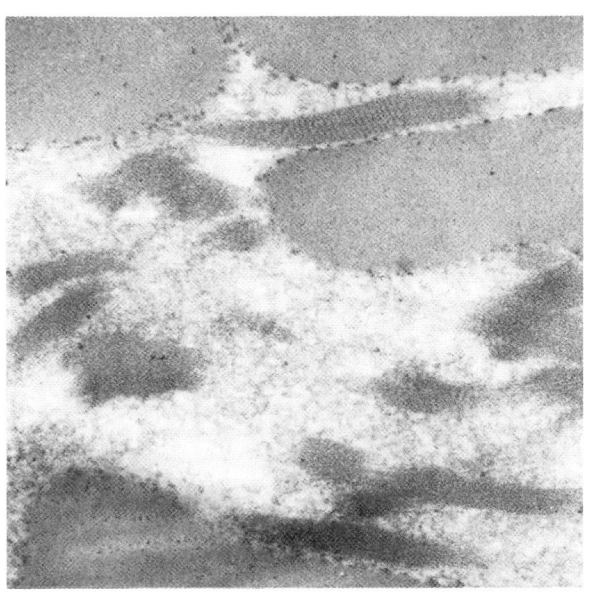

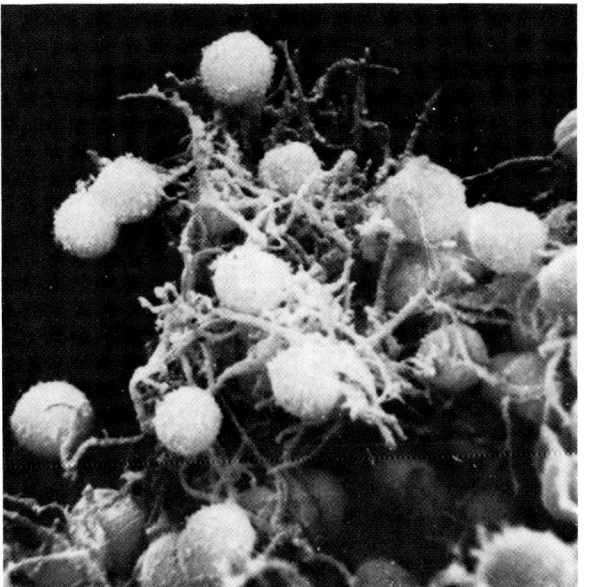

FIGURE 8. Scanning and transmission electronic microscopy of blood clots. Note the periodicity of appr. 180 Å
a) SEXM magnification 500 : 1
b) TEM magnification 24.000 : 1

The results indicate the presence of free plasmin since substrate 2251 is cleaved by plasmin. This is confirmed by the inhibition of the activity in MS by adding the plasmin inhibitor aprotonin. The data are in complete agreement with our previous results. Beller (1971) had observed that plasminogen present in menstrual serum obtained from the uterine cavity was higher than that in vaginal samples because plasminogen was activated (and therefore consumed) to free plasmin.

We are not convinced that the activation of plasminogen to plasmin is entirely due to release of plasminogen activator. This is for two reasons: the concentration of endometrial tissue is rather low compared to myometrium (Glas-Greenwalt et al., 1971) or tissue of the fallopian tube (Astrup et al., 1965); secondly IUD's which are releasing ϵ-amino caproic acid (EACA) fail to reduce spotting (Tauber, 1978).

We expected therefore additional proteolytic activity of unspecific nature deriving from lysosomal activity (Henzl et al., 1972) as indicated by Flowers (1971). As a working hypothesis it may be suggested that these enzymes activate plasminogen.

Whatever the principle mechanism may be, the end result is impressive. The high concentration of fibrinogen degradation products indicate a very effective breakdown of fibrin and most likely also of fibrinogen. Previous data were obtained by the TRCHII method (Mersky et al., 1969; Mersky et al., 1971; Mersky, 1970).

The present results are given in absolute concentration using the Laurell-technique. These data may therefore clarify a previous discrepancy as indicated by Holly (1971). There is little doubt that the large concentration of split products inhibit coagulation by virtue of their anticlotting activity (Bang et al., 1974). That even this second line of defense can fail is indicated by the discrete strands of fibrin.

We have previously demonstrated that the so called clots found in the vagina were aggregates of erythrocytes and not coagulation clots. However, we had observed that some of these "clots" did not lyse upon raising the pH as indicated by Oster. Clottable fibrinogen was never demonstrated by any investigator. Fibrin was found only in low amounts in endometrium by light microscopy.

The present study by scanning and electron microscopy has revealed a discrete network. The strands exhibited a periodicity of 180 Å and it is very likely that this material is indeed fibrin.

We therefore summarize our present concepts on the incoagulability of menstrual blood: During menstruation fibrinogen is dissolved very rapidly by a variety of proteolytic enzymes, among them predominantly plasmin which may be activated by plasminogen activators.

However, since there is less plasminogen activator in endometrial tissue than in the myometrium, it is expected that additional proteolytic enzymes presumably of lysosomal origin add to the breakdown of fibrinogen (fibrinogenolysis). The resulting fibrin(ogen) breakdown products are effective anticlotting agents and prevent further coagulation. There may be an occasional failure of clot inhibition as demonstrated in this study. Plasminogen activators present in the cervix (Beller and Weiss, 1966) may dissolve into these clots and lyse them as a second line of defense. The clots formed in the vagina are the result of a biochemical process whereby a red cell suspension with added mucoid substances forms these structures.

ACKNOWLEDGEMENT

The support of the Deutsche Forschungsgemeinschaft (DFG), Contract No. 648/5) is acknowledged.

REFERENCES

Astrup T.F., Beller, F. K., Glas, P., Rasmussen, J.: Fibrionlytic activity of the human uterine tube. Obstet. and Gynec. 25: 853, 1965.

Bang, N. M., Chang, M.L.: Soluble fibrin complexes. Seminars in Thrombos. 1: 91, 1974.

Beller, F. K.: Observations on the clotting of menstrual blood and clot formation. Am. J. Obstet. Gynec. 111: 545, 1971.

Beller, F.K., Weiss, G.: The fibrinolytic enzyme system in cervical mucus. Fertil. Steril. 17: 654, 1966.

Flowers, Ch. E.: Prepared discussion to paper Beller, F.K., Am. J. Obstet. Gynec. 111:545, 1971.

Glas-Greenwalt, P., Beller, F.K., Astrup, T.: Comparative assays of tissue plasminogen activator in myometrium, cervix and fibromas of the human uterus. Am. J. Obstet. Gynec. 110: 721–725 1971.

Henzl, M.R., Smith, S.E., Boost, G., Tayler; E.T.: Lysosomal concept of menstrual bleeding in humans. J. Clin. Endocrinol. NMetab. 34: 860, 1972.

Holly, R.G.: Prepared discussion to paper Beller, F.K., Am. J. Obstet. Gynec. 111:545, 1971.

Mersky, C., Lalezari, P., Johnson, A.J.: A rapid simple sensitive method for measuring fibrinolytic split products in human serum. Proc. Soc. Exp. Biol. Med. 63: 871, 1969.

Merskey, C., Lalezari, P., Johnson, A.J.: Tanned red cell hemagglutination inhibition immunoassay for fibrogen-fibrin-related antigen in human serum. Scand. J. Haematol. Suppl. 13: 83, 1971.

Mersky, C: Tanned red cell haemagglutination inhibition immunoassay. Recent developments. Workshop on fibrin(ogen) degradation products. Leuven, July 22–25th, 1970.

Oster, G.: Personal communication.

Tauber, P.F.: Ergebnisse einer Blutungsprophylaxe mit Fibrinolyse-Inhibitoren bei intrauteriner Kontrazeption. IUD-Symposium, 17–23th. September 1978, Zermatt, Switzerland.

BACTERIOLOGY OF LOCHIAE

H. A. Hirsch

SUMMARY

Although there have been conflicting reports on the microbial status of puerperal uterus over the past 80 years, there is good evidence that bacteria found in the endometrial cavity represent true colonization.

Colonization of the uterus is established at least by the 3rd post partum day by a variety of microorganisms, mostly anaerobes, in concentrations up to 10^5-10^8/ml.

The species most frequently isolated are T-strains of mycoplasma, diphtheroids, anaerobic cocci and bacteroides species.

Essentially the same flora is found in normal post partum women and in patients with endometritis.

Bacteria causing post partum infections are endogenous to the genital tract.

INTRODUCTION

The early concept that the uterine cavity normally remains sterile post partum (Döderlein and Winternitz 1900) was challenged from the beginning (Burkhardt 1898, Franz 1902). The controversy has continued, and there are re-

Universitäts-Frauenklinik, Tübingen, FRG

cent publications, which confirm Döderlein's findings (Mischell et al. 1966, Spore et al. 1970).

The contradictory results can be explained by the different methods used in obtaining and processing bacteriological specimens and therefore it is necessary to discuss some aspects of the methodology of these investigations.

CRITICAL COMMENTS ON THE METHODS EMPLOYED

Collection of Specimens

The major difficulty in obtaining a satisfactory specimen from the endometrial cavity is to avoid contamination by organisms from the vagina or cervix, which may or may not reflect the situation in the endometrial cavity. Various instruments and procedures have been used to obtain an uncontaminated specimen by loop, aspiration or lavage through the cervix (Peter and Moeseritz 1961, Thomsen and Fromm 1950, Wierdsma and Clayton 1964) by transabdominal uterine aspiration (Ledger et al. 1976) and by transfundal uterine puncture at laparotomy (Mishell et al. 1976, Spore et al. 1970).

Though undoubtedly the risk of cervical contamination is highest in transcervical methods, sterile cultures have been obtained using this technique by several authors (Döderlein and Winternitz 1900, Smorodizeff et al. 1935, Thomsen and Fromm 1950, Tscherne 1938). This may be due to an absence of culturable organisms in the uterus or simply to failure in culturing these organisms.

Transuterine specimen collection avoids cervical contamination. The problem with this technique is the difficulty of assurance that the tip of the needle is placed in the uterine cavity and, since only little fluid is aspirated, the concern, that the uterine cavity itself has not been sampled. A comparison of the two methods in the same patients with endometritis showed both a lower yield of positive cultures (7/19=36.8%) and fewer (11/7) after transabdominal puncture as compared to positive culture in all patients and a mean of 4 isolates (100/25) after transcervical sampling (Ledger et al. 1976)

Processing of the Specimens

The transport as well as the handling and processing of the specimens in the laboratory makes a major impact on the culture results (Peter and Moeseritz 1961, Gibbs et al., 1975). Improvement in these methods resulted in a constantly increasing isolation of fastidious organisms especially anaerobes both in infections and normal flora of the female genital tract.

It has been shown that some methods employed in endometrial culturing considerably decrease the growth of the organisms involved and this may explain the contradictory results to some extent.

B. fragilis had a 10–15 times higher colony count, when diluted with deoxygenated Ringer solution than with saline (Gibbs et al. 1975). Both solutions were used for lavage of the endometrial cavity (Gibbs et al. 1975, Spore et al. 1970).

Anaerobic cultures incubated for two days in the presence of CO_2 grew three different organisms in concentrations of 10^5–10^7/ml, while there was no growth at all under ordinary anaerobic conditions by evacuation without adding CO_2 (Peter and Moeseritz 1961).

In summary there is much evidence, that the puerperal uterus becomes colonized and that appropriate transcervical cultures give a reasonably true picture of the microbiological status of the endometrial cavity. Results from transabdominal cultures which not only yield fewer positive cultures but also fewer organisms per positive culture shed some doubt on this concept. The fact that no organisms were found in some investigations cannot be taken as evidence of a sterile uterine cavity since this may be due to cultural difficulties of fastidious organisms involved. Unfortunately no comparisons of cervical and endometrial cultures are available.

MICROBIAL COLONIZATION OF THE PUERPERAL UTERUS

Species

Numerous studies have shown that there is abundant growth of a variety of organisms in the post partum endometrial cavity. The species most frequently isolated by Gibbs and co-worker (1975) were T-stains of mycoplasma, diphtheroids, anaerobic cocci and (anaerobic) bacteroides species (Table I). Similar results were found by other investigators (Decker 1979, Goblerud et al. 1976, Ledger et al. 1976).

While some authors thought that there may have been a change in organisms in recent years, E. coli, being the most common one isolated (Sweet and Ledger 1973, White and Koontz 1973), others have still found a predominance of anaerobic organisms (Decker 1979, Gibbs et al. 1975, Gibbs et al. 1978a, Gibbs et al. 1978b, Ledger et al. 1976).

Concentration of Organisms

The number of species and the high concentration of organisms in the lower uterine segment before delivery and post partum are shown in Table II. Though quantitative cultures of that kind are not available elsewhere, other investigators have found comparable results with semiquantitative methods (Gibbs et al. 1975). This suggests that the microorganisms in the post partum endometrial cavity do not represent some aberrant bacteria but rather a real colonization.

Dynamics of Uterine Colonization

Peter and Moeseritz (1961) cultured the lower uterine segment of 10 healthy parturients quantitatively before delivery, 3–5 days, 6–9 days and 10–12 days after delivery. They found a disappearance of lactobacilli and a marked rise in aerobic and anaerobic cocci, anaerobic gramnegative rods and anaerobic grampositive rods other than lactobacilli (Table II). Only anaerobes were present in 1–2 logs at 12–24 hours post partum. These represent lower concentrations than on the 3rd day. E. coli, streptococci and yeasts were absent.

Goblerud and coworkers (1976) taking cervical cultures once in every trimester of pregnancy, 3 days after delivery and 6 weeks after delivery, had very similar results. They observed a continuous decline in the average number of an-

TABLE I. Quantitative Frequency of Organisms Found in the Endometrial Cavity of 47 Afebrile Women on the 3rd Post Partum Day*

	Total No.	%	Many	Mod.	Few
Pathogens:					
Aerobic gram-positive					
α-Streptococci	16	34	3	6	7
β-Streptococci, Group A	0	—	—	—	—
β-Streptococci, Group B	0	—	—	—	—
β-Streptococci, not Group A, B, D	4	8.5	0	3	1
γ-Streptococci	8	17	2	3	3
Enterococci (incl. Group D strep.)	4	8.5	0	1	3
S. aureus	0	—	—	—	—
Anaerobic gram-positive					
Peptostreptococci	30	63	14	14	2
Peptococci	26	55	7	12	7
Other anaerobic gram-positive cocci, not further identified	7	14	3	0	4
Cl. perfringens	0	—	—	—	—
Clostridia, other	0	—	—	—	—
Aerobic gram-negative					
E. coli	7	14	1	1	5
Klebsiella	0	—	—	—	—
Enterobacter	1	2	0	0	1
P. mirabilis	0	—	—	—	—
Anaerobic gram-negative					
B. fragilis	5	10	0	4	1
Bacteroides, other	6	13	1	4	1
Fusobacterium	1	2	1	0	0
Nonpathogens:					
S. epidermidis	8	17	5	1	2
Lactobacilli	8	17	3	2	3
Diphtheroids	30	63	13	10	7
Proprionibacterium	8	17	3	2	3
Eubacterium	1	2	0	1	0
Other anaerobic gram-positive non-spore-forming rods	5	10	1	3	1
Mycoplasma:					
T. form	39/46	84			
M. hominis	7/47	15			

* Gibbs et al., 1975.

TABLE II. Flora of the Cervix Just Prior to Delivery and of the Lochiae on the 3rd Day Post Partum*

	Before delivery	Logs of organisms 3rd day post partum
Anaerobic lactobacilli	5, 6, 6, 8, 6	—
Aerobic lactobacilli	5, 4, 5	7
Anaerobic gram+ rods	8, 8, 5, 3,	7, 5, 7, 7, 4, 4
Bacteroides sp.	8	4, 6, 7, 8, 7, 4, 4, 6, 4
Peptococci	6, 4	4, 5, 6, 6, 5, 6
Streptococci	4	7, 4, 3
Proteolytic organisms	4, 3, 4	3, 5, 5, 3, 3, 4, 4, 5
Yeasts	4, 5, 3	—

* From Peter and Moeseritz, 1961.

aerobes during pregnancy followed by a steep rise after delivery. Aerobes remained fairly constant except E. coli, which rose from 5.3% positive cultures in the 3rd trimester to 32.6% after delivery and yeasts, which decreased from 15.89% to 0 respectively. At 6 weeks the organisms had returned to a level similar to that of the first trimester (Figure 1). Mackay and coworkers (1977) found a similar change in the pattern after delivery in perineal and vaginal cultures with a decrease in lactobacilli, common commensals and yeasts and an increase in coliforms and anaerobic cocci.

Origin of Organisms Found in the Endometrial Cavity

Organisms found in the endometrial cavity after delivery (Gibbs et al. 1975, Gibbs et al. 1978, Peter and Moeseritz 1961) are very similar in distribution and concentration to those found in the cervix (Goblerud et al. 1976), vagina and perineum (Mackay et al. 1977).

The same organisms were isolated from the amniotic fluid of afebrile parturients undergoing cesarean section (Table III Dahler et al. 1975). The colonization of the amniotic fluid increased with time after rupture of the membranes (Figure 2) and was higher in patients with internal fetal monitoring. The uterine colonization correlated with an increased maternal infection rate following cesarean section.

CLINICAL CORRELATIONS

Considering the abundant colonization of the puerperal uterus by a wide variety of potentially pathogenic organisms it is not surprising that essentially the same bacteria were found in afebrile women after delivery and in patients with endometritis (Decker and Hirsch 1979, Gibbs et al. 1975) (Table IV). This is also true for patients with infection following cesarean secton with and without internal fetal monitoring (Gibbs et al. 1978a, Gibbs et al. 1978b).

An exception may be group A streptococci which are not normally found in the puerperal uterus.

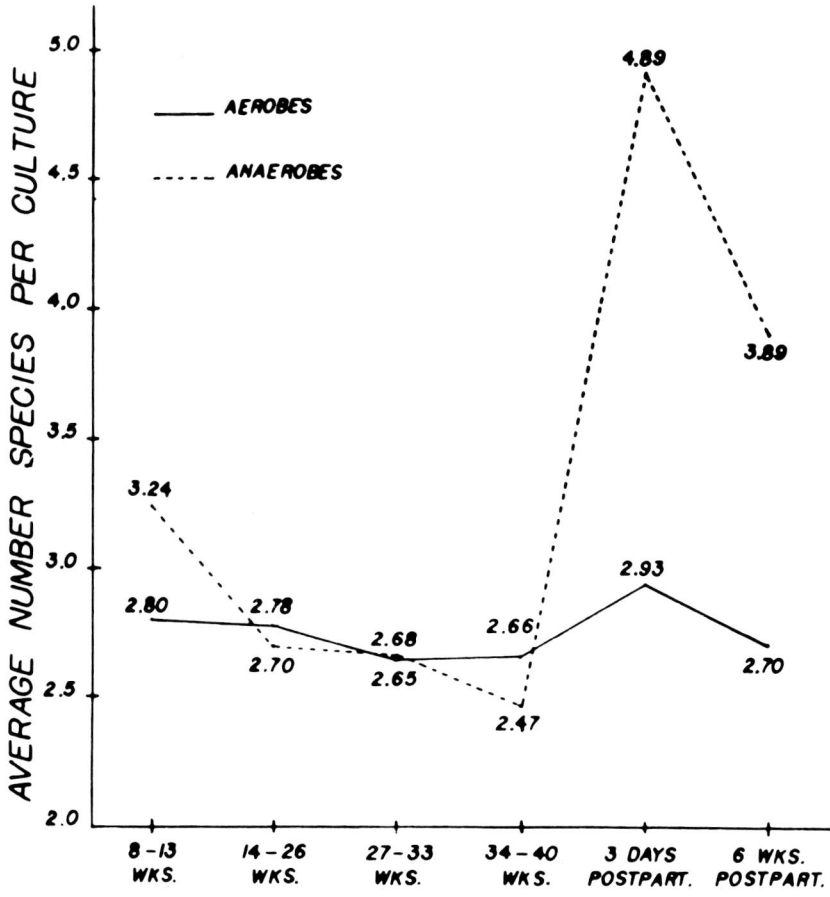

FIGURE 1. The average number of different species of organisms per culture found in each of six study periods during pregnancy and post partum (Goblerud et al. 1976).

TABLE III. Microorganisms Isolated from 77 Amniotic Fluid Specimens Collected During Cesarean Section*

	No.	%
Bacteroides sp.	18	23.4
Anaerobic cocci	3	3.9
Enterobacteria	14	18.2
Streptococci	17	22.1
S. aureus	5	6.5
S. epidermitis	4	5.2
C. vaginale	15	19.5
Yeasts	3	3.9
Grampositive rods	27	35.1

* Dahler et al., 1975.

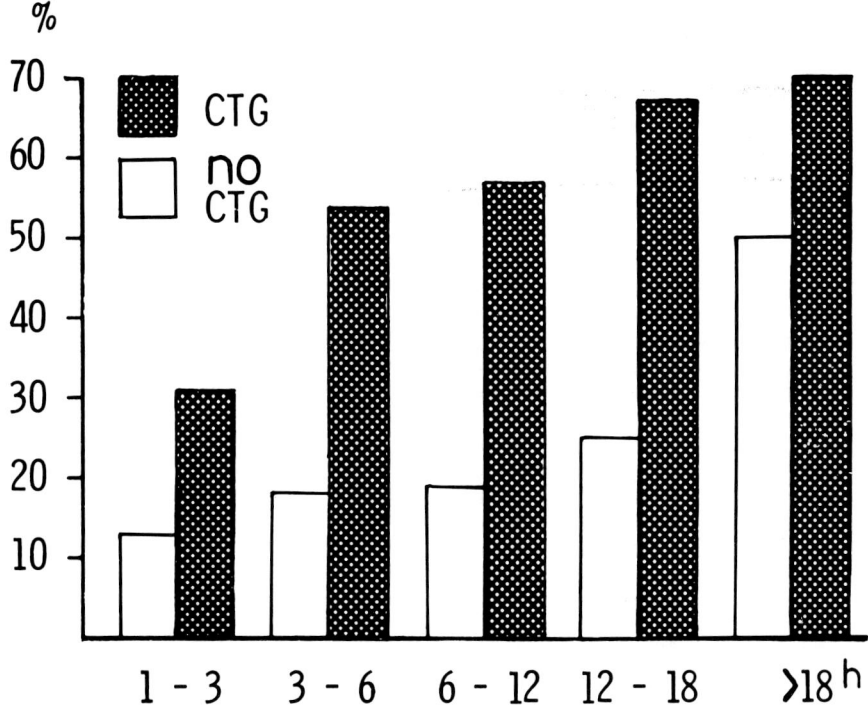

FIGURE 2. Percentage of positive cultures of amniotic fluid specimens sampled during cesarean section in patients with and without internal fetal monitoring (CTG). (Dahler et al. 1975).

TABLE IV. Flora of the Post Partum Cervix From Patients With and Without Fever*

	No fever (52 pts.)	Fever ≥ 38°C 56 (pts.)
Enterobacteria	29	39
Bacteroides sp.	31	45
Peptococci	4	5
Peptostreptococci	8	9
Clostridia	2	5
Enterococci	12	14
Streptococci	14	13
Staphylococci	6	9
C. vaginale	23	27
Mycoplasma	17	29
Ureaplasma	25	32
Yeasts	4	5

* Decker, 1979.

Therefore, bacterial colonization is not apparently a decisive factor in the development of post partum uterine infection. The reason why these women do not become febrile is not known. Changes in host resistance, local or general, seem to be more important. An example is trauma such as the uterine wound by cesarean section, which clearly predisposes to infection.

REFERENCES

Burkhardt, H.: Uber den Keimgehalt der Uterushöhle bei normalen Wöchnerinnen. Zbl. Gynäk. 22: 686–689, 1898.

Dahler, R., Decker, K., Hirsch, H.A.: Bakterielle Besiedelung des Fruchtwassers unter der Geburt. 1. Einfluβ des internen CTG; Sektiomorbidiät. In: Perinatale Medizin IV (eds), Dudenhausen, Saling, Schmidt, Thieme Stuttgart, 1975, pp. 235–236.

Decker, K., Hirsch, H.A.: Unpublished data 1979.

Döderlein, A. and Winternitz, E.: Die Bakteriologie der puerperalen Sekrete. Beiträge zur Geburtshilfe und Gynäkologie 3: 161–174, 1900.

Franz, C.: Zur Bakterilogie des Lochialsekretes fieberfreier Wöchnerinnen. Beiträge zur Geburtshilfe und Gynäkologie 6: 332–349, 1902.

Gibbs, R.S., O'Dell, T.N., MacGreggor, R.R., Schwarz, E.H., Morton, H.: Puerperale endometritis: A prospective microbial study. Am. J. Obstet. Gynecol. 121: 919–925, 1975.

Gibbs, R.S., Facog, Jones, P.M and Wilder, C.J.Y.: Internal fetal monitoring and maternal infection following cesarean section. A prospective study. Obstet. Gynecol. 52: 193–197, 1978a.

Gibbs, R.S., Facog, Jones, P.M., and Wilder, C.J.: Antibiotic therapy of endometritis following cesarean section. Treatment successes and failures Obstet. Gynecol. 52: 31–37, 1978b.

Goblerud, C.P., Ohm M.J., Galask, R.P.: Aerobic and anaerobic flora of the cervix during pregnancy and the puerperium. Am. J. Obstet. Gynecol. 126: 858–865, 1976.

Ledger, W.J., Gee, C.L., Pollin, P.A., Lewis, W.P., Sutter, V.L., Finegold, S.M.: A new approach to patients with suspected anaerobic pelvic infection. Am. J. Obstet. Gynecol. 126: 1–6, 1976.

Mackay, E.V., Khoo, S.K. and Baddeley, A.: A prospective study of the flora of the lower genital tract during pregnancy. Aust. N.Z.J. Obstet. Gynaec. 17: 133–136, 1977.

Mishell, D.R., Jr, Bell, J.H., Good, R.G., and Moyer, D.L.: Bacteriology of postpartum oviducts and endometrium. Am. J. Obstet. Gynecol. 96: 119–126, 1966.

Peter, A., and Moeseritz, E.: Ergebnisse quantitativer Keimbestimmungen aus dem Uterussekret im fieberfreien Wochenbett. Arch. Gynäk. 194: 510–532, 1961.

Smorodinzeff, A.A., Dertschinsky, G.D., Wygodskaja, J.G.: Das Problem der Autoinfektion in der Geburtshilfe. II. Mitt. Neue Ergebnisse auf dem Gebiete der Bakteriologie des Uterus und der Vagina im Puerperium. Arch. Gynäk. 159: 155–165, 1935.

Spore, W.W., Moskal, P.A., Nakamura, R.M., Mishell, D.R.: Bacteriology of postpartum oviducts and endometrium. Amer. J. Obstet. Gynec. 107: 572–577, 1970.

Sweet, R.L., Ledger, W.J.: Puerperal infectious morbidity (A two-year review) Am. J. Obstet. Gynecol. 117: 1093–1100, 1950.

Thomsen, K., and Fromm, E.: Der Keimgehalt des Cavum uteri im Wochenbett. Arch. Gynäk. 177: 111–148, 1950.

Tscherne, E.: Zur Frage der Keimfreiheit der Uterushöhle im normalen Wochenbett. Zbl. Gynäk. 62: 2306–2307, 1938.

White, C.A., Koontz, F.P.: Beta-hemolytic streptococcus infections in postpartum patients. Obstet. Gynec. 41: 27–32, 1973.

Wierdsma, J.G., Clayton E.M.: The effect of certain antibiotics on the normal postpartum intrauterine bacteriologic flora. Am. J. Obstet. Gynecol. 88: 541–544, 1964.

ULTRASTRUCTURAL OBSERVATIONS ON TRANSFORMATION OF DECIDUA INTO ENDOMETRIUM POST PARTUM

H. Wagner, K.W. Schweppe, and F.K. Beller

SUMMARY

The repair mechanism of the endometrium post partum was studied by scanning and transmission electron microscopy. The study comprised 64 lactating and non-lactating patients. In agreement with the few available data on light microscopy the placental site needs more than 14 days of repair. Necrosis is demarked not before day 3 post partum and occurs unrelated to inflammatory processes.

The repair of decidua parietalis is more rapid and is completed as early as 10 days post partum. There is no necrosis involved. The principal mechanism seems to be the transformation of decidua cells to fibroblasts in conjunction with enzymatic activity.

The cervix uteri is completely restored as early as day ten post partum. There was no apparent evidence for differences in lactating and non-lactating women.

INTRODUCTION

The involution of the uterus post partum is an impressive biological accomplishment of the organism whose mechanism is unclear. Hormonal parameters were only recently (Rolland et al., 1975; Delvoye et al., 1978; Crystle, 1973;

Frauenklinik, Abtlg. Geburtshilfe und Gynäkologie, Westfälische Wilhelms-Universität Münster/Westf.

Reyes et al., 1972) elaborated in the puerperal phase and very little information is available regarding morphology and function of decidua, myometrium and cervix uteri.

Williams (1931) extensively reviewed the literature and came to definitive conclusions regarding placental site repair. His statements that inflammatory processes and necrosis are unrelated were important contributions to the understanding of this process. Anderson and Davis (1968) reviewed the literature again and provided data on a large series of post partum hysterectomies studied by light microscopy. Their findings will be discussed in reference to our data on ultrastructure. By animal experiments Brandes and Anton (1969) and Dessouky (1971) assumed that the involution of the myometrium in the puerperium was related to macrophages and liberated enzymes.

The assumption that in the human cervix decidua cells are transformed into fibroblasts thereby restoring the connective tissue structure, according to electronmicroscopic observations of Bani Sacchi and Lo Stumbo (1972), needs further confirmation.

Immediate post partum vacuum aspiration of the cavum uteri revealed incomplete placenta areas and membranes (Rhen et al., 1974; Rolland et al., 1975) correlated endometrium biopsies with lactation, the onset of amenorrhea between 40 and 94 days, and hormonal levels. The first menses observed in 10 subjects during the study were preceded by normal progesterone levels. Endometrial biopsies revealed early and late proliferative changes and secretory transformations.

The first appearance of secretory endometrium as indicated by consecutive endometrial biopsies was the 33rd day post partum (Kava et al., 1968).

Our own ongoing study is concerned with providing answers to the following questions:

1. When is the earliest proliferative change observable?
2. Is there a difference in the endometrial change between lactating and non-lactating women?
3. Is there a correlation between the cessation of lochial excretion and regeneration of the endometrium?

The present paper is concerned with scanning and electron microscopic observations about the involution of decidua in the early post partum period.

MATERIALS AND METHODS

Two hysterectomy specimens were available for study and endometrial biopsies were taken from 64 post partum patients. One uterus was obtained at the third cesarean section and the other uterus was removed because of atonic hemorrhage 16 hours post partum. The uteri were dissected at the left margin and target biopsies under the dissected microscope were taken for electron and scanning electron microscopy (Figure 1).

The endometrial biopsies were taken from volunteers after informed consent on various days of the first days post partum. Placenta insertion was determined before delivery by sonography. The distribution of material is presented in Table I.

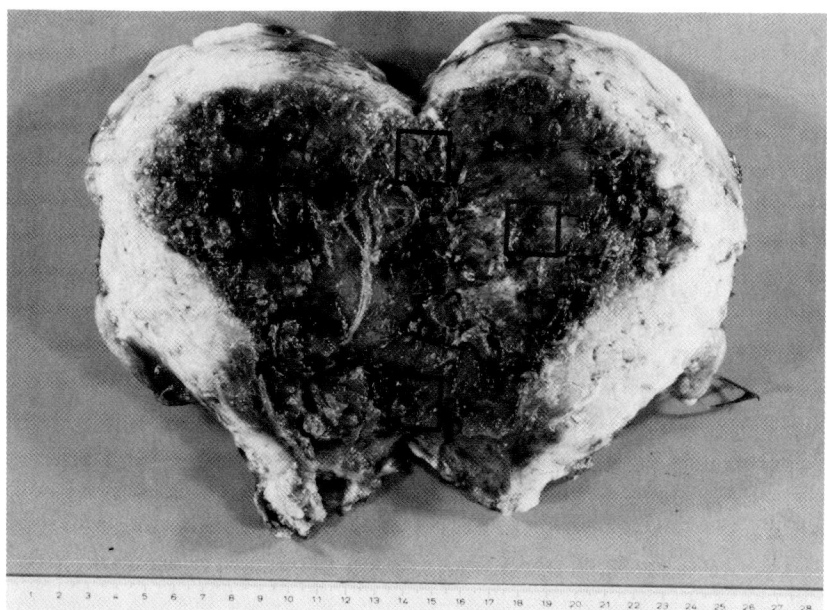

FIGURE 1. Uterus 16 hours post partum opened at the left corner and washed with saline. The placenta site is on the left, the decidua parietalis on the right. The squares mark the areas from which the specimens were taken.

TABLE I. Patients Examined in This Study.

Day p.partum	No. of patients	lactating	non lactating	Age (years)
1	4	3	1	31 - 39
2	7	6	1	16 - 35
3	6	6	-	18 - 35
4	4	2	2	22 - 37
5	9	7	2	23 - 32
6	10	9	1	24 - 39
7	11	9	2	16 - 38
8	6	4	2	21 - 37
9	2	2	-	19 / 26
10	2	-	2	24 / 38
11	1	-	1	31
13	2	1	1	25 / 38
Total	64	49	15	

The material was rinsed immediately in 3% glutaraldehyde to remove tissue parts and blood contamination. The purified tissue was additionally incubated in 3% glutaraldehyde for two hours. The material was then contrasted for 3 hours in Os O_4 1, 33%. Dehydration was performed in increasing alcohol concentration and the material was embedded in Epon. For the pilot study thick sections were prepared using a Porter-Blum-MT1B ultramicrotome, stained with toluidine blue and examined by light microscopy. Ultra thin sections were obtained from special areas and examined by an electron microscope (Philips EM 301) operated at 60 KV. Samples were prepared for scanning electron microscopy as described previously and examined with a Cambridge stereoscan 150.

RESULTS

The quantity and duration of lochia was proportional to the involution of the uterus in puerperal phase. The duration of lochial excretion was 3 weeks. The morphological constituents of lochia corresponded with the common clinical arrangement of lochiae rubrae (first week), lochiae fuscae (beginning of second week), lochiae flavae (end of second week) and lochiae albae (end of third week). Erythrocytes were present with white blood cells, cellular debris and amorphous substances with protein structure (Figure 2). Immediately post partum the walls of the cavum uteri were remarkably smooth. After washing out and removing blood the decidua parietalis appeared as a smooth surface with grayish-red appearance. The placental insertion site, however, showed a rough surface with firmly detached clots. A distinct differentiation could be made by light microscopy and scanning electron microscopy (SEM) between decidua parietalis and placental site. On the first day post partum the decidual structure was preserved. The surface was covered by a smooth epithelial layer. There were scattered epithelial clefts from which bleeding originated. Focal bleedings were present in decidua next to blood vessels filled with hemostatic plugs (Figure 3).

In contrast the placental site revealed parts of decidua with thrombosed and hyalinized vessels especially at the surface. The bleeding areas were multiple and wide.

Thrombi were present on the surface together with necrotic particles of decidua and placenta and membranes composed of a protein- and mucus-like substance (Figure 4).

At the first post partum day, but more pronounced on day 2, there was a disintegration of decidua cells caused by an invasion of polymorphonuclear leucocytes, lymphocytes and macrophages other than erythrocytes. The leucocytes contained numerous osmiophilic granules undergoing discharge. Lysosomes were seen extracellularly. This correlates with the increased enzyme activity of lochia in the first post partum days.*

The surface epithelium was monolayered with wide intracellular clefts (Figure 5).

On the third day post partum there was early shedding of membrane like material consisting of necrotic tissue clots and an amorphic ground substance.

Smooth surfaces were seen below these membranes. Decidual reactions

---

* Ebert, C. et al., pp. 247-256.

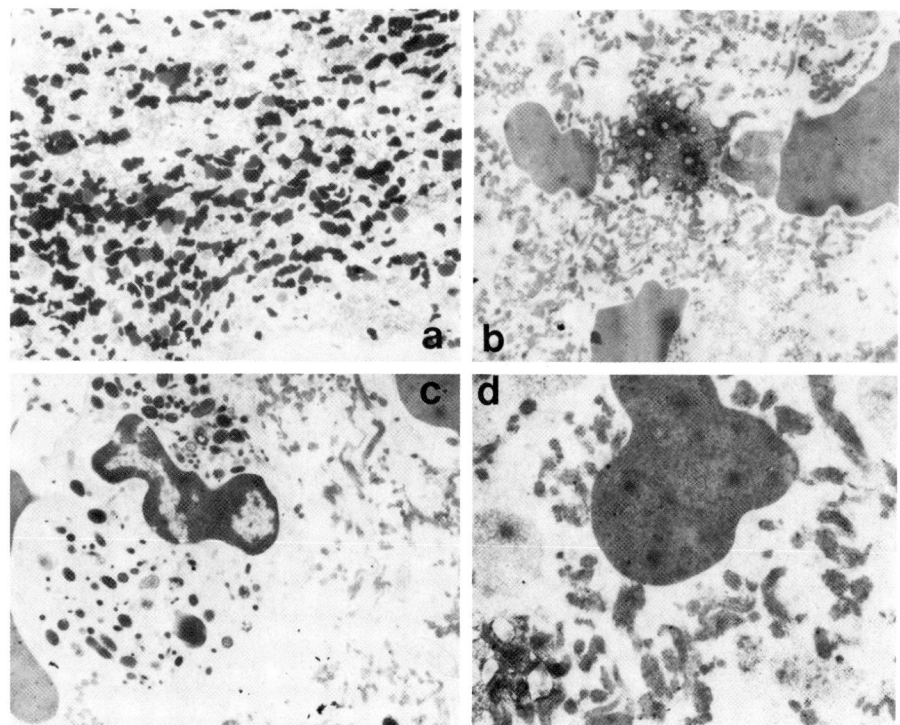

FIGURE 2. The morphologic components of lochia at day 2 post partum. a) Based on a protein-like substance lochia consists of blood cells, cellular debris and various small vesicles. Magnification: 1250 : 1; LM (light microscopy photograph) b) Cellular debris surrounded by erythrocytes (Er) Magnification: 5700 : 1: TEM (transmission electronmicroscopy photograph) c) Polymorphic nuclear leucocyte and small vesicles (arrow). Magnification: 9100 : 1; TEM d) High magnification of the lochia protein like amorphic substance. There is lack of any periodicity. Magnification: 15000 : 1; TEM

were still present at the stroma with bleeding and partial necrosis especially near thrombosed blood vessels. Lacking was a surface epithelium (Figure 6).

At this time there were thrombosed vessels in the decidua parietalis. Macro- and microphages were seen. There seemed to be a regression of decidua cells into fibroblasts. Fibrils were present without any periodicity (Figure 7).

Differentiation into stroma and endometrial surface epithelium increased during the next days with great individual variation. The macro- and microphages decreased. The stroma tissue became more dense and there was a decrease of decidual like cells.

The earliest complete conversion of decidua into endometrium was seen at day 10 post partum in one instance (Figure 8). Reparation of the placental site may need more time; it was not completed on day 13 post partum.

Since we were dealing with biopsy material there was also available material

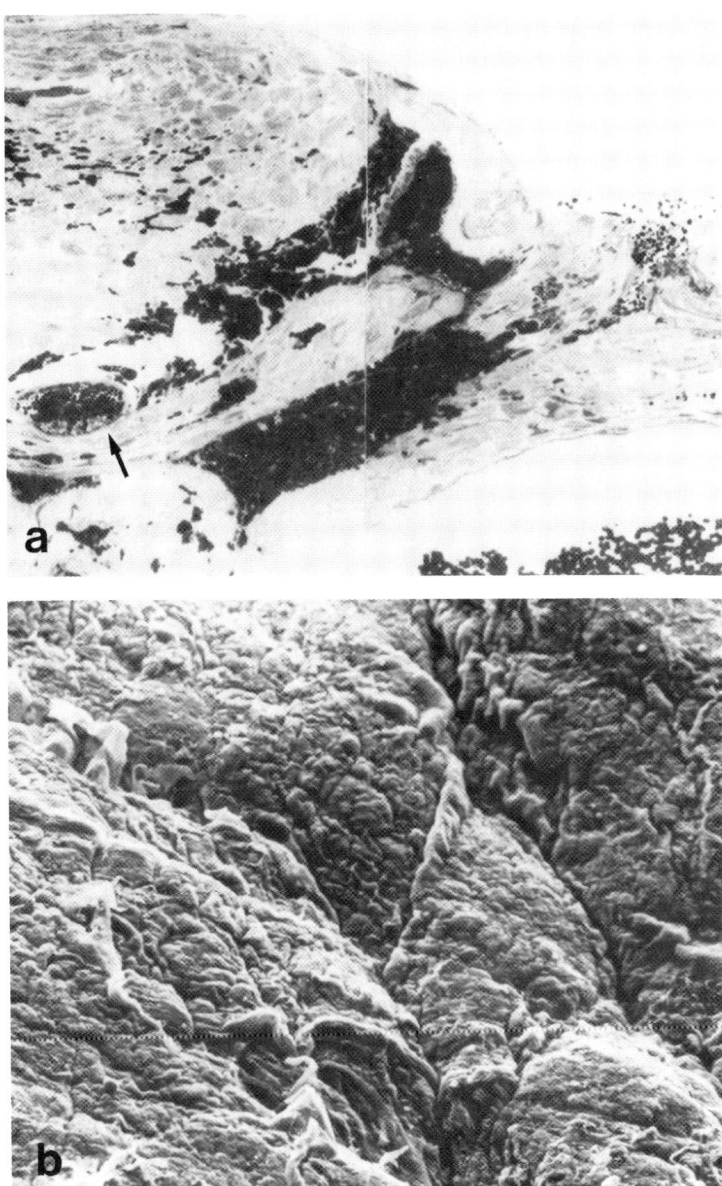

FIGURE 3. Decidua parietalis; day 1 post partum. a) Typical decidua with focal tissue bleeding and vessels well filled with blood cells. Partial thrombosis can be observed (Arrow). The surface is smooth, however small defects appear where blood cells are passing through. Magnification: 500 : 1; LM b) The decidual surface appears smooth with some valley-like regions breaking up at the bottom. The surface is covered with membranes of mucoid material. Magnification: 50 : 1; SEM (Scanning electron microscopic photograph)

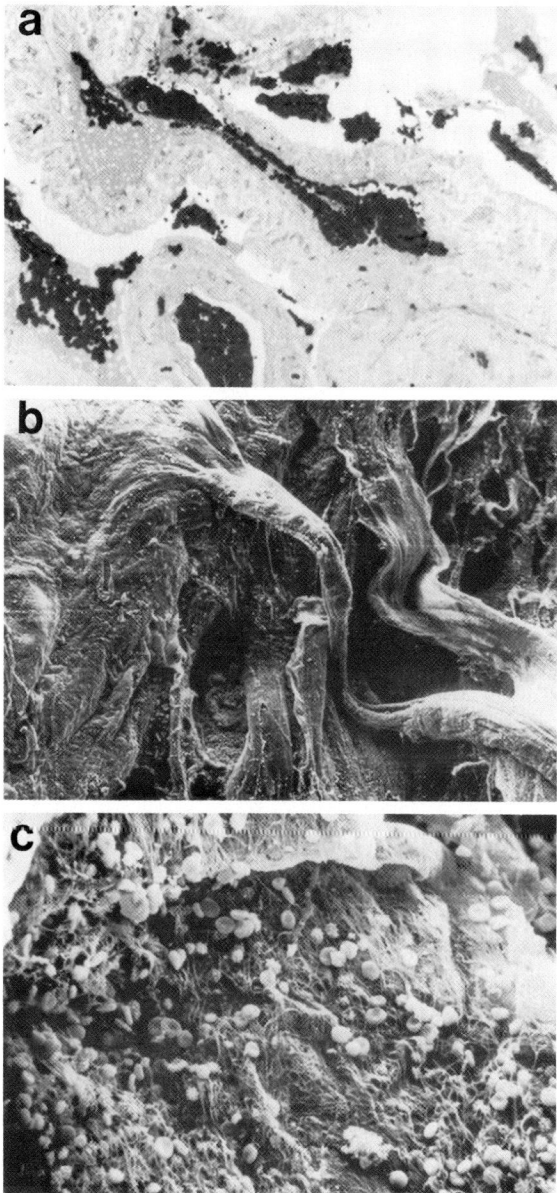

FIGURE 4. Placenta insertion site; day 1 post partum. a) The surface is covered with thrombotic deposits, placental and decidual tissue particles. Multiple bleedings occur in the tissue next to the thrombosed blood vessels. Magnification: 500 : 1; LM b) Membranes of mucus and tissue are characteristic structures of the surface. Magnification: 200 : 1; SEM c) Between the membranes occurs a network of fibrin-like substance, filled with blood cells and cellular debris. Magnification: 500 : 1; SEM

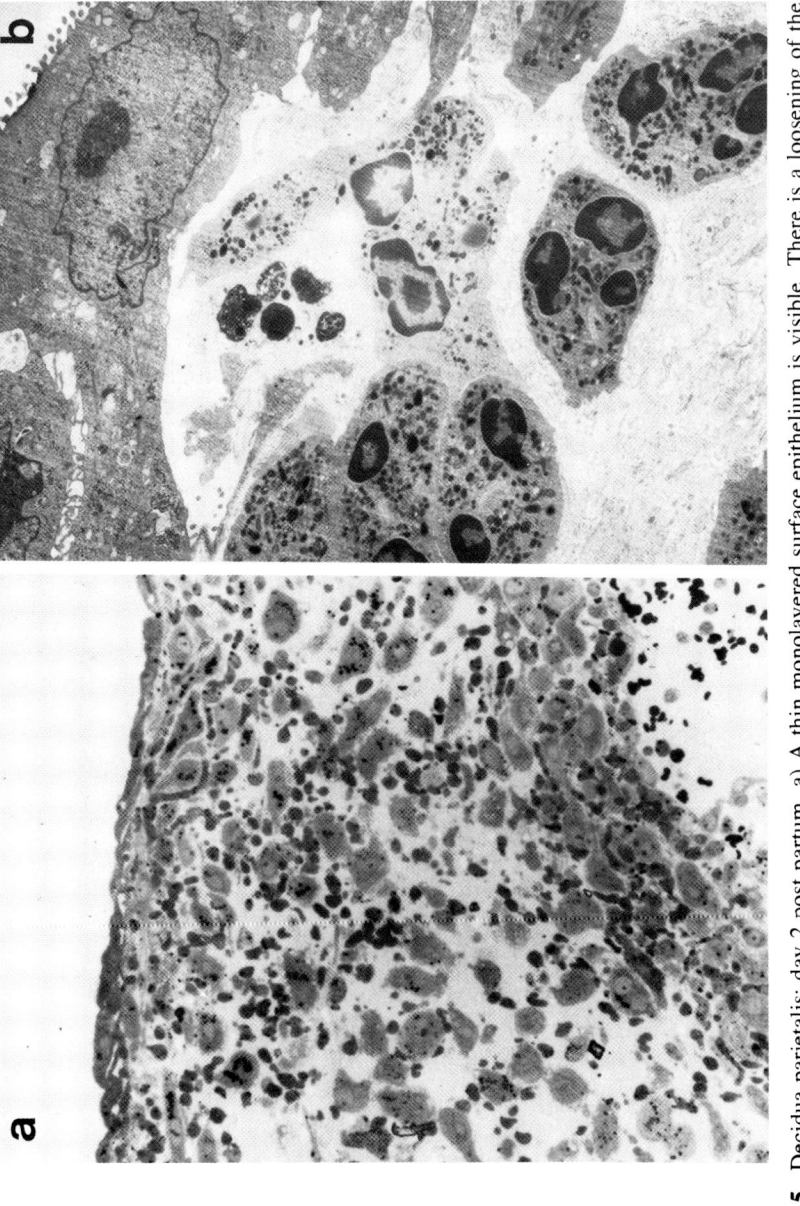

FIGURE 5. Decidua parietalis; day 2 post partum. a) A thin monolayered surface epithelium is visible. There is a loosening of the decidual cells caused by an invasion of white blood cells and phagocytes. Magnification: 780 : 1; LM b) The monolayered surface epithelium with enlarged interepithelial spaces and lots of leucocytes lying subepithelially. Magnification: 3400 : 1; TEM

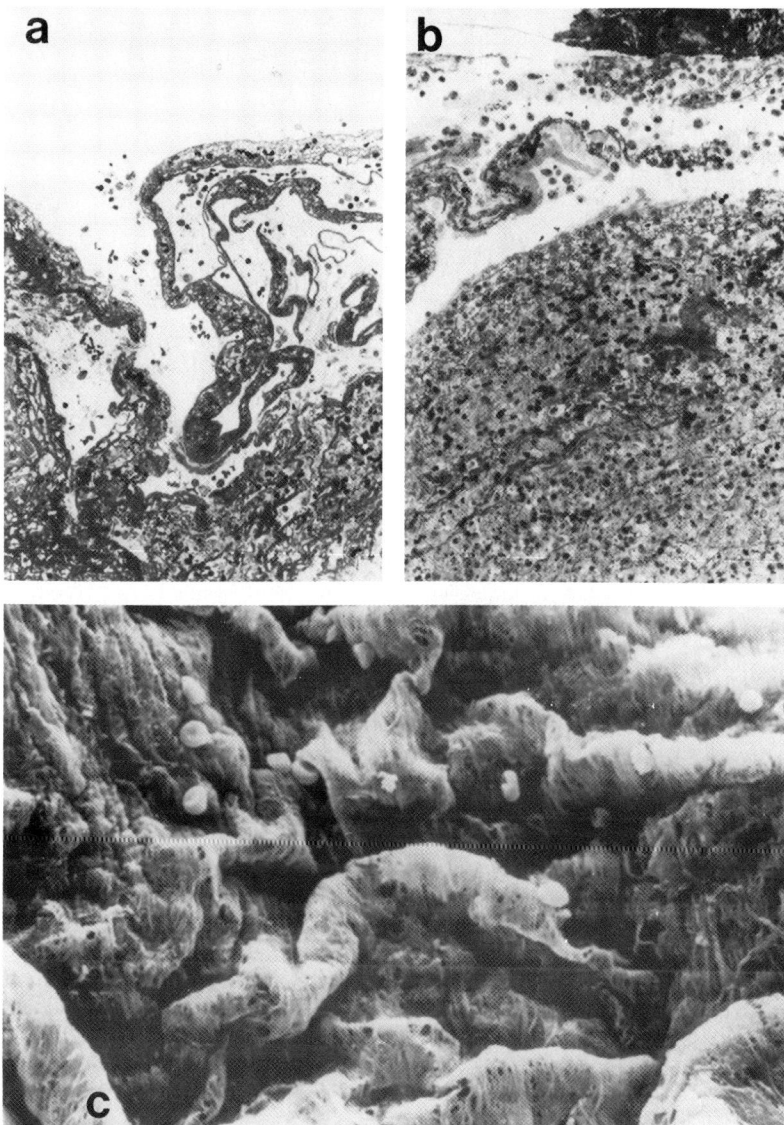

FIGURE 6. Placenta insertion site; day 3 post partum. a) Membrane-like structures consisting of necrotic tissue and thrombotic elements cover the surface. Magnification: 780 : 1; LM b) The lower decidual parts also show various areas of necrosis. Shedding of necrotic material starts. Magnification: 780 : 1; LM c) The shedding of membranes is well demonstrated in this area. Magnification: 500 : 1; SEM

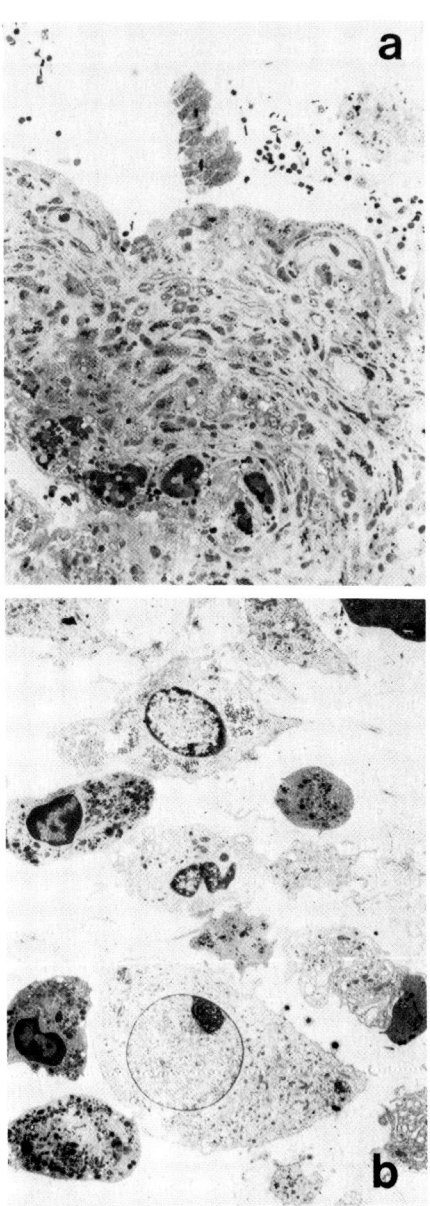

FIGURE 7. Decidua parietalis; day 3 post partum. a) There is thrombosis in the lower vessels, and a beginning of differentiation into surface epithelium and stroma. Magnification: 780 : 1; LM b) Fibroblasts are present beside the decidual and white blood cells. Magnification: 2500 : 1; TEM

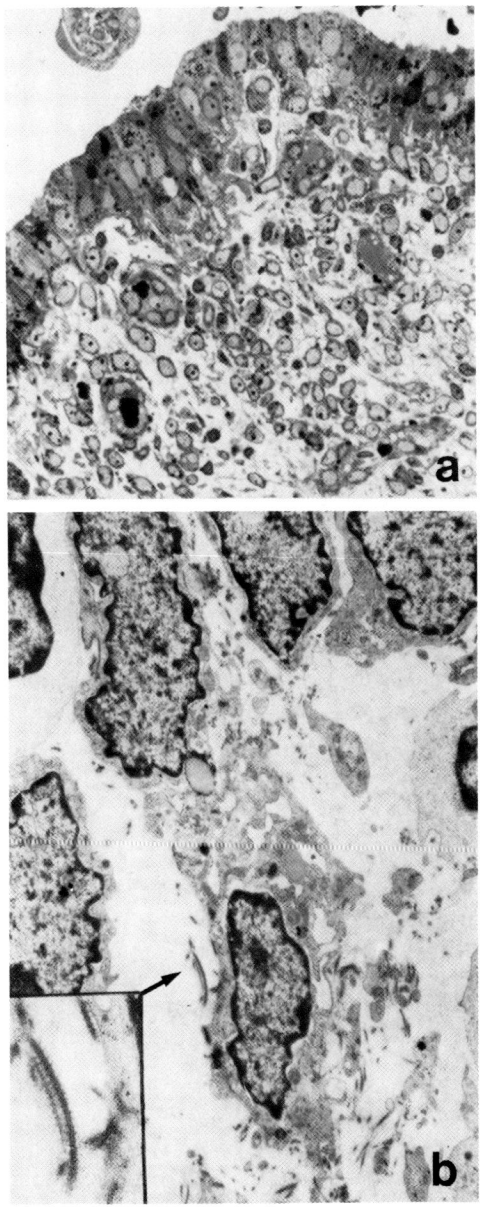

FIGURE 8. Decidua parietalis; day 10 post partum. a) Complete regeneration of endometrium. Magnification: 1250 : 1; LM b) The stroma consists of fibroblasts producing kollagen fibrills. Magnification: 5700 : 1; TEM

from the cervix. At the second day post partum we observed cylindric epithelium of the cervix with multiple areas of degeneration (Figure 9). The decidual transformation corresponded with that of the cavum uteri, especially multiple focal bleeding areas were visible. The stroma and epithelium of the cervix uteri were restored completely at the tenth day post partum with already apical secretion (Figure 10). There was no difference between lactating and non-lactating women.

COMMENTS

The regression of the decidua parietalis proceeds according to our data similar to the description of Bani Sacchi and Lo Stumbo (1972) of the cervix uteri. During the first two days post partum the decidua contained focal bleeding areas, thrombosed vessels and breaks of the surface structure. Necrosis was absent but there was an invasion of leucocytes.

Differentiation into surface epithelium and stroma was apparent on day three. The increasing number of fibroblasts were correlated with a decreased number of decidua cells: The transformation develops in a continuous fashion during the next days.

A complete regular endometrium was first seen in one instance on day ten post partum in agreement with previous data of Williams (1931) and Anderson (1968). The variation in different patients may be partly explained by the small samples of material obtained by biopsy.

The results correlated with the clinical observation that lochiae flavae (means yellowish with very little blood contamination) occur in the beginning of the second week. They are presumably derived from the placental insertion site and not anymore from the decidua parietalis.

We have not seen glands in the decidua like Anderson and Davis (1968), but this may be related to the sampling procedure. There is ultrastructural evidence for the presence of lysosomal enzymes which are present in both lochia and decidua. This correlates with the proteolytic enzyme activity in lochia as presented by Ebert et al.* in this symposium. The placental site repair differs from that of the decidua parietalis. The thrombosis of small and large vessels and the tissue bleeding exceeds that of the decidua. Necrosis develops which is sloughed following the third day post partum. The cellularity of the stroma reveals larger accumulations of polymorphonuclear leucocytes, lymphocytes and micro- and macrophages.

Our material covers up to 13 days post partum. By this time there was no repair mechanism noticed at the placental site.

There is remarkable agreement between the older observations of Williams (1931) Sharman (1953) and Anderson and Davis (1968) obtained by light microscopy, especially the later authors who examined a unique material of post partum uteri following hysterectomies. It is unlikely that such a material will be available again. According to their data the repair of the placental site develops from tongue like protusions of the already regenerated endometrial margia and left over basal endometrium glands.

Taking together the various data in the literature and the results of the present study, one can make the following statements:

> The transformation of decidua cells into fibroblasts seems to be a significant factor in the regeneration of endometrium supported by enzymatic processes.

* Ebert et al., 247–256.

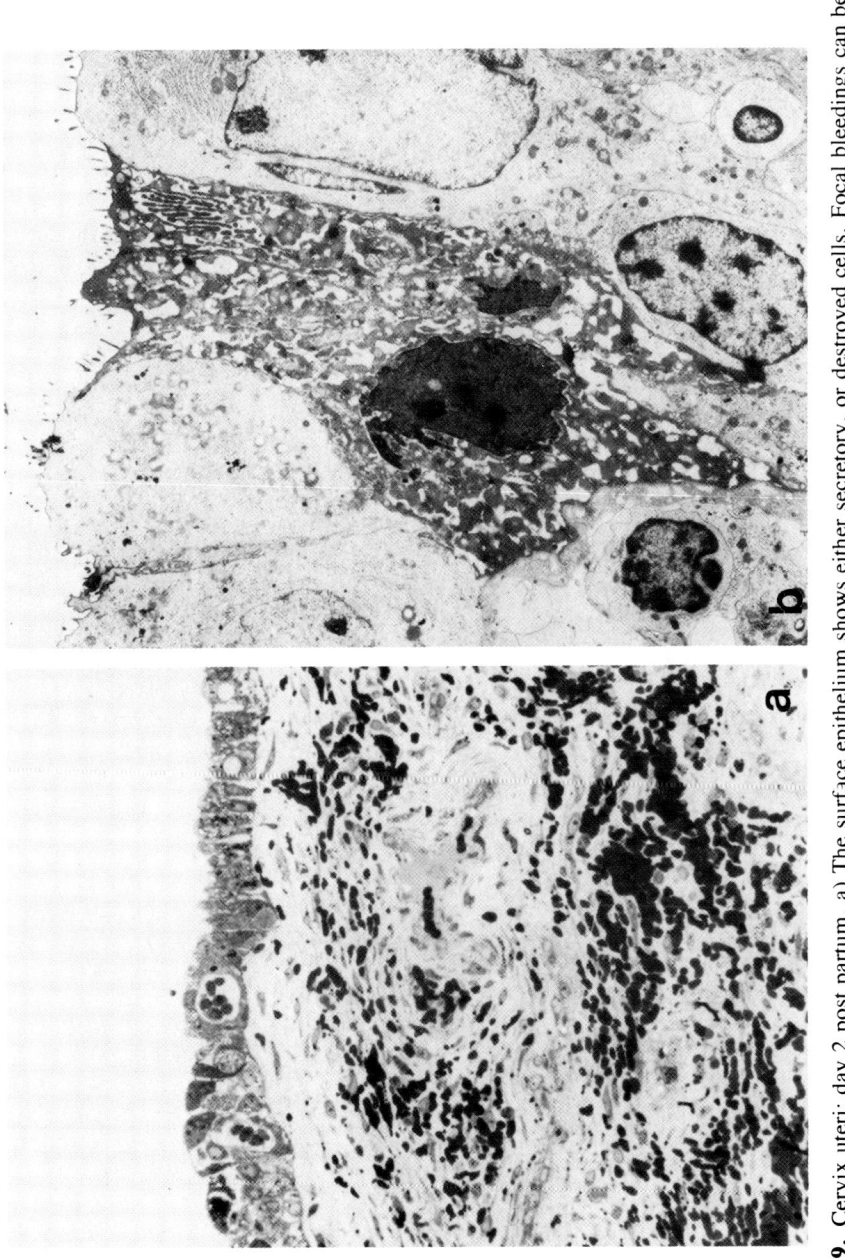

FIGURE 9. Cervix uteri: day 2 post partum. a) The surface epithelium shows either secretory, or destroyed cells. Focal bleedings can be seen in the subepithelial decidual tissue. Magnification: 780 : 1; LM b) Part of the surface epithelium with a necrotic epithelial cell. Magnification: 2500 : 1; TEM

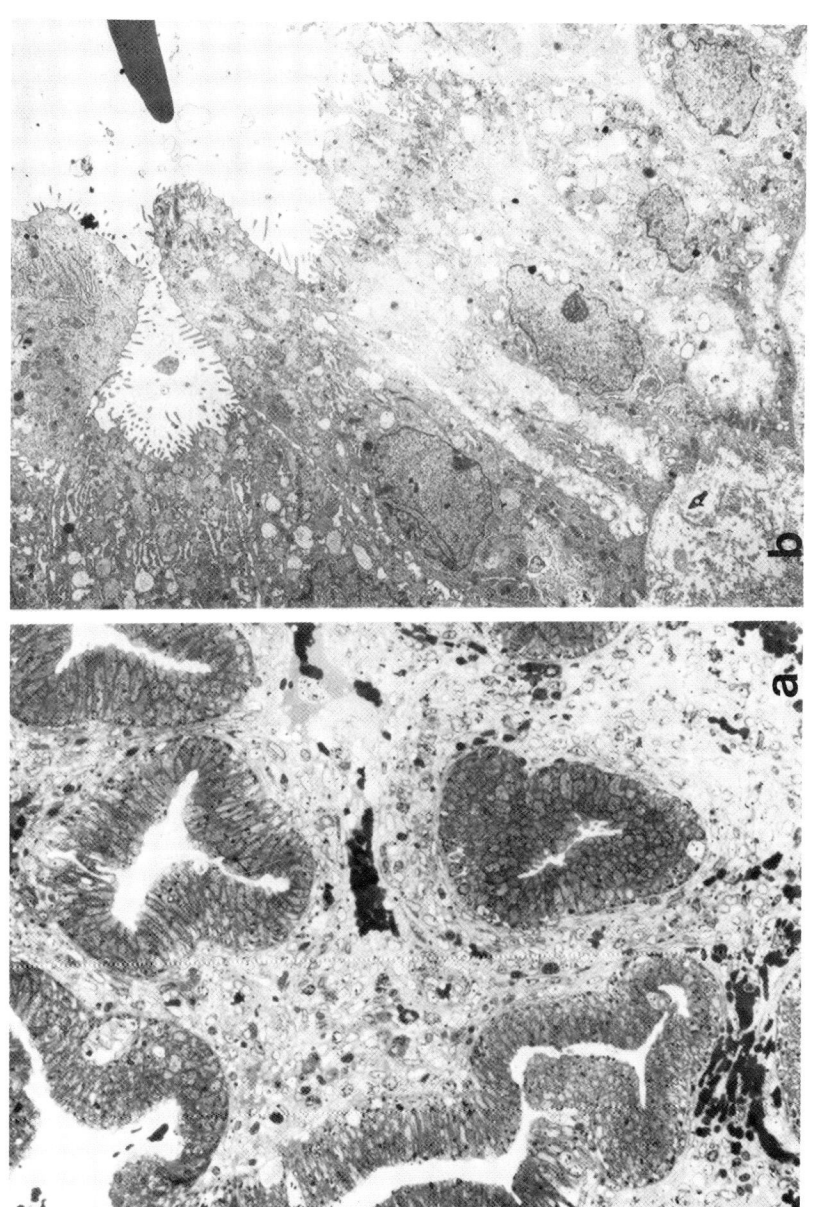

FIGURE 10. Cervix uteri; day 10 post partum. a) Completely regenerated epithelium and stroma. Magnification: 780 : 1; LM b) Secretion of the cervical epithelial cells. Magnification: 1900 : 1; TEM

The earliest endometrial proliferation was present on day 10 in our material and was completed after the first 14 days post partum. The repair processes of placental insertion takes much longer.

The change in the appearance of lochia correlates with the repair processes as evidenced by ultrastructure.

The repair mechanism at the cervix uteri was completed at day 10 since the glandular structure of the cervical canal was already present intact.

There was no evidence for differences between lactating and non-lactating patients which is in agreement with data on lochia by Bernstine and Bernstine (1951).

REFERENCES

Anderson, W.R. and Davis, J.: Placental site involution. Am. J. Obstet. Gynecol. 102:23, 1968.

Bani Sacchi, T. and Lo Stumbo, F.: Comportamento del connettivo del collo uterino umano in gravidanza, travaglio e puerperio. Arch. Ital. Anat. Embriol, 77:237, 1972.

Bernstine, J.B. and Bernstine, R.L.: Lochia. A quantitative study. West. J. Surg. 59:312, 1951.

Brandes, D. and Anton, E.: An electronmicroscopic cytochemical study of macrophages during uterine involution. J. Cell Biol. 41:450, 1969.

Crystle, C.D., Sawaya, G.A. and Stevens, V.C.: Effects of ethinyl estradiol on the secretion of gonadotropins and estrogens in post partum women. Am. J. Obstet. Gynecol. 116:616, 1973.

Delvoye, P., Demaegd, M., Uwayitu-Nyampeta, Robyn, C.: Serum prolactin, gonadotropins and estradiol in menstruating and amenorrhoic mothers during two years lactation. Am. J. Obstet. Gynecol. 130:635, 1978.

Dessouky, A.D.: Myometrial changes in post partum uterine involution. Am. J. Obstet. Gynecol. 110:318, 1971.

Kava, H.W., Klinger, H.P., Molnar, J.J. and Rommey, S.L.: Resumption of ovulation post partum. Am. J. Obstet. Gynecol. 102:122, 1968.

Reyes, R.I., Winter, J.S.D. and Faiman, C.: Pituitary-ovarian interrelationships during the puerperium. Am. J. Obstct. Gynecol. 144:589, 1972.

Rhen, K., Rönnberg, L. and Kannel, L.: Vacuum Aspiration in the delivery room. Acta Obstet. Gynec. Scand, 53:151, 1974.

Rolland, R., Lequin, R.M., Schellekens, L.A. and De Jong, F.H.: The role of prolactin in the restoration of ovarian function during the early post-partum period in the human female. Clinical Endocrinology 4:15, 1975.

Sharman, A.: Post-partum regeneration of the human endometrium. J. Anat. 87:1, 1953.

Williams, J.W.: Regeneration of the uterine mucosa after delivery, with especial reference to the placental site. Am. J. Obstet. Gynecol. 22:664, 1931.

Copyright 1979 by Elsevier North Holland, Inc.
F.K. Beller and G.F.B. Schumacher, eds.
The Biology of the Fluids of the Female Genital Tract

BIOCHEMISTRY OF POST PARTUM FLUID (LOCHIAE)

C. Ebert, K.W. Schweppe, and F.K. Beller

SUMMARY

The concentrations of soluble plasma proteins in lochia were studied in relation to the course of the pueperium. In 60 patients and a total of 70 samples immune assays were performed for Albumin, IgG, IgM, IgA, C_3C, ceruloplasmin and α acidic glycoprotein, prothrombin, FDP, plasminogen, α_2 MG, α_1 AT and AT III.

These proteins were present in concentrations lower than in peripheral venous plasma. The distribution of proteins in lochia did not correspond to those in peripheral venous plasma.

The concentration of fibrinogen degradation products was unusually high (fraction D larger than fraction E) and was even higher than in menstrual serum.

Based on these results it seems unlikely that the plasma proteins originate only from blood constituents derived from placental insertion.

INTRODUCTION

The biochemistry of lochial discharge has received very little attention by obstetricians and biochemists. It is therefore not surprising that neither the origin of lochiae nor their biologic function is known. The microbiology of lochiae will be discussed in another section of the Symposium.

Frauenklinik, Abteilung Geburtshilfe and Gynäkologie, Westfälische Wilhelms Universität, Münster / Westf. FRG

According to Stieve, (1929), lochial discharge contains decidual remnants infiltrated by leucocytes and degraded leucocytes in addition to necrotic tissue debris. Liquefied blood clots are presumed to appear with serum and lymph fractions from the dissolved fibrin coat of the placental bed (Ludwig, 1971; Bernstine et al., 1951).

The present paper is concerned with a study of the biochemical composition of soluble plasma proteins in lochiae and some elements of proteolytic activity.

MATERIALS AND METHODS

Lochiae were obtained from 60 patients with an uneventful post partum course and regular uterine involution. Blood smear, alkaline phosphatase, SGOT, SGPT, serum creatinine as a measure of renal function, sodium, potassium, calcium were within normal limits. Total serum protein and hemoglobin content exceeded 5 and 10 mg per 100 ml, respectively.

All patients routinely received methylergometrin, iron and vitamins. Bromocriptin (5 mg/day) was given for lactation inhibition.

The lochiae samples were taken from the second to the tenth day post partum with informed consent. A speculum was introduced into the vagina and the vagina was swabbed with sterile gauze. The cervix was clamped at 12 o'clock using a tenaculum and then repositioned distally. A sterile disposable catheter of 14 Charriere was introduced into the uterine cavity up to the fundus. Using a 10 ml syringe 200-3500 mg of lochiae discharge were removed.

Preparation of samples:

Following the determination of total weight of the lochia, a small portion was removed, reweighed and subjected to lyophilization. The proportion of non-fluid constituents was determined. The larger sample portion was repeatedly (5-6 times) washed with equal volumes of physiological saline by shaking for 10 min. at room temperature. Between each elution step the samples were centrifuged at 3000 g, the supernatant removed and the sediment added to the next elution step. The combined eluates of a sample were freeze dried, weighed and adjusted to the original volume of the sample. Assays for plasma proteins were performed on these samples. For the determination of proteolytic activity those samples were utilized. from which "lochial serum" could be obtained by centrifugation. This was used for immediate photometric measurement.

Assay for plasma proteins: Albumin, prothrombin, plasminogen, α_2 MG, α_1 AT, AT III, IgG, IgM, IgA, C_3C, ceruloplasmin and α_1 acidic glycoprotein were determined by radial immunodiffusion (Mancini). Partigen-plates (Fa. Behring/Marburg FRG) were used.

Assay for fibrin(ogen) degradation products: The small fibrin-fibrinogen degradation products D and E were determined by the Laurell immuno electrophoresis with specific antibodies (Fa. Behring/Marburg FRG).

The concentrations of antibodies was 1% for anti-D and 2% for anti-E in 1% agarose. Running time: 5 hours at 6 V/cm, running buffer; barbiturate buffer at pH 8.6.

Assay for proteolytic activities: Proteolytic activities were assayed using the chromogenic substrates of Kabi (Kabi Laboratories, Stockholm Schweden) S 2160 (substrate for serin proteases), S 2238 (substrate for thrombin), S 2251 (substrate for plasmin), S 2302 (substrate for kallikrein) and S 2222 (substrate for F Xa).

For the assay 10 μl of lochia were incubated with 590 μl of Tris-buffer pH 7.4 or pH 8.4. Extinction was measured at 405 nm over 30 min. at 37° C after addition of 200 μl of the chromogenic substrate.

RESULTS

The consistency and the blood contamination of the lochial samples varied greatly. The blood fraction decreased during the post partum period.

The proportion of non-fluid constituents in the lochia (cellular material, proteins and mucous material) varied between 9 and 29% dry weight (average 15.7%) after lyophilization of small representative samples. Using physiological saline approximately 10% of the lochial discharge was eluted as soluble components.

Plasmaproteins

The plasma protein concentration in lochial discharge was lower than that of peripheral plasma (see Table I). The protein distribution was similar in samples from various patients, but the distribution differed from peripheral plasma.

Clottable fibrinogen was absent. Addition of fibrinogen and thrombin resulted in a reduced clotting activity.

The concentration of fibrin(ogen) degradation products was very high; for E in the range of 20—350μg/g lochiae and for D 50-2000 μg/g (Figure 1) (Ebert et al. 1979).

The plasma inhibitors AT III, α_2 MG and α_1 AT were low and in the range from 0.06-0.23 mg/g for AT III, 0.2-1.7 mg/g for α_2 for MG and 0.9-1.7 for α_1 AT.

The concentrations remained relatively constant during the post partum course (Figures 2-4).

The immunologically determined plasminogen levels were 0.02-0.8 mg/g. The concentration remained relatively constant until the tenth day post partum. The prothrombin concentrations of 0.20—0.70 mg/g did not change up to the tenth day post partum (Figures 5-6).

Immunoglobulines: IgG increased until the seventh day post partum but was still lower than the plasma concentration in the range from 1.6—6.5 mg/g lochia). IgM levels reached peripheral plasma concentrations (range 0.2—1.5 mg/ml) but did not change during the post partum course. The IgA concentration (0.2—1.0 mg/g) was below peripheral plasma levels (Figures 7-9).

The C_3C component of the complement system displayed (0.2—0.52 mg/g) a course comparable to that of IgA (Figure 10).

The albumin present in lochial discharge was in the range of 6—23 mg/g. The concentration increased slightly during the post partum phase until the eighth day, but remained below the normal blood plasma concentrations (Figure 11). The α_1 acidic glycoprotein concentration in lochiae varied between 0.25—0.7 mg/g; ceruloplasmin was the only plasma protein showing levels at least partly within the normal blood plasma values (0.12-0.36 mg/g) (Figures 12-13).

Proteolytic activities: When lochiae were prepared as described there was no proteolytic activity in the saline soluble sample. It is therefore assumed that the proteolytic activity of the lochial samples was destroyed by lyophilization. There-

TABLE 1. Protein Concentration in Lochine and Peripheral Plasma

protein	concentration in lochiae mg/g lochiae	$\bar{M}$	concentration in plasma mg/100 ml
albumin	6-23	13,8	3500-5500
plasminogen	0,02-0,8	5,2	10-30
prothrombin	0,2-0,7	0,43	5-10
AT III	0,06-0,23	0,14	17-30
α_1 AT	0,9-1,7	1,32	200-400
α_2 MG	0,2-1,7	0,91	175-420
IgG	1,6-6,5	4,1	800-1800
IgM	0,2-1,5	0,85	70-280
IgA	0,20-1,0	0,60	90-450
C_3C	0,2-0,52	0,39	50-120
α_1 acidic glycoprotein	0,25-0,7	0,43	55-140
ceruloplasmin	0,12-0,36	0,25	15-60

fore in the first three days post partum, fresh lochiae were freshly centrifuged and small amounts were used immediately for enzyme assays.

S 2222: this substrate, which is cleaved by F X_a, trypsin, acrosin, F IX_a, kallikrein and subtilisin, did not reveal activity at pH 8.4 neither in lochia nor in peripheral plasma.

S 2251: This substrate is cleaved by plasmin but not by urokinase or kallikrein. A considerable enzymatic activity was demonstrated in lochia samples at 37° C at pH 7.4. The enzymatic activity was equivalent to approximately 1.5 n catalytic units plasmin/ml.

Addition of urokinase increased the activity, whereby the immunologically demonstrable plasminogen was activated to plasmin.

The plasminolytic activity of lochial discharge was inhibited by aprotinin or EACA (Epsilon Amino Capnoic Acid) (Figure 14).

S 2160: Thrombin, trypsin, brinase and papain-like enzymes cleave this substrate. Enzymatic activity was very low in lochia.

S 2238: With this substrate, which is cleaved by thrombin, proteolytic activity was very low, and could be partially inhibited by hirudin (Figure 15).

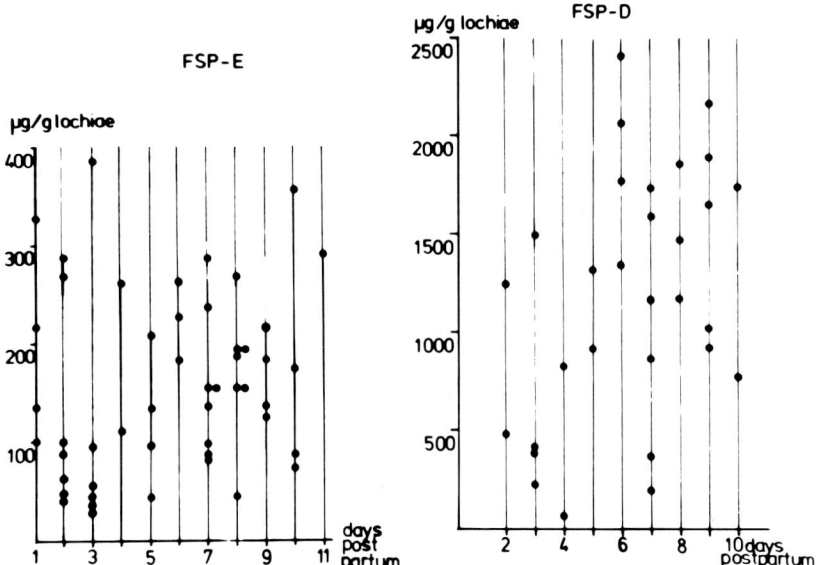

FIGURE 1. Distribution of values of fibrin(ogen) degradation products E und D in lochiae during the postpartum course.

S 2302: The highest proteolytic activity of lochial discharge was found using the chromogenic substrate 2302, which is cleaved by plasma kallikrein. It was not inhibited by hirudin. The enzymatic activities measured with the last three chromogenic substrates indicated an equivalent of approximately 25 IU, thrombin/ml lochial serum.

DISCUSSION

The concentrations of immunologically determined proteins in lochial discharge were lower than the plasma concentrations in peripheral blood. There was little change in the concentration of any constituent during the first ten days of the puerperium.

It is unlikely that the proteins of plasma originate only from blood constituents deriving from the site of placental insertion. They come presumably from lymphatic elements and cellular material.

The concentration of fibrin(ogen) degradation products is very high and corresponds to concentrations of other fluids of the female genital tract, namely menstruation blood (Ebert et al. 1979).*

The post partum concentration of degradation products in plasma also increases after delivery (Bonnar et al, 1969, Stiehm et al. 1970).

The concentration obtained by using anti-D-antibody was much higher than those obtained with an anti-E-antibody. Since anti-D, in contrast to anti-E, leads

*Ebert, C. et al. pp. 247-256.

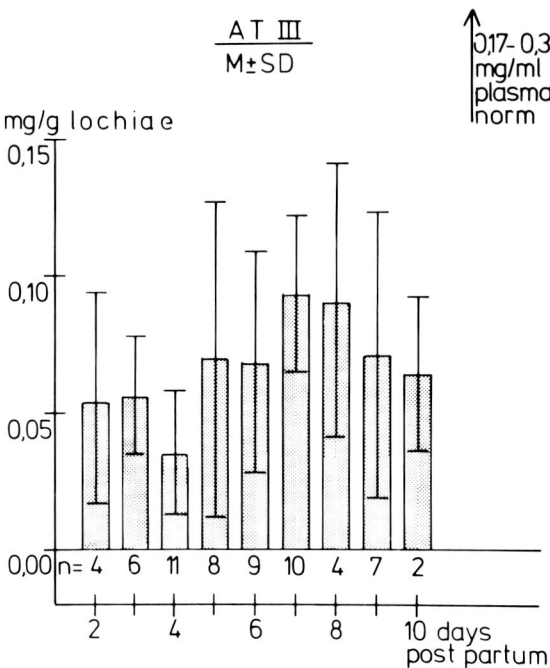

FIGURE 2. Distribution of antithrombin (AT III) concentrations in lochiae during the postpartum course.

FIGURE 3. Distribution of α_1 AT concentrations in lochiae during the peuperium.

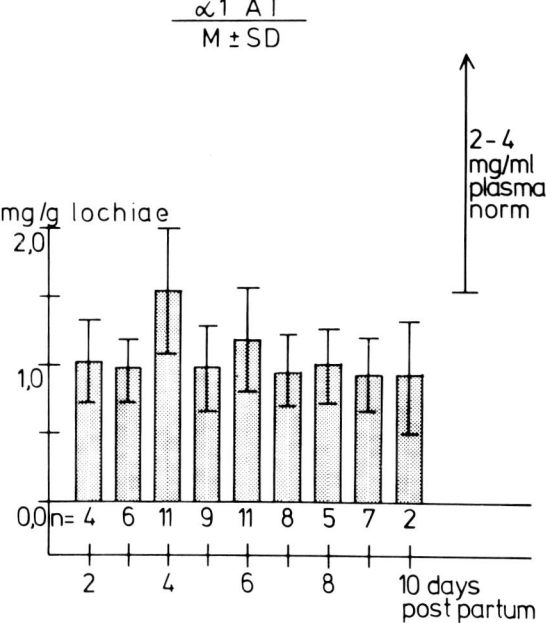

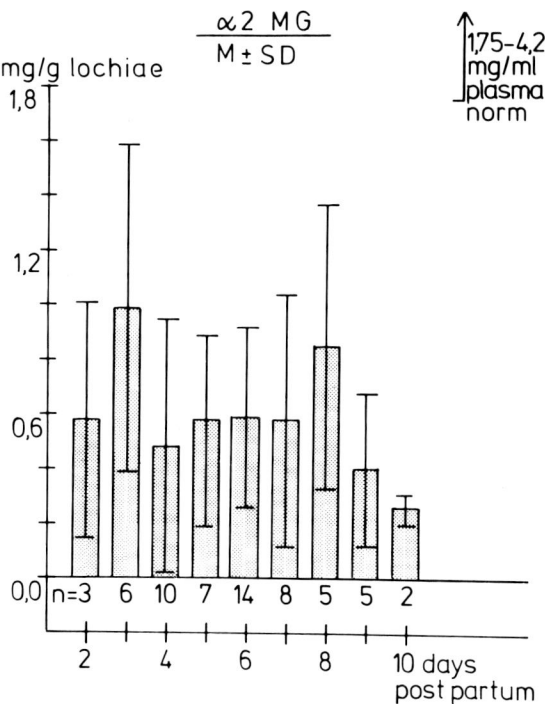

FIGURE 4. Distribution of α_2 MG concentrations in lochiae during the pueperium.

FIGURE 5. Distribution of plasminogen concentration in lochaie during the pueperium.

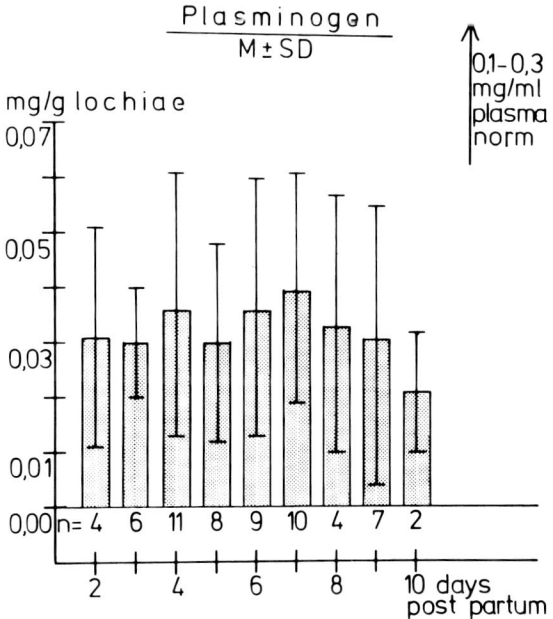

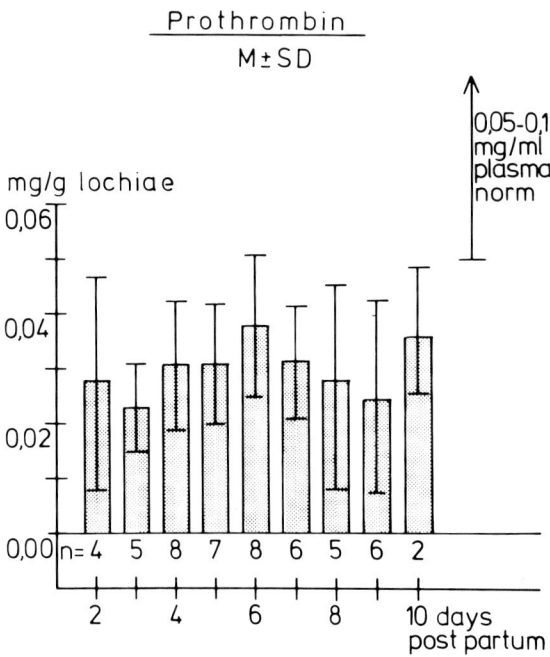

FIGURE 6. Distribution of prothrombin concentrations in lochiae during the pueperium.

FIGURE 7. Distribution of IgG concentration in lochiae during the pueperium.

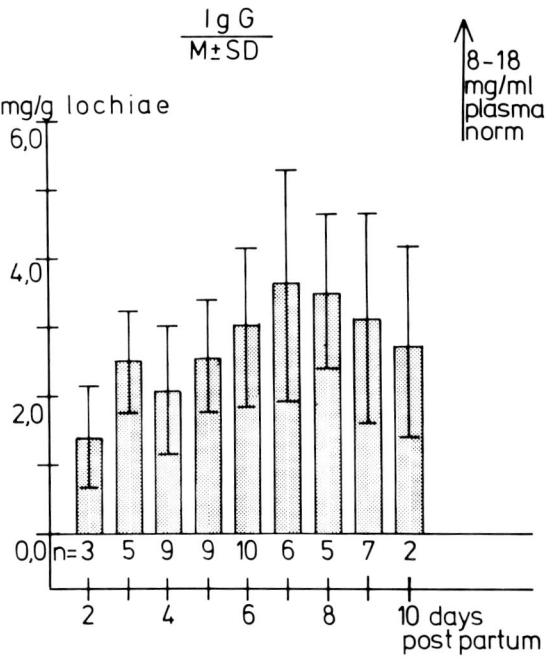

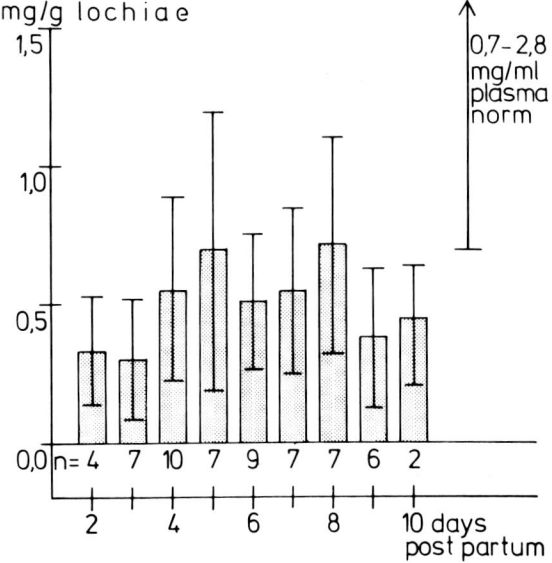

FIGURE 8. Distribution of IgM concentrations in lochiae during the pueperium.

FIGURE 9. Distribution of IgA concentration in lochiae during the pueperium.

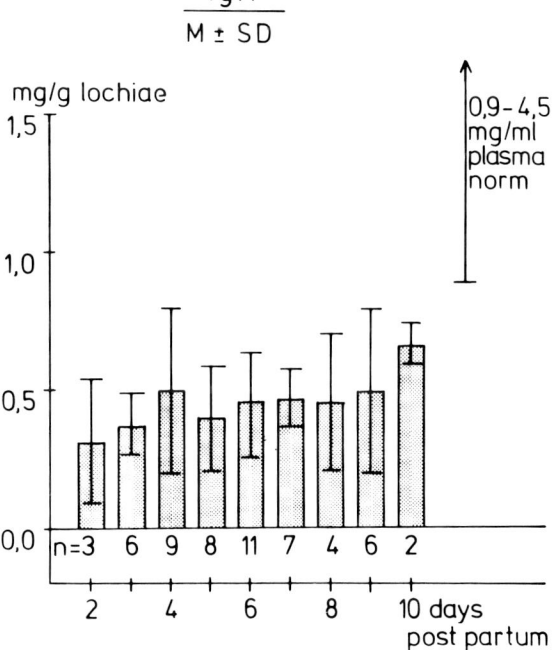

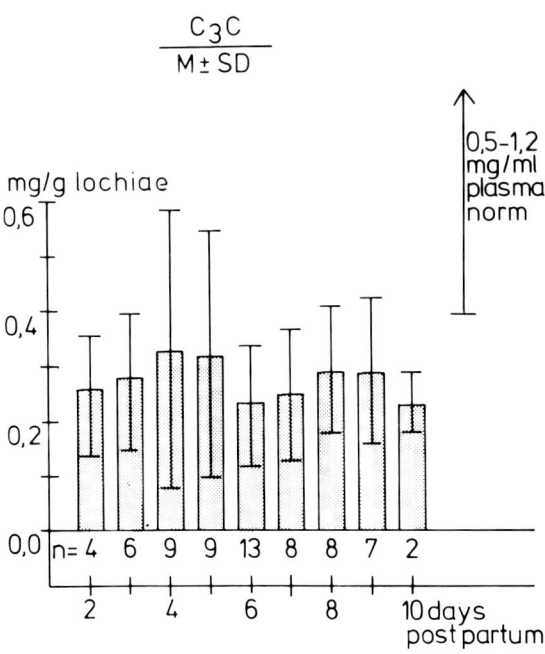

FIGURE 10. Distribution of C_3C concentrations in lochiae during the pueperium.

FIGURE 11. Distribution of albumin concentration in lochiae during the pueperium.

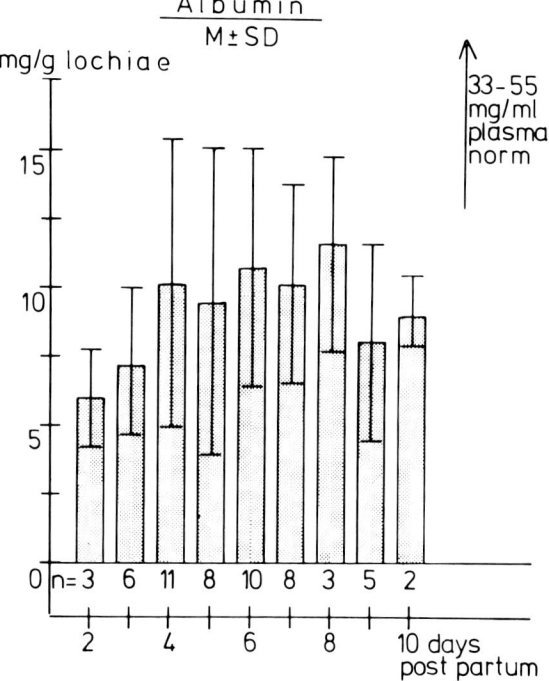

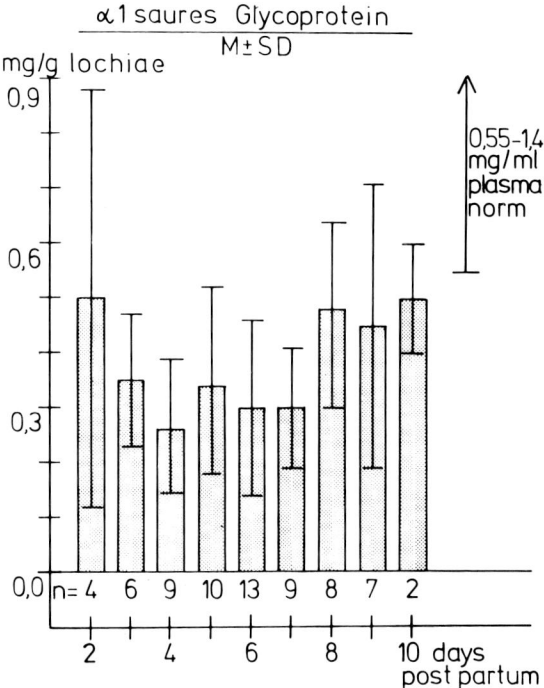

FIGURE 12. Distribution of α_1 acidic glycoprotein concentrations in lochiae during the pueperium.

FIGURE 13. Distribution of ceruloplasmin concentration in lochiae during the puerperium.

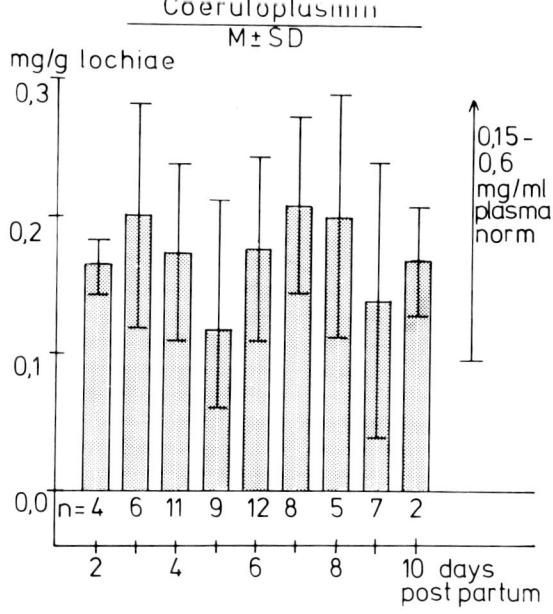

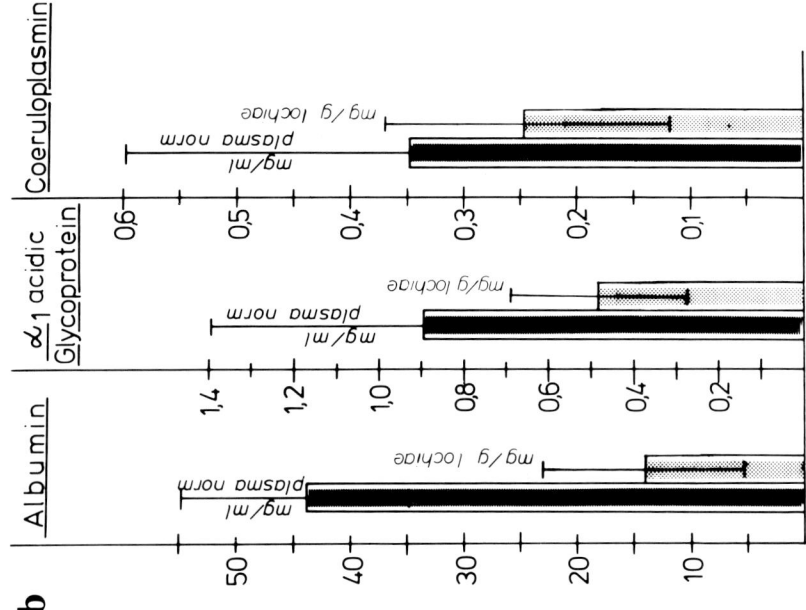

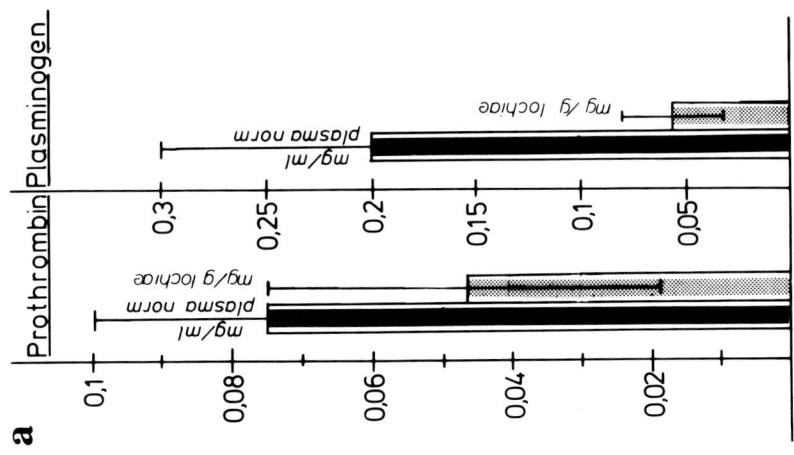

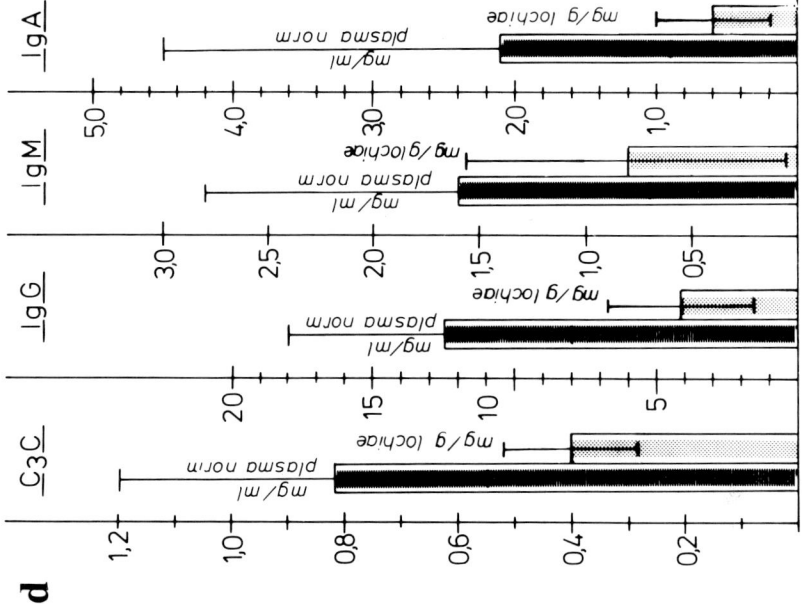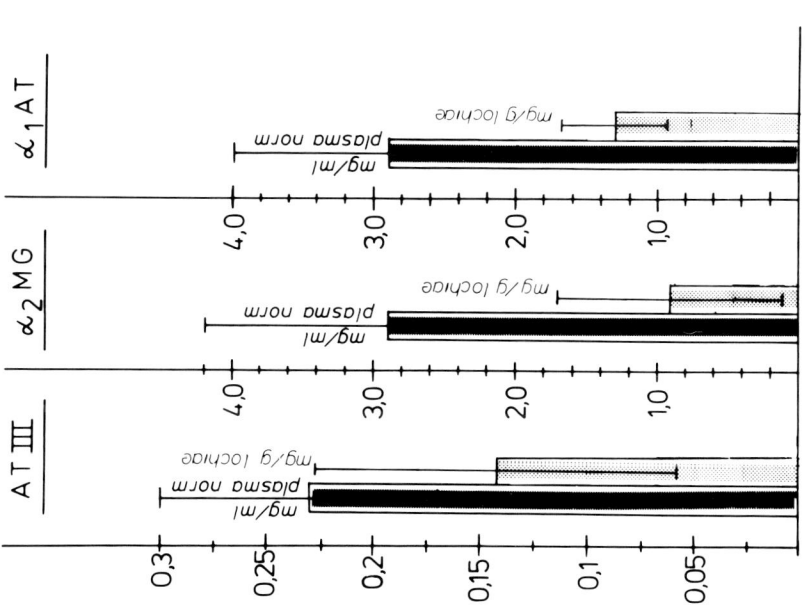

FIGURE 14. Mean values and standard deviations of plasma protein concentrations in lochiae and normal peripheral plasma: **a)** prothrombin and plasminogen; **b)** albumin, α_1 acidic glycoprotein, ceruloplasmin; **c)** C_3C, IgG, IgM, and IgA; **d)** AT III, α_1 MG and α_1AT.

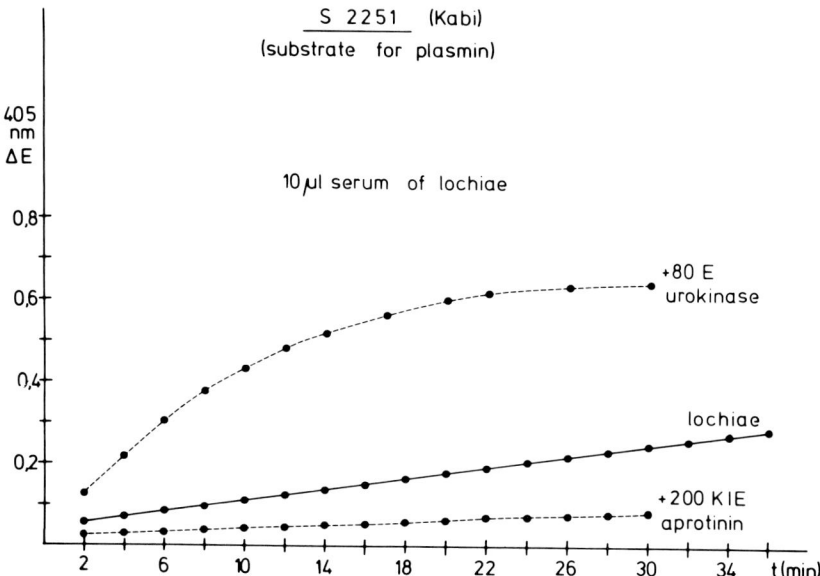

FIGURE 15. Cleavage kinetics of substrate S 2251 (substrate for plasmin) in lochiae. The activity is nearly completely inhibited by aprotinin. Urokinase added increased the activity.

FIGURE 16. Cleavage kinetics of substrate S 2238 (substrate for thrombin) of three different lochial samples. Addition of hirudin did not inhibit the enzymatic activity completely (samples b without and with addition of hirudin).

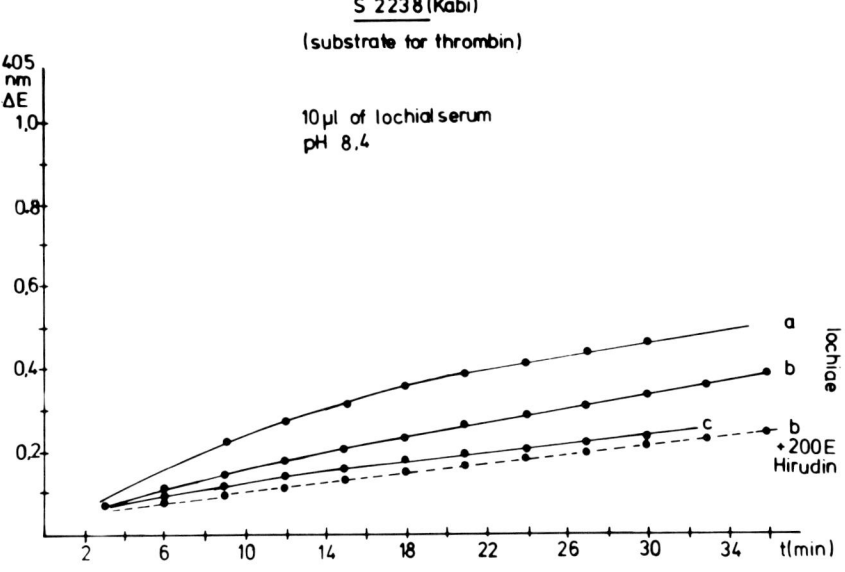

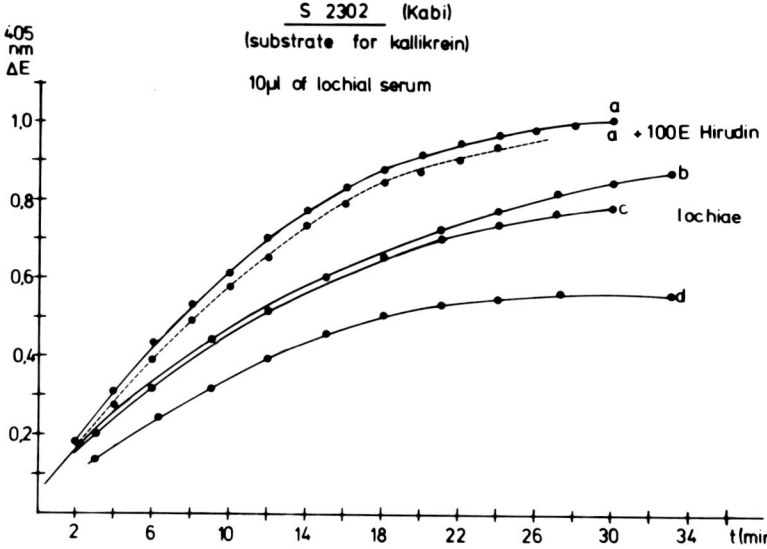

FIGURE 17. Cleavage kinetics of substrate S 2302 (substrate for kallikrein) of four different lochial samples. Addition of hirudin did not inhibit the enzymatic activity (samples a without and with addition of hirudin).

to cross reaction with fibrinogen and other fibrinogen derivatives, this suggests that components other than fibrinogen are involved.

After defibrination at 56°C, the concentrations of degradation products determined with anti-D did not change. Clottable fibrinogen was not present at any time. Adding fibrinogen to lochial samples induced clotting with thrombin only slowly. This is believed to be the result of the inhibitory activity of the split products (Bang and Chang 1974). The ratio of the immunoglobulins IgG and IgA in relation to albumin corresponds approximately of that of plasma. IgM is slightly increased, the same is true for the complement components of C_3C.

The concentrations of α_1 acidic glycoprotein and especially ceruloplasmin are high in comparison to other proteins, and are only slightly below those in peripheral plasma.

The fibrinolytic-plasmin activity present in lochial discharge explains the high concentration of degradation products. Plasminogen, which can be activated by urokinase, is found in lower quantities than in peripheral plasma. In addition the presence of free plasmin indicates activation and consumption of plasminogen. α_2 MG is present in approximately 20% of peripheral venous plasma. Since it is a potent inhibitor of plasmin, it is suggested, in agreement with the data of Gallimore and Fareid (1979), that a part of α_2 MG is bound to free plasmin.

The proteolytic activity, which cleaves the substrates S 2302 and 2238, is predominantly thrombin. However, hirudin, a potent thrombin inhibitor, does not change the activity. This suggests that there are other, as yet undetermined, proteolytic enzymes present which cleave these substrates. These are most likely related to the leucocyte proteases from cells which migrate to the placental insertion area.

REFERENCES

Bang, N.M., Chang, M.L.: Soluble fibrin complexes. Seminars in Thrombos. 1, 91 (1974).

Bonnar, J., Davidson, J.F., J.F., Pidgeon, C.F., McCol, G.P., Douglas, A.S.: Fibrin degradation products in normal and abnormal pregnancy and partituration. Br. med. J. 3, 137 (1969).

Bernstine, J.B., Bernstine, R.L.: Lochia. quantitative study. West. J. Surg. 59, 312 (1951).

Ebert, Ch., Beller, F.K., Schweppe, K.-W., Wagner, H.: Biochemistry of menstrual blood. Referat: International workshop on Biology of the Fluids of the female Genital Tract (1979).

Gallimore, M.J., Fareid, E.: Studies of human plasma inhibitors of plasmin, plasma kallikrein, trypsin, thrombin and urokinase using chromogenic substrate assays. In: Chromogenic Peptide Substrates. Ed. M.F. Scully and V.V. Kakkar, Churchill Livingstone, Edinburgh London and New York, 1979 S. 248.

Ludwig, H., Metzger, H.: Das uterine Placentabett post partum im Rasterelektronenmikroskop, zugleich ein Beitrag zur Frage der extravasalen Fibrinbildung. Arch. Gynäk. 210, 251 (1971).

Stiehm, E.R., Kennan, A.L., Scheible, D.T.: Split products of fibrin in maternal serum in the perinatal period. J. Am. Obstet. Gynecol. 108, 941 (1970).

Stieve, H.: Der Halsteil der menschlichen Gebärmutter, seine Veränderungen während der Schwangerschaft, der Geburt und des Wochenbetts und ihre Bedeutung. Z. mikr. anat. Forsch. 17, 371 (1929).

Part III:
OVIDUCT

MORPHOLOGY OF THE FALLOPIAN TUBE

C. J. Pauerstein and C. A. Eddy

SUMMARY

This paper discusses the morphology of the Fallopian tube, in the following order: 1) General anatomic relationships of the tube to other pelvic viscera. 2) The regional anatomy of the intramural segment, uterotubal junction (UTJ), isthmus, ampullary-isthmic junction (AIJ) and ampulla. 3) The vascular anatomy, including arterial supply and venous and lymphatic drainage. 4) The neuroanatomy, including the intrinsic adrenergic innervation. 5) the epithelium, including light microscopy, scanning electron microscopy, and a brief discussion of transmission electron microscopy of the tube. Finally, the responses of the epithelium to various physiologic hormonal conditions are discussed.

INTRODUCTION

The morphology of the Fallopian tube may be considered in relation to surrounding structures, in relation to the anatomic regions and component cells and tissues of the tube, or in relation to tubal function. We will attempt to utilize each of these approaches in a manner appropriate to an orderly exposition.

Center for Research and Training in Reproductive Biology, Department of Obstetrics and Gynecology, The University of Texas Health Science Center at San Antonio, San Antonio, Texas

We will begin our discussion of tubal anatomy by recalling to your minds the first accurate description by Gabriele Fallopius in 1561:

"This seminal duct originates from the cornua uteri; it is thin, very narrow, of white color, and looks like a nerve. After a short distance it begins to broaden and to coil like a tendril, winding its folds almost up to the end. There, having become very broad, it shows an extremitas of the nature of skin and color of flesh, the utmost end being very ragged and crushed like the fringe of wornout clothes. Further, it has a great hole which is held closed by the fimbria which lap over each other. However, if they spread out and dilate, they create a kind of opening which looks like the flaring bell, the brazen tube. Because the course of the seminal duct, from its origin up to its end, resembles the shape of this classic instrument, whether the curves are existing or not, I named it tuba uteri."

The Fallopian tube is a pelvic organ, except during pregnancy. The proximal end of the oviduct opens into the uterine cavity, at its lateral and superior angle, posterior to the mid-coronal plane. The distal orifice of the tube opens into the pelvic cavity. The tube is enclosed within the leaves of the broad ligament and this portion of the peritoneum with its enclosed structures is designated the "mesosalpinx." The superior aspect of the tube is apposed to the intestine and pelvice peritoneum. At its uterine insertion, the oviduct is related to the origin of the round ligament anteriorly and inferiorly and to the suspensory ligament of the ovary posteriorly and inferiorly. Laterally, the inferior surface of the tube approximates the surface of the ovary, and the mesosalpinx is continuous with the infundibulopelvic ligament. The epoophoron, a mesonephric vestige, is located in the mesosalpinx between the ampulla and the ovary, whereas the paroophoron, also a mesonephric remnant, lies inferior to the tubal isthmus, near the utero-tubal junction. The fimbriated end of the tube encroaches upon the medial surface of the ovary to which it is attached by the fimbria ovarica (Figure 1).

The extrauterine portion of the Fallopian tube ranges from 8 to 15 cm in length with an average length of 11 cm.

REGIONAL ANATOMY

The oviduct is usually described as divided into 5 anatomic regions: the intramural or interstitial portion contained in the wall of the uterus; the isthmic portion immediately distal to the uterotubal junction (UTJ); the ampullary-isthmic junction (AIJ), the ampulla and the infundibulum, which terminates in the fimbriated end (Figure 2).

Intramural Segment

The interstitial portion of the tube may follow a simple straight or curved course to the endometrial cavity or it may take a tortuous route within the uterine wall. Tubal epithelial folds may extend to the uterine cavity or may end several millimeters short of the cavity. Ciliated mucosa of intermediate type, between that of the endometrium and that of the oviduct, is noted in the transition between the tubal lumen and the uterine cavity (Hermstein and Neustadt, 1924). The transition zone between the endometrial cavity and the endosalpinx is characterized by a

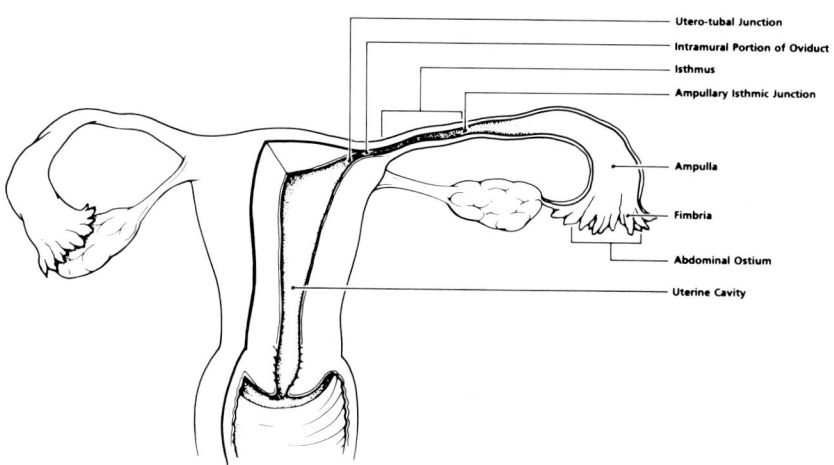

FIGURE 1. Drawing demonstrating the general anatomic relationships of the oviduct. See text for explanation.

FIGURE 2. Gross anatomy and histology of the human oviduct. Light photomicrographs (above) and scanning electron photomicrographs (below) at various levels. Note differences in ciliation, lumen size from fimbria to uterus. (From: Eddy, C.A. and Pauerstein, C.J. Tubal reproductive function and the development of reversible sterilization techniques. In: Reversal of Sterilization, Sciarra, J.J., Zatuchni, G.I., Speidel, J.J., (eds), Harper and Row, 1978).

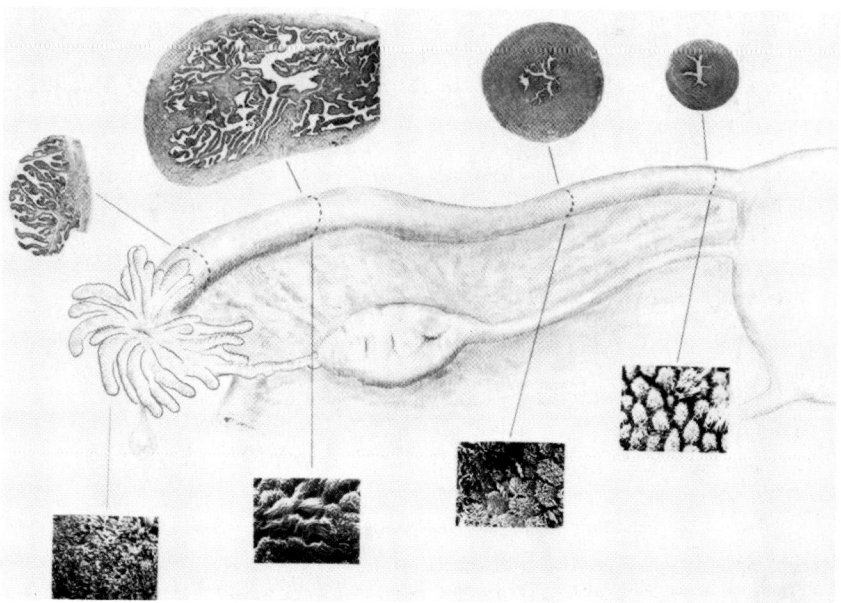

marked increase in the number of ciliated cells, and by changes in the shape of the secretory cells (Fadel et al., 1976).

The musculature of the intramural portion of the tube contains a layer of inner longitudinal muscle, immediately below the epithelium, a middle layer of circular muscle, which is arranged in a spiral, and an outer longitudinal layer below the peritoneal covering. A most complete description of the musculature was given by Vasen (1959, 1959a), who reported that each of the three layers of the uterine wall was continuous with the tubal musculature without interruption. He defined a sub-peritoneal layer with longitudinal fibers, which was especially prominent on the superior aspect of the tube, a vaso-muscular layer with the fibers paralleling the long axis of the vessels, and an inner autochthonous layer, which was composed of four systems of bundles arranged in spirals. On examination of cross sections this spiral arrangement gave the appearance of three zones within the autochthonous layer, an outer and inner zone which were parallel to the long axis of the tube and a middle zone which appeared circular in cross section. Although Vasen was unable to define any sphincter muscle in the fallopian tube he claimed that the sub-peritoneal muscular layer of the uterus formed a loop of muscle tissue around the distal end of the tubal lumen. He also noted vascular rings in the vaso-muscular layer, which could close the distal portion of the intramural segment of the fallopian tube when distended with blood.

Isthmus

The isthmus begins at the uterotubal junction and extends distally for 2 to 3 cm. It contains the heaviest musculature of any portion of the extrauterine tube. The inner longitudinal muscle layer of the interstitial portion of the tube disappears in the isthmus about 2.5 cm distal to the UTJ (Williams, 1891). The outer longitudinal muscle continues into the broad ligament. The bulk of the myosalpinx originates from the Mullerian duct as an autochthonous layer composed of four systems of bundles arranged in spirals. In cross section one sees three zones: an outer and inner zone parallel to the axis of the tube, and a middle zone, which appears circular (Vasen, 1959) (Figure 3). The isthmus contains the narrowest lumen of any segment of the oviduct. Measurements on fixed and frozen tissue indicate an average luminal diameter at the isthmus of 400 microns (range 100 microns to 1 mm). The mucosa at the cornual end of the tube is usually arranged into four primary folds.

Ampullary-Isthmic Junction

The ampullary-isthmic junction (AIJ) can be identified by the change in consistency of the tubal wall. The thick wall of the isthmus feels cord-like, whereas the thin musculature of the ampulla offers less resistance to palpation. An abrupt transition of the patterns of the mucosal folds can be seen at the AIJ, after perfusion of the lumen with methylene blue (Eddy et al., 1977) (Figure 4).

Ampulla

The ampulla is the longest portion of the human Fallopian tube, measuring 5 to 8 cm in length. The ampullary luminal diameter varies from 1 to 2 mm at its junction with the isthmus to more than 1 cm near its distal end. A defined inner

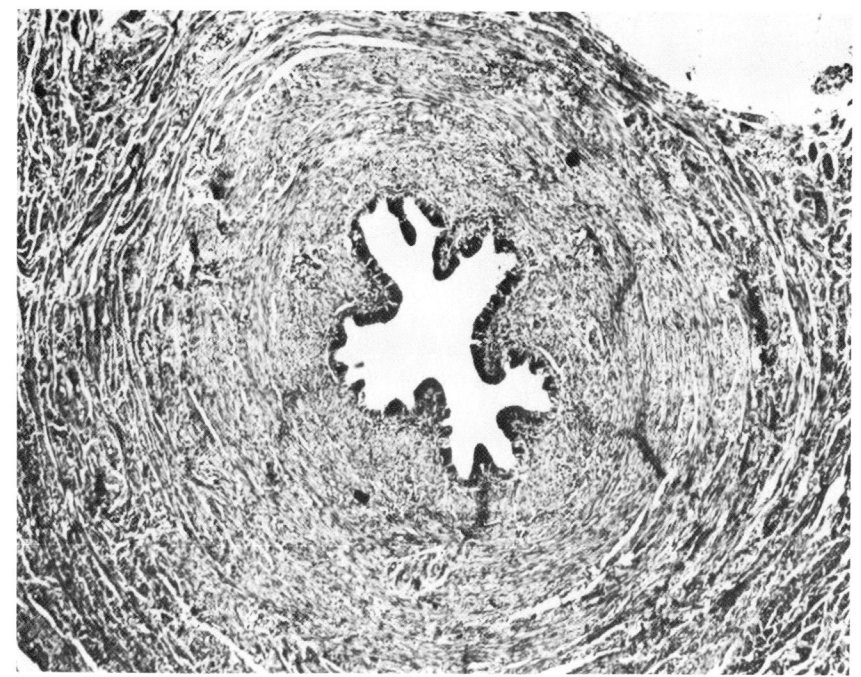

FIGURE 3. Section through the tubal isthmus, near the tubo-uterine junction, showing the well-defined inner longitudinal muscle layer and the four primary folds of the mucosal pattern.

FIGURE 4. Surface topography of the endosalpinx in the region of the ampullary-isthmic junction. Note changes in the mucosal fold pattern from isthmus (left) to ampulla (right).

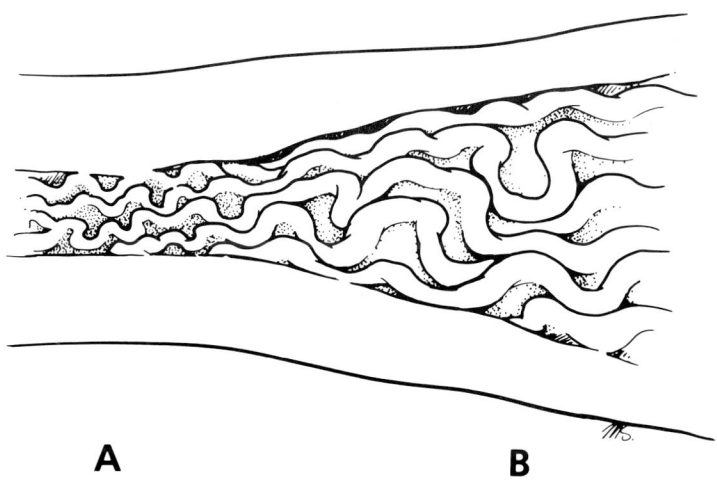

A   B

longitudinal musculature is lacking in the ampulla, but the inner longitudinal musculature is contained as scattered muscle bundles dispersed within the lamina propria of the complex mucosal folds seen in this area (Figure 5).

Infundibulum

The infundibulum is the trumpet shaped distal portion of the oviduct terminating in the fimbriated end surrounding the abdominal ostium of the tube. As the anatomic connection between fimbria and distal ampulla, the infundibulum is the site of the transition from ovum pick-up to ovum transport. One of the fimbriae, the ovarian fimbria is attached to the ovary. It is possible that this attachment is essential to the normal mechanism of ovum pick-up. In the usual mechanism of ovum pick-up, the tube is brought into opposition with the ovary. Westman (1926, 1959) stated that the infundibular portion of the tube is brought into apposition with the ovary at the time of ovulation by movement of the tubal musculature. Decker (1951) demonstrated this movement of the tube toward the ovary via laparotomy and culdotomy. Stange (1952a) stated that the musculature nearest the tubal fimbria became longitudinally oriented at the base of the fimbria ovarica and by union with the sub-peritoneal musculature formed the "musculus attrahens tubae" which, extending into the cranial pole of the gonad, drew the

FIGURE 5. Section through the ampulla, demonstrating the complex pattern of the mucosal folds. The musculature is comparatively thin, and it is difficult to distinguish well-defined circular and longitudinal muscle layers.

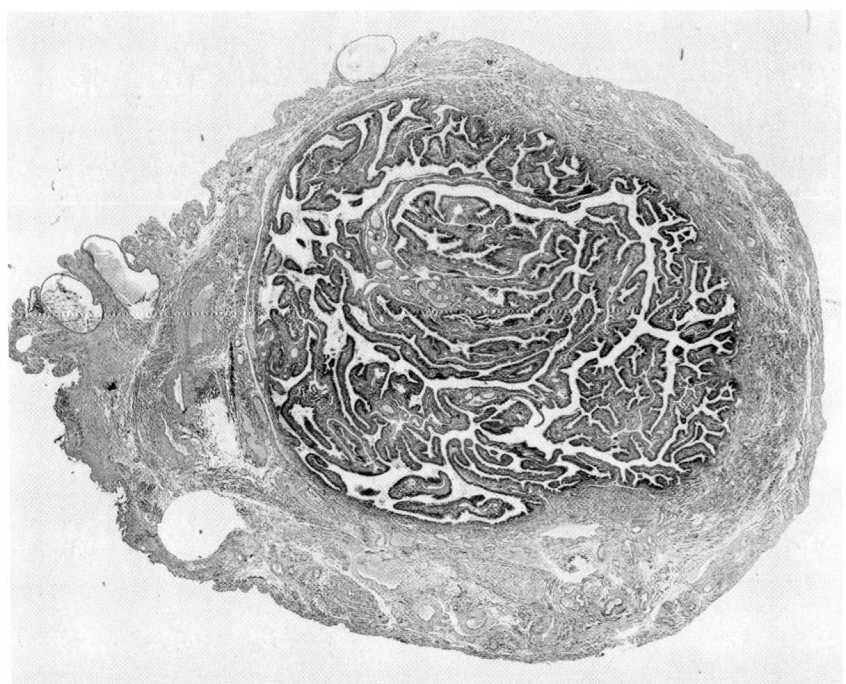

tube near the ovary as the musculature of the epoophoron raised the ovary toward the tube.

The autochthonous musculature of the tube ends at the abdominal ostium after establishing contact with the fibers of the musculo-vascular layer. The rearranged bundles may form a sphincter at the abdominal ostium of the tube. The functional muscle ridge of this infundibular sphincter is formed by a grouping of the fiber bundles and muscle sheaths of the vasculo-muscular layer (Horstmann, 1952; Stange, 1952, 1952a). During ovum pick-up, the densely ciliated fimbria are brought into close contact with the cumulus mass surrounding the ovum, and the ovum is thus conducted into the tubal ostium (Stange, 1952; Westman, 1926, 1959) (Figure 6).

VASCULAR ANATOMY

The arterial blood supply of the fallopian tube is derived from the uterine and ovarian arteries. The relative contributions of each vary greatly in individual women. Generally, the uterine supplies the medial two-thirds of the tube, and the ovarian artery the remainder. However, either artery alone may supply the entire tube. It is very likely that autoregulation shunts the blood supply under varying physiologic conditions. The ovarian and uterine arteries may yield either two or three arterial branches to the Fallopian tube (Borell and Fernstrom, 1953; Lapina, 1963; Pitchuev, 1961). Synthesis of the experimental data suggested the following

FIGURE 6. Mechanism of ovum pick-up. Contraction of tubal and ovarian ligaments at ovulation brings ovary and fimbria into close apposition.

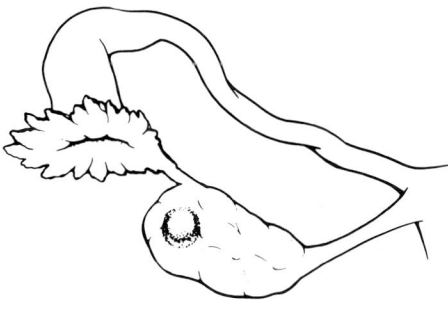
BEFORE OVULATION

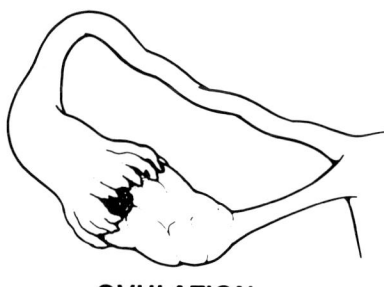
OVULATION

schema of tubal blood flow: (Figure 7). The uterine artery ascends and near the cornu sends a branch (A) which supplies the cornu and the interstitial portion of the tube. It then splits into two trunks, one of which (B) supplies the medial portion of the tube, while the other (C) anastomoses with the ovarian artery. The terminal portion of B then anastomoses with a tubal branch of the ovarian artery. The ovarian artery divides into two trunks, one of which (D) supplies the ovary and anastomoses with the ovarian branch of the uterine artery, while the other (E) supplies the distal portion of the tube. Either the uterine or the ovarian artery may send a second trunk to the oviduct (broken lines).

The venous drainage follows the arterial supply. Gatsalov (1963, 1964) reported interconnected capillary networks in the mucosa, muscularis and subserosa. The network in the mucosal folds drained to a plexus located between the mucosa and the muscularis. The muscularis plexus received veins from the mucosa and submucosa as well as those of the muscle layer. These intrinsic veins were located between the bundles of circular muscle. The serosal capillary network was dense in the isthmus and sparse in the ampulla. The three venous plexuses became confluent in the subserous connective tissue where the extrinsic drainage of the tube originated.

FIGURE 7. Diagrammatic representation of the arterial blood supply to the tube. A, cornual branch of uterine artery; B, isthmic branch of uterine artery; C, ovarian branch of uterine artery; D, ovarian artery; E, ampullary branch of ovarian artery.

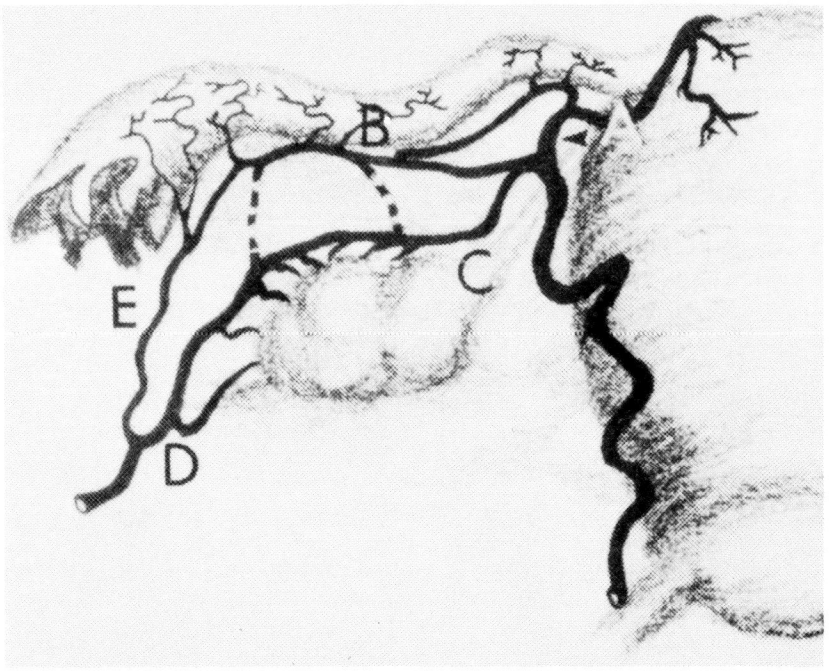

LYMPHATICS

The lymph vessels of the tube drain to the aortic or lumbar nodes. The lympatics of the tube follow the course of the ovarian and uterine lymphatic drainage. Lymphatic vessels from the tube combine and then pass, in the broad ligament to the lymphatic network near the hilum of the ovary, and thence to the aortic nodes (Reiffenstuhl, 1964). Gatsalov has studied the intrinsic lymphatic systems of the human tube (1963a, 1964a). The lymphatics of the serosal system are more delicate in the isthmus and more variable in the ampulla. A thick network is present in the utero-tubal angle. All lymphatic vessels drain into a subserous plexus. The mucosal lymphatic drainage varies with the segment of the tube considered. The isthmic mucosa drains into the lymph capillaries of the muscular layer. The ampullary mucosal lymph drains directly into the lymphatics of the muscular layer through an anastomotic system, and also into the subserous connective tissue. A lymphatic capillary system was noted in the mucosa, the muscularis and the serosa. In addition an intramural plexus was noted. The structure of these plexuses varied from segment to segment. During reproductive life the lymphatic drainage of the muscularis is composed of a three dimensional network of lymph capillaries in the circular and longitudinal muscle.

In summary, three lymphatic networks drain the mucosa, muscularis and serosa respectively. Upon emerging from the intrinsic system of the tube, the lymphatic vessels combine, enter the mesosalpinx and run upward in the broad ligament to the para-aortic nodes.

NEUROANATOMY

The autonomic innervation of the tube is both sympathetic and parasympathetic (Figure 8). Some of the sympathetic preganglionic fibers which arise from T10 to L2 terminate in the inferior mesenteric ganglion. From this ganglion postganglionic fibers pass via the hypogastric plexus to the Fallopian tube. The isthmus and a portion of the proximal ampulla are supplied by fibers from the hypogastric plexus. Other sympathetic preganglionic fibers from T10 and T11 synapse in the celiac, aortic, and renal ganglia, and send postganglionic fibers to the fimbriae and distal ampulla of the oviduct.

In addition to postganglionic fibers which originate in the inferior mesenteric ganglia ("long adrenergic neurons"), the hypogastric nerve carries preganglionic fibers that supply ganglia located near the vagina. Postganglionic fibers originating in these peripheral ganglia have been called "short adrenergic neurons." The intrinsic adrenergic innervation of the myosalpinx is derived about equally from both long and short neurons. A rich distribution of adrenergic nerve terminals has been identified in the circular muscle of the isthmus and at the ampullary-isthmic junction of the human Fallopian tube. In contrast, the adrenergic supply to the smooth muscle cells of the ampulla is sparse (Brundin and Wirsen, 1964; Owman, Rosengren and Sjöberg, 1967) (Figure 9).

The afferent innervation of the tube, which carries pain sensation, accompanies the sympathetic nerves and is derived from T11 and T12 and the upper lumbar nerves. The afferent visceral fibers travel from the tube to the central

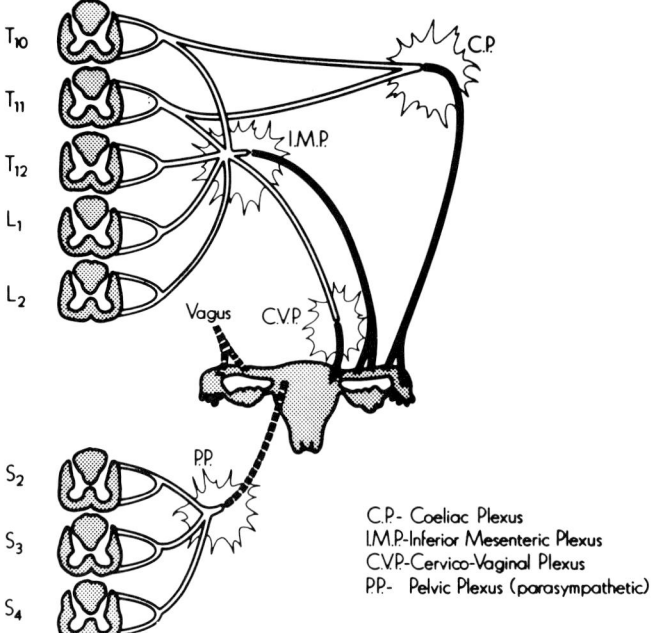

FIGURE 8. Diagram of autonomic innervation to oviduct. Parasympathetic supply on left, sympathetics on right. Preganglionic fibers are shown in white, sympathetic postganglionics in solid black, and parasympathetic postganglionics in broken black lines. (From: Pauerstein, C.J. The Fallopian Tube: A Reappraisal. Zuspan, F.P. (ed), Lea & Febiger, 1974.)

nervous system via the autonomic system. Sensory nerves from the fimbria and ampulla may travel to the spinal cord via the ovarian plexus and splanchnic nerve.

The parasympathetic supply to the tube is also dual. The distal portion of the tube is supplied by vagal fibers from the ovarian plexus. The sacral parasympathetic fibers, derived from S2, S3 and S4, are conveyed to the terminal ganglia of the pelvic plexuses. From these ganglia short postganglionic fibers supply the interstitial portion of the isthmus.

EPITHELIUM

Four cell types have been described in the epithelium of the Fallopian tube: a ciliated cell, a secretory cell, an intercalary or "peg" cell, and an "indifferent" cell (Figure 10). The latter two types may represent exhausted secretory cells or deciliated cells.

The ciliated cell is relatively square in contour and contains finely granular cytoplasm. The central nucleus is large in comparison with cytoplasmic volume and is round or oval in shape. The cilia are about 7 microns long and are attached to a refractile row of basal granules located beneath the cell membrane. They ex-

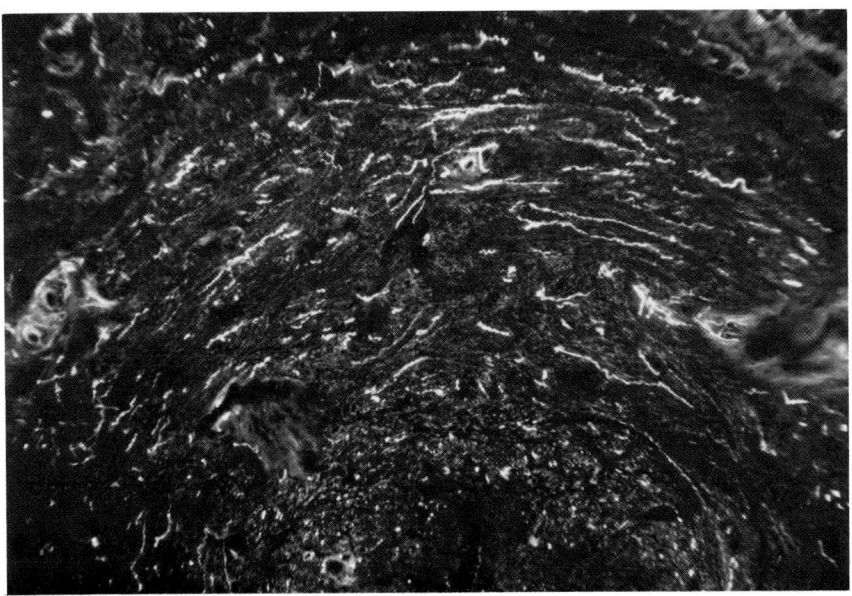

FIGURE 9. Transverse section of tubal isthmus viewed with fluorescence microscopy after treatment with formaldehyde gas. The catecholamines on the adrenergic nerve fibers fluoresce and appear white on the photomicrograph.

hibit the classic structural arrangement of two central filaments and nine double lateral filaments (Figure 11).

Ciliated cells are more densely distributed on the apices of the epithelial folds, and non-ciliated cells are found in greater numbers in the crypts formed between folds, and at the bases of the folds. Although some authors (Ferenczy et al., 1972) have reported a fairly uniform distribution of ciliated cells along the length of the tube, others report a progressive decrease in the percentage of ciliated cells from the fimbriae to the isthmus (Patek et al., 1972; Critoph and Dennis, 1977).

These debates may have become moot, since the question of distribution of ciliated cells was thought important in relation to their putative role in gamete transport. Recent reports of normal fertility in women suffering from the immotile cilia syndrome (Figure 12) cast serious doubt upon the necessity for cilia to human reproduction. This syndrome is characterized by a congenital defect in the dynein arms of the cilia (Afzelius et al., 1978). This cilial defect has been demonstrated in the endocervical cells (Bleau et al., 1978) and in the tubal ciliated cells (Jean et al., 1979) of fertile women.

Secretory cells contain a more granular cytoplasm. The darker oval nucleus is oriented with its long axis parallel to the long axis of the cell, and its position in the cell varies with the phase of the cycle. Secretory cells vary in appearance during the menstrual cycle but are distinguishable from ciliated cells at any time. The cytoplasm is darker and contains fine granules, and the endoplasmic reticulum is spread out irregularly. The mitochondria appear smaller than those in ciliated cells and as well-developed Golgi field can be discerned (Figure 13).

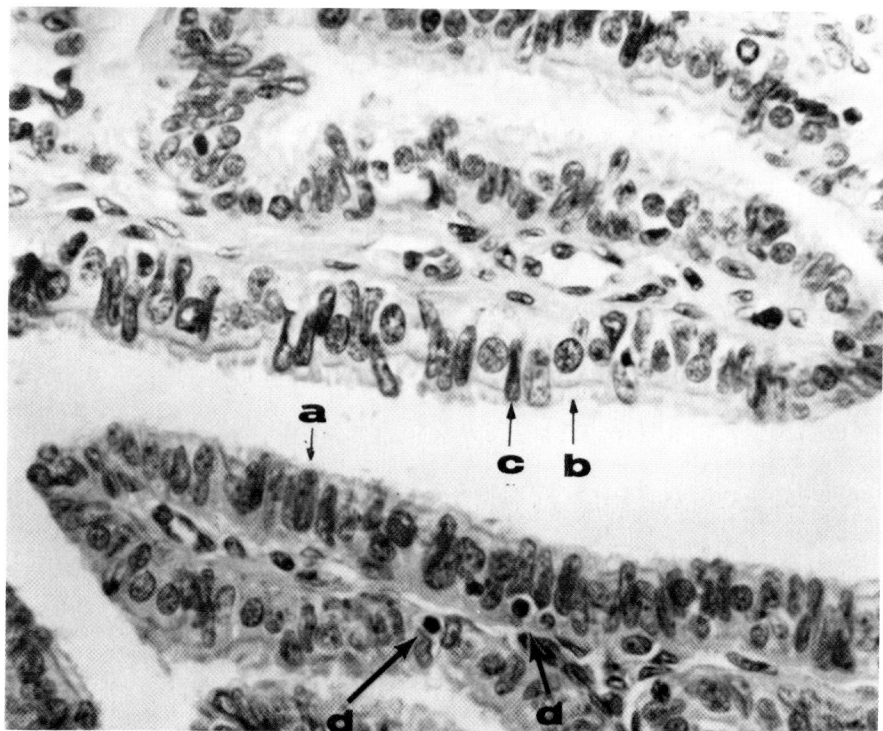

FIGURE 10. Characteristic cell types in tubal epithelium: a, secretory; b, ciliated; and c, intercalary.

Physiologic Responses of Epithelium

Mitotic figures rarely occur in the epithelium of the normal adult human tube. Amitotic renewal of the epithelium has been suggested, as has the presence of a "reserve" cell from which the epithelium is produced. This question remains unresolved. In contrast, fetal Fallopian tubes demonstrate mitotic activity. The genesis of the human oviduct follows a pattern similar to that seen in the hamster, rat, mouse, and guinea pig. Both ciliated and secretory cells can be identified in the five-month fetus.

In the newborn, ciliated and secretory cells are well developed, as is secretory activity. The advanced differentiation seen at birth suggests that the human fallopian tube responds to hormonal influence *in utero*. Experimental evidence for this is lacking, however.

In the adult, tubal epithelium undergoes morphologic changes during the ovarian cycle, pregnancy, the puerperium and the menopause.

Changes During the Ovarian Cycle

During the proliferative phase of the cycle (Figure 14), the epithelium attains its greatest height (30 microns) and the secretory and ciliated cells are of equal height, so that the lumenal border of the epithelium is regular. During the

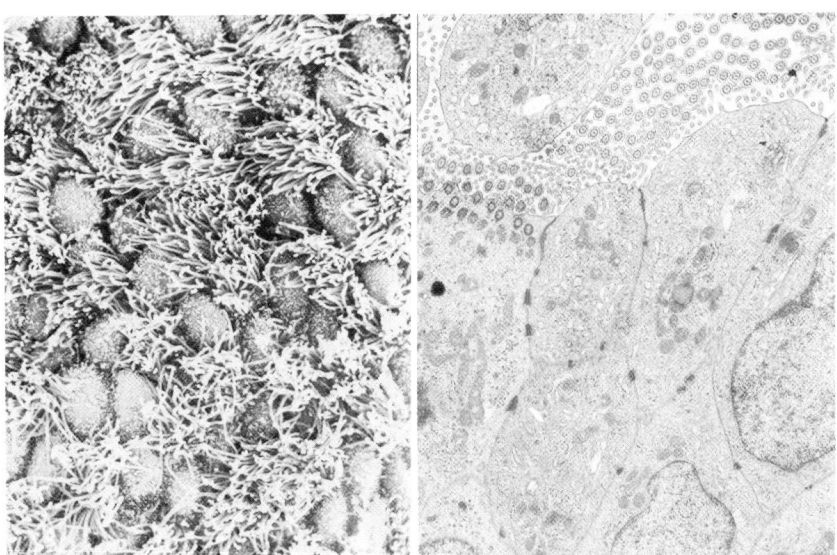

FIGURE 11. Ciliated epithelium of human oviduct. Scanning electron photomicrograph (left) and transmission electron photomicrograph (right) demonstrating ciliated cells interspersed among secretory cells.

luteal phase, the ciliated cells become broader and lower, and the secretory cells protrude above the level of ciliated cells, forming a dome or cupola. Late in the secretory phase, the domed extremity may break into the tubal lumen, extruding cytoplasm. A marked irregularity of the border is seen, due to diminution in the height of non-ciliated cells. Secretory cells frequently occur in clusters at the summits of the folds with their nuclei often so closely packed that they give the impression of a single giant nucleus. During menstruation, the cells become lower, and cytoplasmic and nuclear extrusion is complete. The intercalary cell is most prominent during the premenstrual and menstrual periods. Immediately after menstruation, the tubal epithelium becomes very low (10 to 15 microns). Ciliated cells are shorter and narrower than in the interval phase, and secretory cells assume a narrow cylindrical shape, so that they superficially resemble ciliated cells. Peg cells are less obvious.

Studies with the scanning electron microscope reveal marked changes in size and profile of the secretory cells. Immediately after menstruation, the secretory cells begin to show early protrusion. The apices are flat, and covered with microvilli. At midcycle, the protrusions increase to form a dome, and the cells assume a polyhedral columnar shape. Their apices reach the tips of the cilia of the adjacent ciliated cells. After ovulation, holes appear in the cell membranes of the apices. These holes coalesce, and allow the release of intracellular materials into the lumen. Just prior to menses, cellular integrity is repaired. The secretory cells again appear flattened and polygonal in shape, with distinct cell boundaries. Ciliated cells do not undergo a morphologic cycle (Ludwig and Metzger, 1978).

The secretory cells undergo definite ultrastructural changes during the ovarian cycle. Early in the proliferative phase, the secretory cells display a compact

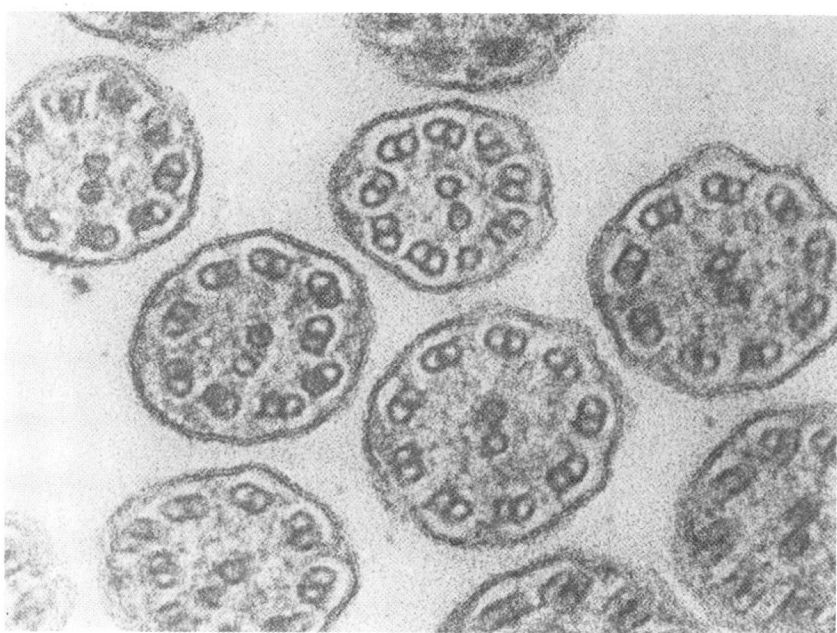

FIGURE 12. Transmission electron photomicrograph of individual cilia from oviduct of patient suffering "Immotile Cilia Syndrome." Note absence of dynein arms in axial filaments. (From: Jean, Y. et al. Fertility of a woman with nonfunctional ciliated cells in the fallopian tubes. Fertil. Steril. 31:349, 1979.)

Golgi apparatus, a limited endoplasmic reticulum, and diminished mitochondria. Later, the mitochondria, endoplasmic reticulum, and Golgi apparatus become more prominent. On about day 10, Palade granules become numerous, and the cells increase in height. At the end of this phase, the cell surface is domed, and secretory granules appear beneath the cell membrane and near the lumen.

During the luteal phase, the endoplasmic reticulum dilates, and numerous secretory droplets and granules appear. The Golgi apparatus expands, and the mitochondria decrease in number. In the mid-luteal phase, some secretory cells rupture and extrude their contents. Late in the cycle, liposomes appear in increased numbers. Secretory function is more prominent in the isthmus than in the ampulla.

There is disagreement as to specific changes in the ultrastructural morphology and distribution of the ciliated cells during the cycle. Our best inference is that human tubal epithelium does not undergo cyclic ciliation-deciliation. Some changes, such as increase in size, number of cytoplasmic granules, and mitochondria, may occur in ciliated cells as the cycle progresses. Some renewal of ciliated cells does occur, but there is no evidence for transformation of ciliated into secretory cells, nor for cyclic desquamation of ciliated cells, nor for estrogen dependent ciliogenesis (Patek and Nilsson, 1973).

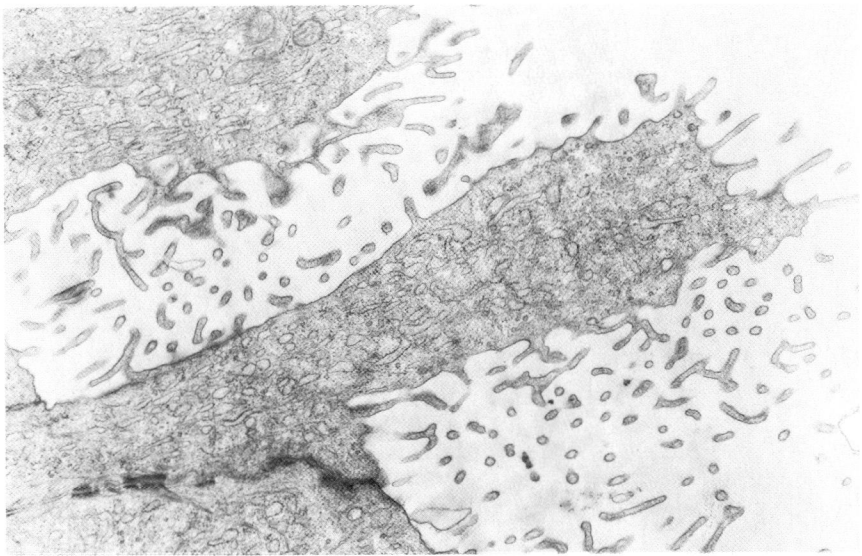

FIGURE 13. Transmission electron photomicrograph of tubal secretory cells. (From: Seki, K. et al. Deciliation in the puerperal fallopian tube. Fertil. Steril. 29:75, 1978.)

Pregnancy and the Puerperium

In pregnancy, the changes seen at menstruation continue. The epithelium remains low. There is some evidence of extrusion of nuclei by non-ciliated cells. Lipid droplets appear in ciliated cells, and secretory cells display further enlargement of the endoplasmic reticulum. Patek et al., (1973) reported no degeneration nor decreased numbers of ciliated cells in later pregnancy, as did Seki et al., (1978) (Figure 15).

The former authors also reported no deciliation in specimens taken from 72 to 120 hours postpartum. In contrast, Seki et al., (1978) found progressive deciliation in specimens removed from 62 to 112 hours after delivery (Figure 16). Non-ciliated cells were in the resting stage at term, and secretory activity returned during the puerperium. Earlier studies that employed classic histologic techniques (Andrews, 1951) reported extension of nuclei and cytoplasm from the secretory cells during the puerperium. The ciliated cells decreased in size and number. In those that remained, the cilia were smaller and fewer in number. Two weeks after delivery, the epithelium resembled that of the late postmenopause. Exogenous estrogen antagonized these puerperal changes, and within 48 hours induced proliferation of both ciliated and secretory cells, especially the former. Progesterone alone did not change the normal puerperal histology, but when given in combination with estrogen, progesterone inhibited estrogen-induced growth.

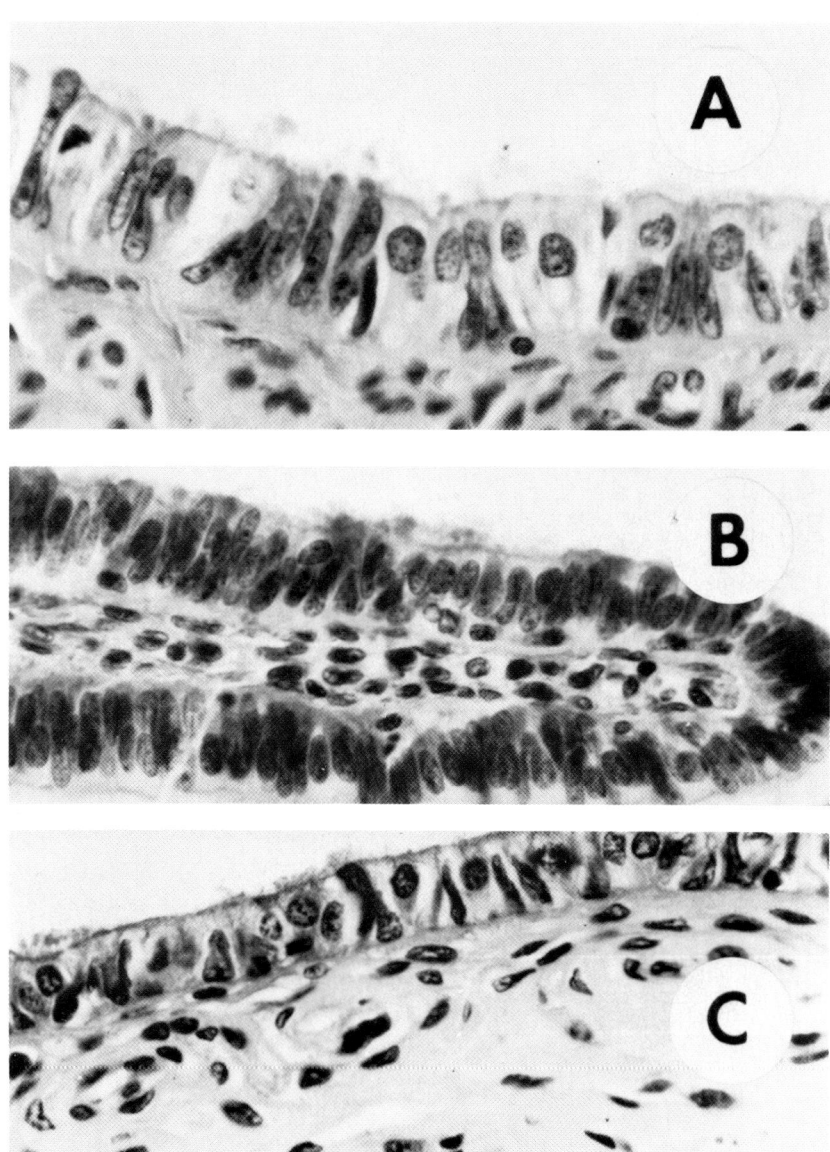

FIGURE 14. A, Uniform height of ciliated and secretory cells in proliferative phase. B, luteal phase, showing protrusion of secretory cells above ciliated cells. C, low epithelium of postmenstrual phase.

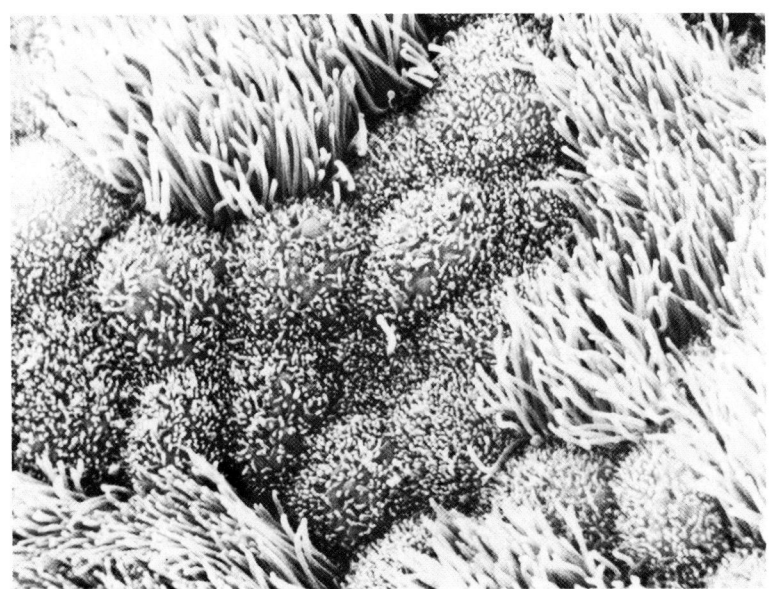

FIGURE 15. Ampulla of fallopian tube at cesarean section. Note microvilli on secretory cells and single cilia on several cells. (From: Seki, K. et al. Deciliation in the puerperal fallopian tube. Fertil. Steril. 29:75, 1978.)

FIGURE 16. Transmission electron photomicrograph of oviduct 55 hours post partum. Note sparse ciliation with single prominent striated rootlet in longitudinal section. (From: Seki, K. et al. Deciliation in the puerperal fallopian tube. Fertil. Steril. 29:75, 1978.)

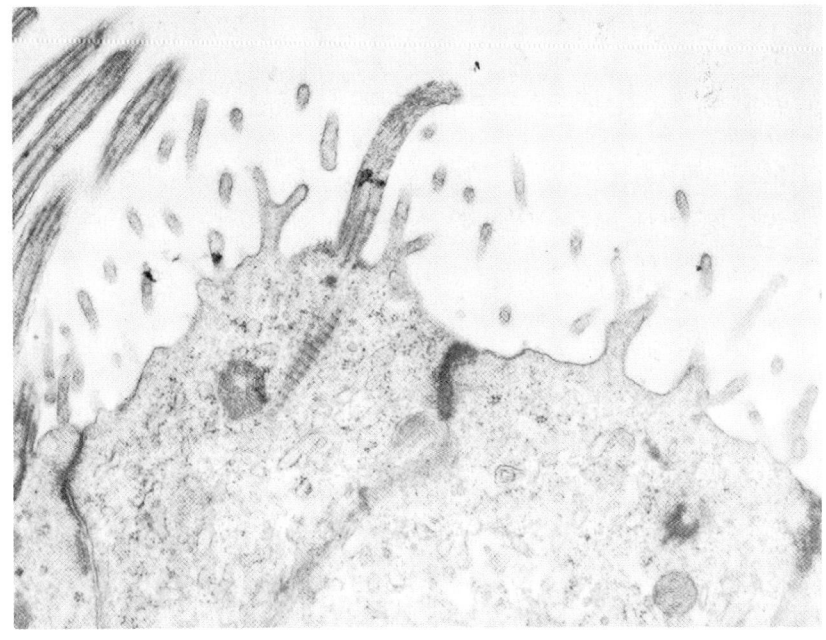

The Menopause

There is some disagreement concerning the appearance of the endosalpinx after the menopause. Some reports have noted an atrophy which affects both the ciliated and non-ciliated cells, but others have noted little or no atrophic change until age 60. Significant secretory function apparently ceases after the menopause, but ciliated cells persist without significant regression until the late postmenopause, when deciliation may become more apparent, particularly on the fimbria (Patek et al., 1973). A recent study with the scanning electron microsope revealed no significant deciliation in tubes from women as much as 30 years postmenopausal. It is possible that sufficient estrogen production to maintain the ciliated cells occurs in many postmenopausal women, although the non-ciliated cells become inactive.

REFERENCES

Afzelius, B.A., Camner, P. and Mossberg, B.: On the function of cilia in the female reproductive tract. Fertil. Steril. 29:72-74, 1978.

Andrews, M.C.: Epithelial changes in the puerperal fallopian tube. Am. J. Obstet. Gynecol. 62:28-37, 1951.

Bleau, G., Richer, C.-L. and Bousquet, D.: Absence of dynein arms in cilia of endocervical cells in a fertile woman. Fertil. Steril. 30:362-363, 1978.

Borell, U. and Fernstrom, I.: The adnexal branches of the uterine artery. Acta. Radiol. 40:561–582, 1953.

Brundin, J. and Wirsen, C.: The distribution of adrenergic nerve fibers in the rabbit oviduct. Acta. Physiol. Scand. 61:203–204, 1964.

Critoph, F.N. and Dennis, K.J.: The cellular composition of the human oviduct epithelium. Brit. J. Obstet. Gynecol. 84:219–221, 1977.

Decker, A.: Culdoscopic observations on the tubo-ovarian mechanism of ovum reception. Fertil. Steril. 2:253–259, 1951.

Eddy, C.A., Antonini, R., Jr. and Pauerstein, C.J.: Fertility following microsurgical removal of the ampullary-isthmic junction in rabbits. Fertil. Steril. 28:1090–1093, 1977.

Fadel, H.E., Berns, D., Zaneveld, L.J.K., Wilbanks, G.D. and Brueschke, E.E.: The human uterotubal junction: A scanning electron microscope study during different phases of the menstrual cycle. Fertil. Steril. 27:1176–1186, 1976.

Ferenczy, A., Richart, R.M., Agate, F.J., Purkerson, M.L. and Dempsey, E.W.: Scanning electron microscopy of the human fallopian tube. Science 175:783–784, 1972.

Gatsalov, M.D.: The intraorganic venous circulation of the circulation of the human uterine tube. Arkh. Anat. 44:87–92, 1963.

Gatsalov, M.D.: The lymphatic system of the mucous membrane of the human fallopian tube. Akush. Ginek. (Sofiia) 39:85–90, 1963a.

Gatsalov, M.D.: The lymphatic system of the serous membrane of the fallopian tube in humans. Sborn. Nauch. Trud. Severo-Ostetinsk Med. Inst. 11:166–172, 1964.

Gatsalov, M.D.: The anatomy of the intrinsic veins of the human fallopian tube. Sborn. Nauch. Trud. Severo-Ostetinsk Med. Inst. 11:180–185, 1964a.

Hermstein, A. and Neustadt, B.: Intramural portion of the oviduct. Z. Geburtsh. Gynaek. 88:43–60, 1924.

Horstmann, E.: The musculature and vascular architecture of the human oviduct. Z. Zellforsch. 37:415–454, 1952.

Jean, Y., Langlais, J., Roberts, K.D., Chapdelaine, A. and Bleau, G.: Fertility of a woman with nonfunctional ciliated cells in the fallopian tubes. Fertil. Steril. 31:349–350, 1979.

Lapina, Z.V.: Certain developmental peculiarities of tubo-ovarian circulation in women. (Abstract). Excerpta Medica, Sect. I, 17:941, 1963.

Ludwig, H. and Metzger, H.: Surface iconography of the human fallopian tube. In: Reversibility of Female Sterilization, I. Brosens, R. and Winston, R. (eds), Academic Press, London, pp. 31–43, 1978.

Owman, C., Rosengren, E. and Sjoberg, N.O.: Adrenergic innervation of the human female reproductive organs: A histochemical and chemical investigation. Obstet. Gynecol. 30:763–773, 1967.

Patek, E., Nilsson, L. and Johannisson, E.: Scanning electron microscopic study of the human fallopian tube. Report I. The proliferative and secretory stages. Fertil. Steril. 23:459–465, 1972.

Patek, E. and Nilsson, L.: Scanning electron microscopic observations on the ciliogenesis of the infundibulum of the human fetal and adult fallopian tube epithelium. Fertil. Steril. 24:819–831, 1973.

Patek, E., Nilsson, L. and Hellema, M.: Scanning electron microscopic study of the human fallopian tube. Report IV. At term gestation and in the puerperium. The effect of a synthetic progestin on the postmenopausal tube. Fertil. Steril. 24:832–843, 1973.

Pitchuev, V.P.: Vascularization of the fallopian tubes under normal and pathological conditions. Arkh. Anat. 40:94–100, 1961.

Reiffenstuhl, G.: The Lymphatics of the Female Genital Organs. J. B. Lippincott Co., Philadelphia (1964), p. 165.

Seki, K., Rawson, J., Eddy, C.A., Smith, N.K. and Pauerstein, C.J.: Deciliation in the puerperal fallopian tube. Fertil. Steril. 29:75–83, 1978.

Stange, H.H.: Comparative morphologic studies on human fallopian tube in extreme functional states; question of existence of infundibular sphincter. Zbl. Gynaek. 74:1176–1182, 1952.

Stange, H.H.: Functional morphology of the fimbriate end of the human oviduct and the epoophoron. Arch. Gynaek. 182:77–103, 1952a.

Vasen, L.C.L.M.: The intramural part of the fallopian tube. Int. J. Fertil. 4:309–314, 1959.

Vasen, L.C.L.M.: On the Musculature of the Intramural Part of the Fallopian Tube and Its Functional Significance. Dijkstrsa's, Groningen (1959a).

Westman, A.: A contribution to the question of the transit of the ovum from the ovaries to the uterus in rabbits. Acta Obstet. Gynecol. Scand. 5, Suppl. 3:1–104, 1926.

Westman, A.W. Studies of the function of the fallopian tube. Int. J. Fertil. 4:20 201–207, 1959.

Williams, J.W. Contributions to the normal and pathologic histology of the fallopian tube. Am. J. Med. Sci. 102:377–388, 1891.

Copyright 1979 by Elsevier North Holland, Inc.
F.K. Beller and G.F.B. Schumacher, eds.
The Biology of the Fluids of the Female Genital Tract

TUBAL TRANSPORT

R. J. Blandau, R. Bourdage, and S. Halbert

SUMMARY

Although the anatomical configuration of the various subdivisions of the oviducts may vary greatly in different species the basic mechanisms of gamete transport are remarkably similar in all mammals so far studied. The fimbriae of rats, mice and hamsters are similar in their anatomic configurations. They are diminutive in relation to the size of the ovaries but the action of muscles and cilia transport the ovulated eggs into the oviducts efficiently. In rabbits, cats, monkeys and women the fimbriae are expansive and at ovulation form ovarian bursae whose ciliated surfaces are in close contact with the ovarian surfaces. Ciliary activity is responsible for egg transport from the ovarian surface into the ampulla. Ampullar transport of the ovulated eggs varies with the species—in some ciliary activity is primarily the propelling force—in others both muscle contractility and ciliary action transport the eggs in cumulus to the ampullar-isthmic junction—the site of fertilization. The epithelium lining of the isthmus varies dramatically in different species. Ciliated cells are almost absent in the isthmi of rats and guinea pigs. Dual ciliated pathways are present in the isthmus of rabbits and pigs, while in primates the mucosal folds are well ciliated and all of the cilia beat in the direc-

University of Washington, School of Medicine, Department of Biological Structure, Seattle, Washington

tion of the uterus. The directionality of the contractions of the isthmus varies according to the endocrine status of the animal. During the immediate preovulatory period the luminal contents are transported into the ampullae by vigorous antiperistaltic contraction waves. During the luteal phase the pro-ovarian contractions of the isthmus are replaced by segmental undulating contractions that gradually propel the fertilized eggs towards the uterus.

INTRODUCTION

This paper reviews some of the anatomical and physiological characteristics of the oviducts of several species that are essential in gamete transport, fertilization, and segmentation. Since gamete transport in the oviduct may be influenced by smooth muscle contractions, ciliary activity, the hydrodynamics of luminal fluids and the hormonal status of the animal, accurate knowledge of the function of each must be determined if we are to understand the complexity of transport mechanisms.

Studies on gamete transport have emphasized oviductal muscular contraction as the primary effector of gamete transport throughout the tube. A variety of miniature intraluminal and extraluminal transducers have been developed and applied to the oviducts to assess motility and, indirectly, transport. Techniques for short and long term monitoring of electrical activity of the oviductal musculature throughout the cycle and under various hormonal influences have been applied, and the data from these collated. The roles of ions, hormones, and various pharmacological agents, such as adrenergic drugs, and the multitude of prostaglandins in addition to drugs that specifically inhibit muscle activity are being and have been evaluated (for an extensive review see Harper et al., 1976). All of these techniques have led to the accumulation of a large body of data on oviductal contractile activity; their relevancy to gamete transport in any specific species is yet to be determined.

A complete description of normal gamete transport mechanisms is not available for any animal. Without such critical observations, quantitative analytical studies on the basic mechanism of tubal transport cannot be properly interpreted. Gamete transport in the living animal at different times of the estrus or menstrual cycle, is astonishing in its complexity and in the variety of ways nature accomplishes her end in order to assemble the gametes within the ampulla to continue life's processes.

EGG TRANSPORT FROM THE OVARIES TO THE OSTIAE OF THE OVIDUCTS IN A VARIETY OF MAMMALS

The anatomical configuration of the fimbriae of the infundibuli in relationship to the ovaries is different in different animals. The variation determines the manner in which the eggs are transported by means of the fimbriae into the ampullae (Beck and Boots, 1974). In the mouse, hamster and rat the fimbriae are diminutive and are in contact with only a very small part of the ovary (Figure 1). In these animals no fimbrial bursae partially or completely enclose the ovaries. How then are eggs, which are ovulated at some distance from the fimbriae (and most of them are), transported into the oviducts? The ovulatory process can be observed directly in living animals, and the movements of the eggs in cumuli can be fol-

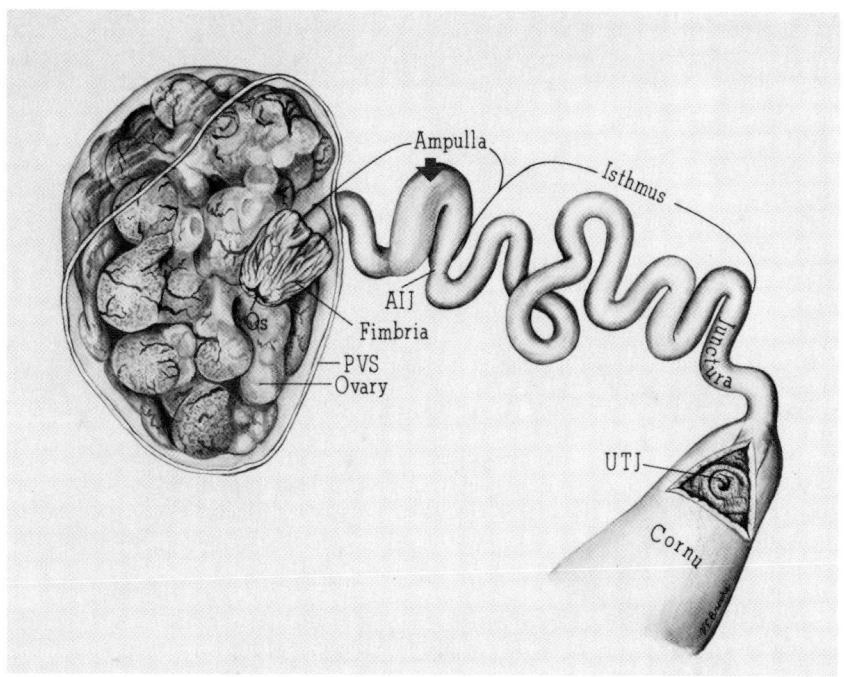

FIGURE 1. A drawing of the appearance of the ovary and oviductal components in rat during estrus. Note the diminutive fimbria in relationship to the size of the ovary; the periovarial sac (PVS) completely enclosing the ovary; the dilated second loop of the ampulla (arrow); the constricted ampullar isthmic junction (AIJ); the extensive coils of the isthmus; the junctional segment and the intramural portion ending in the uterotubal junction (UTJ).

lowed. In the rat, mouse and hamster the ovaries are completely enclosed in a thin transparent periovarial sac. The fimbriae penetrate the periovarial sac, are attached to it, and extend for a very short distance into each periovarial space. At about the time of ovulation the periovarial-peritoneal slit, which is the only opening between the periovarial sac and the peritoneal cavity, is closed so that fluids accumulate within the periovarial space and distend the membrane (Alden, 1942; Kellogg, 1941). The origin of these fluids and how they are retained within the periovarial space are unknown. At least 50% of the surface cells of the fimbria are ciliated (Figure 2a, b). Each cilium has at its tip a ciliary crown (Figure 3). All of the fimbria cilia beat in the direction of the osteim of the oviduct. At ovulation the eggs are surrounded by a number of layers of compacted cumulus cells similar to a bolus. The eggs are shed free into the periovarial space. It should be emphasized that they do not adhere to the rupture site. Bleeding from the stigmal area is very rare indeed. At intervals during the period of ovulation the contractions of muscular mesovarium shifts the position of the ovary within the periovarial sac and displaces the ovulated eggs. When the eggs in their cumulus masses are gradually moved into the vicinity of the fimbria, fluid convection currents move them toward it; they come in contact with the cilia of the fimbria and

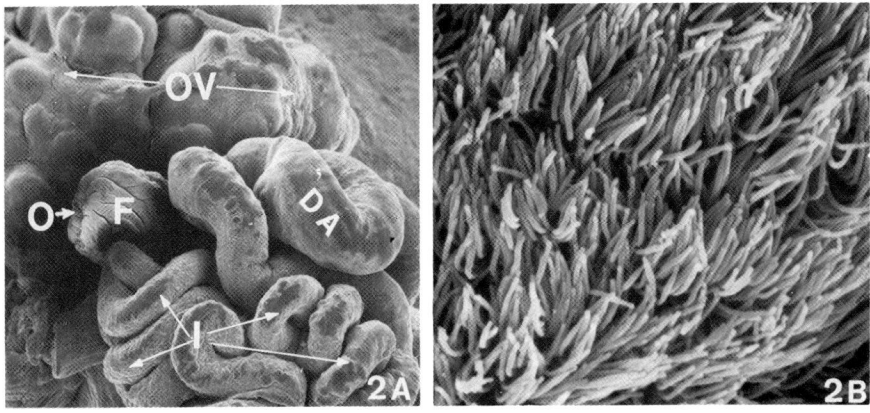

FIGURE 2. Scanning electron micrographs of the ovary and oviduct of the rat at the time of ovulation. (A) The periovarial sac has been dissected away revealing the ovary and fimbria (see Figure 1). (B) A scanning electron micrograph of the ciliated surface of the fimbria. F = Fimbria. O = Osteim of fimbria. Ov = Ovary. DA = Dilated ampulla. I = Isthmus.

FIGURE 3. Electron micrographs of longitudinal sections through several single cilia from the fimbria of the rat revealing the ciliary crowns (arrow). Original mag. X 41,000.

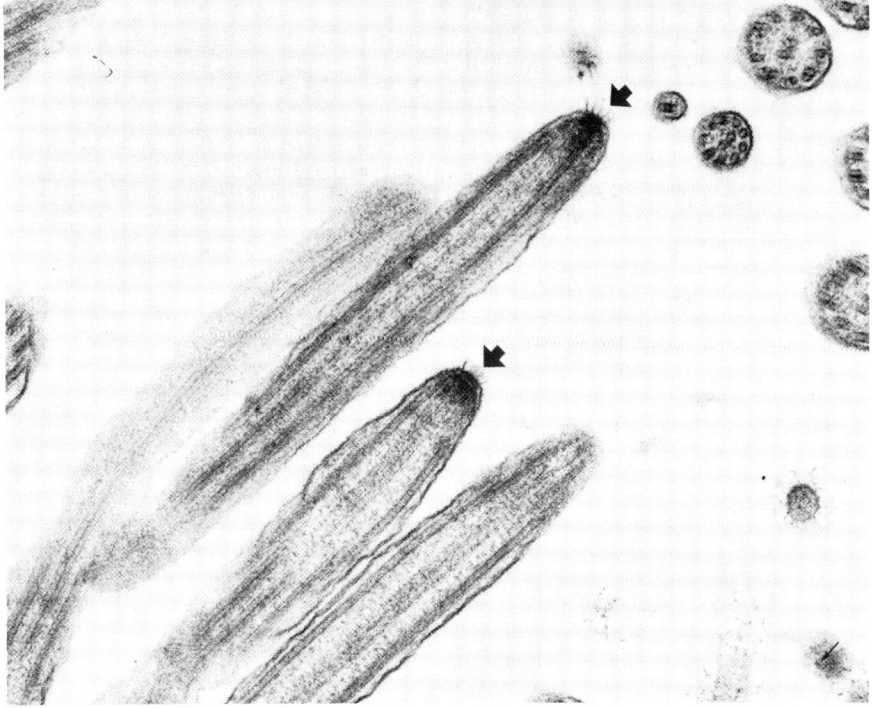

they are carried forward rapidly and enter the osteim. Does this seem to be an inefficient way to transport ovulated eggs? Not if you have observed the manner by which they reach the fimbria and the rapidity with which they are then transported into the ampulla. It is an impressive sight.

Once the eggs in cumulus have entered the osteim they are moved along for several millimeters by ciliary action alone, after which they enter the first convoluted loop of the ampulla and are transported rapidly by a series of peristaltic waves, repeated approximately every 2 seconds. They then enter the dilated ampulla (Figure 4). The dilation of this ampullar loop is caused by an accumulation of fluid that is retained by an efficient valve-like constriction of the muscles of the ampullar-isthmic junction (Figure 1). The movements of the ovulated eggs in cumulus can be readily observed through the thin muscular walls of this dilated loop. Mild peristaltic and antiperistaltic contractions drive the cumulus masses containing the eggs backward and forward until they accumulate eventually near the ampullar-isthmic junction where they are compacted into a single ball of cells. Even though the mucosal lining of the dilated ampulla has a significant number

FIGURE 4. Frozen and stained sections from the first and second loops of the ampulla of a rat in heat. A_1 cross-section through the first loops; A_2 cross-section of the dilated ampulla containing several ovulated eggs (arrows). X50.

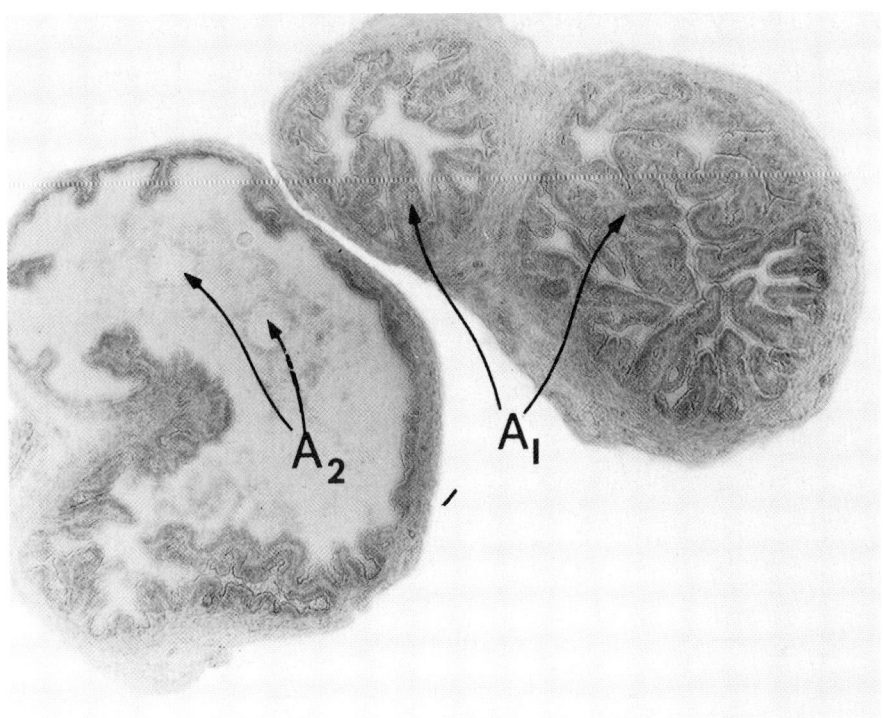

of ciliated cells, these play only a minor role in the forward movement of the cumulus masses. Thus in the rat, muscle contractions are primary in the transport of eggs through this segment.

FIMBRIAL AND AMPULLAR EGG TRANSPORT IN THE CAT AND RABBIT

The fimbriae of the cat are considerably thicker and much more muscular than those of the rabbit. Rhythmic muscular contractions displace the cat fimbriae over the ovarian surface in such a way as to seem to massage them. Otherwise the fimbrial and ampullar egg transport in the rabbit and cat are similar. The fimbriae of the rabbit form ovarial bursae that, at the time of ovulation, almost completely enclose the ovaries (Figure 5). Approximately one-half of the surface epithelial cells facing the ovaries are ciliated, and all of the cilia beat toward the ostea of the oviducts. The cilia of the cat and rabbit fimbriae possess ciliary crowns similar to those illustrated for the rat in Figure 3. It is suggested that these

FIGURE 5. Drawing of the various subdivisions of the rabbit oviduct. The fimbria forms a bursa enclosing the ovary at the time of ovulation. The ampulla and isthmus is divided equally by isthmo-ampullar constriction. The muscular mesotubarium superius contracts vigorously at the time of ovulation displacing the fimbria over the surface of the ovary.

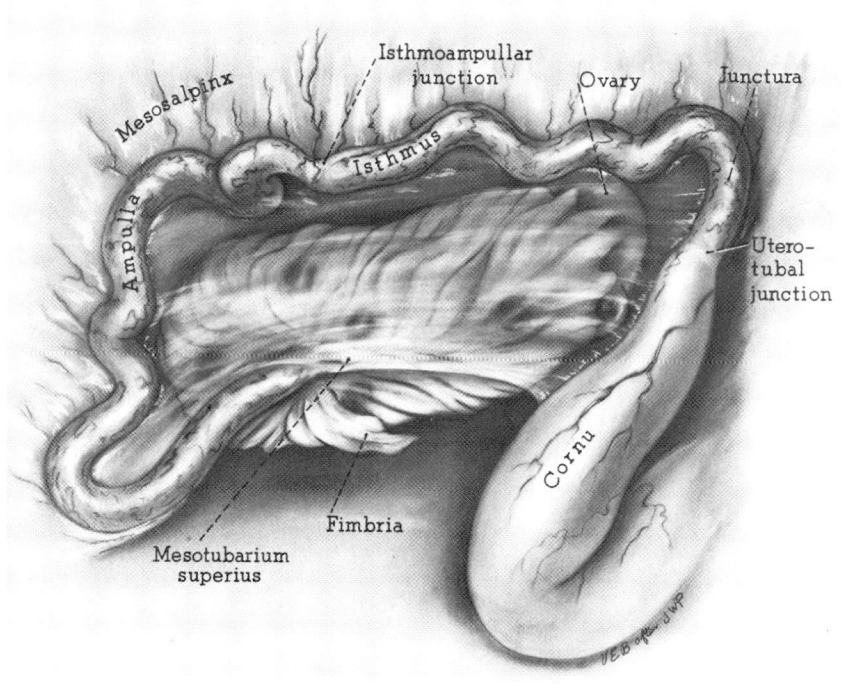

ciliary crowns play an important physical role in egg transport (Anderson and Hein, 1977). The ovulated cumulus masses in both the cat and rabbit are exceedingly sticky, and remain adherent to the site of rupture. They must be pulled from the ovarian surface by the action of fimbrial cilia. The sticky matrix of the ovulated eggs, particularly in the cat, may be pulled out into long strands as the eggs are gradually carried into the osteim. After the eggs enter the osteim they are transported exclusively by ciliary action for the first few millimeters. The complex mucosal folds of the ampulla are lined by numerous ciliated cells (Figure 6a, b). All of the cilia beat in the direction of the ampullar-isthmic junction.

Observation on the transport of freshly recovered, then supravitally stained cumulus masses, through the ampulla in the living rabbit reveal that both contractile activity of the musculature and ciliary action propel the eggs forward. It is difficult to determine precisely which is the primary propelling force. When the ampullary muscles are paralyzed by the intravenous infusion of isoproterenol (Isoprel hydrochloride, Winthrop), a B-receptor agonist, the cumulus masses are transported by the cilia alone at the same rate as that obtained when muscle-

FIGURE 6A. A frozen cross-section of a rabbit ampulla that was quick-frozen in Freon cooled to the temperature of liquid nitrogen. Note the complexity of the mucosal folds. F = a longitudinal section through a segment of the fimbria. X12.

FIGURE 6B. A scanning electron micrograph of a small section of a mucosal fold showing the arrangement of the ciliated and secretory cells. X3000.

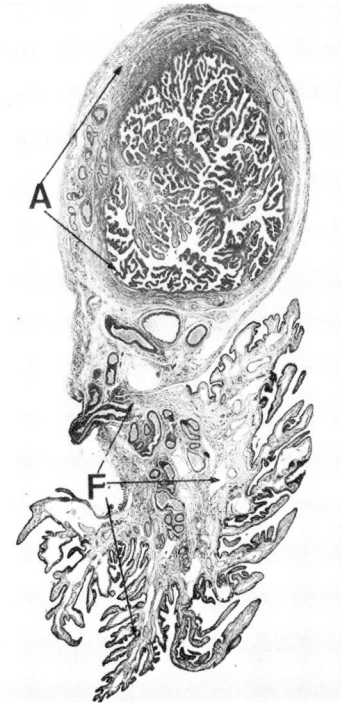
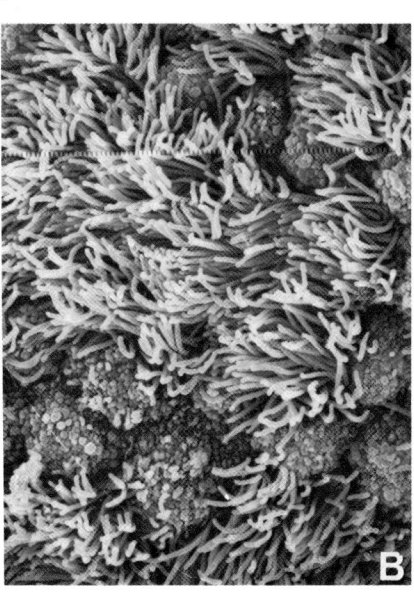

induced movements are also acting (Halbert et al., 1977). Under normal conditions the cilia may act as a "ratchet" that stabilizes the cumulus mass so that it is not regurgitated (Verdugo et al., 1976).

AMPULLARY TRANSPORT OF EGGS IN MONKEYS AND WOMEN

Observations on cumulus mass transport in the ampullae of living Macaca nemestrina at mid-cycle and in human oviducts removed surgically at mid-cycle do not show the segmental, peristaltic muscle contractions of rodents, rabbits and cats (unpublished observations). The fimbriae in the pigtail monkey are fluted and fringed and at the time of ovulation form significant bursae in which the ovaries are almost completely enclosed. More than one-half of the surface cells are ciliated, all beating in the direction of the ostia. The cilia of the primate fimbriae do not appear to possess the ciliary crowns of other species, which may account for the somewhat slower egg transport over the fimbriae in primates. The fringed, fluted and lansiform mid-cycle human fimbriae are the most complex of any mammalian species we have observed. The mucosal folds of the ampullae in both monkey and human are very extensive, so much so in appropriately prepared frozen sections, they may completely fill the lumen. Thus there is only a potential space in this segment of the oviduct in both monkeys and women (Figures 7a, b and 8a, b). In the several primates we have examined, all of the cilia in the ampullae beat toward the ampullar-isthmic junctions. We are convinced from many observations that the eggs in cumulus are transported primarily by ciliary activity. In both monkeys and women it requires approximately 30 minutes for the eggs in cumulus to be transported through the ampullae to reach the ampullar-isthmic constriction. The diverse pathways the cumulus masses take as they move in and about the complex mucosal folds may partially account for the length of time of the passage.

The primary function of the fimbria and ampulla then is to transport the ovulated eggs from the ovary to the ampullar-isthmic junction, the normal site of fertilization. As is obvious from the description of the natural history of this phenomenon in the several species mentioned, transport is accomplished efficiently and in a relatively short period of time after ovulation by the action of cilia and in some species by the action of both cilia and muscles, their predominance in this process depending upon the species (Gaddum-Rosse and Blandau, 1976).

GAMETE TRANSPORT THROUGH THE ISTHMUS

Witness the paradox in gamete transport in the isthmus: spermatozoa must ascend to the site of fertilization in the ampulla during the preovulatory period and the fertilized eggs must be transported 24 to 48 hours later, in the opposite direction to reach the uterus. The contractile activity of the isthmus of the oviduct at various times in the reproductive cycle is perhaps the most complex of any tubular system in the body. Its function is strictly under hormonal control. In addition to the contractile variations there are marked differences in the cellular configuration of the mucosal lining in various species. In the rat and guinea pig there are very few ciliated cells, and these are confined primarily to the proximal isthmic segment. The surfaces of the remaining cells have very long and complex microvilli that appear to completely fill the lumen (Figure 9). In the rabbit and

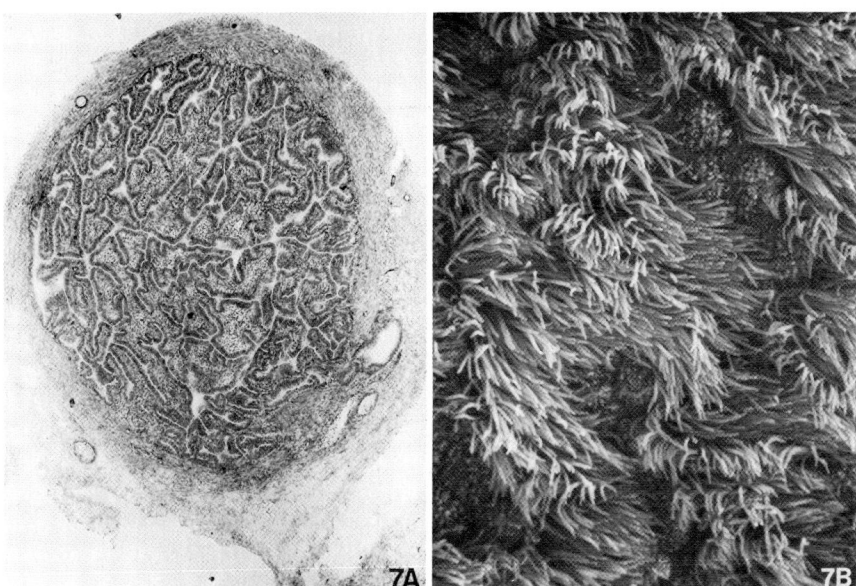

FIGURE 7A. A frozen cross-section of a Macaca nemestrina ampulla that was quick-frozen in Freon cooled to the temperature of liquid nitrogen. The mucosal folds almost completely fill the ampullar lumen. X56.

FIGURE 7B. A scanning electron micrograph of a small section of one of the mucosal folds of the ampulla showing the large number of ciliated cells and a few of the secretory cells. X4100.

pig, dual ciliated pathways are present in which the ciliated cells are arranged in rows on the tips of the folds and in the recesses between them. The cilia beat simultaneously in two directions; upward toward the ovary and downward toward the uterus (Table I). These dual ciliated pathways do not appear to participate in sperm transport but seem to be involved in the even application of the oölemmal membranes that are applied to the zonae pellucidae as the eggs move through this segment. The cilia in the isthmi of monkeys, women, cows and sheep beat only toward the uteri (Gaddum-Rosse and Blandau, 1976). The mucosal folds of the isthmi of monkeys and women are not as complex as those of the ampullae and they do not possess as many ciliated cells (Figures 10 and 11).

MUSCULAR CONTRACTILE ACTIVITY OF THE ISTHMUS DURING THE PREOVULATORY AND POSTOVULATORY PERIOD

Observations on the contractile activity of the isthmi *in vivo* in the preovulatory period in rats, guinea pigs, rabbits, monkeys and *in vitro* observations on the isthmi of women reveal antiperistaltic contractile waves that propel the contents of the lumen in a pro-ovarian direction into the ampullae. The most dramatic pro-ovarian contraction waves may be observed in the rat during this pro-

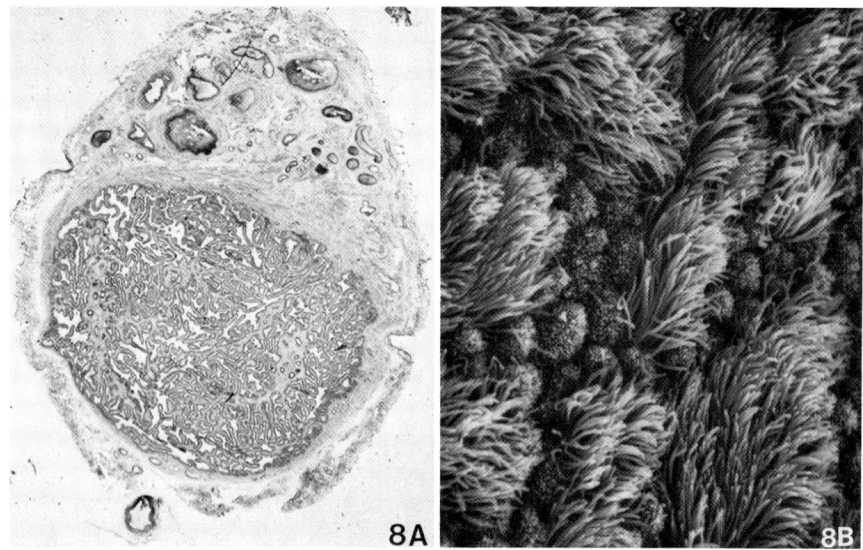

FIGURE 8A. A frozen cross-section of the human ampulla from a surgical specimen at mid-cycle. The ampulla was quick-frozen in Freon cooled to the temperature of liquid nitrogen. The mucosal folds are more complex than those of the pigtailed monkey (Figure 7A) and almost completely fill the lumen. X11.

FIGURE 8B. A scanning electron micrograph of the surface of one of the mucosal folds. Note the arrangement of the ciliated cells with the intervening secretory cells. X4000.

cedure. The uterotubal junction in the rat is cannulated with a very fine polyethylene tube held in place with tissue glue and then small boluses of stained mineral oil are inserted into the junctura region, minute boluses of oil may be observed moving intact through the entire isthmus in approximately 3-5 seconds. When the boluses reach the ampullar-isthmic junction they are propelled past this constriction into the ampulla where they are retained. As increasing amounts of oil are transported through the isthmus, the ampulla may become greatly distended without regurgitating any of the oil into the isthmus. We have been impressed repeatedly with the competency of the ampullar-isthmic constriction during the preovulatory and ovulatory periods.

Similar pro-ovarian contractile waves have been observed, both *in vivo* and *in vitro*, in blood perfused preparations in rabbit isthmi. Although the rate of proovarian progression of the boluses of oil is somewhat slower in these animals than that observed in the rat, it nevertheless is moved forward continuously and efficiently (unpublished observations). During each antiperistaltic contraction wave the lumen is completely occluded. This complete occlusion carries its contents forward as a continuous column. Similar transport has been observed in human oviducts removed at surgery during the mid-cycle. The transport of the oil boluses in the human isthmus is slower and more gentle than it is in the other mammals we have examined.

Our observations have led us to conclude that the transport of the luminal

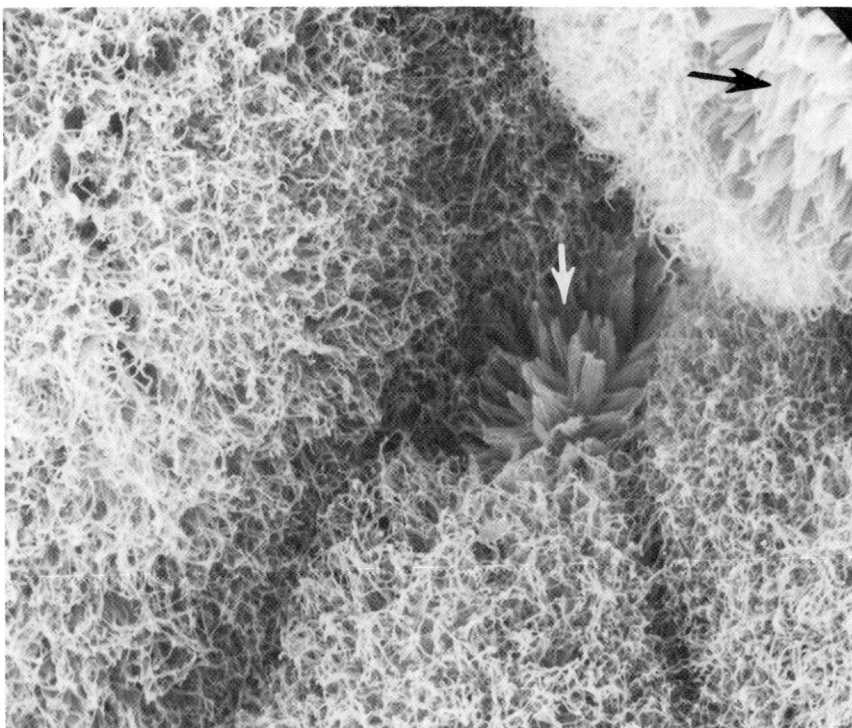

FIGURE 9. A scanning electron micrograph of a portion of the upper isthmus from a rat at the time of ovulation. Note the complexity of the microvilli projecting from the cells of the mucosa and the occasional ciliated cell (arrows).

contents of the isthmus during the preovulatory and ovulatory period is principally pro-ovarian; that the rate of transport varies in different species but that the antiperistaltic contraction we have observed in a variety of species is the primary mechanism for the transport of spermatozoa into the ampullae. Since ciliated cells are almost absent from the isthmi of some species, it is very unlikely that ciliary activity plays any significant role in sperm transport through this oviductal segment. During the postovulatory or early luteal phase of the cycle, the contractile activity of the isthmus changes dramatically from principally pro-ovarian to a segmental, undulatory pattern that shuttles the denuded eggs backward and forward from loop to loop. How the eggs finally reach the junctura region near the uterus and are expelled into the uterus is unknown.

QUANTITATIVE EVALUATIONS OF ISTHMIC TRANSPORT USING OPTOELECTRONIC TRANSDUCERS

Quantitative descriptions of the motility of the isthmi of anesthetized animals have been obtained by analyzing 16 mm motion picture films taken of this process. These observations have been extended to intact, awake rabbits by implanting optoelectronic transducers in the animals (Halbert et al., 1975; Blandau et

TABLE I. Comparative Studies of Ciliary Currents in Various Mammalian Oviducts.

	Direction of Ciliary Beat			
Animal	Fimbria of Infundibulum	Ampulla	Isthmus	Ciliary Crowns
Rat	All Cilia Beat Towards Ostium of Oviduct	All Cilia Beat Towards Ampullar-Isthmic Junction	No Ciliated Pathways	Present
Guinea Pig				?
Rabbit			Dual Ciliated Pathways ↑↓	Present
Pig				?
Cat			Cilia Beat Towards Uterus	Present
Sheep				?
Hamster				?
Cow				?
Monkey				Absent
Man	↓	↓	↓	Absent
	Ostium of Oviduct	Ampullar-Isthmic Junction	Uterus	

FIGURE 10. A frozen cross-section of a human isthmus that was quick-frozen in Freon cooled to the temperature of liquid nitrogen. Note that the mucosal folds are not as complex as those of the human ampulla prepared in the same manner (Figure 8). There also are not as many ciliated cells in this segment of the oviduct.

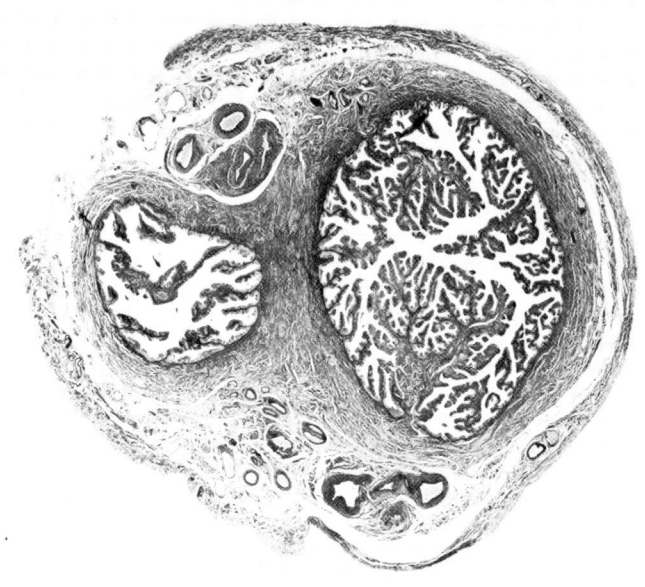

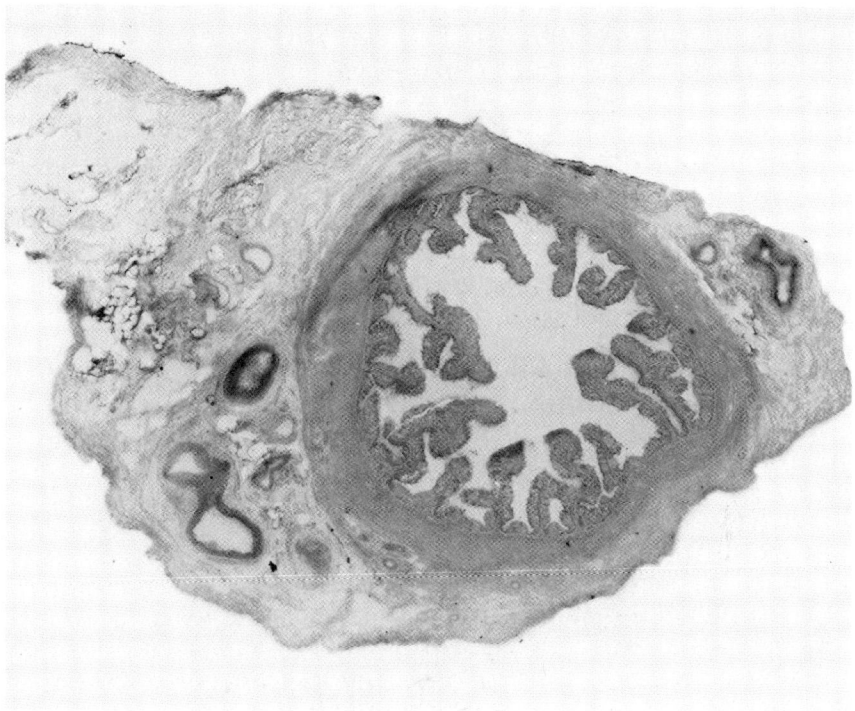

FIGURE 11. A frozen cross-section of a Macaca nemestrina isthmus prepared from a quick-frozen Freon liquid nitrogen cooled tissue. Note that the isthmus is a very muscular organ with a relatively sparse ciliated mucosa.

al., 1975). When closely-spaced pairs of sensors are applied externally to the isthmi, contractile activity may be recorded and the resultant data analyzed by computer to give the speed and direction of propagation of contraction waves at each sensor (Halbert et al., 1977), in addition to the frequency of contractile events (Bourdage 1978) (Figure 12). Within a few hours following an ovulation-inducing injection of luteinizing hormone, continuous monitoring of the oviductal sensors shows that the frequency of isthmic contractions increase 20-30%. During this time the contraction waves propagate uniformly in the pro-ovarian direction at a speed of about 3mm/sec (Figure 12). Twenty to 35 hours after ovulation the contraction frequency declines slowly to reach a plateau of 30-50% below the estrous control level. During the postovulatory period the contraction wave propagation changes to a random collection of pro-ovarian and prouterine waves of widely varying speeds. The data recorded in this period correspond with the segmental contractions and pendular motility patterns observed and recorded cinematographically in the exposed oviducts of anesthetized rabbits. This dramatic change in isthmic muscular activity appears to provide an explanation for the seemingly contradictory direction and speed of the rapid sperm transport through the isthmus prior to ovulation and the slow progress of the fertilized ovum in the opposite direction a few hours later.

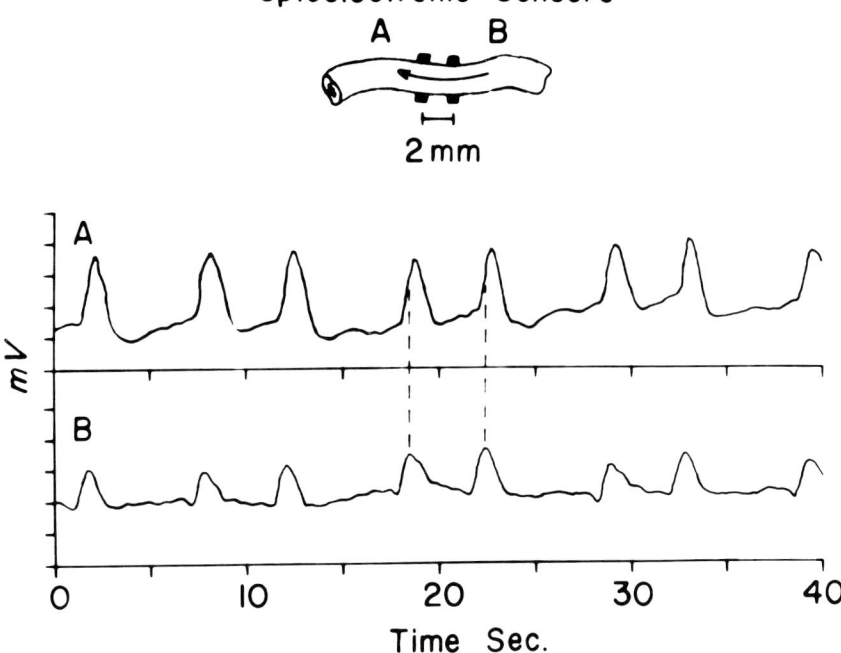

FIGURE 12. Signals from two sensors (A and B) placed on the mid-isthmus with a 2 mm separation. Records of isthmic contractions taken 4 hours after 100 μg LH (preovulatory). Eight contractions propagating through the sensors in a pro-ovarian direction at an average velocity of 5 mm/sec. The dashed line serves to emphasize the phase shift between the two signals. These extraluminal sensors allow us to quantitate the direction and rate of contraction propagation during the pre- and postovulatory periods.

At 70-80 hours following LH stimulation, the frequency of isthmic contractions returns to the control level. Perhaps this relative increase in activity and change in motility pattern facilitates transport of the fertilized eggs into the uterine horns.

ACKNOWLEDGEMENTS

Unpublished studies referred to in this paper were supported by Program Project Grant HD-03752 from the National Institutes of Health.

I am grateful for the photographic skills of Roy Hayashi and the technical assistance of Lynn Langley and Dorothy Patton.

REFERENCES

Alden, R.H.: The periovarial sac in the albino rat. Anat. Rec. 83, 421–434 (1942).

Anderson, R.G.W., Hein, C.E.: Distribution of anionic sites on the oviduct ciliary membrane. J. Cell Biol. 72, 482–492 (1977).

Beck, I.R. and Boots, L.R.: The comparative anatomy, histology and morphology of the mammalian oviduct. In: Johnson, A.D. and C.W. Foley, (eds.): The Oviduct and Its Functions. New York, Academic Press 1–51 (1974).

Blandau, R.J., Boling, J.L., Halbert, S.A., Verdugo, P.: Methods of studying oviductal physiology. Gynecol. Invest. 6. 123–145 (1975).

Bourdage R.J.: Oviductal smooth muscle: Relation of frequency of contractions to gamete transport. Anat. Rec. 190, 344 (1978).

Gaddum-Rosse, P., Blandau, R.J.: Comparative observations on ciliary currents in mammalian oviducts. Biol. Reprod. 14, 605–609 (1976).

Halbert, S.A., Boling, J.L., Blandau, R.J., Ringo, J.A.: An optoelectronic instrument for chronic monitoring of oviduct contractions. Conference on Engineering in Medicine and Biology 17 319, (1975).

Halbert, S.A., Tam, P.Y., Blandau, R.J.: Egg transport in the rabbit oviduct: The role of cilia and muscle. Science 191, 1052–1053 (1976).

Halbert, S.A., Verdugo, P., Boling, J.L., Blandau, R.J.: *In vivo* studies of contraction wave propagation and its role in sperm and egg transport in the oviductal isthmus of rabbits. Biophys. J. 17, 266a (1977).

Harper, M.J.K., Pauerstein, C.J., Adams, C.E., Coutinho, E.M., Croxatto, H.B., and Paton, D.M., eds: Ovum Transport and Fertility Regulation. Scriptor, Copenhagen 1976.

Kellogg, M.P.: The development of the periovarial sac in the white rat. Anat. Rec. 79, 465–477 (1941).

Verdugo, P., Blandau, R.J., Tamp, P.Y., Halbert, S.A.: Stochastic elements in the development of deterministic models of egg transport. In: Harper, M.J.K., Pauerstein, C.J., Adams, C.E., Coutinho, E.M., Croxatto, H.B., and Paton, D.M. (eds.): Ovum Transport and Fertility Regulation. Copenhagen, Scriptor, 126–137 (1976).

Copyright 1979 by Elsevier North Holland, Inc.
F.K. Beller and G.F.B. Schumacher, eds.
The Biology of the Fluids of the Female Genital Tract

TUBAL SECRETIONS

L. Mastroianni, Jr., and K. J. Go

SUMMARY

Oviduct fluid provides an environment in which the initial phases of reproduction occur. Tubal fluid affords the proper conditions for sperm capacitation, the fertilization process, cleavage of the ovum and the nuturing of the developing zygote. Several methods of tubal fluid collection have been developed by which the biochemical and physiological properties of these secretions can be assessed. Variations in tubal fluid volume, protein and electrolyte content, and ability to support sperm capacitation and embryo development correlate with hormonal status. Several regulatory components are present in the tubal fluid which may modulate gamete and embryo function.

INTRODUCTION

The mammalian oviduct is a dynamic organ, with a critical role in the preparative events culminating in fertilization. By provision of a chemically balanced environment within its lumen, the oviduct creates an optimum medium in which the spermatozoon achieves fertilizing ability (capacitation) and in which the ovum

Division of Reproductive Biology, Department of Obstetrics and Gynecology, University of Pennsylvania School of Medicine, Philadelphia, Pennsylvania, U.S.A.

is prepared for fertilization. The tubal environment also provides the milieu in which the developing embryo resides during the first three post-fertilization days.

In general, oviductal fluid is looked upon as a combination of an active secretion and a transudate. The secretory function of the endosalpinx has been recognized for many years, as evidenced by morphological changes during the course of the menstrual cycle. Fluctuations in tubal fluid volume are, in part, brought about by transudation. In addition, various biochemical constituents of tubal fluid have been identified which play pivotal roles in reproduction.

METHODS OF EVALUATION OF THE TUBAL ENVIRONMENT

The oviductal environment has been evaluated in a number of species, including rabbit (Hamner and Williams, 1965; Holmdahl and Mastroianni, 1965; Shapiro et al., 1971), ewe (Restall and Wales, 1966; Iritani et al., 1969; Roberts et al., 1976), sow (Iritani, 1974), hamster (Noske and Daniel, 1974), mare (Engle, 1975), bovine (Perkins, 1974; Stanke et al., 1974; Roberts et al., 1975), mouse (Borland et al., 1977), monkey (Mastroianni et al., 1961a, 1969, 1970; Marcus and Saravis, 1965) and human (Lippes et al., 1972; David, 1973; Shams et al., 1977). Methods of collection of tubal fluid have been devised in an effort to recover physiologically unaltered specimens. The most recent of these involves continuous collection of fluid via cannulation. Hamner and Williams (1965) have devised an internally placed collecting system which allows collection of oviductal fluid continuously at body temperature. This has been useful in evaluating the effect of a changing hormonal status on tubal contents. Others have devised an external system for collection of tubal fluid which was then refined to include refrigeration such that tubal fluid could be collected continuously at approximately 3°C (Mastroianni et al., 1961a; Holmdahl and Mastroianni, 1965). These methods offer a distinct advantage over those used earlier which involved the ligation of the oviduct near the uterotubal junction and at the fimbriated end. The tubal fluid contained by the ligatures could be recovered for evaluation.

The effectiveness of these various collections methods has been evaluated. There is a distinct difference, for example, between fluid collected continuously and fluid collected by the ligation method. The addition of refrigeration to an external collecting chamber results in the preservation of certain substrates. When refrigerated and non-refrigerated specimens are compared in the same animal, there are differences, especially in the glucose content (Mastroianni et al., 1973). This suggests that the refrigeration system substantially decreases the level of contamination of the specimen contained in the chamber.

The effect of continuous collection on the oviductal epithelium immediately adjacent to the cannula has been studied by electron microscopy. No histological alterations, even at the ultrastructural level, are observed in sections of the oviduct after as long as two weeks of cannulation (Mastroianni and Nicosia, unpublished results, 1976). Others have also reported no significant changes in fluid which could be related to the presence of a cannula (Sloan and Johnson, 1974). These experiments notwithstanding, there is no method of collection which will absolutely insure that there has been no effect of the collection system on tubal contents.

A somewhat more physiologic approach involves the use of probes to evaluate the tubal environment. An intraluminal probe was first used to assess the changes in oxygen content within the rabbit tubal lumen in association with ovulation (Mastroianni and Jones, 1965). These methods were extended to the monkey, and probes were used to evaluate changes in pH, carbon dioxide and oxygen tension within the oviductal lumen in that species (Maas et al., 1976, 1977). In the mouse, microprobes have been devised to evaluate electrolyte content (Borland et al., 1977).

EFFECT OF HORMONAL STATUS ON TUBAL SECRETIONS

In several species, including rabbit, bovine, rhesus monkey and human, dramatic changes in the volume of tubal fluid occur in association with ovulation. When fluid is collected continuously in the rabbit, there is a decrease in the rate of accumulation of fluid following ovulation to about 50% of the estrous rate (Mastroianni and Wallach, 1961). Estrogen causes an increase in fluid accumulation in the castrate, and progesterone in the presence of estrogen inhibits fluid production (Mastroianni et al., 1961b). A pattern similar to that seen in the rabbit has been observed in the ewe and bovine (Perkins, 1974; Roberts et al., 1975). The rate of human tubal fluid production increases significantly during the late proliferative phase of the menstrual cycle, reaching a maximum at the time of ovulation (Lippes et al., 1972; Shams et al., 1977). In the rhesus monkey, there is a substantial increase in the rate of fluid production immediately prior to ovulation (Mastroianni et al., 1970). In these spontaneously ovulating species, this increase coincides with the estrogen surge which occurs during the menstrual cycle. Thus, it appears that tubal fluid is present in greatest concentration at a time when it is most important in terms of reproduction: during sperm migration and fertilization.

CYCLIC ALTERATIONS IN PROTEIN CONTENT

The protein pattern observed in tubal fluid varies according to the hormonal status of the female. In some species, certain oviduct-specific proteins appear after ovulation. A β-glycoprotein has been observed in postovulatory human tubal fluid (Moghissi, 1970). A protein not found in serum was observed migrating behind transferrin in postovulatory rhesus monkey fluid (Mastroianni et al., 1970). Several proteins were identified in rabbit oviductal fluid which were not found in serum (Urzua et al., 1970; Feigelson and Kay, 1972). Small amounts of protein were detected in bovine tubal fluid which were not observed in serum (Roberts et al., 1975). A protein band similar to that observed in the rhesus monkey appearing in the β-globulin region has been observed in the hamster during the first six days of pregnancy (Noske and Daniel, 1974). In contrast, the polypeptide environment in the rabbit oviduct, as evaluated by two-dimensional gel electrophoresis, appears unchanged during the first six days of pregnancy (Tucker and Schultz, 1977). It is possible, however, that the method used was not sensitive enough to detect subtle changes in the polypeptide content or of proteins outside the measured pH range. The physiological significance of such changes in protein constituents, if any, remains to be elucidated.

PREPARATION OF SPERMATOZOA

Sperm deposited into the female reproductive tract are not capable of fertilization. Capacitation, the ability to fertilize, is acquired during residence in the female tract. Oviductal fluid may participate in this important preparative stage and in the subsequent events involving the acrosome reaction and binding of spermatozoa to the egg.

When incubated in oviduct fluid, sperm achieve a higher level of oxygen consumption, with a resulting increase in metabolism (Hamner and Williams, 1963). This increase in respiration rate has been attributed to the presence in the tubal fluid of bicarbonate ion (Hamner and Williams, 1964; Storey, 1975). It is thought to be related to capacitation and the acrosome reaction, as suppression of respiration results in the retardation of these two events (Rogers et al., 1979).

An osmolarity higher than that of plasma facilitates capacitation *in vitro* (Brackett and Oliphant, 1975), and electrolytes present in the tubal fluid may afford the optimum ionic environment for this phase of sperm preparation (Brackett and Mastroianni, 1974). The calcium concentration in tubal fluid increases after ovulation in the monkey (Mastroianni and Stambaugh, 1974) and rabbit (Holmdahl and Mastroianni, 1965). Ca^{2+} has been shown to be necessary for capacitation (Singh et al., 1978) and binding of sperm to egg (Saling et al., 1978). Experiments examining the competition of Mg^{2+} with Ca^{2+} for binding by sperm suggest that the Mg^{2+}/Ca^{2+} ratio in the reproductive tract may be an important modulator for the timing of the acrosome reaction (Rogers and Yanagimachi, 1976). The Mg^{2+}/Ca^{2+} ratio is very low in the oviduct fluid of species in which the acrosome reaction occurs in the oviduct.

The ability of the oviduct to support sperm capacitation shows some dependence on the hormonal state of the female and can be modified by estrogen and progesterone. The mechanism by which this effect is mediated is not known. A synergistic relationship between uterine and oviductal fluid in capacitation has been proposed (Hunter and Hall, 1974). The oviduct, however, is by itself capable of initiating and completing capacitation and is endowed with a higher innate basal capacitating ability than the uterus. In the rabbit, the capacitating ability of the oviduct is diminished after ovariectomy, but can be restored by estrogen. Capacitation is not significantly disturbed in the oviducts of intact progesterone-dominated females. The basal capacitating activity of the oviduct persists in progesterone-treated ovariectomized females (Bedford, 1970).

The efficiency of capacitation in the rabbit oviduct has been studied as a function of estrus and pseudopregnancy (Brown and Hamner, 1971). Oviduct fluid collected during estrous and throughout pseudopregnancy supports capacitation. There is, however, some depression in the number of eggs fertilized in pseudopregnancy fluid, suggesting that progesterone domination has some adverse effects on sperm well-being. The ability of the oviduct to effect capacitation is also dependent on the concentration of sperm in the oviduct, with unphysiologically high concentrations overwhelming its capacitation potential.

Another parameter of sperm fertilizing ability is motility. Sperm motility is reduced or enhanced as a function of location in the rabbit female reproductive tract (Overstreet and Cooper, 1975). Motility of isthmic sperm is dramatically decreased in contrast to the motility of uterine sperm. Ampullar sperm, however, often show motility greater than that of uterine sperm. Differential changes in acrosomal morphology also occur as a function of site of sperm recovery. Ampullar sperm show lifted or missing acrosomal caps most frequently. In contrast, motile sperm from the uterus or isthmus do not display these changes in acrosomal morphology. These effects may be related to the varying segmental composition of oviduct fluid in this species (David et al., 1969).

The role that the oviductal milieu plays in the conservation of sperm motility is being investigated. The possibility that macromolecules, such as albumin, may be important in this process has been suggested. Serum albumin exerts a preservative and protective action on sperm motility *in vitro* (Harrison et al., 1978). Albumin is a major protein of tubal fluid (Mastroianni et al., 1970; Moghissi, 1970; Urzua et al., 1970; Feigelson and Kay, 1972).

Clearly, oviduct fluid contains the necessary components to confer fertilizing ability on sperm. No single component of tubal fluid alone can effect capacitation. Rather, the oviduct contributes to this critical phase by providing the proper conditions of osmolarity, pH, metabolic substrates, and electrolytes in appropriate ratios.

PREPARATION OF THE OVUM

The freshly ovulated ovum of the rabbit, monkey, human and other mammals is surrounded by a mass of cumulus cells, a more densely arranged inner layer of corona cells, and the zona pellucida. The corona cells have pseudopod-like processes which project into the zona pellucida. The tubal environment causes gradual dispersal of the cumulus, and the separation of the corona cells from each other and from the zona pellucida (Zamboni et al., 1965). The component in tubal fluid responsible for this effect is bicarbonate ion (Stambaugh et al., 1969). Bicarbonate is present in significant amounts and is thought to occur through active secretion (Vishwakarma, 1962). The mechanism by which the cumulus cells are dispersed has not, as yet, been elucidated. Hyaluronidase, an enzyme capable of effecting this action, has not been reported in tubal fluid. It is, however, present in the sperm acrosome and may be released in proximity to the cumulus to effect dispersion (Metz et al., 1972).

THE EFFECT OF THE TUBAL ENVIRONMENT ON THE EMBRYO

Embryos transferred prematurely from the oviduct to the uterus fail to develop properly and implant, indicating that exposure to the oviductal environment is important for embryo survival (Chang, 1950). The effects of oviduct fluid on the developing zygote have been studied in an attempt to isolate factors which may play a role in embryonic maintenance and preparation for implantation.

Specific components from the oviduct are incorporated into the egg. The zonae of unfertilized and fertilized hamster eggs contain components of oviductal origin, as demonstrated immunologically. These zona components are retained in the unfertilized egg, but disappear during the course of embryogenesis (Fox and Shivers, 1975).

A high-molecular-weight (73,000 daltons) acidic glycoprotein has been isolated from rabbit oviduct fluid. This is thought to be a component of the mucin coat normally deposited around the tubal embryo (Shapiro et al., 1974). Three sulfur-containing macromolecules have been isolated in the rabbit. Two are present under all hormonal states and are common to serum, and an additional, apparently oviduct-specific component appears during progesterone domination. All three macromolecules may contribute to the mucin coat (Hanscom and Oliphant, 1976).

The influence of oviduct fluid on rabbit embryo development has also been assessed *in vitro* by culture of embryos in oviduct fluid, and *in vivo*, by transfer of embryos to oviducts under various hormonal conditions. The *in vitro* culture experiments suggest that the oviduct synthesizes and secretes a factor particularly active on Days 2, 8 and 9 after ovulation which significantly enhances development through blastocyst expansion (Kille and Hamner, 1973). The oviducts of ovariectomized females support normal cleavage of zygotes through the 32-cell stage. In the ampullae of estrogen-treated, ovariectomized females, however, embryo development is significantly impaired. An estrogen-induced protein of low molecular weight (<10,000 daltons) is implicated as the inhibitory factor (Stone and Hamner, 1977; Stone et al., 1977).

TUBAL FLUID CONSTITUENTS
Enzyme Inhibitors

Inhibitors of enzymes have been described in oviduct fluid. Acrosin, a proteolytic enzyme bound to the inner membrane of the acrosome, is implicated in the fertilization process. It is suggested that acrosin facilitates sperm penetration through the zona pellucida (Stambaugh and Buckley, 1969; Stambaugh and Smith, 1976). Several inhibitors of acrosin and trypsin have been isolated in the oviduct fluid of rhesus monkey (Stambaugh et al., 1974). The concentrations of these inhibitors vary during the menstrual cycle. They are present at high levels before ovulation, decrease to significantly lower levels around the time of ovulation, and rise again within one to three days after ovulation. A total of six proteinase inhibitors is found, five of which inhibit acrosin from rhesus monkey sperm. These include α_1-antitrypsin, α_2-macroglobulin, α_1-antichymotrypsin. Two others with isoelectric points of 5.8 and 3.3 remained unidentified. Recently, acrosin inhibitors with acidic isoelectric points have been identified as secretory IgA in the tubal fluid of both rhesus monkey and rabbit (Go et al., 1978, 1979).

Rabbit oviduct fluid contains at least four inhibitors of trypsin (McLaughlin and Hamner, 1975). Total inhibitor concentration varies with hormonal state of the female, with low levels at estrus and high levels several days after ovulation.

These enzyme inhibitors may play a role in the regulation of fertilization by preventing the fertilization of an ovum at other than the optimum time in the life of the gamete. The inhibitors may also afford the oviductal lumen protection from the released proteolytic enzymes from degenerating spermatozoa.

Trace Elements

The concentration of trace elements in human tubal fluid has been measured. Several of these are known to act as enzyme co-factors and may participate in the function of such oviductal enzymes as carbonic anhydrase and alkaline phosphatase. Zn^{2+} and Mn^{2+} appear at fairly constant levels in the human endosalpinx in each phase of the menstrual cycle (Patek and Hagenfeldt, 1974). Mg^{2+} reaches its highest level during the proliferative phase and decreases at ovulation (Kadi, 1978).

Steroid Hormones

Free steroid hormones have been measured in rhesus monkey oviduct fluid (Wu et al., 1977). The concentrations of estrone, testosterone and progesterone increase to greater than plasma levels after ovulation, suggesting that some steroids appear in tubal fluid by active secretion. The influence of this high free steroid concentration on fertilization and early embryogenesis is not, as yet, well understood.

Prostaglandins

Prostaglandins may be involved in the physiological control of oviductal motility and thus may have a role in the timing of ovum entry into the uterus (Spilman and Harpa, 1975). $PGF_{2\alpha}$, which stimulates muscular activity in humans, has been identified in human tubal fluid (Ogra et al., 1974). Its concentration is high before and after ovulation, substantially exceeding serum levels, suggesting synthesis by the oviduct.

Immunoglobulins

The oviduct as an immunologically responsive organ has been evaluated. Several investigators have sought to identify immunologically reactive components in tubal fluid. IgG and IgA immunoglobulins and the secretory component associated with local immunoglobulin secretion have been identified in the human oviduct (Lippes et al., 1970; Rebello et al., 1975). The levels of IgG, IgA and IgM in rabbit oviduct fluid are 4%, 24% and 2% of serum levels, respectively (Oliphast et al., 1977). IgA is present in the highest concentration, suggesting a local immune response. Complement component C_3 is also present, but no complement activity is demonstrated, suggesting that some of the other components of complement do not penetrate into the oviductal lumen from the serum due to large molecular size.

Oviductal immunoglobulins may have antifertility effects. They can bind to sperm membranes and cause immobilization and agglutination (Beer and Neaves, 1978) or inhibit the activity of proteolytic enzymes important for fertilization (Arnon, 1974; Go et al., 1978, 1979). Elevated levels of immunoglobulins, particularly secretory IgA, correlate with infertility in women (Wong, 1978). A greater understanding of the immunological capacity of the oviduct may provide insights into some causative factors of infertility.

CONCLUSION

The oviduct, by a combination of active secretion and transudation, elaborates a complex fluid. The tubal fluid contains a spectrum of biologically active constituents, enabling the oviduct to prepare the gametes for fertilization and sustain the developing zygote during its transport to the uterus. Through a study of the environment provided by the oviduct, we may achieve greater insights into the regulation of infertility and the causes of infertility.

REFERENCES

Arnon, R.A.: Enzyme inhibition by antibodies. In: Karolinska Symposia on Research Methods in Reproductive Endocrinology, 7th Symposium, Karolinska Institutent, Stockholm (1974), pp. 133–138.

Bedford, J.M.: The influence of estrogen and progesterone on sperm capacitation in the reproductive tract of the female rabbit. J. Endocrinol. 46:101–200, 1970.

Beer, A.E. and Neaves, W.B.: Antigenic status of semen from the viewpoints of the female and male. Fertil. Steril. 29:3–22, 1978.

Borland, R.M., Hazra, S., Biggers, J.D. and Lechene, C.P.: The elemental composition of the gametes and preimplantation embryo during the initiation of pregnancy. Biol. Reprod. 16:147–157, 1977.

Brackett, B.G. and Oliphant, G.: Capacitation of rabbit spermatozoa *in vitro*. Biol. Reprod. 12:260–274, 1975.

Brackett, B.G. and Mastroianni, L., Jr.: Composition of oviductal fluid. In: The Oviduct and Its Functions. Eds.: A.D. Johnson, C.W. Foley, Academic Press, New York, 1974, pp. 133–159.

Brown, S.M. and Hamner, C.E.: Capacitation of spermatozoa in the female reproductive tract of the rabbit during estrus and pseudopregnancy. Fertil. Steril. 22:92–97, 1971.

Chang, M.C.: Development and fate of transferred rabbit ova or blastocysts in relation to the ovulation time of recipients. J. Exp. Zool. 114:197–216, 1950.

David, A.: Chemical composition of human oviduct fluid. Fertil. Steril. 24:435–439, 1973.

David, A., Brackett, B.G., Garcia, C.-R. and Mastroianni, L., Jr.: Composition of rabbit oviduct fluid in ligated segments of the Fallopian tube. J. Reprod. Fert. 19:285–289, 1969.

Engle, C.C. and Foley, C.W.: Influence of mare uterine tubal fluids on the metabolism of stallion sperm. Amer. J. Vet. Res. 36:1149–1152, 1975.

Feigelson, M. and Kay, E.: Protein patterns of rabbit oviductal fluid. Biol. Reprod. 6:244–252, 1972.

Fox, L.L. and Shivers, C.A.: Immunologic evidence for addition of oviductal components to the hamster zona pellucida. Fertil. Steril. 26:599–608, 1975.

Go, K.J., Mastroianni, L., Jr. and Stambaugh, R.: The presence of secretory IgA specific for acrosin in rhesus monkey (*Macaca mulatta*) oviduct fluid. Fed. Proc., 37:1474, 1978. (Abstract).

Go. K.J., Mastroianni, L., Jr. and Stambaugh, R.: Antibodies from oviduct fluid which inhibit acrosin. Proc., 12th Annual Meeting. Society for the Study of Reproduction, August 1979, Quebec City. Canada (Abstract 155, p. 89A).

Hamner, C.E. and Williams, W.L.: Effect of the female reproductive tract on sperm metabolism in the rabbit and fowl. J. Reprod. Fert. 5:143–150, 1963.

Hamner, C.E. and Williams, W.L.: Identification of sperm stimulating factor of rabbit oviduct fluid. Proc. Soc. Exp. Biol. Med. 117:240–243, 1964.

Hamner, C.E. and Williams, W.L.: Composition of rabbit oviduct secretions. Fertil. Steril. 16:170–176, 1965.

Hanscom, D.R. and Oliphant, G.: Hormonal regulation of incorporation of ^{35}S into macromolecules of oviduct fluid. Biol. Reprod. 14:599–604, 1976.

Harrison, R.A.P., Cott, H.M. and Foster, G.C.: Effect of ionic strength, serum albumin and other macromolecules on the maintenance of motility and the surface of mammalian sperm in a simple medium. J. Reprod. Fert. 52:65–73, 1978.

Holmdahl, T.H. and Mastroianni, L., Jr.: Continuous collection of rabbit oviduct secretions at low temperature. Fertil. Steril. 16:587–595, 1965.

Hunter, R.H.F. and Hall, J.P.: Capacitation of boar sperm: synergism between uterine and tubal environments. J. Exp. Zool. 188:203–214, 1974.

Iritani, A.: Secretion rates and chemical composition of oviduct and uterine fluid in sows. J. Anim. Sci. 39:582–588, 1974.

Iritani, A., Gomes, W.R. and Vademark, N.L.: Secretion rates and chemical composition of oviduct and uterine fluids in ewes. Biol. Reprod. 1:72–76, 1969.

Kadi, M.S.M.Y.: Trace elements study of human fallopian tube fluid. M.D. Thesis, University of Alexandria, 1978.

Kille, J.W. and Hamner, C.E.: The influence of oviductal fluid on the development of one-cell rabbit embryos *in vitro*. J. Reprod. Fert. 35:415–423, 1973.

Lippes, J., Enders, R.G., Pragay, D.A. and Bartholomew, W.R.: The collection and analysis of human fallopian tube fluid. Contraception 5:85–103, 1972.

Lippes, J., Ogra, S., Tomasi, T.B. and Tourville, D.R.: Immunohistological localization of IgG, IgA, and IgM, secretory piece, and lactoferrin in the human female genital tract. Contraception 1:163–168, 1970.

Maas, D.H.A., Storey, B.T. and Mastroianni, L., Jr.: Oxygen tension in the oviduct of the rhesus monkey. Fertil. Steril. 27:1312–1317, 1976.

Maas, D.H.A., Storey, B.T. and Mastroianni, L., Jr.: Hydrogen ion concentration and carbon dioxide content of the oviduct fluid of the rhesus monkey. Fertil. Steril. 28:981–985, 1977.

Marcus, S.L. and Saravis, C.A.: Oviduct fluid in the rhesus monkey: A study of its protein components and its origin. Fertil. Steril. 16:785–794, 1965.

Mastroianni, L., Jr. and Jones, R.: Oxygen tension within the rabbit fallopian tube. J. Reprod. Fert. 9:99–102, 1965.

Mastroianni, L., Jr. and Stambaugh, R.: The secretory function of the primate oviduct. In: Physiology and Genetics of Reproduction, Part B. Eds.: E.M. Coutinho, F. Fuchs, Plenum Publishing Corp., New York, 1974, pp. 25–34.

Mastroianni, L., Jr., and Wallach, R.C.: Effect of ovulation and early gestation on oviduct secretions in the rabbit. Amer. J. Physiol. 200:815–818, 1961.

Mastroianni, L., Jr., Shah, U. and Abdul-Karim, R.: Prolonged volumetric collection of oviduct fluid in the rhesus monkey. Fertil. Steril. 12:417–424, 1961a.

Mastroianni, L., Jr., Urzua, M. and Stambaugh, R.: Protein patterns in monkey oviductal fluid before and after ovulation. Fertil. Steril. 21:817–820, 1970.

Mastroianni, L., Jr., Urzua, M. and Stambaugh, R.: The internal environmental fluids of the oviduct. In: The Regulation of Mammalian Reproduction. Eds.: S.J. Segal, R. Crozier, P.A. Corfman, R.G. Condliffe. Charles C. Thomas, Springfield, 1973, pp. 376–381.

Mastroianni, L., Jr., Beer, F., Shah, U. and Clewe, T.H.: Endocrine regulation of oviduct secretions in the rabbit. Endocrinology 68:92–100, 1961b.

Mastroianni, L., Jr., Urzua, M., Avalos, M. and Stambaugh, R.: Some observations on fallopian tube fluid in the monkey. Amer. J. Obstet. Gynecol. 103:703–709, 1969.

McLaughlin, C. and Hamner, C.E.: Preliminary characterization of rabbit oviduct fluid trypsin inhibitors. Biol. Reprod. 12:556–565, 1975.

Metz, C.B., Seiguer, A.C. and Castro, A.E.: Inhibition of the cumulus dispersing and hyaluronidase activities of sperm by heterologous and isologous anti-sperm antibodies. Proc. Soc. Exp. Biol. Med. 140:776–781, 1972.

Moghissi, K.S.: Human fallopian tube fluid. I. Protein composition. Fertil. Steril. 21:821–829, 1970.

Noske, I.G. and Daniel, J.C., Jr.: Changes in oviduct fluid in golden hamster. J. Reprod. Fert. 38:173–176, 1974.

Ogra, S.S., Kirton, K.T., Tomasi, T.B. and Lippes, J.: Prostaglandins in the human fallopian tube. Fertil. Steril. 25:250–255, 1974.

Oliphant, G., Randall, P. and Cabot, C.L.: Immunological components of rabbit oviduct fluid. Biol. Reprod. 16:463–469, 1977.

Overstreet, J.W. and Cooper, G.W.: Reduced sperm motility in the isthmus of the rabbit oviduct. Nature (London) 258:718–719, 1975.

Patek, E. and Hagenfeldt, K.: Trace elements in the human fallopian tube epithelium. Int. J. Fertil. 19:85–88, 1974.

Perkins, J.L.: Fluid flow of the oviduct. In: The Oviduct and Its Functions. Eds.: A.D. Johnson, C.W. Foley, Academic Press, New York, 1974, pp. 119–132.

Rebello, R., Green, F.H.Y. and Fox, H.: Study of the secretory-immune system of the female genital tract. Brit. J. Obstet. Gynaec. 82:812–816, 1975.

Restall, B.J. and Wales, R.G.: The fallopian tube of the sheep. III. The chemical composition of the fluid from the fallopian tube. Austral. J. Biol. Sci. 19:687–698, 1966.

Roberts, G.P., Parker, J.M. and Symonds, H.W.: Proteins in the luminal fluid from the bovine oviduct. J. Reprod. Fert. 45:301–313, 1975.

Roberts, G.P., Parker, J.M. and Symonds, H.W.: Macromolecular components of genital tract fluids from the sheep. J. Reprod. Fert. 48:99–107, 1976.

Rogers, B.J. and Yanagimachi, R.: Competitive effect of magnesium on the calcium-dependent acrosome reaction in guinea pig spermatozoa. Biol. Reprod. 15:614–619, 1976.

Rogers, B.J., Chang, L. and Yanagimachi, R.: Glucose effect on respiration: possible mechanism for capacitation of guinea pig spermatozoa. J. Exp. Zool. 207:107–112, 1979.

Saling, P.M., Storey, B.T. and Wolf, D.P.: Calcium-dependent binding of mouse epididymal spermatozoa to the zona pellucida. Develop. Biol. 65:515–525, 1978.

Shams, A., Rizk, M.A., Toppozada, H.K., Khowessah, M.M., Abul-Enin, M., Said, S., Habib, Y.A. and Kira, L.H.: Human tubal fluid collection via vagina and its quantitative variations during the menstrual cycle. J. Reprod. Med. 18:61–65, 1977.

Shapiro, S.S., Brown, N.E. and Yard, A.S.: Isolation of an acid glycoprotein from rabbit oviduct fluid and its association with the egg coating. J. Reprod. Fert. 40:281–290, 1974.

Shapiro, S.S., Jentsch, J.P. and Yard, A.S.: Protein composition of rabbit oviductal fluid. J. Reprod. Fert. 24:403–408, 1971.

Singh, J.P., Babcock, D.F. and Lardy, D.H.: Increased calcium-ion influx is a component of capacitation of spermatozoa. Biochem. J. 172:549–556, 1978.

Sloan, M.H. and Johnson, A.D.: The influence of a cannula in the rabbit oviduct. J. Reprod. Fert. 37:149–153, 1974.

Spilman, C.H. and Harpa, M.J.K.: Effects of prostaglandins on oviductal motility and egg transport. Gynecol. Invest. 6:186–205, 1975.

Stambaugh, R. and Buckley, J.: Identification and subcellular localization of the enzymes effecting penetration of the zona pellucida by rabbit spermatozoa. J. Reprod. Fert. 19:423–432, 1969.

Stambaugh, R. and Smith, M.: Sperm proteinase release during fertilization of rabbit ova. J. Exp. Zool. 197:121–125, 1976.

Stambaugh, R., Noriega, C. and Mastroianni, L., Jr.: Bicarbonate ion: the corona cell dispersing factor of rabbit tubal fluid. Biol. Reprod. 1:223–227, 1969.

Stambaugh, R., Seitz, H.M. and Mastroianni, L., Jr.: Acrosomal proteinase inhibitors in rhesus monkey oviduct fluid. Fertil. Steril. 25:352–357, 1974.

Stanke, D.F., Sikes, J.D., DeYoung, D.W. and Tumbleson, M.E.: Proteins and amino acids in bovine oviductal fluid. J. Reprod. Fert. 38:493–496, 1974.

Stone, S.L. and Hamner, C.E.: Hormonal and regional influences of the oviduct on the development of rabbit embryos. Biol. Reprod. 16:638–646, 1977.

Stone, S.L., Richardson, L.L., Hamner, C.E. and Oliphant, G.: Partial characterization of hormone-mediated inhibition of embryo development in rabbit oviduct fluid. Biol. Reprod. 16:647–653, 1977.

Storey, B.T.: Energy metabolism of spermatozoa. IV. Effect of calcium on respiration of mature epididymal spermatozoa of the rabbit. Biol. Reprod. 13:1–9, 1975.

Tucker, E.B. and Schultz, G.A.: Temporal changes in proteins of oviduct and uterine fluids during the preimplantation period in the rabbit. Biol. Reprod. 17:749–759, 1977.

Urzua, M.A., Stambaugh, R., Flickinger, G. and Mastroianni, L., Jr.: Uterine and oviduct fluid protein patterns in the rabbit before and after ovulation. Fertil. Steril. 21:860–865, 1970.

Vishwakarma, P.: The pH and bicarbonate-ion content of the oviduct and uterine fluids. Fertil. Steril. 13:481–485, 1962.

Wong, W.P.: Sperm antibody activity in human fallopian tube fluid. Fertil. Steril. 30:740, 1978. (Abstract)

Wu, C., Mastroianni, L., Jr. and Mikhail, G.: Steroid hormones in monkey oviduct fluid. Fertil. Steril. 28:1250–1256, 1977.

Zamboni, L., Hongsanand, H. and Mastroianni, L., Jr.: Influence of tubal secretion on rabbit tubal ova. Fertil. Steril. 16:117–184, 1965.

TUBAL SECRETION—ULTRASTRUCTURE RELATED TO ENDOCRINOLOGY

M. Mall-Haefeli, K.S. Ludwig, U.M. Spornitz, A. Uettwiler, and I. Werner-Zodrow

SUMMARY

Ultrastructural changes of the epithelium of the tubal mucosa were correlated with phases of the menstrual cycle as defined by hormonal variables.

The administration of gestagens resulted in a deviation of morphology, which was correlated with endocrine data of the same patient.

INTRODUCTION

Estrogens and progesterone are known to affect tubal function and mucosal ultrastructure. Interpretation of various findings with respect to the influence of estrogens and progesterone as reported in the literature is, however, impeded for a number of reasons:

1) It was not always clearly stated which region of the oviduct was investigated.
2) It is difficult to compare results from different mammalian species with one another.
3) The cycle phase of a patient is mostly determined on the basis of the number of days which have elapsed since the last menstruation.

Sozialmedizinischer Dienst der Frauenklinik und des Anatomischen Instituts der Universitaet Basel/Switzerland

To avoid these difficulties in this study only the ampullary region of the oviducts was examined. Light and electron microscopic examination were performed and hormonal profiles were obtained.

Available for study were 35 patients, admitted for sterilization in most instances. Daily determination of serum LH, FSH, E_2 and progesterone was done on the day of operation and one to two days preceding and following the operation. Hormonal profiles, compared to standard profiles established in our clinic (Figure 1) allowed differentiation between early and late follicular and early late luteal phases. An electron micrograph representative of the early follicular phase (Figure 2) reveals a ratio of ciliated to non-ciliated cells of 0.9:1.0 and little evidence for secretory activity. The synthetic apparatus of the cells was poorly developed and there were no secretory granules. Basal secretion as evidenced by the presence of small electron-transparent vesicles, present in both ciliated and non-ciliated cells, was minimally present.

In the late follicular phase (Figure 3) the ratio of ciliated to non-ciliated cells

FIGURE 1. Hormonal profiles. From M. Mall-Haefeli et al. (1974).

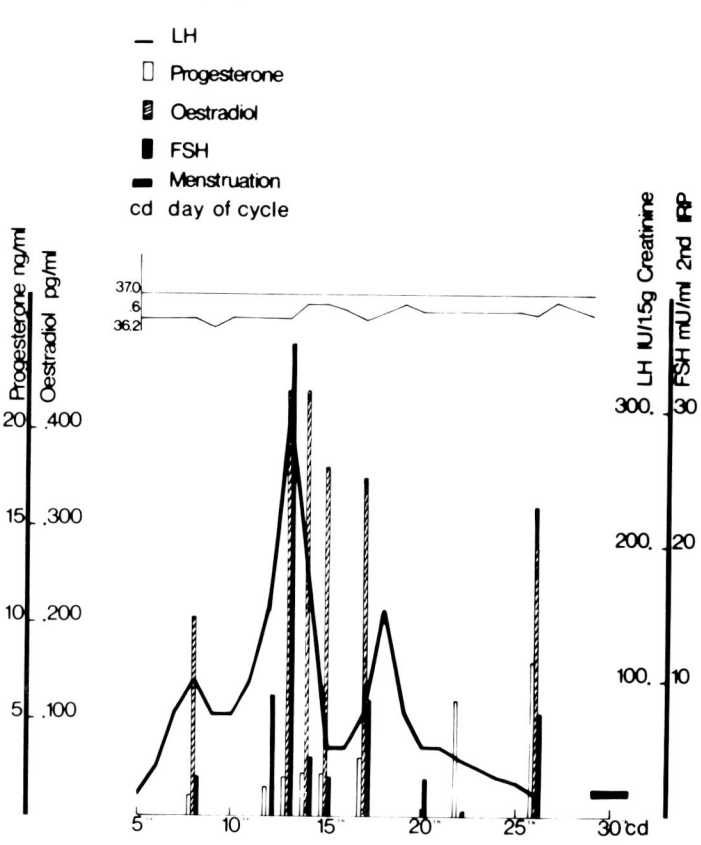

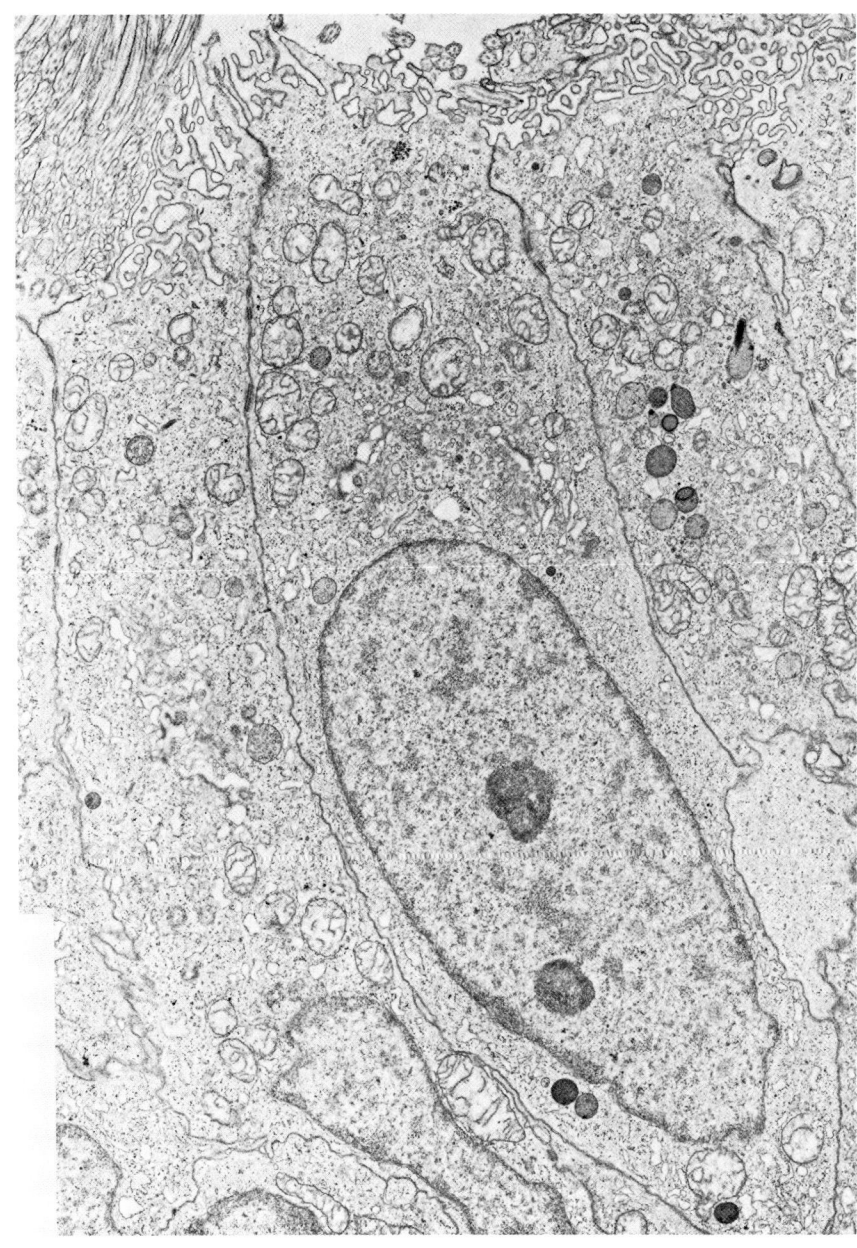

FIGURE 2. Tubal epithelium in the early follicular phase

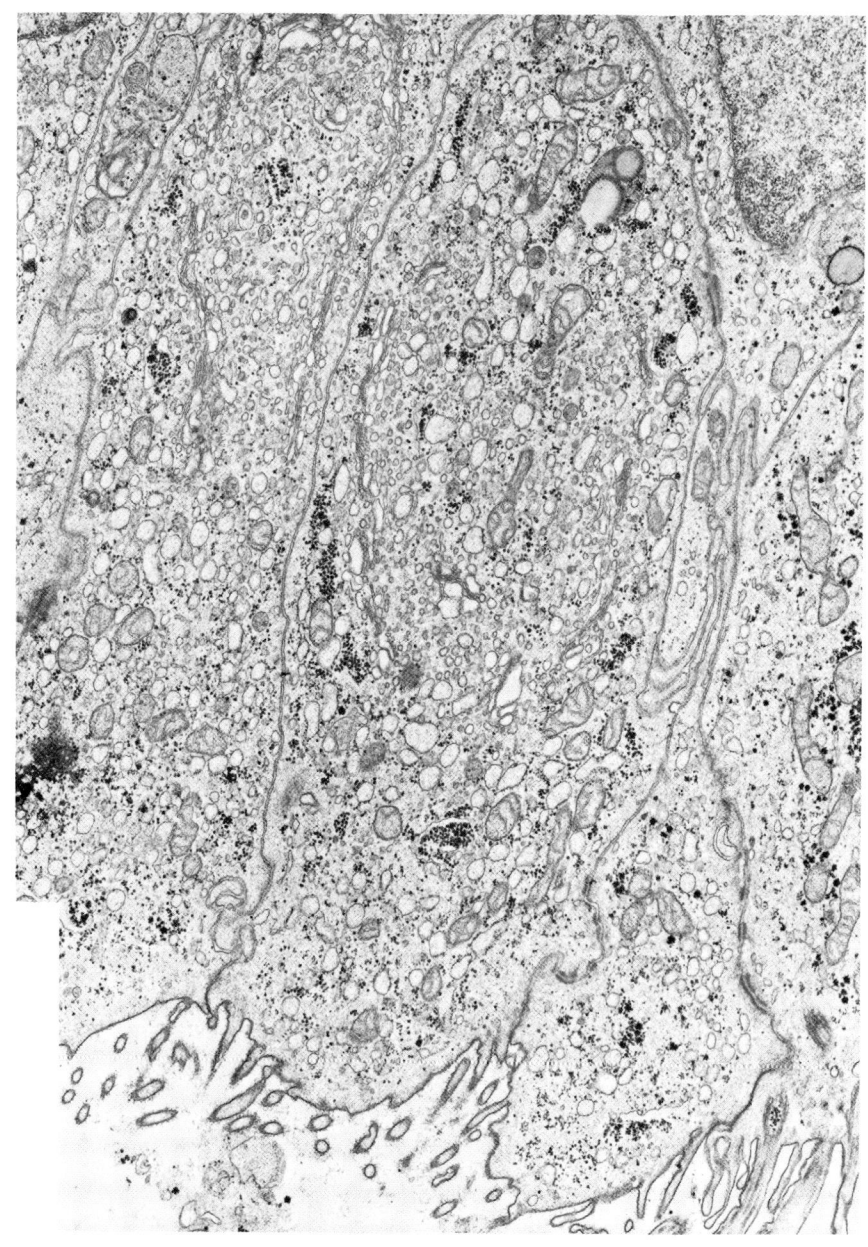

FIGURE 3. Tubal epithelium in the late follicular phase

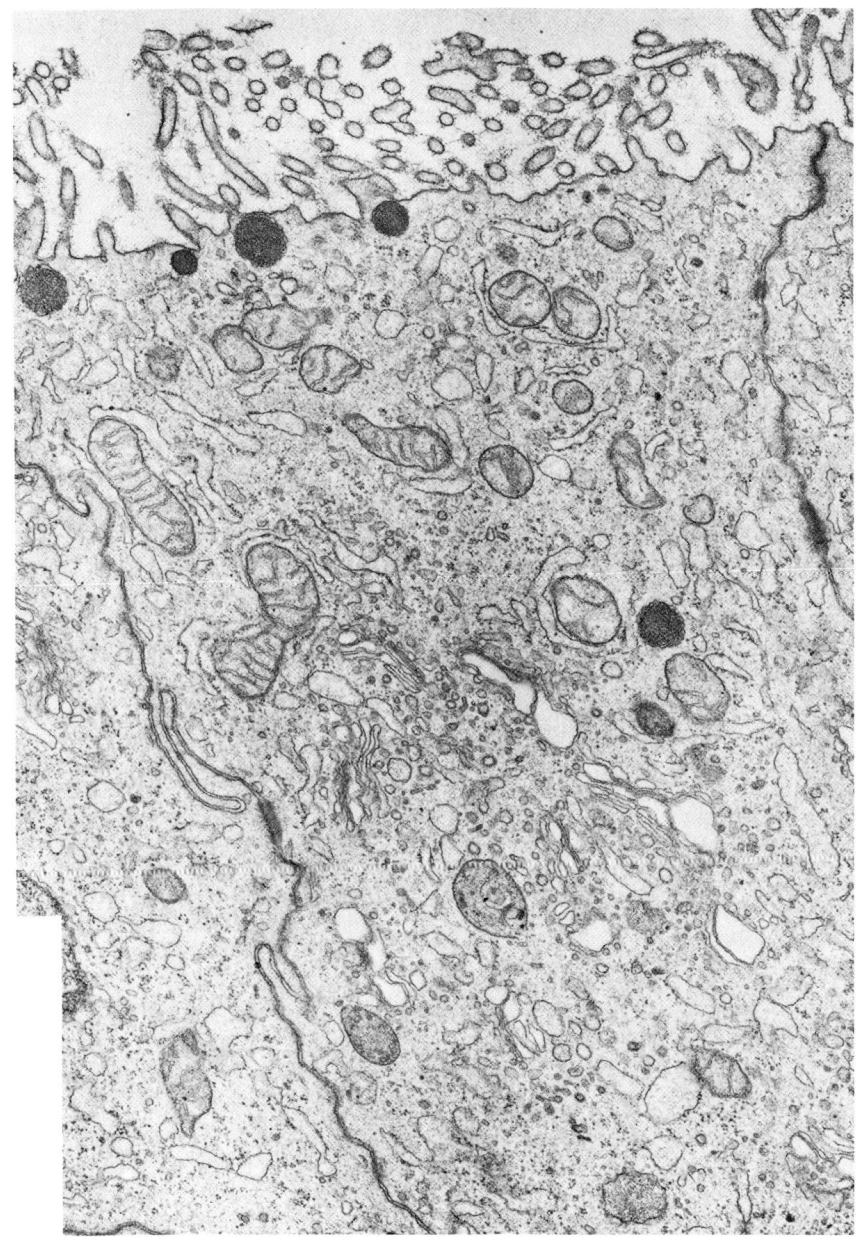

FIGURE 4. Tubal epithelium at the very early luteal phase

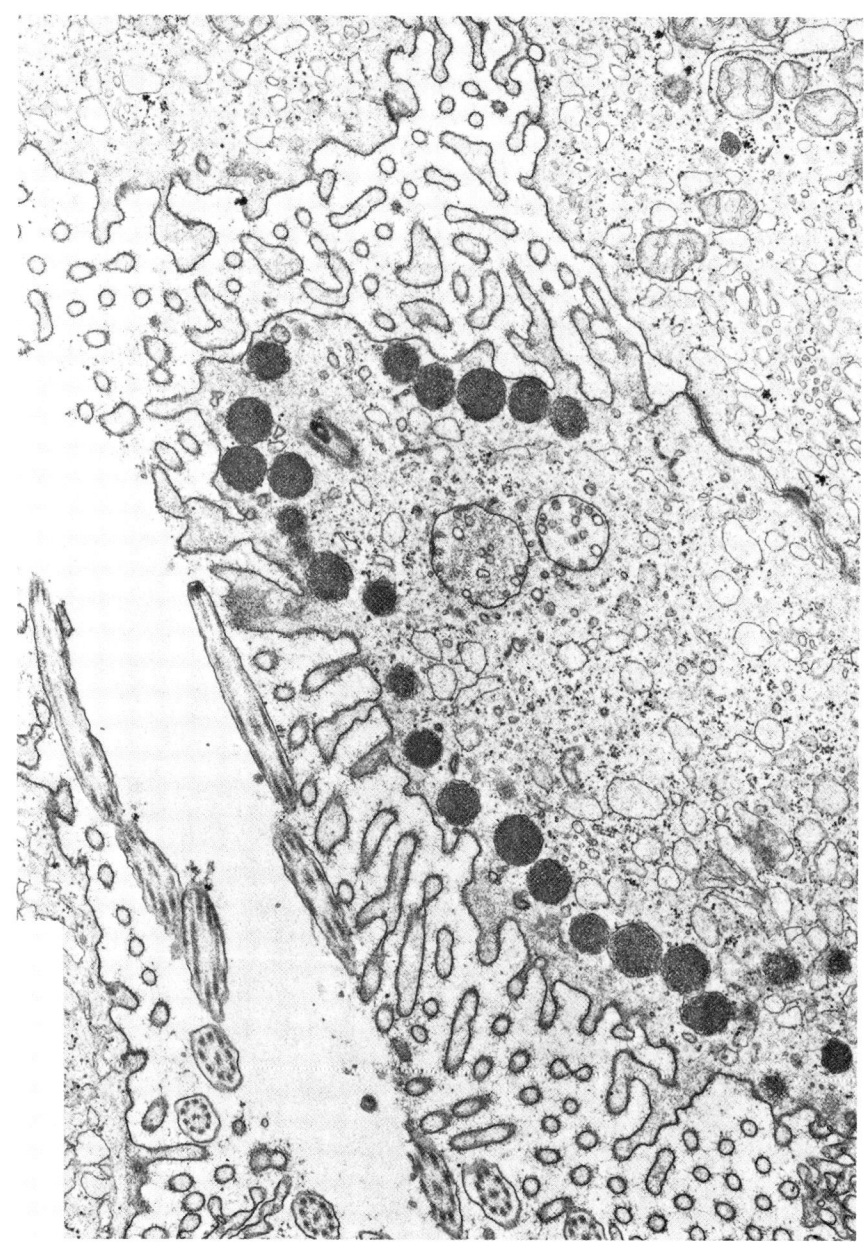

FIGURE 5. Epithelial cells at mid-luteal phase

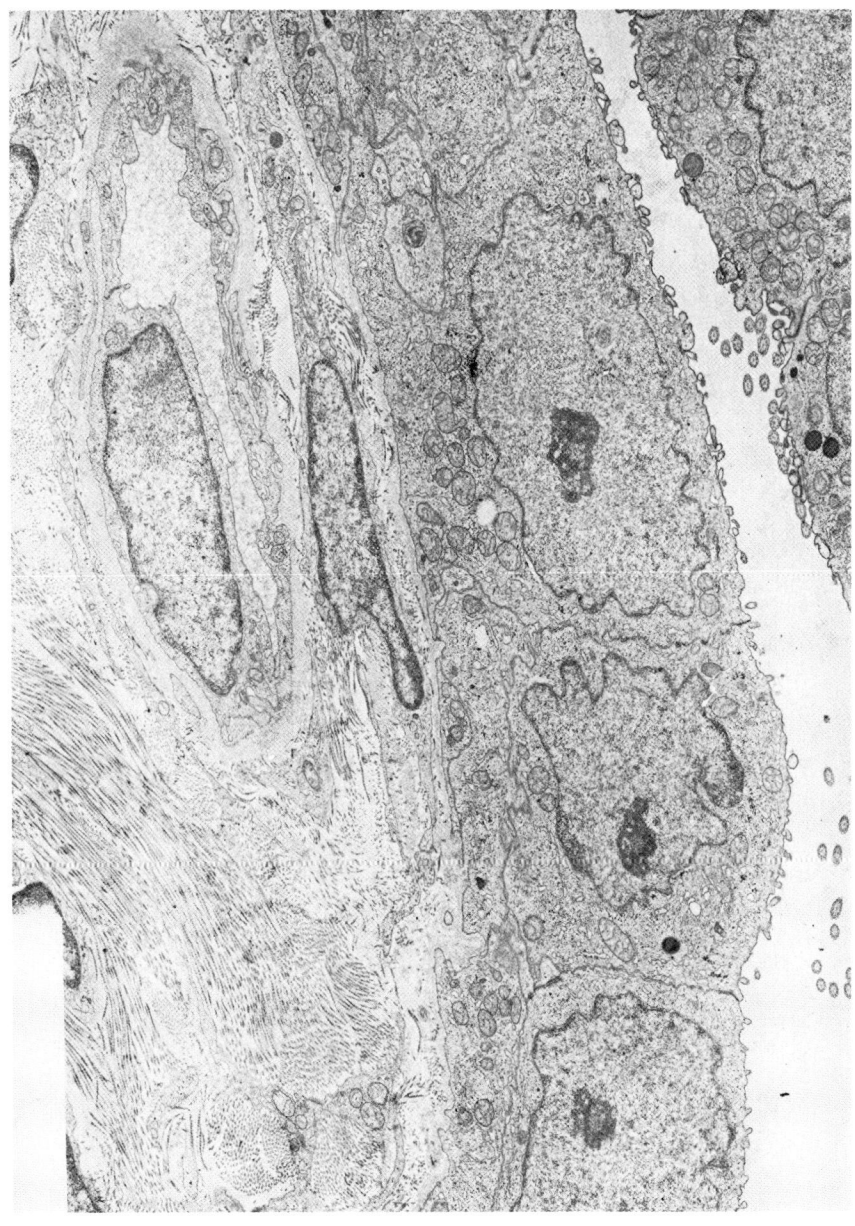

FIGURE 6. Oviduct at the menopause

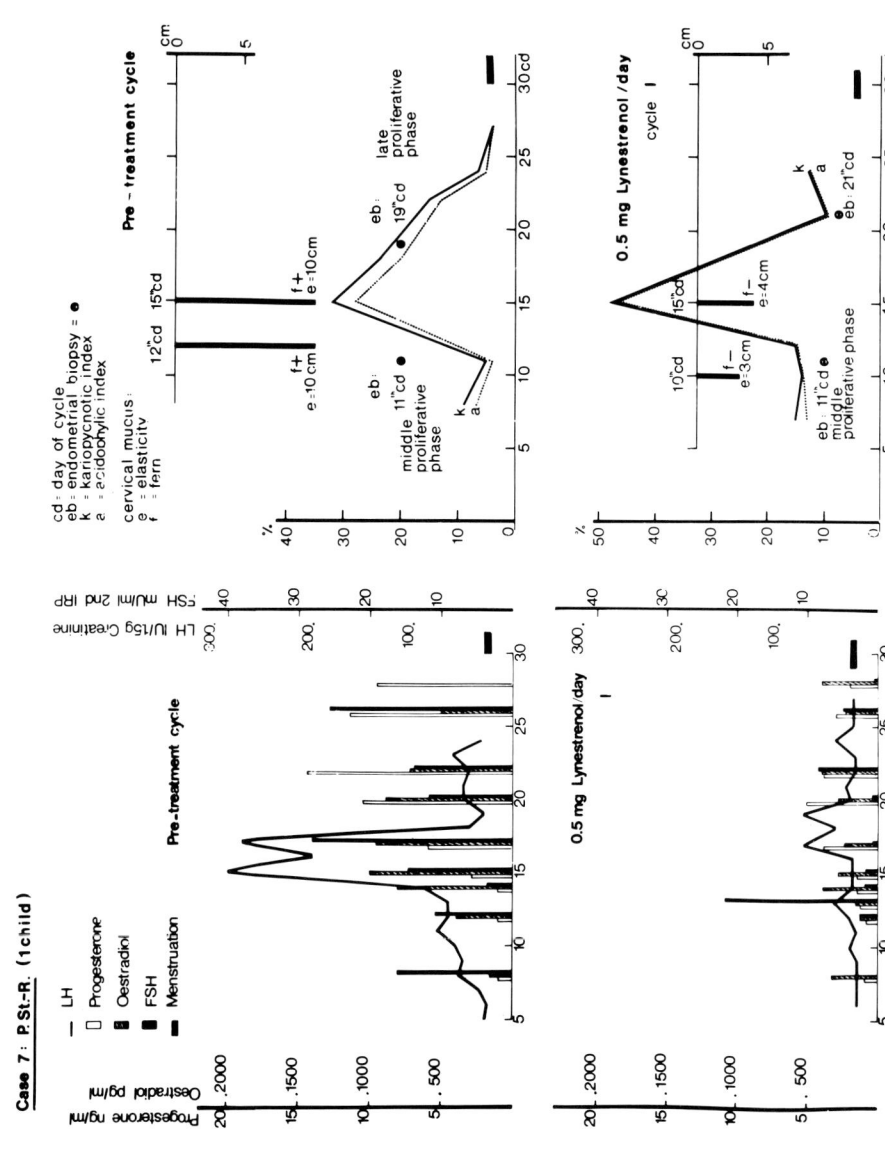

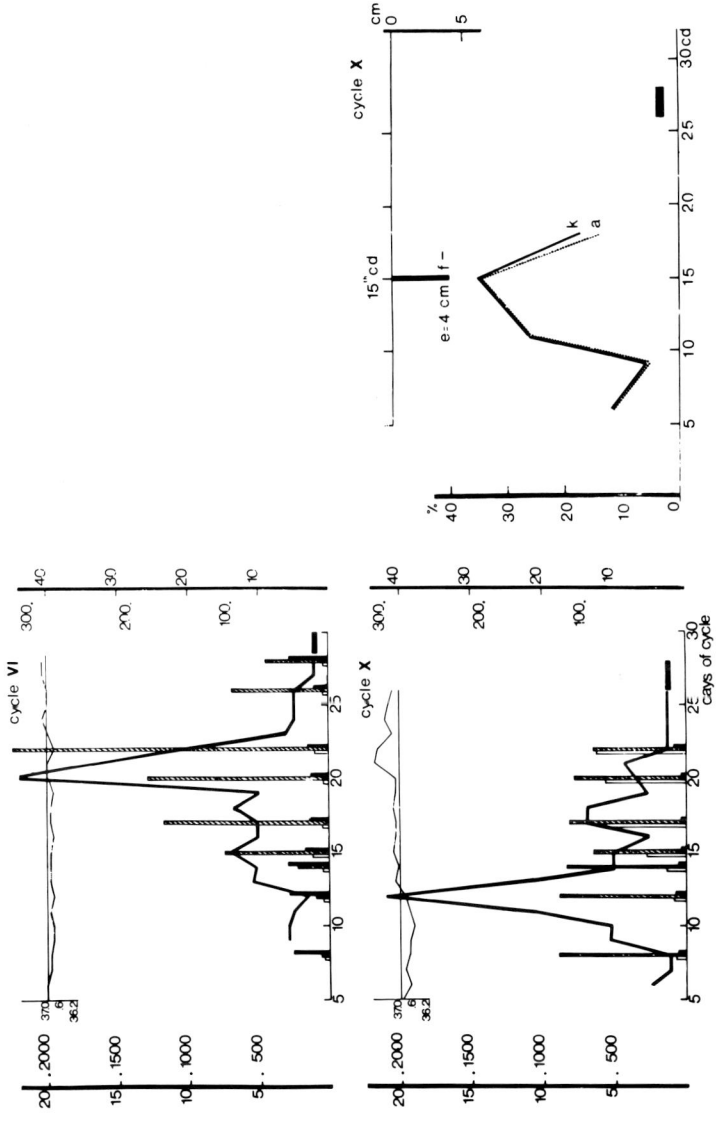

FIGURE 7. Hormonal profile of control cycle and 3 cycles under low dose progesterone therapy (minipill). From Mall-Haefeli et al. (1974)

was 1.4:1.0. The rough endoplasmic reticulum and particularly the Golgi-apparatus were very prominent reflecting a high activity of synthesis of the epithelium. There are numerous prosecretory granules in the region of the Golgi-apparatus and basal secretion was also elevated.

Tissue taken from a patient in the very early luteal phase of the cycle is depicted in Figure 4. At this time the ratio of ciliated to non-ciliated cells was 2.0:1.0. The rough endoplasmic reticulum and the Golgi apparatus were both very active. Several secretory granules of the dark type were already present. The nuclei of the non-ciliated cells were lobated which can also be taken as a sign of increased activity. The basal secretion of both cells types was elevated.

Epithelial cells taken from a patient in the mid-luteal phase of the cyle are seen in Figure 5. The ratio of ciliated to non-ciliated cells was 2:1. Numerous secretory granules of the dark type were present, indicating a very high secretory activity. The endoplasmic reticulum was relatively inactive while the Golgi-apparatus was slightly enlarged. Basal secretion in the form of small vesicles was maximal.

Oviducts taken at caesarian section revealed a wide variety of morphology. The ultrastructure of the epithelial cells reflected various phases of the cycle ranging from hyperactivity to almost complete inactivity. Thus the morphology of the epithelium at term did not correspond to a single phase of the cycle. The hormonal values of these patients revealed the expected high steroid concentrations.

The susceptibility of the oviduct to hormonal stimulation can best be documented in cases where this stimulation is missing.

The epithelium of a postmenopausal oviduct from a woman with low steroid values is shown in Figure 6. No ciliated cells were seen and the height of the epithelium was only half of that in cycling women. The overall appearance of the cells suggested a low level of activity; the Golgi-apparatus was very small and the endoplasmic reticulum was barely discernible in most cells. There appears to be, however, still a minimal basal secretion (Spornitz et al., 1977).

Treatment with a progestational agent (lynestrenol Exlutona^R) given continuously in low dose (0.5 mg per day) resulted in drastic changes in the morphology of the oviduct and in the hormonal profiles of the patients. The steroid secretion was in some patients extensively suppressed, the steroid peaks delayed or advanced with associated changes in the length of the cycle phases or in the cycle itself.

Morphologically we encountered changes which appeared to be dependent to a large extent on the duration of the treatment with lynestrenol rather than on the actual phase of the cycle. Essentially these changes take the following course:

While the synthesis of secretory products was continued for some time, the actual process of secretion appeared to be inhibited. Toward the end of the first month of treatment this led to the accumulation of secretory material within large lysosomes which were located in the apical portions of the cells. Shortly after the process of synthesis had been blocked these accumulations disappeared. At the same time a marked ciliogenetic activity started which resulted in a change of the ratio of ciliated to non-ciliated cells from the original 1:1 to about 1:3. One of the huge lysosomes resulting from this inhibition of the discharge of secretory products from the cells is seen in Figure 8. The beginning of ciliogenesis on the luminal surface of the cells is obvious.

During the first 10 to 12 months of treatment with Exlutona the synthesis

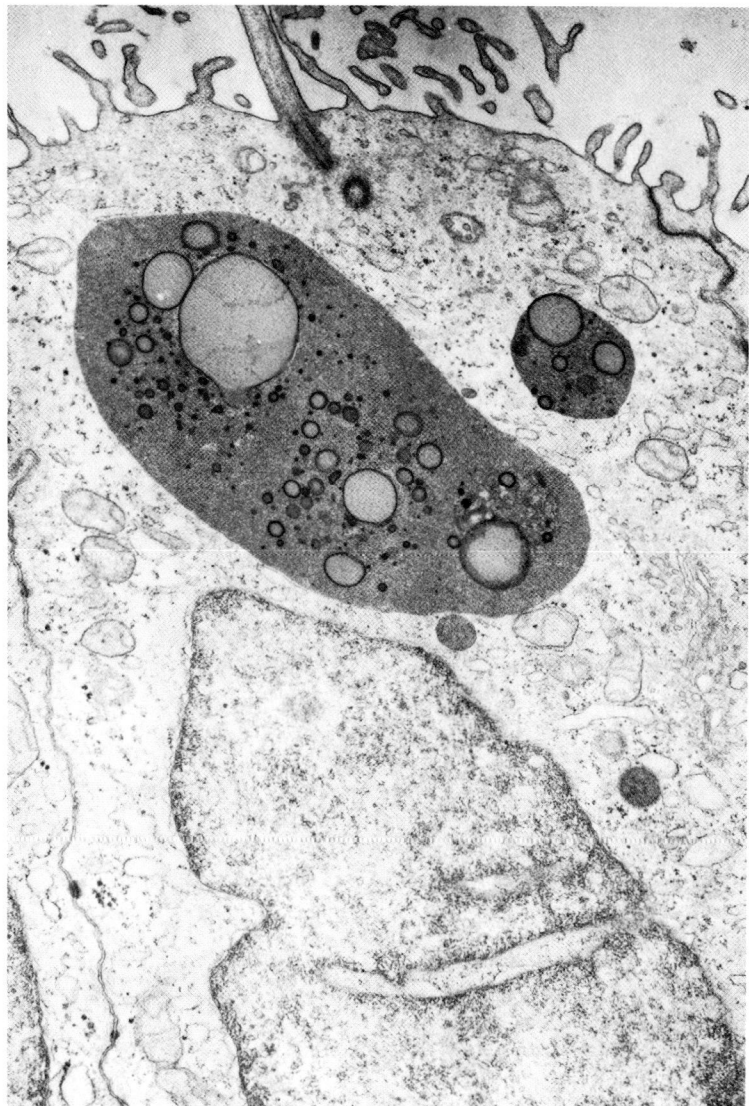

FIGURE 8. Electronmicroscopy under application of low dose progesterone

and the secretory activity of the non-ciliated cells seemed to be almost completely suppressed. After prolonged treatment there was a moderate recovery of the secretory activity.

The hormonal pattern of cycles from women carrying a Progestasert IUD are given in Figures 9 and 10. Under the progesterone IUD the first postinsertion cycle was almost invariably normal, from the fourth month on, however, about half

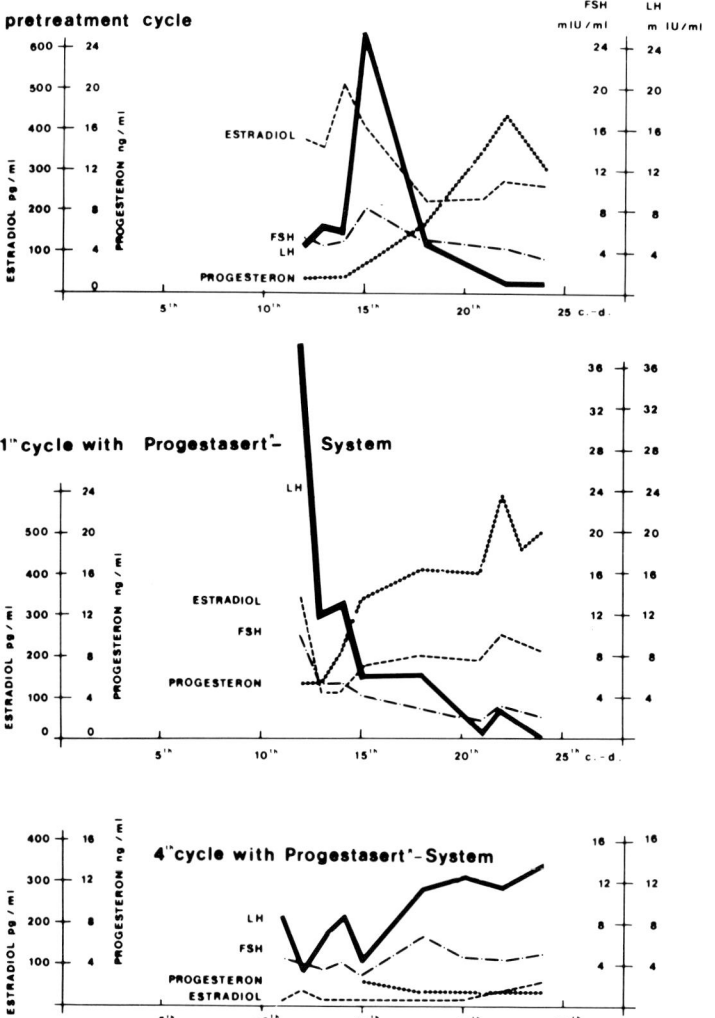

FIGURE 9. Hormonal profile before and during application of the minipill. From Mall-Haefeli et al. 1977

HORMONE-PROFILE WITH PROGESTASERT^R-SYSTEM

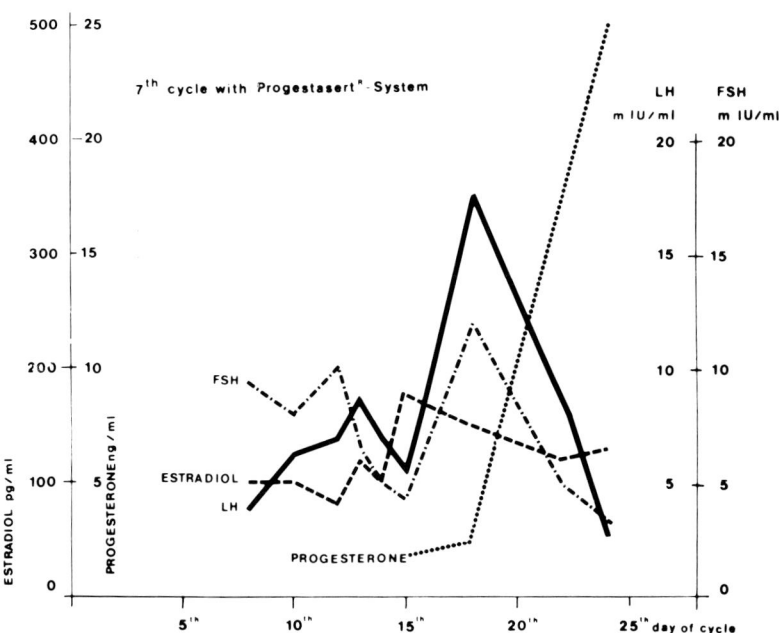

FIGURE 10. Hormonal profile during the 7th cycle under the minipill

of the cycles were anovulatory and showed the lowered steroid values characteristic for this condition.

From the morphological point of view the tubal epithelium appeared to be unaltered under the Progestasert IUD in large areas. The ratio of ciliated to non-ciliated cells, however, remained at about 1.0:1.0 throughout the cycle.

A cell which contains an excessive number of secretory granules is demonstrated in Figure 11. This response was typical for some cells under the progesterone IUD. In certain areas both the ciliated and non-ciliated cells contained large numbers of lysosomes comparable to those found during the first trimester of pregnancy. There were numerous granules present immediately beneath the plasma membrane.

In conclusion we consider knowledge of the hormonal profile a prerequisite for interpretation of any morphologic changes associated with specific phases of the cycle. Particularly under experimental conditions that are capable of inducing alterations in the hormonal status, like the administration of progesterone or other steroids; a careful determination of the actual phase of the cycle seems therefore to be necessary.

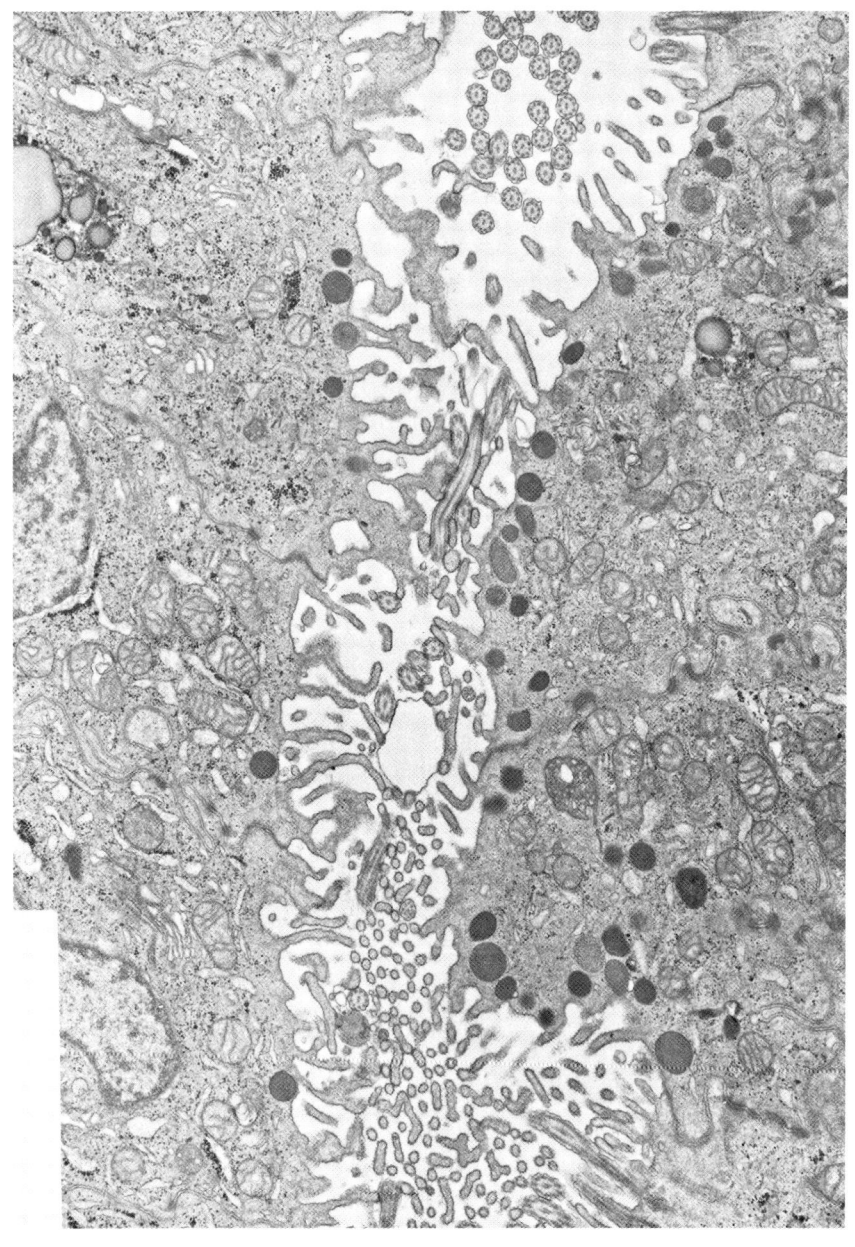

FIGURE 11. Ultrastructure of a Fallopian tube under treatment with progesterone

REFERENCES

Mall-Haefeli, M., Ludwig, K.S., Uettwiller, A., The Mechanism of Low Dose Progestogen Therapy Clinical Trials Journal 1974, 11, No. 2, 93–109.

Mall-Haefeli M., Der gegenwärtige Stand der Intrauterin-Pessare Das Progestasertsystem Geburtshilfl.-gynäk. Praxis II. Internationales Münsteraner Gespräch über geburtshilflich-gynäk. Praxis. Veranstaltet von der Frauenklinik der Westfälischen Wilhelms-Universität, Münster, 1976 Hrsg. von F.K. Beller und H. D. Böttcher Georg Thieme Verlag Stuttgard 1977.

Mall-Haefeli et al., Endokrinologische und histologische Untersuchungen zur Tubenphysiologie, In: Gynäkologie und Geburtshilfe, Hrsg. H. Husslein Verlag H. Egermann, Wien, 1977.

Spornitz et al., Morphologic alterations in the eptithelium of the human oviduct induced by a low dosis gestagen. Arch. Gynäk. 223:269–281, 1977.

Copyright 1979 by Elsevier North Holland, Inc.
F.K. Beller and G.F.B. Schumacher, eds.
The Biology of the Fluids of the Female Genital Tract

ULTRASTRUCTURAL CHANGES IN THE HUMAN OVIDUCT EPITHELIUM DURING THE PUERPERIUM AND LACTATION

C. Oberti,* J. Zanartu,** G. Vasquez,* I. Brosens,* and B. Robertson†

SUMMARY

The human oviduct undergoes marked changes during the puerperium and lactation. At the end of pregnancy the thickness of the epithelium and the percentage of ciliated cells are both reduced and, if amenorrhoea persists, there is a further decrease in the percentage of ciliated cells. With the resumption of ovarian activity a new type of cell, the villous cell, can be identified. The villous cell, which may derive from a resting deciliated cell, would appear to be the immediate precursor of the ciliated cell and to be responsible for the consequent increase in thickness of the mucosa. Further studies of the mechanism of ciliogenesis in the human oviduct would be of value in the investigation of cases of infertility related to tubal defects and in contraceptive technology.

Dr. Brosens was unable to present this paper. The editors believe that the content is sufficiently important to be included in the transcript.

  * The Unit for the Study of Human Reproduction, Department of Obstetrics and Gynecology, Katholieke Universiteit, Leuven, Belgium.
 ** Department of Obstetrics and Gynecology, University of Chile, Santiago, Chile.
  † Department of Histopathology, St. Georges Hospital Medical School, London, England.

INTRODUCTION

Light and electron microscopy studies of the human oviduct have shown changes to occur in the epithelium during the menstrual cycle and during and after pregnancy. In the puerperium the height of the epithelium is only about 12 microns (Andrews, 1951) and the proportion of ciliated cells is much lower than in the oviduct of the normal non-pregnant woman. The observations that administration of estrogens to castrated monkeys (Brenner, 1967 a & b; Brenner and Anderson, 1973) can induce ciliogenesis and that stilbestrol given to women post partum (Andrews, 1951) increases the number of ciliated cells in the oviducts have led to the assumption that estrogens are largely responsible for the growth of ciliated cells in the female genital tract; the assumption is supported by the fact that progestogens (Andrews, 1951), potent anti-estrogens, inhibit the estrogenic effect on tubal epithelium. The mechanism of ciliogenesis in the oviduct, however, is not understood.

Halbert and his collaborators (1976) have demonstrated experimentally the important role of the ciliated cells in ovum transport while Odor and Blandau (1973) have shown that, in the rabbit, effective transport of the ovum over the fimbrial surface and in the ampullary segment is maintained only in the presence of more than 60 per cent ciliated cells.

This study is concerned primarily with the changes in the epithelium of the human oviduct post partum in women who were lactating.

MATERIALS AND METHODS

The material comprises biopsies taken from 18 women at the time of tubal sterilization in the following circumstances:

Controls

Six young, fertile women requesting sterilization had biopsies taken at midcycle.

Group 1.
Four women had biopsies taken either at the time of caesarean section or during the week following delivery while being sterilized.

Group 2.
Six women with post partum amenorrhoea who were lactating had biopsies taken at the time of sterilization three to four months after delivery.

Group 3.
Two women who were lactating but each had had one menstruation and had biopsies taken four months after delivery at the time of sterilization.

The women in the control group and in groups 2 and 3 were sterilized at the Department of Obstetrics and Gynecology, University of Chile. In these cases salpingectomy was performed and mucosal biopsies were selected immediately under the stereomicroscope from the ampullary and infundibular parts of the oviduct and fixed in a mixture of acrolein, paraformaldehyde and glutaraldehyde. The women in group 1 were sterilized at the Department of Obstetrics and Gynecology, Katholieke Universiteit Leuven; a small mucosal biopsy from the infundibulum in each case was fixed in glutaraldehyde.

All biopsies were subsequently post-fixed in osmic acid and embedded in Epon. Selected semi-thin sections were stained with iron haematoxylin to demonstrate cytoplasmic organelles such as mitochondria and centrosomes. Toluidine blue and methylene blue were used also as general staining methods to select areas of blocks for ultramicrotomy. Ultrathin sections were cut on an LKB ultramicrotome and examined in the Zeiss EM9-2S electronmicroscope.

Stained semithin sections were used to measure and count the various types of oviduct epithelial cells (see below) and percentages of each type were calculated on the basis of counts of 500 cells in each case. The mean height of the mucosa was calculated from random measurements on semi-thin sections using a calibrated eye-piece.

OVIDUCT EPITHELIUM

In order that accurate, reproducible counting could be achieved it was necessary to define, as precisely as present knowledge permits, the different types of cell in the mucosa. The two principal types universally recognized are ciliated and non-ciliated cells. The majority of the latter are considered to be secretory cells but a minority have been called the "peg" or intercalated cells ((Stiftchenzellen in the German literature).

Recently, Oberti and Gomez-Rogers (1972) have described another type of non-ciliated cell which they call the villous cell. Although all non-ciliated cells possess surface microvilli of variable number and height, usually undetectable on light microscopy, the villous cell possesses abundant, long surface villi imparting to the cell a distinct brush border easily seen in semithin sections. The controversial basal or reserve cells (Odor, 1974), sometimes equated with the "peg" cells were few in number. They comprise about 5 per cent of the total cells of tubal epithelium (Van Bogaert et al., 1978) and, being basal or parabasal, could be ignored in the morphometric part of this study. Thus only the ciliated, secretory and villous cells forming the bulk of the mucosa were counted.

RESULTS

Light Microscopy

The data on the height of the epithelium and on the percentages of ciliated, secretory and villous cells in each of the 4 groups are collated in Table I.

In the control group, women with normal menstrual cycles, the mean height of the tubal epithelium in mid-cycles was 24.7 microns and the surface epithelium was composed of 61 per cent ciliated and 39 per cent secretory cells but no villous cells (Figure 1). In contrast the parturient women in group 1 had tubal epithelium only 11.3 microns in height, 33.7 per cent of the cells being ciliated and 66.3 per cent secretory, again with no villous cells. The women in group 2, lactating for three to four months with amenorrhoea, also had low epithelium at 9.5 microns and even less ciliated cells at 11.0 per cent with more secretory cells at 89.0 per cent and no villous cells (Figure 2).

A difference from group 2 is noted in group 3, lactating women who, how-

TABLE I. Height of Oviductal Epithelium and Percentages of Ciliated Secretory and Villous Cells in Normal Cycles and During Post Partum and Lactation

	Number of cases	Height of epithelium (microns)	Ciliated cells (%)	Secretory cells (%)	Villous cells (%)
CONTROL GROUP Normal midcycle	6	24.7 (± 0.9)*	61.0 (± 6.1)	39.0 (± 6.0)	0
GROUP 1 Immediate post partum	4	11.3 (± 0.8)	33.7 (± 11.4)	66.3 (± 11.4)	0
GROUP 2 Post partum and lactation (3-4 months)	6	9.5 (± 1.3)	11.0 (± 1.4)	89.0 (± 1.4)	0
GROUP 3 First post partum menstrual cycle	2	19.1 (± 0.6)	17.7 (± 0.9)	76.8 (± 3.0)	5.5 (± 2.3)

* Standard deviation in brackets

ever, had had each one menstruation. Here the epithelium is higher at 19.1 microns with 17.7 per cent ciliated cells, 76.8 per cent secretory cells and 5.5 per cent villous cells (Figure 3). The difference for epithelial height and percentages of ciliated cells between the control group and groups 1 and 2 are statistically highly significant ($P < 0.001$).

From the light microscopy studies it was apparent that the increase in mean height of the oviduct epithelium in lactating women who had menstruated (group 3) was due to the appearance of the villous cells, which imparted a degree of pseudostratification to the mucosa, coupled with an increased percentage of ciliated cells. At the light microscope level the villous cells are larger than the other cells with a round, lightly stained nucleus and translucent cytoplasm. Many such cells are seen in the parabasal region of the mucosa, at which stage they look relatively undifferentiated, but with the acquisition of cytoplasmic organelles and the development of luminal microvilli they then appear to surface between neighbouring cells (Figure 4). These cells were found at intervals in the mucosa at the bottom, sides and top of the plicae of the fimbriae and ampullary segments of the oviducts.

Ultrastructure

Electronmicroscopy, particularly on the material from group 3, was used to characterize better the cell types of the mucosa and to provide evidence for the histogenesis of the villous cell and for the mechanism of ciliogenesis. In a typical villous cell the surface villi are seen to be much longer than the somewhat stunted, irregular microvilli of neighbouring secretory cells; the nucleus is round with finely dispersed chromatin and basally situated. In the supranuclear zone there are numerous centrosomes in various stages of development associated with abundant large mitochondria (Figure 5).

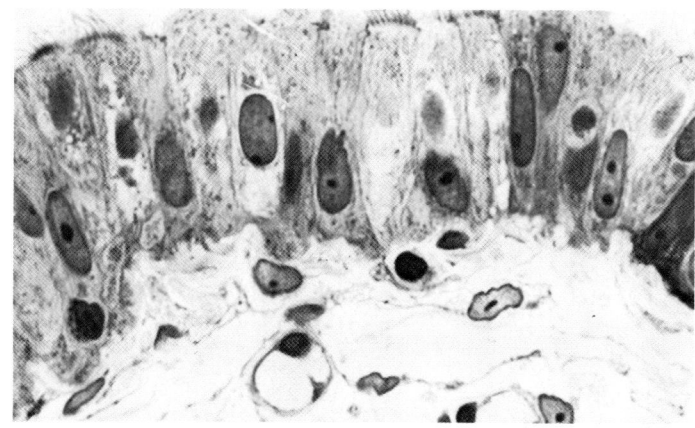

FIGURE 1. Human tubal mucosa from the fimbrial region at mid-cycle. Columnar epithelium with ciliated and secretory cells. Height of mucosa 25 microns. Toluidine blue x 1,000.

FIGURE 2. Fimbrial epithelium during 4th month of post partum lactation with amenorrhoea. Cuboidal epithelium of light and dark cells. Height of mucosa 9.5 microns. Toluidine blue x 1,000.

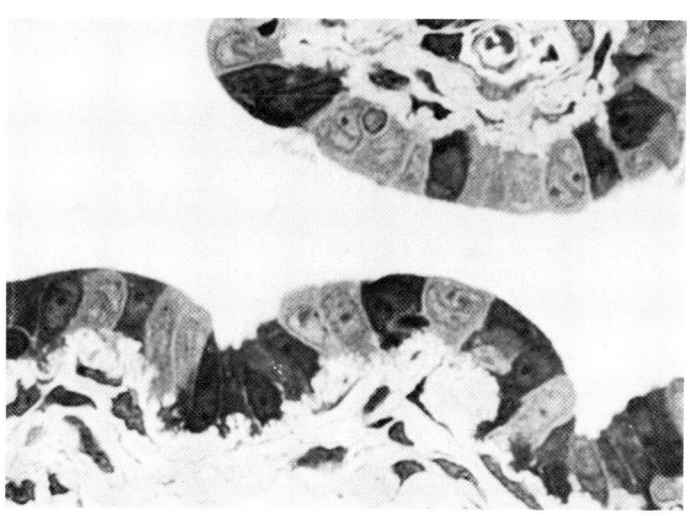

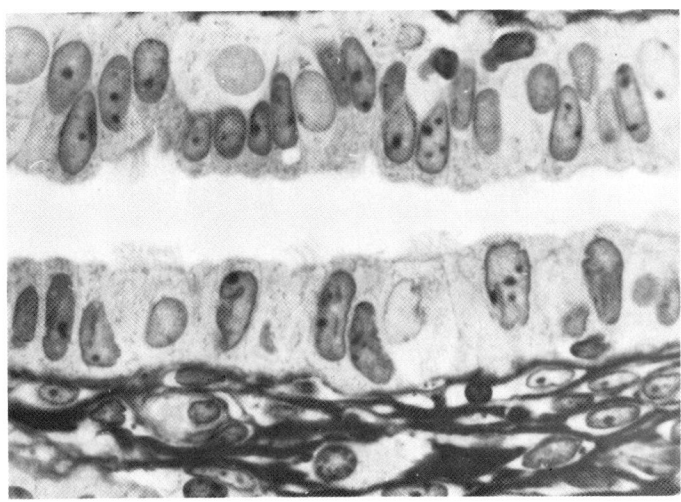

FIGURE 3. Fimbrial mucosa during 4th post partum month but post menstruation showing increase in numbers of ciliated cells. Height of mucosa 19 microns. Ferric-hematoxylin x 1,000.

FIGURE 4. Mucosa adjacent to Fig. 3. Villous cell (arrow) surfacing between two secretory cells. Developing villous cell (V) in the parabasal position. Stromal collagen darkly stained. Ferric-hematoxylin x 1,000.

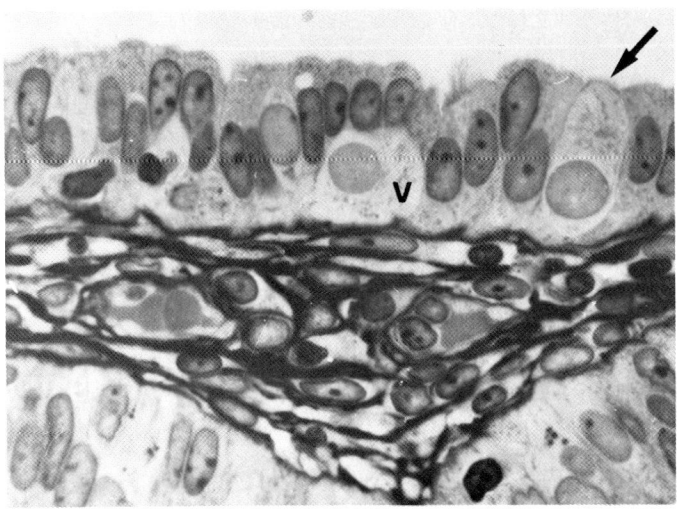

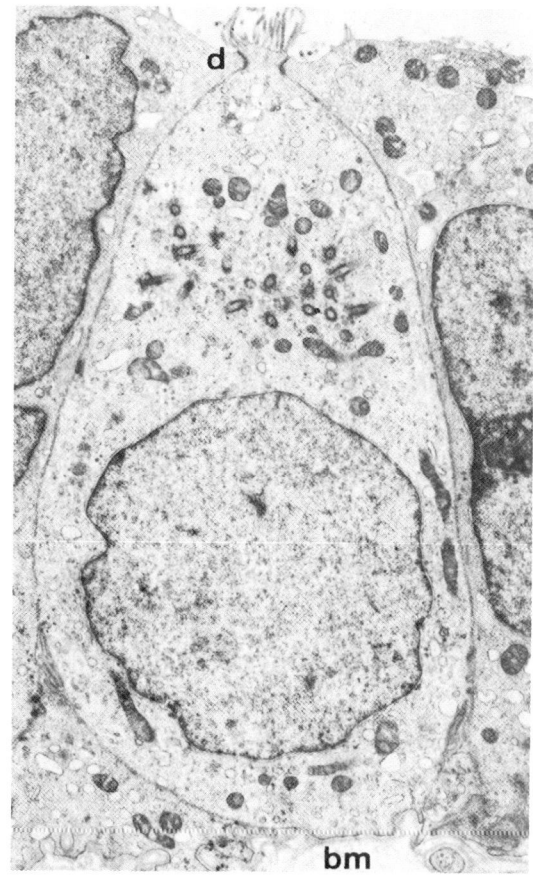

FIGURE 5. Villous cell in the ampulla. Long surface microvilli forming brush border. Apical aggregation of centrosomes with surrounding mitochondria. Cell junctions (d) and convoluted basement membrane (bm). Electronmicrograph (Em) × 11,000.

In their early stage of development the centrosomes consist of aggregates of granular material and microfilaments which come to be arranged in centriolar configuration into a ring of nine triplet microtubules (Figure 6). In the more differentiated cell the centrioles are seen to be near the cell surface beneath the origin of the villi and aligned as basal bodies. At this stage the cell is partly villous and partly ciliated (Figure 7). Random sections occasionally showed a composite picture (Figure 8) of basal, para-basal and surface cells encompassing most of the cell types encountered in the tubal mucosa. Neither by light microscopy nor by electronmicroscopy were mitoses seen in any cell.

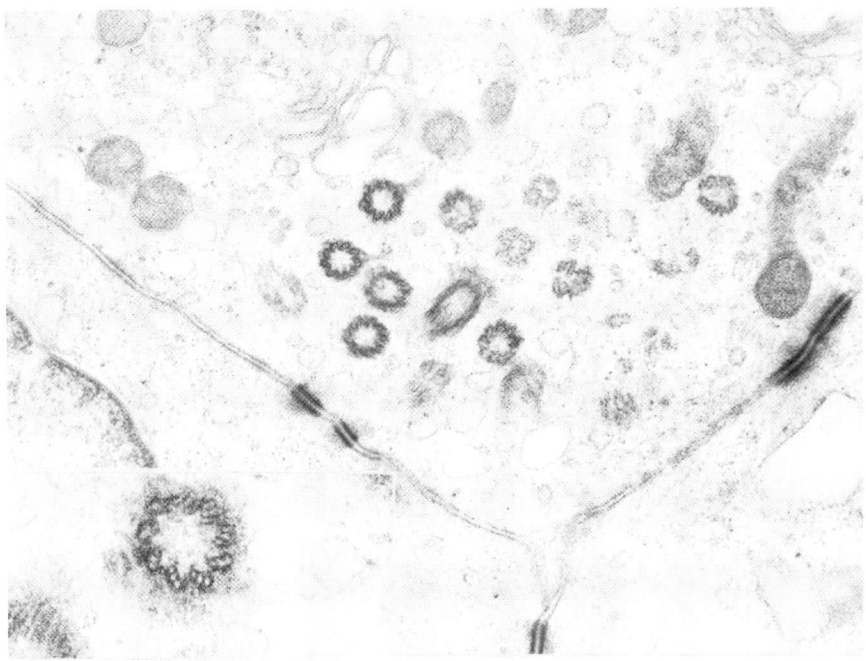

FIGURE 6. Villous cell showing various stages of centriolar development. Desmosomes connecting adjacent cells. Inset gives the detail of the ring of nine triplet microtubules. Em x 30,000

DISCUSSION

Holtzbach (1908) was the first to describe cyclical changes in human tubal epithelium during the menstrual cycle and more detail was added by Novak and Everett (1928). Snyder (1924) in his study included a description of the human tubal epithelium in late pregnancy. Recent studies (Clyman, 1966; Vasquez and Brosens, 1976) however, indicate that there is little, if any, change in the percentage of ciliated cells in the human oviduct throughout the menstrual cycle in contrast to the sequence of events in the endometrium (More and Masterton, 1975). It is known (Seki et al., 1978) that there is marked deciliation of the tubal epithelium in the post-menopausal woman, presumably due to cessation of ovarian estrogenic stimulation. Our study, like that of others, shows that the tubal epithelium immediately post partum is low and the percentage of ciliated cells is markedly reduced when compared with the oviduct of the normal non-pregnant woman. With prolonged post partum amenorrhoea associated with lactation of the epithelium is even lower and the percentage of ciliated cells further reduced but as soon as ovarian function is resumed, as indicated by menstruation, the mucosa increases in height and the percentage of ciliated cells rises, both phenomena being associated with the appearance of villous cells. This recently described cell (Oberti and Gomez-Rogers, 1972) in the human oviduct would appear to have much in common with the "clear cell" associated with ciliogenesis in the human endome-

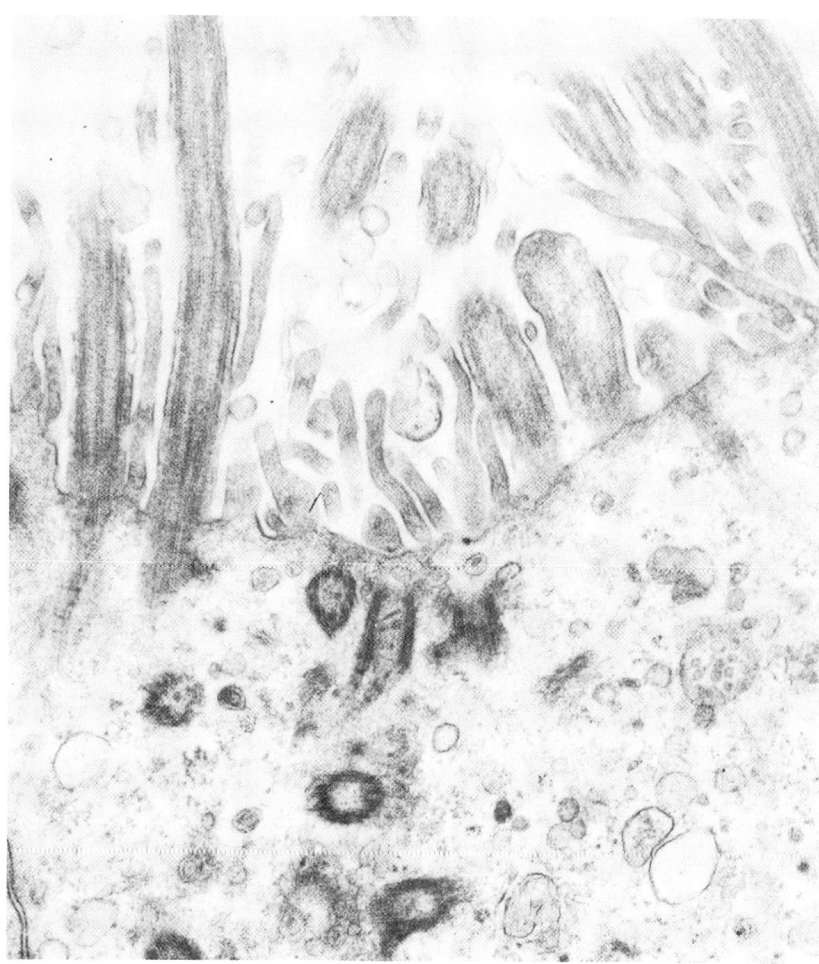

FIGURE 7. Differentiating villous cell with a mixture of surface villi and cilia. The centrioles are near the apex of the cell, some aligned as basal bodies. Em x 30,000.

trium (More and Masterton, 1975) and the "light cell" subserving a similar function in the oviduct of the rhesus monkey (Brenner, 1969). A characteristic feature of these three cell types is the development of supranuclear or apical structures resembling centrioles associated with numerous mitochondria and the development of long surface villi. The concomitant appearance of similar cells with a mixture of villi and cilia and associated basal bodies and centrioles is strong evidence, if short of proof, that the villous cell is a precursor of the ciliated cell.

The origin of the villous cell in the human oviduct must, for the moment, remain conjectural. Many have assumed that either the intercalated cells or the basal cells act as "reserve" cells to refurbish the tubal mucosa but, since cell turnover in the epithelium of the oviduct in the normal fertile woman would appear to be

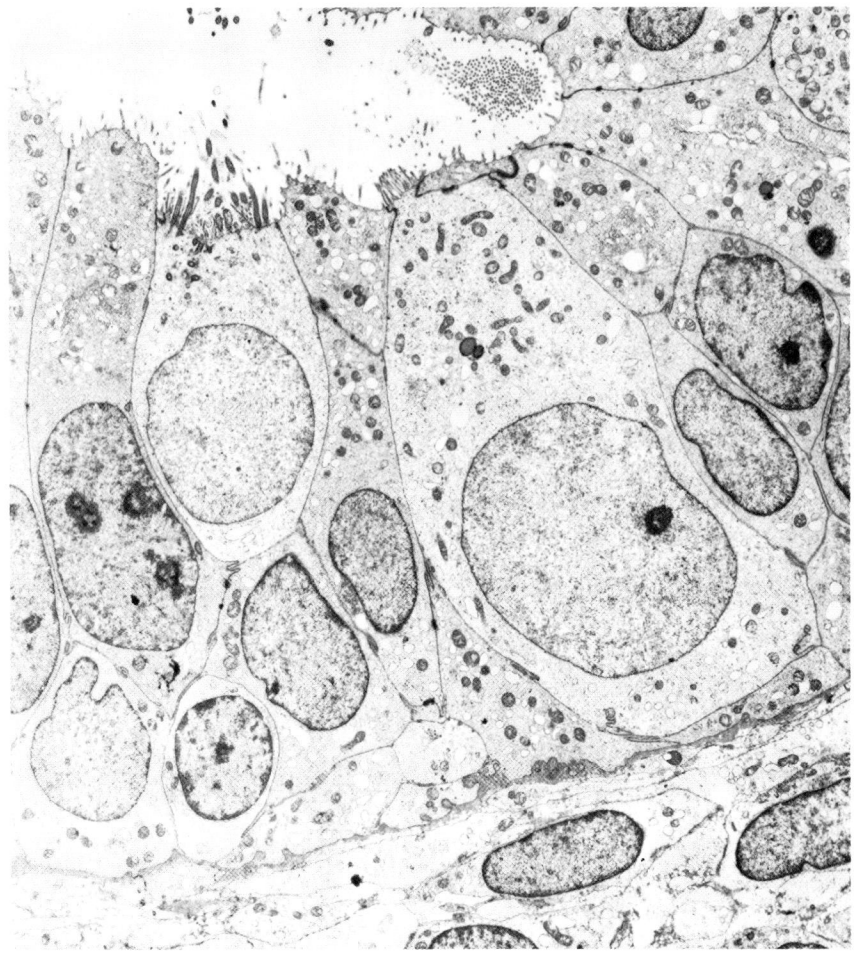

FIGURE 8. Human tubal mucosa: post partum lactation but post menstruation. Pseudostratification with a mixture of basal, parabasal and surface cells including differentiating villous cells, a partially ciliated cell and secretory cells. Em x 11,000.

very low, the evidence that such cells develop into ciliated and non-ciliated cells is, to say the least, unconvincing. Odor (1974) has challenged the whole concept of a basal, reserve cell in the endocervix and oviduct. Basing her arguments on ultrastructural evidence from the rabbit cervix and oviduct in experimental conditions, she concludes that such cells are lymphocytes which have migrated into these mucosae. Estrogen administered to castrated animals was followed by mitotic activity in mature secretory cells, but not in ciliated cells, of the tubal mucosa. The finding of lymphocytes in the basal layer of rabbit secretory mucosae, a well recognized feature of human mucosae, is probably irrelevant to the argument other than to exclude such cells as precursors of secretory or ciliated cells. It cannot be concluded from Odor's work that regenerative changes in human tubal mucosa are identical with, or even analogous to, those of the rabbit oviduct.

The oviduct in the post menopausal era is deciliated but reciliation will occur only if an Estrogenic stimulus is provided and amenorrhoea, apart from pregnancy, implies pathology of one form or another. The morphologic findings of our study certainly indicate a progenitor of the oviduct ciliated cell but if the existence of a reserve cell is to be denied and cell turnover is low then the only explanation remaining for the phenomenon of reciliation of the mucosa is that when a cell is deciliated it is not shed but enters a refractory or resting phase (Seki et al., 1978) in the parabasal position until there is sufficient Estrogenic stimulation to reactivate ciliogenesis. The low plasma oestriols and deciliated tubal mucosa of the lactating parturient woman and the increase in ciliated cells consequent upon resumption of the ovarian activity are in keeping with this hypothesis.

Our observations give strong support to the widely held view that estrogens are the key promoters of ciliogenesis in the female genital tract, a view that is based, amongst other things, on studies of the human endometrium (More and Masterton, 1975), of the human oviduct in the proliferative phase of the menstrual cycle (Oberti and Gomez-Rogers, 1972) and on experimental studies in castrated female monkeys given estrogen replacement therapy (Brenner, 1967 a).

Women who lactate following parturition are subfertile which is attributable, at least in part, to the marked reduction in the percentage of ciliated cells in the oviducts, particularly in view of the observation (Halbert et al., 1976) that, even when the muscularis of the oviduct is paralyzed by isoproteronol, ovum transport is unimpaired provided the percentage of ciliated cells remains optimal. Another factor may be the increased percentage of non-ciliated cells many of which are probably not true secretory cells, but as we have suggested, resting deciliated cells. Although we did not attempt to assess the secretory activity of the mucosa we suspect that the altered hormonal milieu of the oviducts post partum leads to an alteration in the quantity of tubal fluid which would probably also inhibit fertility.

It is evident from this preliminary study of the human post partum oviduct that much useful information could be gained from such easily obtainable material. We are ignorant of many of the factors involved in promotion and inhibition of the growth and development of the oviduct mucosa and of the significance of changes in the epithelium in relation to infertility of tubal origin. A better understanding of the biology of the tubal mucosa would also benefit research in contraceptive technology.

ACKNOWLEDGEMENTS

Supported in part by the Ford Foundation (grant to C.O.) and in part by the Fonds voor Wetenschappelijk Geneeskundig Onderzoek (N.F.W.O. grant no. 20035 to I.B.).

REFERENCES

Andrews, M.C. Epithelial changes in the puerperal fallopian tube. Am. J. Obstet. Gynecol. 62:28–37, 1951.

Brenner, R.M. Electronmicroscopy of estrogen effects on ciliogenesis and secretory cell growth in rhesus monkey oviduct. Anat. Rec. 157:218–219, 1967 a.

Brenner, R.M. Ciliogenesis during the menstrual cycle in rhesus monkey oviduct. J. Cell Biol. 35:16A, 1967b.

Brenner, R.M. Renewal of oviduct cilia during the menstrual cycle of the rhesus monkey. Fertil. Steril. 20:599–611, 1969.

Brenner, R.M., Anderson, R.G.W. Endocrine control of ciliogenesis in the primate oviduct. In: Handbook of Physiology, Section 7, Endocrinology II, Part. 2. Ed. R.O. Greep and E.B. Astwood. Williams and Wilkins Co., Baltimore. pp. 123–139, 1973.

Clyman, M.J. Electronmicroscopy of the human fallopian tube. Fertil. Steril. 17:281–301, 1966.

Halbert, S.A., Tam, P.Y., Blandau, R.J. Egg transport in the rabbit oviduct: The roles of cilia and muscle. Science 191:1052–1053, 1976.

Holtzbach, E. Vergleichende anatomische Untersuchungen über die Tubenbrunst und die Tubenmenstruation. Z. Geburtsh. Gynaek. 61:565–580, 1908.

More, I.A.R., Masterton, R.G. The fine structure of the human endometrial ciliated cell. J. Reprod. Fertil. 45:343–348, 1975.

Novak, E., Everett, H.S. Cyclical and other variations in the tubal epithelium. Am. J. Obstet. Gynecol. 16:499–530, 1928.

Oberti, C., Gomez-Rogers, C. De novo ciliogenesis in the human oviduct during the menstrual cycle. In: Biological Reports: Basic and Clinical Studies. Ed. J.T. Velardo and B.A. Kasprow. Pan American Congress of Anatomy III, New Orleans. pp. 241–248, 1972.

Odor, D.L. The question of "basal" cells in oviductal and endocervical epithelium. Fertil. Steril. 25:1047–1061, 1974.

Odor, D.L., Blandau, R.J. Egg transport over the fimbrial surface of the rabbit oviduct under experimental conditions. Fertil. Steril. 24:292–300, 1973.

Seki, K., Rawson, J., Eddy, C.A., Smith, N.K., Pauerstein, C.J. Deciliation in the puerperal fallopian tube. Fertil. Steril. 29:75–83, 1978.

Snyder, F.F. Changes in the human oviduct during the menstrual cycle and pregnancy. Bull. Johns Hopkins Hosp. 35:141–146, 1924.

Van Bogaert, L.J., Maldague, P., Staquet, J.P. The percentage of granulocyte-like cells in human oviduct epithelium. Br. J. Obstet. Gynaecol. 85:373–375, 1978.

Vasquez, G., Brosens, I. Fimbrial microbiopsy. J. Reprod. Med. 16:171–178, 1976.

Copyright 1979 by Elsevier North Holland, Inc.
F.K. Beller and G.F.B. Schumacher, eds.
The Biology of the Fluids of the Female Genital Tract

ANALYSIS OF HUMAN OVIDUCTAL FLUID FOR LOW MOLECULAR WEIGHT COMPOUNDS

J. Lippes

SUMMARY

It has been demonstrated that it is possible to safely collect human oviductal fluid (HOF). Without complications, we have done so on 47 occasions from 63 attempts, a success rate of about 75%. Studies of electrolytes in human oviductal fluid reveal that sodium is on average 9.7 meg./L., but drops to about 7.5 meq./L. after ovulation. Calcium, on the other hand, increases its concentration from 7.8 mg.% in human oviductal fluid before ovulation to 9.4 mg.% after ovulation. Glucose apparently drops slightly with ovulation.

A definite relationship exists between electrolytes in the patient's serum compared to their level in HOF. Sodium remains the same in serum and HOF. Potassium and chloride levels are consistently higher in HOF, while calcium, phosphorus and magnesium levels appeared to be consistently lower in HOF than in serum. Glucose in human oviductal fluid is approximately one-half the serum level. With high pressure liquid chromatography and UV absorbance, 12 cyclic compounds have been identified. Other peaks were observed but not identified. Some of these compounds may be utilized by the oviductal embryo to form nucleic acids

Department of Obstetrics and Gynecology, School of Medicine, State University of New York at Buffalo, Buffalo, New York

and proteins. More investigations in this area are needed in order to completely understand the functions of the human oviduct and the physiologic roles of HOF constituents.

INTRODUCTION

The recent success of Steptoe and Edwards with *in vitro* fertilization and transfer of a human ovum (Steptoe and Edwards 1978) has aroused renewed interest in the physiological events which occur in the human oviduct. The secretions of the human oviduct probably play important physiologic roles in sperm capacitation, fertilization, cleavage and early embryogenesis. Although a technique to collect human oviductal fluid (HOF) has been known since our presentation in 1969 (Lippes et al. 1972), few investigators have pursued the collection of HOF in quantities sufficient for biochemical analyses (Lippes 1975). What are the components of HOF? What are the physiological roles which these secretory products play? Which of these components are under endocrine control? How do these events correlate with the processes of capacitation, fertilization and embryogenesis? In finding answers to these questions, the first step is the collection of HOF. The second step is a biochemical analysis of the constituents of HOF. This paper will limit itself to an analysis of some low molecular weight compounds found in HOF.

MATERIALS AND METHODS

Collection of Human Oviductal Fluid

Multiparous patients electing to be sterilized, volunteered as study subjects. Our original surgical technique involved the placement of Foley catheters in the fimbriated ends of the oviducts, coincidental to a Pomeroy technique for elective sterilization. Because Foley catheters could be deflated and removed, just as surgical drains, this operation is a one time surgical procedure which has been shown to be safe on more than 60 cases we have operated to this date.

When we first presented some aspects of this material in 1969, we utilized a Pfannenstiel incision, which was 8 cm. in length. (Lippes et al. 1972). Foley catheters were placed in the fimbriated ends of the oviducts. The balloons were distended. The catheters were held in place with a retaining suture at the fimbriated ends of the fallopian tubes which encircled the tube just lightly enough to retain the distended balloon and catheter tip, but not enough to interfere with the blood supply to the oviducts. The ends of the catheters were brought out through peritoneal puncture wounds, lateral to the Recti muscles. See Figures 1A, 1B and 1C. They were then connected to collecting bags at the distal ends of the incision.

Recently, we have altered this technique because of the popularity of minilaparotomy sterilization. The "minilap" incision is only two and one half to three and one half cm. in length. With such a small incision, Foley catheters inserted in the oviducts are now brought out in the midline through the incision but avoiding the extra puncture wounds which we formerly made in the peritoneum. See Figure 1D. This change in surgical technique allows us to collect HOF while using the popular minilap incision for female sterilization. While the catheters are in place, HOF is collected in transfusion transfer bags placed beneath the surgical dressings. Postoperatively, HOF is withdrawn from the bag at 12 hour intervals. Patients usually leave the hospital on the second postoperative day. Foley catheters are deflated and removed on the day of discharge.

After collection, the fluid is spun down in sterile test tubes and the sediment is examined for leukocytes and bacteria. The supernatant HOF is sterilized by being forced through milipore filters. It is then placed in sterile tubes and frozen for future biochemical analyses. While the HOF is collected, daily serum samples are obtained from the same patient for determining the levels of estrogen, progesterone, and Lh so that we may correlate the endocrine control of the menstrual cycle with the varying levels of the constituents of HOF.

At convenient times, samples of tubal fluid were thawed and run through high pressure filtration with nitrogen gas forcing HOF samples through an Amicon filter. This separated low molecular weight compounds (those less than 2000 molecular weight) from the proteins in HOF.

Analytical Methods

In this study, we present an analysis of the low molecular weight compounds. Electrolytes and glucose were determined by standard techniques (Andreasen 1967; Baginski et al. 1964; Bowers et al. 1968; Chilcote and Wasson 1958; Cotlove et al. 1958; David et al. 1973; Kadish and Sternbeng 1969; Zall et al. 1956; Zettner 1964). HOF was examined by high pressure liquid chromatography and recording ultraviolet (UV) absorbance of the low molecular weight compounds present in HOF according to the method of Scott (Scott 1968; Scott et al. 1967). HOF low molecular weight compounds were separated with a heated, high pressure anion exchange column into which the HOF was eluted with an acetate buffer of gradually increasing concentrations. Compounds were identified with a UV spectrophotometer, the individual constituents being identified by previous experience in recognition of their retention times.

RESULTS

1. Microscopic examination of HOF sediments were free of leukocytes or bacteria during the first 48 hours of collection. After 48 hours, leukocytes were seen in HOF sediments. Therefore, we no longer collect fluid after the second day.
2. Success of collection and volumes of human oviductal fluid:

Our first report reviewed 37 attempts to collect HOF. Of the first 37 cases we were successful in collecting HOF in 28. Since that report we have operated an additional 26 cases and were successful in collecting fluid in 19 more, making a successful collection rate of 75% (47 of 63 cases). In all cases the largest volumes of HOF were collected around the time of ovulation. One patient in the new series produced 24 ml. of HOF from two oviducts in a 24 hour period. This is the largest single sample we have yet recovered from a patient in one day. Ta-

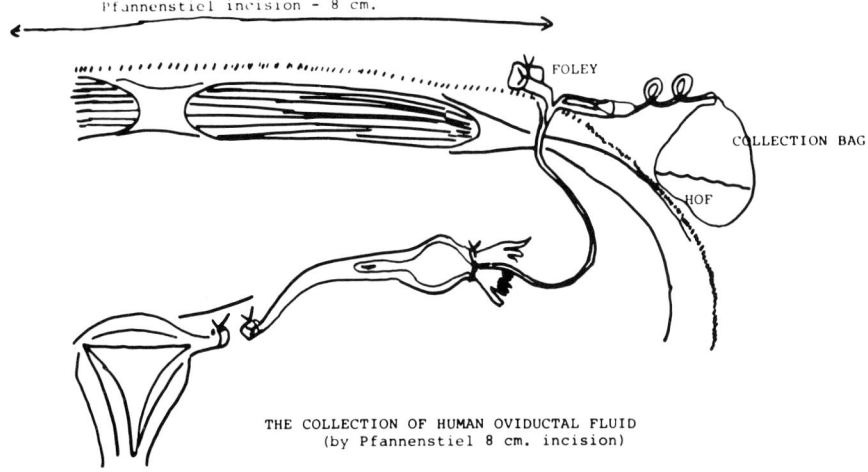

FIGURE 1A. The collection of human oviductal fluid (by Pfannenstiel 8 cm. incision).

FIGURE 1B. Inflated Foley catheter in oviduct retained by purse string suture.

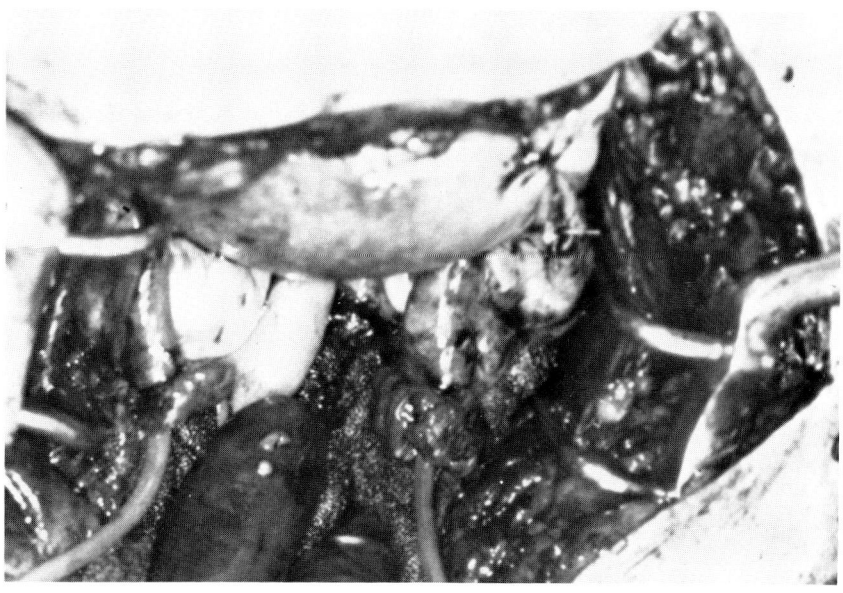

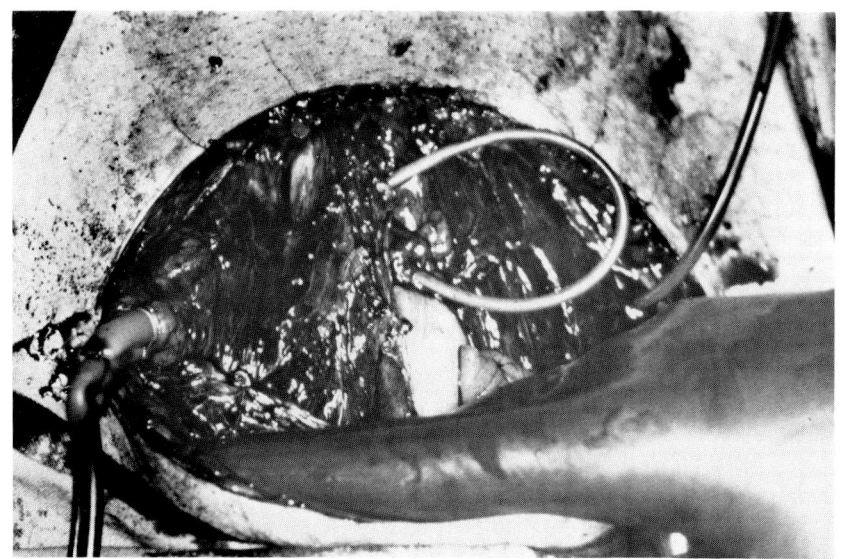

FIGURE 1C. Foley catheter being drawn out lateral to rectus muscle.

FIGURE 1D. Collection of human oviductal fluid (25 mini-lap incision).

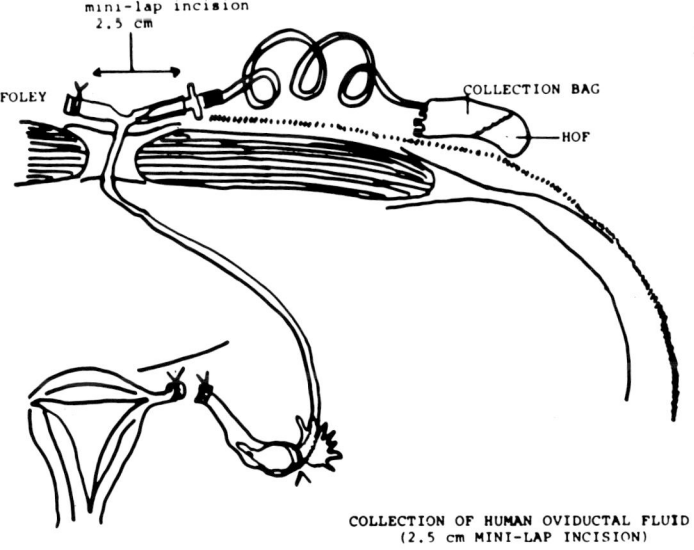

TABLE I. Electrolytes and Glucose in HOF and Serum

	Na*	K*	Cl*	Ca**	P**	Mg **	Glucose**
HOF sample case #1 collected on Day 16 of cycle	139	7.5	115	9.2	3.7	1.1	48
Serum	136	4.4	105	9.9	4.0	1.6	94
HOF sample case #2 collected on Day 13 of cycle	142	9.4	117		3.5	1.3	41
Serum	139	4.2	98			1.8	104

* Na, K, Cl in meq./L
**Ca, P, Mg and Glucose in mg.%

ble I provides examples of electrolyte levels found in human oviductal fluids from two patients and compares these values with electrolyte levels found in the patient's serum on the same day. This sample data confirms our own previous work (Lippes 1975; Lippes et al. 1972) which had been confirmed by the data on electrolytes by David et al. (1973). There was a consistent relationship between the electrolytes and glucose levels of the patient's serum and the electrolytes and glucose levels in HOF (see Table I):

1. Sodium levels did not vary at all, remaining constant both in human oviductal fluid and in serum, at 140 meq./L. ±3.

2. Chloride and potassium were *always* higher in HOF than in serum. On the other hand, calcium, phosphorus and magnesium were always lower than the levels found in human serum. In HOF, the level of glucose consistently appeared to be about one-half of the level found in the patient's serum. Because it was reasonable that the constituents of human oviductal fluid might be under endocrine control, averages of biochemical data from samples taken preovulatory and postovulatory were compared. See Table II. Again, there were no changes in the levels of sodium in human oviductal fluid either before or after ovulation. On the other hand, while potassium appeared to drop approximately 2 meq./L after ovulation, calcium apparently rose 2 mg.% after ovulation from its level prior to ovulation. Glucose appeared to drop by about 14 mg.% after ovulation.

By radioimmunoassay the level of PGF_2 alpha in the oviductal fluid ap-

TABLE II. Variation of Electrolyte Concentrations in HOF with Ovulation

	Na*	K*	Cl*	Ca**	Glucose**
Preovulatory Average	139.5	9.7	119.6	7.8	58.0
Postovulatory Average	139.0	7.5	116.1	9.4	44.4

* Na, K, Cl in meq./L
**Ca and Glucose in mg.%

peared to drop from 7.12 ng/ml before ovulation to 5.0 ng/ml after ovulation (Lippes 1975).
3. High pressure ultraviolet chromatography. See Figures 2A and 2B.
(Compounds identified by this technique include:)

A. Uric acid
B. Xanthine
C. Hypoxanthine
D. Uracil
E. Urocanic acid
F. 5 Acetylamino–5 amino–3 methyl uracil
G. N'methyl–2-pyridone–5-carboxamide
H. Creatinine
I. Pseudouridine
J. Uridine
K. Tyrosine
L. 6 methyl amino purine

Table III lists the concentration of some of the components above, found in a single sample of HOF on cycle day 7, remote from ovulation. Table IV lists levels of compounds in HOF on day 15. On day 7, uric acid is approximately 8.5—10 μg/ml while Xanthine and Hypoxanthine are only traces. From a single sample on day 15, Hypoxanthine was found to be approximately 20–25 μg/ml and Xanthine was determined to be 9 μg/ml. In the same sample, uric acid was 13 μg/ml. See Table IV.

DISCUSSION

The level of glucose is probably not important. Glucose is not needed for energy requirements during cleavage and early embryogenesis. The new mammalian embryo requires lactate and pyruvate for energy in its early stages of development in the oviduct (Brinster 1965). The changes in potassium and calcium would make one think that the human oviductal mucosa, especially the secretory cells, are physiologically involved in active ion transport (Brunton, 1972; Brunton and Brinster 1971). These changes also could be a reflection of oviductal smooth muscle activity and/or the known increase in ciliary activity which occurs after ovulation. Here, prostaglandin may be important. Carsten (Carsten 1972; Carsten 1969) has pointed out the role of prostaglandin in regulating uterine muscular contractions by the transport of calcium. In all probability, similar physiologic phenomena are occurring in the human oviduct. Substantiating this, we have reported (Lippes 1975; Ogra et al. 1974) that there is a change in the level of PGF$_2$ alpha in human oviductal fluid after ovulation. By immunofluorescence (Ogra et al. 1974) it was shown that prior to ovulation, prostaglandins were found in the oviductal mucosa while after ovulation, prostaglandins were seen in the lamina propria. (See Figures 3A and 3B.)

UV absorbance will detect cyclic compounds. The following 12 metabolites which are discussed represent only a small portion of low molecular weight compounds in HOF.

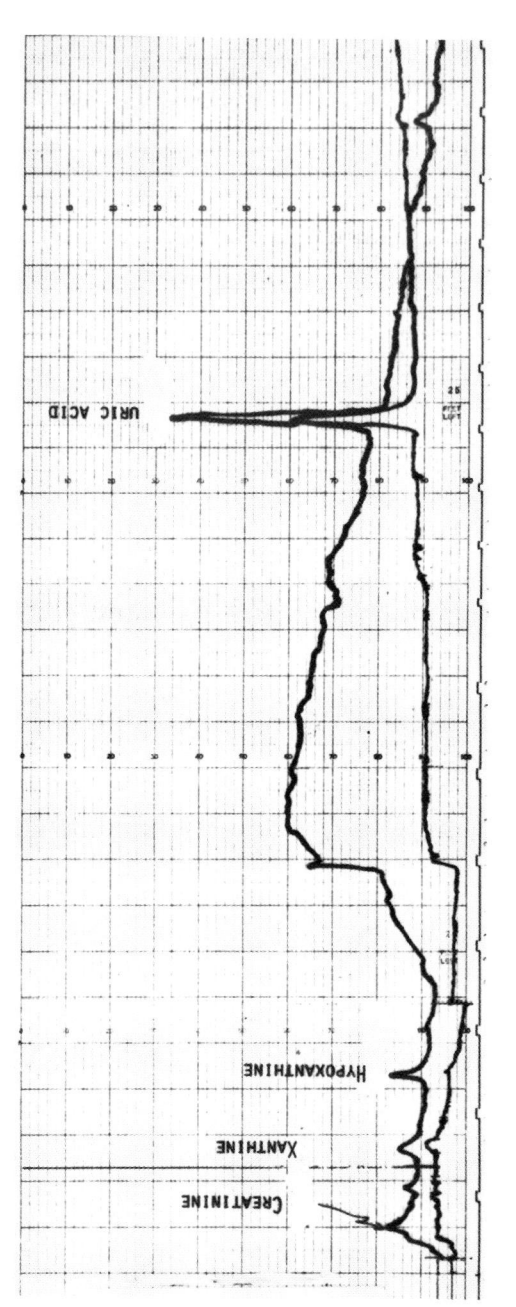

FIGURE 2A. High Pressure Ultraviolet Chromatography at Day 7

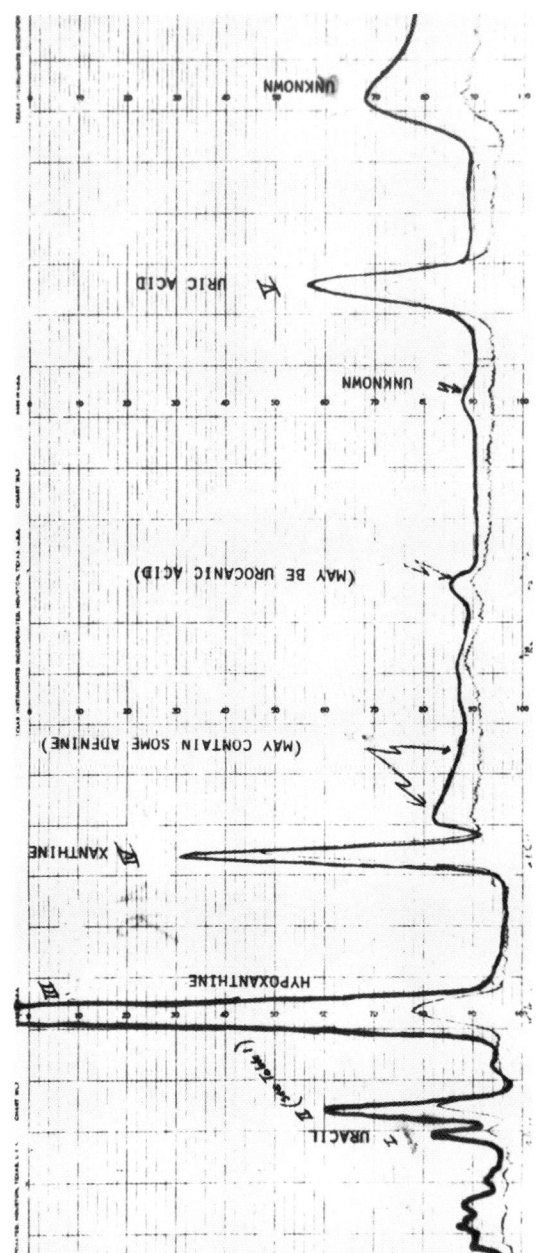

FIGURE 2B. High Pressure Ultraviolet Chromatography at Day 15

TABLE III. Concentration of Compounds From Ultraviolet and Carbohydrate Analyses on Day 7 of Cycle

Compound	Concentration in HOF μg/ml	Usual Blood Conc. μg/ml
Uric Acid	8.5–10	27.5
Hypoxanthine	0.2	not reported
Xanthine	trace	not reported
Glucose	5–7	900
Mannose	0.1	not reported
Fructose	3.8	0–10

TABLE IV. Compounds in HOF on Day 15 of Cycle

Peak No.	Compound	Approx. Quantification (μg/ml)
I	Uracil	1
II	5-Acetylamino-6-Amino-3-Methyl Uracil	trace
III	N'-Methyl-2-Pyridone-5-Carboxamide	trace
IV	Hypoxanthine	20–25
V	Xanthine	9
VI	Uric Acid	13

7 Major and 13 Minor Peaks Observed

TABLE V. Compounds in HOF and Blood Serum on Day 13

Compound	Approx. Concen. (μg/ml)	
	Tubal Fluid[a]	Blood Serum[b]
Creatinine	—	0.4
Pseudouridine	—	0.6
Uridine	2	0.2
Tyrosine	—	11(?)[c]
Hypoxanthine	20–25	0.9
6-Methyl Amino Purine	—	1.4(?)[c]
Urocanic Acid	—	0.5
Uric Acid	10–13	27

[a] Minor and 1 Major Peak
[b] Minor and 1 Major Peak
[c] Identification is tentative

1. *Uric acid*—the presence of uric acid in HOF appears to be relatively constant. The quality or level of this substance probably is a reflection of serum uric acid. Since Xanthine was found in HOF, uric acid could be an end product of purine metabolism. It is not a reusable metabolite. Uric acid was found as a major peak in all HOF samples tested by liquid chromatography with UV.

2. *Xanthine*—is a metabolite of purine interconversion. It is converted to uric acid and therefore is not reusable. Xanthine probably plays no role in tubal physiology.

3. *Hypoxanthine*—is another product which is a metabolite of purine interconversion. This could be a transudate from serum or a metabolite from an epithelial cell degradative process. It is available for salvage by conversion to a nucleotide. Therefore, it could be used in early embryogenesis for the formation of nucleic acids.

It is interesting to note that hypoxanthine and Xanthine appear to be major constituents of HOF around ovulation, (See Table V) but only traces of these metabolites are found in HOF samples collected remote from ovulation. The quantity of these compounds may be under endocrine control. This would suggest that the cleaving embryo may possibly use hypoxanthine for nucleotide formation.

4. *Uracil*—is one of the three main pyrimidines found in nucleic acids. It can be found in degradation of purines as well. The importance of uracil in the structure of RNA is well known. HOF contains measurable quantities of uracil. The availability of uracil in HOF for the morula to produce RNA is a reasonable explanation for its presence.

5. *Urocanic acid*—is usually derived from the amino acid, histidine. It is eventually metabolized to glutamic acid. Such an amino acid could be a protein building block in early embryogenesis.

6. *5 Acetylamino-5-amino-3 methyl uracil*—is a metabolite of a ribonucleotide. It can be used, as is uracil, for RNA production.

7. *N' methyl-2-pyridine-5-carboxamide*—is a metabolite of niacin.

8. *Creatinine*—is a metabolite found in blood, muscle and urine. Quantities found in HOF probably represent transudation from blood.

10. *Uridine*—is known in many biochemical processes which includes the synthesis of DNA and pyrimidine nucleotides. Uridine is also involved in the metabolism of sucrose, glycogen, mucopolysaccharides and lipopolysaccharides, to name a few. Any of these might be a biochemical role for uridine in the human oviduct.

11. *Tyrosine*—is an aromatic amino acid found in many proteins. It is found in plasma at levels of 0.8–2.5 $\mu g/100$ ml. To find it in HOF, was, therefore, not surprising.

12. *6 methyl amino purine*—can be utilized to form a purine nucleotide and such a compound can be incorporated into nucleic acids. It obviously could be used or reused by the cleaving morula.

By gas chromatography 65 peaks have been observed (Lippes 1975). See Figure 4. More investigation in this area is needed, because HOF is obviously a complex and dynamic medium.

Further research with this and other techniques analyzing HOF holds promise of eventually revealing the complete composition of HOF. Such data could be utilized to improve artificial media for *in vitro* fertilization and culture of human eggs, with the possibility of improving results with ovum transfer in cases

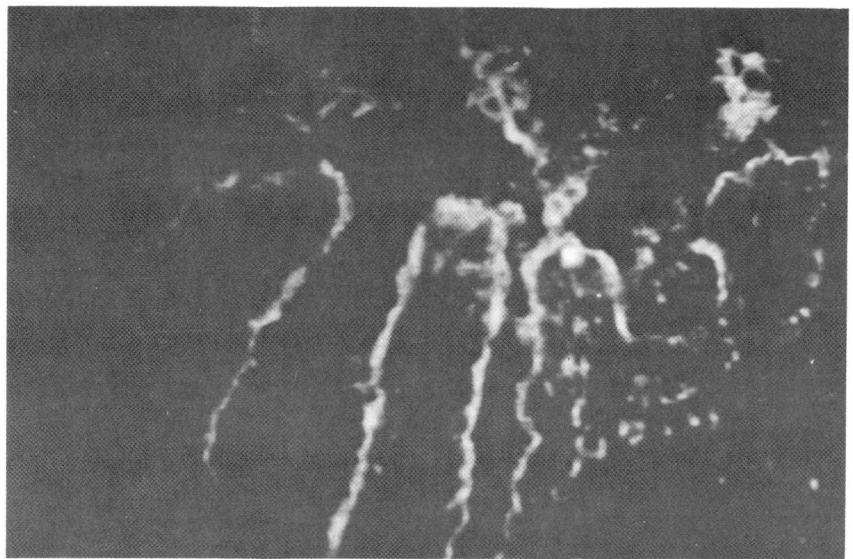

FIGURE 3A. Immunofluorescence of PGF$_2$ Alpha seen in Human Oviductal Mucosa before Ovulation (Reprinted courtesy of Ogra, Kirton, Tomasi and Lippes and the American Fertility Society)

FIGURE 3B. Immunofluorescence of PGF$_2$ Alpha in the Lamina Propria of the Human Oviduct after Ovulation (Reprinted courtesy of Ogra, Kirton, Tomasi and Lippes and the American Fertility Society)

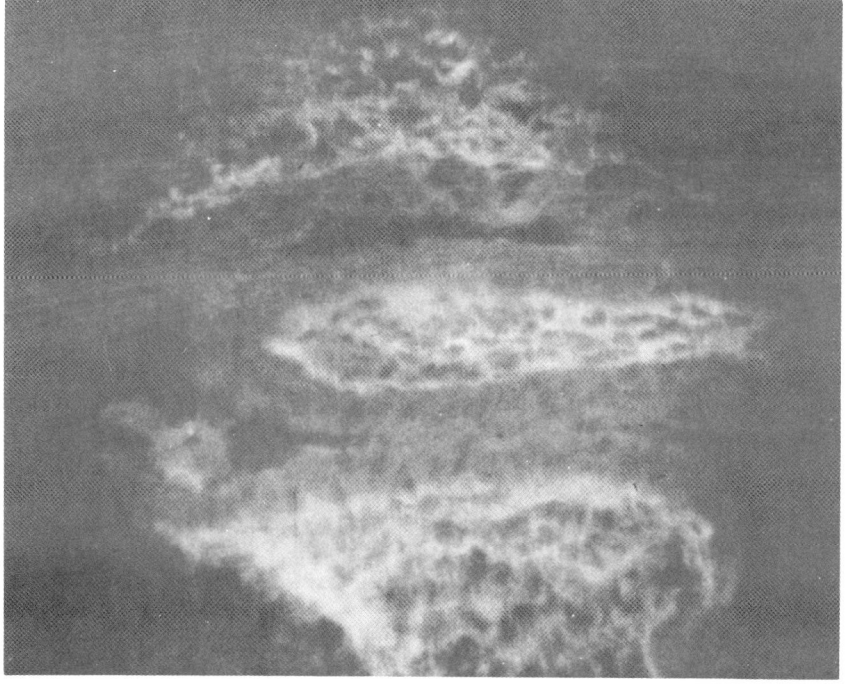

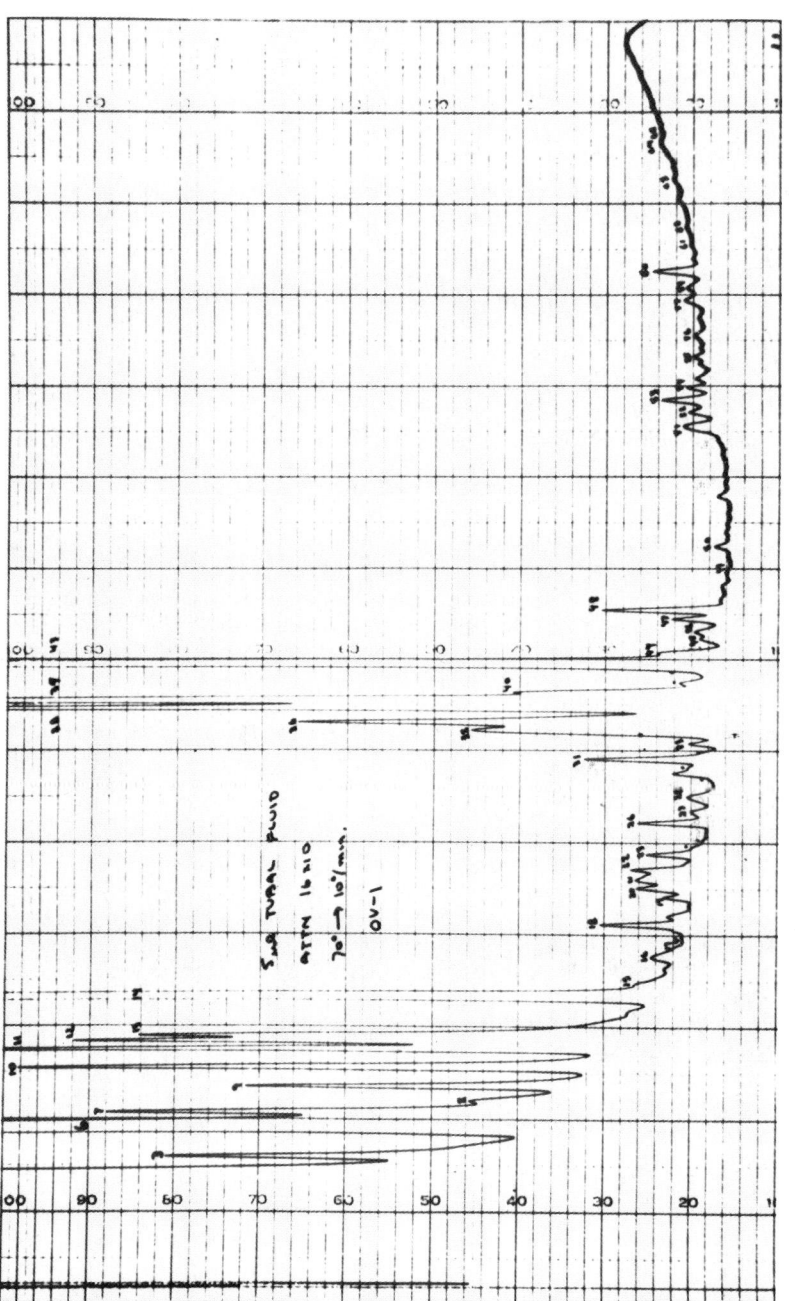

FIGURE 4. Gas Chromatography Demonstrating 65 Peaks in HOF around the Time of Ovulation (Courtesy of Appleton, Century & Crofts and Jack Lippes).

of infertility. The availability of early embryos might aid in advancing human genetic engineering. Perhaps we may be able to prevent certain inherited metabolic defects by a process of superovulation, *in vitro* fertilization, followed by zygote selection.

An understanding of the constituents of HOF may provide us with clues for the development of safer and more natural contraceptives.

ACKNOWLEDGEMENTS

We acknowledge with gratitude the aid of Drs. Charles D. Scott and John E. Mrochek, of the Oak Ridge National Laboratories, with the Gas Chromatographic Analysis and the high pressure liquid chromatography of some samples of human oviductal fluid.

REFERENCES

Andreasen, E.: On the determination of magnesium in serum and urine by the titan yellow method. Scand. J. Clin. Lab. Invest. Suppl. 9(2):138, 1967.

Baginski, E., Epstein, E. and Zak, B.: Automation of methods for the determination of serum phosphoris. Clin. Chem. Acta 10:76, 1964.

Bowers, G.N., Smith, S.B. and Feldman, F.J.: A study of factors affecting the determination of calcium in serum by atomic absorption spectroscopy. Clin. Chem. 14:846, 1968 (Abstr.)

Brinster, R.L.: Studies on the development of mouse embryos *in vitro* II. The effect of energy source. J. Exp. Zool. 158:59, 1965.

Brunton, W.J.: Ion transport by the isolated rhesus monkey oviduct and stimulation by human seminal plasma and prostaglandin-E_1. Biol. Reprod. 5 (Abstract 1):105, 1972.

Brunton, W.J., Brinster, R.L.: Acitive chloride transport in the isolated rabbit oviduct. Am. J. Physiol. 221:658, 1971.

Carsten, M.E.: Prostaglandin's part in regulating uterine contraction by transport of calcium. In: Southern, E.M.E. (ed): The Prostaglandins clinical applications in human reproduction. Mt Kisco, N.Y. Futura Publishing 1972, pp. 59–66.

Carsten, M.E.: The role of calcium binding by sarcoplasmic reticulum in the contraction and relaxation of uterine smooth muscle. J. Gen. Physiol. 53:414–426, 1969.

Chilcote, M.E. and Wasson, R.D.: A new micro method for the colorimetric determination of calcium in serum or urine. Clin. Chem. 4:200, 1958.

Cotlove, E., Trantham, H.V. and Bowman, R.L.: An instrument and method for automatic, rapid, accurate and sensitive titration of chloride in biologic samples. J. of Lab. and Clin. Med. 51:461, 1958.

David, A., Serr, D.M. and Czernobilsky, B.: Chemical composition of human oviductal fluid. Fertil. Steril. 24:435, 1973.

Kadish, A.H., Sternberg, J.C.: Determination of urine glucose by measurement of rate of oxygen consumption. Diabetes 18:467, 1969.

Lippes, J.: Applied physiology of the uterine tube. Obstetrics and Gynecology Annual 1975, pp. 119–166.

Lippes, J., Enders, R.G., Pragay, D.A., Bartholomew, W.R.: The collection and analysis of human fallopian tubal fluid. Contraception 5:85, 1972.

Ogra, S.S., Kinton, K.T., Tomasi, T.B., Jr., Lippes, J.: Prostaglandins in the human fallopian tube. Fertil. Steril. 25:250, 1974.

Scott, C.D.: Analysis of urine for its ultraviolet absorbing constituents by high pressure anion-exchange chromatography. Clin. Chem. 14:521, 1968.

Scott, C.D., Attrill, J.E., Anderson, N.G., Automatic high resolution analysis of urine for its ultraviolet absorbing constituents. Soc. Pro. Med. 125:181, 1967.

Steptoe, P.C., Edwards, R.G.: Birth after the reimplantation of a human embryo. Lancet 2:3, 1978.

Zall, D., Fisher, D., Garner, M.D.: Photometric determination of chlorides in water. Analytical Chem. 28:1665, 1956.

Zettner, A.: Principles and applications of atomic absorption spectroscopy. Advances Clin. Chem. 7:1, 1964.

SPECIFIC ANTIBODIES IN OVIDUCT SECRETIONS OF THE RHESUS MONKEY

G.F.B. Schumacher, S.L. Yang, and K.H. Broer*

SUMMARY

Rhesus monkeys were immunized with a model antigen, which permits quantitative determination of low level antibodies in small volumes of biological fluids. T4-coliphages were used for this purpose and rhesus monkeys were immunized either systemically by injection or by local application to the upper vagina and ectocervix. The very sensitive phage neutralization method was used to determine the level of specific antibodies in oviductal secretion and in serum.

The technique of Mastroianni was used for oviductal fluid collection. Laparotomy was performed on each monkey to insert a perforated stainless steel cannula at the fimbrial end of each tube, which was then connected with a refrigerated collecting chamber by thin polyethylene tubing which lead through the abdominal wall. The monkeys were kept for 6-13 days in a restraining chair. Multiple injections of human menopausal gonadotrophin (HMG) (followed by a single dose of human chorionic gonadotropin (HCG)) were administered to induce ovulation.

The determinations of specific antibody titers both in serum and oviductal fluid indicate that there is 10 to 40 fold less antibody in oviductal fluid as compared to serum. There is a significant decrease of the antibody level of oviductal

---

Department of Obstetrics and Gynecology and Divisional Committee on Immunology, The Univeristy of Chicago, Pritzker School of Medicine, Chicago, Illinois
  * Recipient of a Reproductive Biology Research Stipend by the "Deutsche Forschungs-Gemeinschaft", Bonn-Bad Godesberg, FRG. Present Address: Universitäts-Frauenklinik, köln, FRG

secretions after the HMG injections followed by an increase beginning usually between the 2nd and 3rd day after the HCG injection. The serum values do not show this pattern. Although the specific antibody level is significantly higher in serum and in oviduct fluid of systemically immunized animals as compared to locally immunized the pattern appears to be very similar.

GENERAL CONSIDERATIONS AND PURPOSE

The fertilization process takes place in the environment of oviductal secretions which provide under physiological circumstances the optimal conditions for gamete transport and sperm-egg interaction. Many aspects of the function of the mammalian oviduct and its secretions have been investigated and reviewed in recent years (Hafez and Blandau, 1971; Harper et al., 1976; Lippes, 1975; Beier, 1974; Hafez, 1973; Mastroianni Jr. et al., 1973; Mastroianni Jr., 1976). There is a problem in collecting oviductal fluid in its native state, since all methods involve in one way or another surgical methods and the introduction of collecting devices may induce inflammatory reactions. There is probably no ideal way to obtain tubal secretions particularly if longitudinal studies for the investigation of hormonal effects are desired. Therefore, applying methods which cause the least amount of tissue trauma of the oviduct and of the adjacent tissues may be the best one can do with respect to near-normal conditions. A variety of methods for collection of oviductal fluid in laboratory and farm animals is referenced in a review by Hafez (1973). Studies in humans have been done at the time of sterilization or hysterectomy (Moghissi, 1970; Lippes, 1975) however, the number of days of collection is limited for obvious reasons.

There seems to be agreement among most investigators with respect to the proteins in mammalian oviduct fluid that there are oviduct specific proteins present in addition to a variety of serum proteins. The latter show disparity in the relative amounts of protein components which are common to oviductal secretion and to serum. This indicates that there is most probably a selectivity in the transudation from the blood into the tubal secretion.

Data on immunoglobulins or specific antibodies in mammalian oviduct secretions are rather scarce. Shapiro et al. (1971) immunized rabbits with yeast alcohol dehydrogenase as model antigen. Although serum antibodies could be demonstrated after 3 weeks, no antibodies could be demonstrated in tubal fluid during a follow-up of 10 weeks. Behrman (1969) reported that no appreciable amounts of specific antibodies could be found in rabbit oviductal secretions after immunization with rabbit semen, although the titer in the corresponding sera was very high. Recently, Oliphant et al. (1977) presented data on the level of immunoglobulins in rabbit Fallopian tubal fluid. The authors found that throughout the entire pseudopregnancy cycle only 10 percent of the level of total immunoglobulins present in serum appeared in the oviductal fluid. An increase up to approximately 20 percent was observed during the first 3 days after HCG injection. Of the serum levels only 4 percent IgG, 25 percent IgA and 2 percent IgM were found in the tubal secretion. Information on immunoglobulins in human tubal fluid (Lippes, 1975) indicates that there is a relatively low level of immunoglobulins present, mainly IgG. IgA and IgM are not always detectable. Immuno-histochemical studies on the human oviduct revealed that IgG, IgA and "secretory piece" were present in stroma and villi of the uterine tube, IgM was usually absent except in preovulatory stages (Lippes et al., 1970). Rebello et al. (1975) have shown with fluorescent antibody techniques identifying IgG, IgA or IgM producing lymphocytes that no such cells were present in the tissues of the human oviduct. Immunoglobulin producing cells were seen to some extent in the endometrium, but in larger numbers in the endocervical tissues. There are indications that a local immune system is functional in the internal female genital tract (Behrmann and Liebermann, 1973; Schumacher and Yang, 1977; Cinader and de Weck, 1976), but there may be considerable differences between the different compartments of the genital tract (i.e. vagina, cervix, corpus, Fallopian tubes).

The idea of interfering with the process of fertilization by immunization against acrosomal enzymes of spermatozoa is an intriguing one since enzyme inhibition by specific antibodies can be demonstrated *in vitro*. However, information on specific antibodies in oviduct secretions and their changes in concentration during the cycle, especially at the time of possible fertilization, is lacking. Since longitudinal studies with continuous collection of tubal fluid can not be done in humans, rhesus monkeys were immunized with a model antigen, which permits quantitative determination of low level antibodies in small volumes of biological fluids. T4-coliphages were used for this purpose and rhesus monkeys were immunized either systemically by injection or by local application to the upper vagina and ectocervix.

MATERIALS AND METHODS

Animals

Nine healthy female rhesus monkeys (macaca mulatta) were used in the experiments. The animals showed menstrual bleedings in regular intervals (average 27 days). The immune response to systemic or local (vaginal) immunization with T4-coliphages was previously studied by comparing the titer of neutralizing antibodies in cervical mucus and in serum (Schumacher and Yang, 1977; Yang and Schumacher, 1979). These animals received booster immunizations before the collection of tubal fluid. This was successfully accomplished in 7 of 9 rhesus monkeys under investigation. In 5 instances a second course of tubal fluid collection could be completed. Twenty to thirty milligram of phencyclidine-HCL (Bio-ceutic Lab. Inc., St. Joseph, Missouri) was administered subcutaneously to the animals as a tranquilizer before surgery. During the laparotomy the animals received an intravenous infusion. Pentobarbital i.v. was used for anesthesia. A combination of benzathine and procaine penicillin G of 1.2 million units was given i.m. on the day of surgery.

Antigens

T4-coliphages (abortive type) were used for immunization. The phages were prepared from a stock solution (N69-N104) courteously provided by Dr. R. Haselkorn, Dept. of Biophysics and Theoretical Biology, University of Chicago. The culturing was done in large subcultures (15 liters) of strain B, non-suppressor type of E. coli. Purification was accomplished by differential centrifugation and cesiumchloride step gradient ultracentrifugation (see Yang and Schumacher, 1979).

Immunization Procedure

1. Systemic: Alum-precipitated antigens (Kabat and Mayer, 1961) were injected subcutaneously 3 times per week for 6 weeks (10^{12} plaque forming units (PFU) of T4-phages in 1.0 ml per injection) following the same scheme used for local immunization (18 applications). However, only 3 injections were given in 2-3 day intervals for boosting.
2. Local: A Dispo-Plug (Scientific Products, Chicago, Illinois) plastic sponge (1.5 x 2.0 cm cylinders) was injected with 1 ml antigen solution (10^{12} PFU of phage particles) before each application and placed in the upper part of the vagina against the ectocervix. Subsequently, a parafilm covered sponge and a plain sponge were introduced into the vagina to hold the carrier in its position. The antigen carrier and the other plugs were replaced 3 times per week for 6 weeks (primary immunization: 18 antigen applications). For booster immunization only 10 applications were given. The booster courses were applied 2 1/2 to 5 months after the previous immunization course (primary or booster). Studies with H^3—labelled T4-coliphages revealed that >90% of the phage particles were absorbed from the sponge plug within 48 hours.

Determination of Specific Antibodies

Antibodies to T4-coliphages were quantitatively assessed by the phage neutralization test (Adams, 1959), expressing the antibody titer in terms of the "K-value", the velocity constant of phage neutralization. Each sample or sample dilution was tested in duplicate (for details of the procedures see Yang and Schumacher, 1979).

Collection of Oviduct Fluid

The technique of Mastroianni et al. (1970) with some minor modifications was used for oviductal fluid collection. Laparotomy was performed on each monkey to insert a perforated stainless steel cannula of 10 mm length and 1.5 mm width with a circular groove into the fimbrial end of each tube. The cannulas were fixed by a ligation over the circular groove and connected with a refrigerated collecting chamber by thin, sterilized polyethylene tubing lead through the abdominal wall. The tubing was rinsed with 0.9% NaCl solution containing 100 units of heparin per ml. The oviducts were ligated at the utero-tubal junction. The collecting chamber consisted of two separate small jacketed test tubes. The jackets were connected with each other and armed with two nipples to allow a continuous flow of cooling fluid delivered by a refrigerated cooling bath with circulating pump (Haake, Type FK, Saddle Brook, N.Y.). The stoppers of the two collecting chambers were armed each with a short stainless steel needle connected with the polyethylene tubing, a longer stainless steel needle for withdrawal of the collected fluid once a day and another short needle with a cotton filter for air-escape. The chamber was sterilized before use and embedded in styrofoam for insulation. The device was fixed to the lower abdominal wall by nylon sutures anchored under the fascia using a silastic button. By this arrangement the tubal fluid could be collected from each side separately. The monkeys were kept for 6-13 days in a restraining chair without tranquilizer medication. The animals received orange juice/water, oranges, bananas, apples or tomatoes together with standard food pellets in small portions several times a day.

Multiple injections of human menopausal gonadotrophin (HMG) followed by a single dose of human chorionic gonadotrophin (HCG) were given to induce ovulation. The HMG injections (75 I.U. FSH and 75 I.U. LH) were initiated 3-8 days after the beginning of the menstrual bleeding and surgery was usually performed 2-5 days after the beginning of the HMG treatment. HCG (500 I.U.) was given after 5-8 injections of HMG. Oviductal fluid was collected daily from each side and also blood specimens were drawn from the leg veins. At the end of the experiment another laparotomy was performed to cut off and remove the polyethylene tubing, check the proper position of the stainless steel cannula, and to observe evidence of ovulation from the gross appearance of both ovaries. After several months (3-4) the experiment was repeated successfully in several monkeys by relaparotomy, reconnecting the cannula with polyethylene tubing lead through the abdominal wall and connection with the refrigerated collecting device. The reconnection of the cannula in situ did, surprisingly, not present serious problems, since adhesions were found to be only minimal or moderate. At the end of the second collection cycle, the oviducts were removed in a few instances for histological evaluation.

RESULTS

The results of these experiments present an almost uniform pattern. Figure 1 and Figure 2 are representative examples obtained in two animals during two collection cycles each. The graphs show the levels of specific antibodies against T4-coliphages in serum and in tubal fluid during and after treatment with gonadotrophins. The left scale is applicable to the serum values and the right scale to the tubal fluid.

Figure 1 represents an animal (Nancy) which was originally immunized by local applications of T4-phages to the vagina showing a weak response only at that time (see Yang and Schumacher, 1979). This monkey was immunized systemically several weeks before the collection of tubal fluid by injection of alum-precipitated T4-phages, resulting in a good antibody response with serum K-values (titer) of >2000. During the first collection cycle the serum levels of T4-antibodies show only uncharacteristic variations with K-values around 1800. The second cycle shows a lower level of K-values in the vicinity of 800 ten weeks later. In contrast, the K-values of the tubal fluid present a characteristic pattern which appears to be related to the treatment with gonadotrophins. However the level of antibodies is more than one order of magnitude lower than in serum. The K-values of phage neutralization decrease towards the end of the HMG treatment and one to two days after the HCG injection to minimal values and increase again in subsequent days. The differences between highest and lowest values are characterized by a factor of 4-5 and higher which cannot be explained by tubal fluid dilution, since the increase in volume is less than two fold. The amount of fluid produced during the second cycle shows a reduced volume.

Figure 2 represents an animal (Faye) which was immunized only by vaginal application of T4-phage antigen. The previous courses of immunization, applying plain phages without alum as an adjuvant were followed by a very weak response in this animal compared to others (see Yang and Schumacher, 1979, and

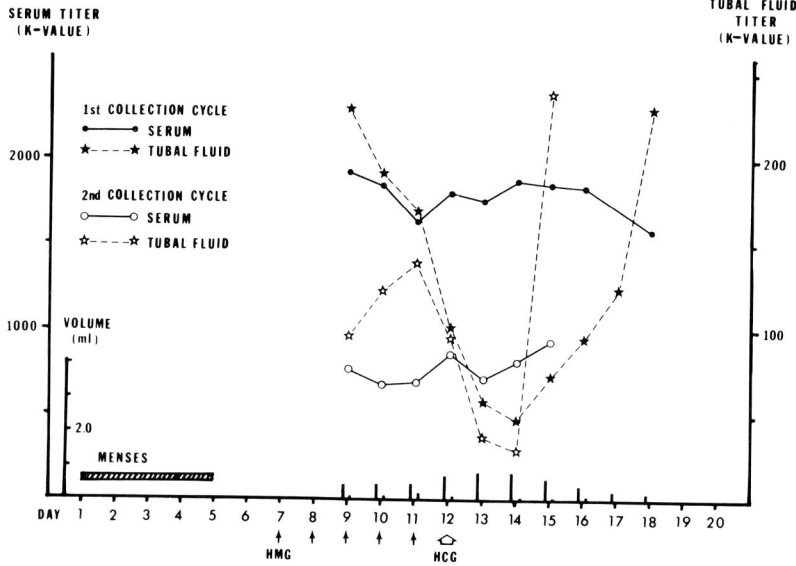

FIGURE 1. Phage neutralization antibody titer (K values) in serum and tubal fluid of monkey Nancy during 2 collection cycles. The monkey was immunized first locally (intravaginal applications) and later systemically (subcutaneous injections) by T4 antigens. Dots and open circles represent antibody titers in serum, solid and open stars represent antibody titers in tubal fluid. The second collection cycle was initiated 10 weeks after the first one. The serum titer decreased during this period of time considerably. The animal received 5 injections of HMG (75 I.U. FSH and 75 I.U. LH) followed by one injection of HCG (500 I.U.). The changes of the K-values in tubal fluid are characteristic and representative for this series. The volume recordings show significantly reduced amounts of fluid production during the second collection cycle.

Schumacher and Yang, 1977). The phage neutralization test is so sensitive, however, that the serum samples were still to be 1/5 diluted whereas the tubal fluid was used undiluted for the test. If one compares the results of these experiments depicted in Figures 1 and 2, one recognizes that the serum K-values of the systemically immunized animal (Figure 1) are approximately 10^4 times higher than those of the locally immunized animal (Figure 2). However, the proportions between the values of serum and tubal fluid are similar, i.e. the antibody levels are approximately one order of magnitude lower in the oviductal secretion. The courses of the K-values in tubal fluid show the same pattern during the first and during the second cycle of collection except that the minimum of the first cycle occurs one day after HCG, whereas the mimimum of the second cycle appears two days after HCG. The differences between the highest and the lowest levels of antibodies are again characterized by a factor 4-5, whereas the increase in volume is also less than two fold.

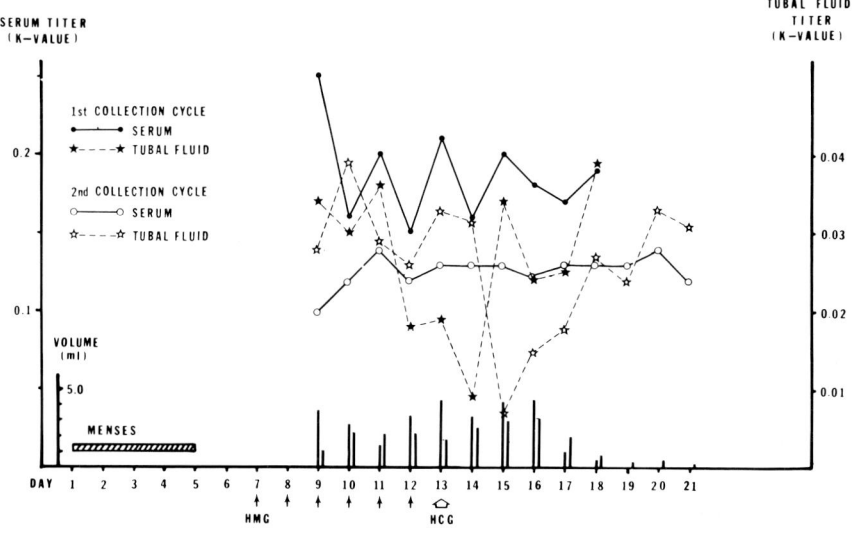

FIGURE 2. Phage neutralization antibody titers (K values) in serum and tubal fluid of monkey Faye. The monkey was immunized and boostered locally by intravaginal application of T4 antigens. Dots and open circles represent antibody titers in serum, solid and open stars represent antibody titers in tubal fluid. The level of antibodies in serum and tubal fluid is drastically lower than in the experiment in Figure 1. This animal received 6 injections of HMG (75 I.U. FSU and 75 I.U. LH) followed by one injection of HCG (500 I.U.). The pattern of changes of the K-values in tubal fluid is very similar to the pattern in Figure 1. The volume of tubal fluid collected is greater in this animal during both collecting cycles, however somewhat smaller during the second collection cycle.

At the time of relaparotomy corpora lutea were recognized to be present. Histological confirmation was obtained in one case after removal of the ovary (experiment in Figure 1 after the second cycle of tubal fluid collection).

The appearance of the tubal fluid was yellowish—clear in most instances of this series of animal experiments. Occasionally some contamination with red cells was obvious and the degree of contamination was assessed by counting the red cells. Only the tubes with clear fluid were used for evaluation. In three instances the number of red blood cells was slightly more than 100,000/mm^3, which may still be considered a very low degree of contamination with blood. In one case a leak was found between the cannula and the tube on one side. The fluid collected from this side was considered to be contaminated with peritoneal fluid and not evaluated. It showed between 600 and 6000 WBC/mm^3. (In the other experiments most specimens were free of WBC, a few contained <50 WBC/mm^3.) It may also be of interest to mention that hemolytic complement was absent in all specimens of 9 investigated collection cycles except for the last 3 specimens of the second cycle of monkey Faye (Figure 2). The quantity of hemolytic complement was in the vicinity of 10 percent of the serum complement activity. Tubal fluid specimens and serum were tested for complement by a radial diffusion in gel method (Kallestad Lab., Inc., Chaska, Minn.). Four other specimens each from the two sides (left and right) did not show complement activity, when tested immediately after collection. All other tubal fluid specimens were tested after storage at -35°C. Therefore, a loss of weak complement activity by freezing and thawing can not be ruled out, since rhesus monkey serum shows a considerable reduction of hemolytic complement after freezing and thawing. The observations indicate, however, that it is highly unlikely that appreciable amounts of hemolytic complement are present in rhesus monkey tubal fluid under physiological conditions.

The finding of weak complement activity in 3 specimens led to the search for C-reactive protein (CRP) known to be an indicator of inflammatory reactions. Double diffusion tests in agar gel using anti-human CRP-serum which cross-reacts with rhesus monkey CRP intensively (Schumacher, unpublished) revealed weak positive CRP tests in the 3 specimens showing low complement activity but not in the other samples of the same collecting cycle. The subsequent testing of all specimens from 9 collecting cycles revealed weakly positive CRP tests in more than half of the samples except the first cycle of monkey Faye (Figure 2). The CRP appeared in some instances during the first few days and in others toward the end of the collecting cycles and may be a result of increased circulating CRP usually observed after surgery (Schumacher, 1960).

The histopathological evaluation of one tube excised after the second collection cycle in one animal shows very little infiltration of inflammatory cells in the walls of the tube throughout its length. However, multiple suture granulomata could be found in the immediate vicinity of the ligatures. From the histopathological point of view the tissue reaction could only be considered as very mild. In this case the CRP was present in all tubal fluids collected prior to the excision of the tube. However, the bacteriological tests on the last two samples were negative. Further investigations are in progress to determine whether or not the appearance of CRP and hemolytic complement can be used as an indicator for the degree of a local inflammatory reaction in the Fallopian tubes.

DISCUSSION AND COMMENTS

Oviductal fluid collected from rhesus monkeys under the conditions described in this communication may be close to normal in uncomplicated experiments. However, the influence of some minor local irritation caused by the surgical trauma itself, by the presence of a stainless steel cannula in the ostium and of polyethylene tubing in the abdomen, and by the ligation of the tube at the uterotubal junction, has to be taken into consideration. The treatment with gonadotrophins in order to provoke ovulation may also cause some effects deviating from the pattern of a normal spontaneous menstrual cycle. However, one would expect that the effects would not be entirely dissimilar.

The levels of circulating hormones are under investigation and the expected data may help to assess the situation along with further studies on the inflammatory proteins of tubal fluid with respect to the influence of possible local irritation. However, one would expect that inflammatory stimuli would most probably increase the level of immunoglobulins unless ovarian steroid hormones could counteract or enhance this process.

With these considerations in mind one may draw the following conclusions:

1. The levels of specific antibodies in oviductal fluid are on an average basis approximately 10 times lower than the serum values.
2. Tubal fluid antibodies show under treatment with gonadotrophins (HMG and HCG) a characteristic decrease and increase in concentration by a factor of approximately 4-5. The minimum was usually observed on the 2nd day after HCG.
3. There is a drastic difference between the serum antibody levels after systemic and after vaginal immunization by a factor of 10^3-10^4. However, the pattern in tubal fluid under treatment with gonadotrophins is very similar except that the difference between serum and tubal fluid appears to be less pronounced after local immunization. The latter may be related to local immune mechanisms and needs further confirmation.
4. The level of specific antibodies in tubal fluid is, relative to the serum values, slightly higher during the second collection cycle compared with the first one. The volume of tubal fluid produced was also noted to be lower during the second cycle. Both observations may be related to the degree of inflammatory changes due to surgery and foreign body reaction.

The evaluation of these conclusions under the considerations discussed above allows one to speculate that the level of antibodies in native tubal fluid without possible artifacts caused by the collection method is probably even lower than reported in this communication. If the periovulatory period is characterized by such extremely low concentrations of specific antibodies, the chances of immunological interference with the fertilization process are rather slim unless the titer is very high in the circulating blood. Furthermore, the susceptibility of the tubes to bacterial infections in humans may be seen in the light of a rather limited humoral immune response in this organ considering the results of this study. Local immunization by placing T4-phages intravaginally resulted, in most instances, in an immune response with higher antibody titers in cervical mucus than in serum (Scnumacher and Yang, 1977; Yang and Schumacher, 1979). This observation together with the morphological findings of Rebello et al. (1975), describing a lack of immunoglobulin producing cells in the human Fallopian tubes as opposed to the endocervical tissues indicates that the cervix is most probably more intimately involved in the local immune response than the oviducts.

ACKNOWLEDGEMENTS

We would like to thank Dr. R. Haselkorn of the Dept. of Biophysics and Theoretical Biology of the University of Chicago for providing stock solutions of the T4-coliphages and for his helpful advice in culturing and purification of the phages.

We also thank Dr. F. Reale, Section of Gynecologic Pathology, Depts. of Obstetrics and Gynecology and Pathology of the University of Chicago for the preparation and histopathological evaluation of the tissue sections.

We are indebted to Dr. P.S. Tobias, of our laboratory, for building the collection chambers. The skillful technical assistance in the animal experiments by Mr. William Jemison, the technical laboratory assistance by Mrs. Margaret Crawford and the help of Mrs. Evelyn Jackson in preparing the manuscript is gratefully acknowledged.

The work was supported in part by Ford Foundation Grant #690-0108A, WHO Project #73119 and the Mother's Aid Research Fund of the Chicago Lying-in Hospital.

REFERENCES

Adams, M.H. (Ed.): Bacteriophages. Interscience Publisher, New York, 1959, pp. 463–464.

Behrman, S.J.: Immunology of oviductal secretions. In: The Mammalian Oviduct. Eds.: E.S.E. Hafez and R.J. Blandau. Univ. of Chicago Press, Chicago and London, 1969, pp. 357–372.

Behrman, S.J., Lieberman, M.E.: Biosynthesis of immunoglobulins by the human cervix. In: The Biology of the Cervix. Eds.: R.J. Blandau and K. Moghissi. Univ. of Chicago Press, Chicago and London, 1973, pp. 235–249.

Beier, H.M.: Oviductal and uterine fluids. J. Reprod. Fert. 37, 221–237 (1974).

Cinader, B., deWeck, A.: Immunological response of the female reproductive tract—WHO Workshop 1975. Scriptor, Copenhagen, 1976.

Hafez, E.S.E., Blandau, R.J.: The Mammalian Oviduct. University of Chicago Press, Chicago and London, 1971.

Hafez, E.S.E.: Endocrine control of the structure and function of the mammalian oviduct. In: Handbook of Physiology, Sect 7, Endocrinol., Vol. II, Part 2, Eds.: Greep, R.O. and Astwood, E.B. American Physiological Society, Washington, D.C., 1973, pp. 97–122.

Harper, M.J.K., Pauerstein, C.J., Adams, C.E., Coutinho, E.M., Croxatto, H.B. and Paton, D.M.: Ovum Transport and Fertility Regulation. Scriptor, Copenhagen, 1976.

Kabat, E.A., E.A., Mayer, M.M.: Experimental Immunochemistry, Charles C. Thomas, Publisher, Springfield, Ill., 1961.

Lippes, J.: Applied physiology of the uterine tube. Obstet. Gynecol. Ann. 4, 119–166 (1975).

Lippes, J., Ogra, S., Tomasi, T.B., Jr. and Tourville, D.R.: Immunohistological localization of gamma G. gamma A, gamma M, secretory piece and lactoferrin in the human female genital tract. Contraception 1, 163–183 (1970).

Mastroianni, Jr., L: Potentials for fertility regulation at the tubal level. Contraception 13, 447–459 (1976).

Mastroianni, Jr., L., Urzua, M., and Stambaugh, R.: Protein patterns in monkey oviductal fluid before and after ovulation. Fertil. Steril. 21, 817–820 (1970).

Mastroianni, Jr., L., Urzua, M. and Stambaugh, R.: The internal environment fluids of the oviduct. In: The Regulation of Mammalian Reproduction, Eds.: Segal, S.J., Crozier, R., Corfman, Ph.A., Condliffe, P.G. Thomas, Ch. C. Publisher, Springfield, Ill., 1973, pp. 376–384.

Moghissi, K.S.: Human fallopian tube fluid: I. Protein composition. Fertil. Steril. 21, 821–829 (1970).

Oliphant, G. Randall. P. and Cabbot, C.L.: Immunological components of rabbit Fallopian tube fluid. Biol. Reprod. 16, 463–469 (1977).

Rebello, R., Green, F.H.Y. and Fox, H.: A study of the secretory immune system of the female genital tract. Brit. J. Obstet. Gynec. 82, 812–816 (1975).

Schumacher, G.F.B.: Über den Ablauf von Serumveränderungen bei traumatischer Entzündung. Verh. Dtsch. Ges. inn. Med. 66, 875 (1960).

Schumacher, G.F.B., Yang, S.L.: Cyclic changes of immunoglobulins and specific antibodies in human and rhesus monkey cervical mucus. In: The Uterine Cervix in Reproduction. Eds.: Insler, V. and Bettendorf, G.. Thieme, G. Publ., Stuttgart, 1977, pp. 187–203.

Shapiro, S.S., Jentsch, J.P. and Yard, A.S.: Protein composition of rabbit oviductal fluid. J. Reprod. Fert. 24, 403–408 (1971).

Yang, S.L., Schumacher, G.F.B.: Immune response after vaginal application of antigens in the rhesus monkey. Fertil. Steril. 1979 (in press).

Copyright 1979 by Elsevier North Holland, Inc.
F.K. Beller and G.F.B. Schumacher, eds.
The Biology of the Fluids of the Female Genital Tract

STUDIES ON THE PROTEIN CONTENT OF HUMAN OVIDUCTAL FLUSHINGS

D.H.A. Maas

SUMMARY

Oviductal flushings of 48 patients were studied for protein content and protein composition. In menopausal women and during non-gestational amenorrhoea only a basal secretion of proteins could be recorded in the oviduct. After estrogen treatment and during the preovulatory phase of the cycle an increased amount of soluble protein was measured. The highest values were found after ovulation and during pregnancy, suggesting a progestational influence on the proteins released into the oviductal lumen. Acrylamide electrophoretic separation of these proteins resulted in three major protein bands: albumin, transferrin and a postalbumin fraction (Rm_{Alb} 0,67 - 0,70). This postalbumin appeared in almost every sample of oviductal fluid, and showed a higher relative percentage than did transferrin. A comparable protein band was found in the sera of 18 patients, mostly menopausal women, with concentrations smaller than that of transferrin.

INTRODUCTION

The mammalian oviduct provides the environment for fertilization and early embryo development. Detailed knowledge of the composition of tubal fluid may be important in performing *in vitro* fertilization and for studies in reproductive bi-

Frauenklinik, Medizinische Hochschule, Hannover, Frg

ology. Data about oviductal secretions in the rabbit, sheep, cow and monkey are available (Hafez and Blandau, 1969), but only limited information exists about human tubal fluid, especially its protein content (Maas, 1976). In the present investigations we have measured the protein content and protein composition of several human tubal flushings, which were obtained from selected patients who underwent laparotomy and salpingo-hysterectomy.

MATERIALS AND METHODS

The oviductal fluid of 48 patients between the age of 15 to 74 years was studied. Surgery was performed for various diseases of the female genital tract—mostly fibroids and prolapsed uteri. Six groups of patients were formed, on the basis of menstrual history: 6 patients were in the preovulatory and 9 in the post ovulatory phase. When the last menstruation was not clear, plasma progesterone values were obtained to indicate the pre- or postovulatory phase. Two women were pregnant and 6 were amenorrhoic for 8 weeks to 7 months for various non-gestational reasons. The menopausal women were grouped into those with (N = 11) and without (N = 14) hormonal treatment. Only normal Fallopian tubes were studied. Immediately after exstirpation of the adnexa the oviducts were isolated, cleared of blood by rinsing with water and dried with paper. Then the oviducts were flushed with 5ml physiological saline from the fimbrial end. Blood contaminated samples were discharged. After centrifugation at 3000 rpm for 5 minutes, the protein content in the supernatant was determined by the method of Lowry et al. (1951). The flushings were concentrated by lyophilization and reconstituted with minimal volumes of distilled water. Disc gel electrophoretic protein separation was performed, according to Davis using the HAVANNA type apparatus (DESAGA co. Heidelberg, W. Germany) with gel tubes of 4 mm diameter and 120 mm length (Davis, 1964). Gels were stained with amido black in 7% acetic acid and scanned in a Zeiss Spectrophotometer at 575 nm. Disc gel electrophoretic separation was performed also on serum samples of each patient.

RESULTS

Flushing the oviducts resulted in the recovery of 0,006 to 0,294 mg protein per oviduct. The average protein content in the preovulatory phase of the menstrual cycle was 0,084 mg. This was significantly lower than that obtained after ovulation (0,156 mg/p < 0,05) (Table I). The amounts recovered from pregnant women were at the same high level, whereas during non-gestational amenorrhoea and during menopause the protein values were lower than in the preovulatory phase of cycle. Estrogen treatment in menopausal women caused a slight increase in the protein content up to the values seen preovulatory.

Electrophoretic analysis was performed on 46 oviductal flushings. In one case no protein-band was detectable while in all other samples at least an albumin peak was present. Because of this permanent appearance of albumin we have chosen the relative mobility to albumin for evaluating our electropherograms.

In all serum electropherograms the second highest peak was transferrin with a relative mobility of Rm_{Alb} 0,53 ± 0,02. A comparable transferrin band was present in 39 oviductal flushings with a Rm_{Alb} of 0,54 ± 0,03.

Besides some minor peaks which appeared irregularly a broad protein band between albumin and transferrin was found in 41 of the 46 electropherograms. This postalbumin band was resolved in our gels with an average relative mobility of 0,67 to 0,70; and differences between the groups of patients were not apparent (preovluatory phase of cycle Rm_{Alb} 0,66 − 0,70; postovulatory phase of cycle Rm_{Alb} 0,62 − 0,76; amenorrhoea Rm_{Alb} 0,64 − 0,75; pregnancy Rm_{Alb} 0,61 − 0,86; menopause without hormonal treatment Rm_{Alb} 0,60 − 0,75; menopause with estrogen treatment Rm_{Alb} 0,65 − 0,79).

Figure 1 and Figure 2 present the gels and electropherograms of two menopausal women − 59 and 57 years of age. In the tubal fluid of both patients the albumin peak, transferrin peak and that of the postalbumin fraction are discernible. In the serum of the first patient (M.R.) no protein band comparable to the postalbumin was visable, while a protein with the same relative mobility was detected in the other patient's serum (H.F.). A corresponding postalbumin band was found in 18 women, predominantly menopausal women and patients with non-gestational amenorrhoea (in 15 of 26 cases). It was present only in 3 of the 15 cycling women.

TABLE I. The Average Protein Content of Tubal Flushings in the Various Patient Groups

PROTEIN CONTENT OF HUMAN OVIDUCTAL FLUSHINGS

Preovulatory phase of cycle

    10.-15. day   n= 6 $\bar{x}$ = 0,084 ± 0,063 mg

Postovulatory phase of cycle

    16.-33. day   n= 9 $\bar{x}$ = 0,156 ± 0,087 mg

Amenorrhoea

    8 weeks - 7 months

                      n= 6 $\bar{x}$ = 0,053 ± 0,031 mg

Pregnancy

    10. week   n= 2   0,126 / 0,127   mg

Menopause

    2 - 32 years past last menstruation
    no estrogentherapy

                 n= 14 $\bar{x}$ = 0,058 ± 0,035 mg

        with estrogentherapy

                 n= 11 $\bar{x}$ = 0,075 ± 0,059 mg

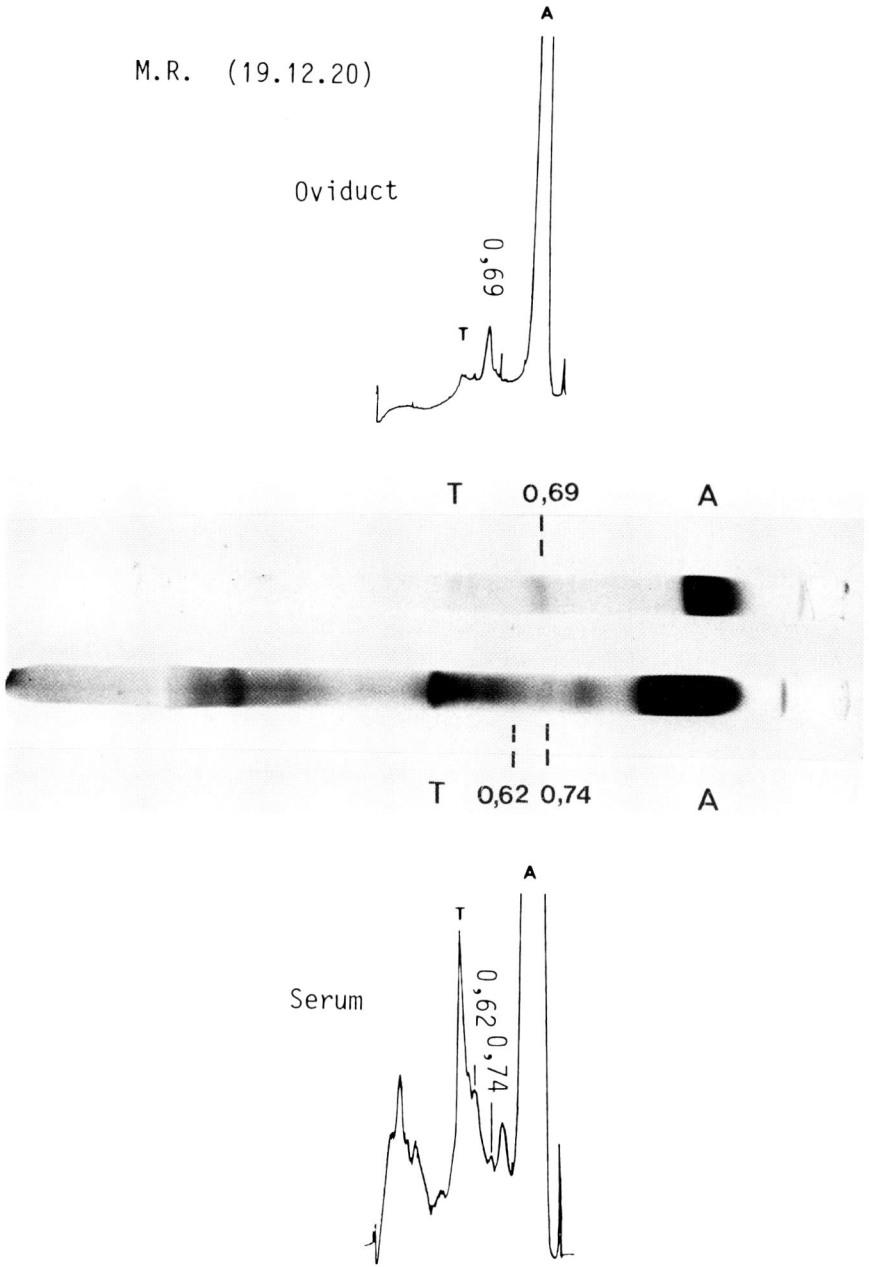

FIGURE 1. Polyacrylamide-disc-gels and electropherograms of the tubal fluid and serum of a 59 year old menopausal women. (A: albumin; T: transferrin)

DISCUSSION

The protein content of the oviductal fluid of cycling women increased from values of 0,084 mg before to 0,156 mg per oviduct after ovulation. During pregnancy similar high values were found, whereas during non-gestational amenorrhoea and during menopause the protein content was lower than it was in the preovulatory phase of the cycle.

During estrogen treatment the protein concentration of the tubal fluid was slightly higher than that without hormones, but the difference was not statistically significant. It is suggested that there might be a basal secretion of proteins in the tubal lumen, which can be stimulated by estrogen treatment and that may occur at a much higher rate under progesterone dominance.

An increase in the protein content of human oviductal fluid after ovulation was observed by David et al. (1973) and Lippes et al. (1972). Since we were unable to measure the volume of the tubal fluid, no direct comparison is possible.

The electrophoretic separation of the proteins in the tubal fluid resulted in three major bands: albumin, transferrin and a postalbumin fraction. This latter protein appeared in almost every sample of tubal fluid, and showed a higher peak than transferrin. A protein band with a comparable relative mobility was found in 18 sera, preferentially in those of the menopausal women. Whether these proteins in tubal fluid and in serum are identical will have to be shown by immunological methods.

Acrylamide disc gel electrophoretic investigations on human tubal fluids with particular attention to characteristic secretory proteins was reported by Beier et al. (1970), Moghissi (1970) and Beier and Beier-Hellwig (1973). Lippes et al. (1972) used for his study classical agarose electrophoresis and described an elevation of the β-globulin-fraction compared to the blood serum β-globulin of the same patients. Moghissi (1970) and Beier et al. (1970) demonstrated a characteristic posttransferrin fraction, that had no counterpart in the serum, and Moghissi (1970) indicated that this protein might be a glycoprotein based on PAS-staining. Beier et al., (1970) reported on characteristic pre- and postalbumin bands, that were not found in comparable amounts in the corresponding serum. An oviduct-specific protein was described by Noske and Feigelson (1976), using immunological means and antirabbit uteroglobin-antibodies. There was cross reaction in 4 specimens of human oviduct material, however, the specificity of this cross-reaction needs further study. There is no evidence for the presence of a uteroglobin-like protein in the oviduct or uterine secretions of the human.

The possibility that hemoglobin contamination may account for the major postalbumin fraction described in the present study cannot be eliminated. Preliminary results on epithelium homogenates indicate that the postalbumin fraction may be released by these cells. Immunohistology will be required to answer this question of cytological localization (Figure 3).

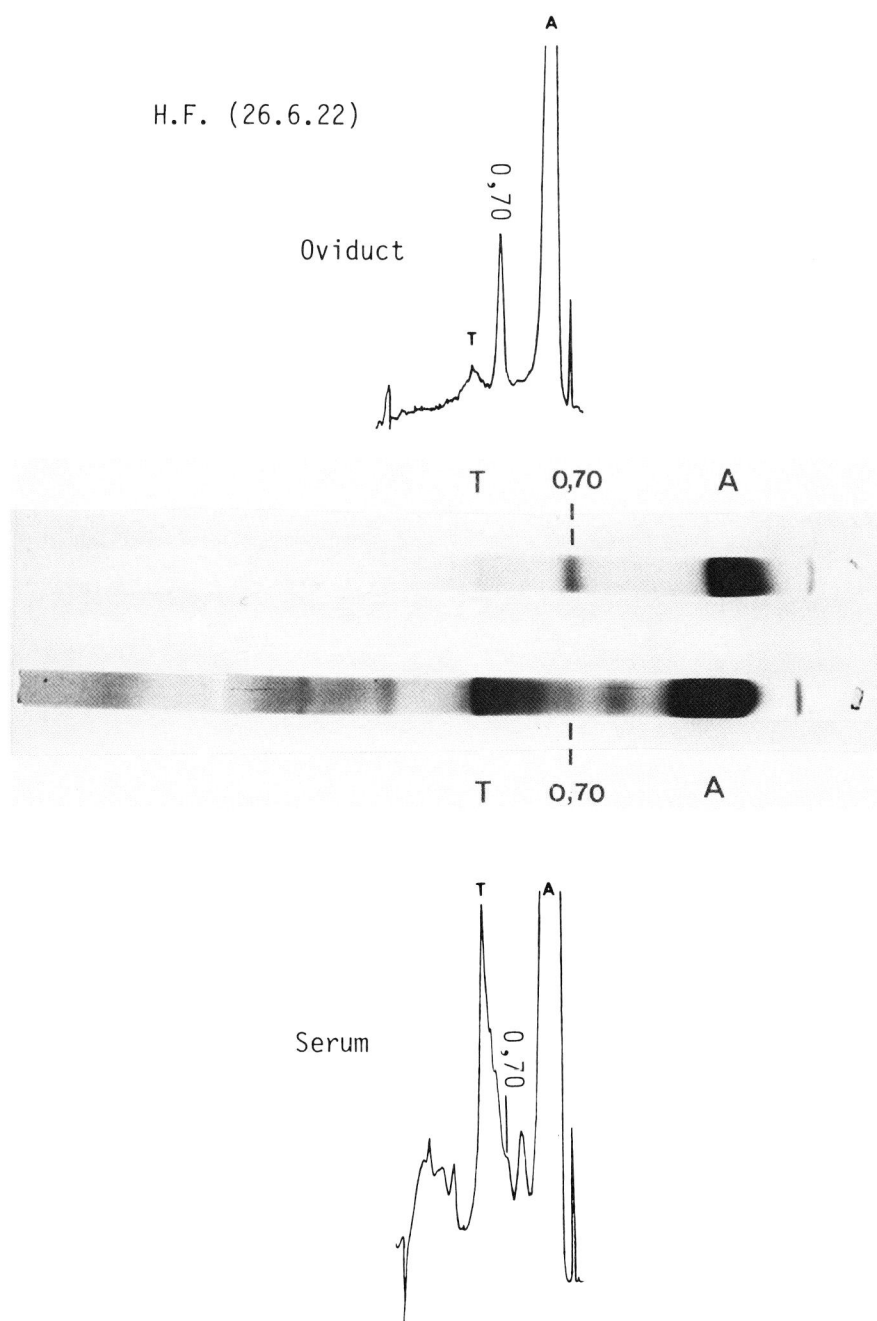

FIGURE 2. Polyacrylamide-disc-gels and electropherograms of tubal fluid and serum of a 57 year old menopausal woman. (A: albumin; T: transferrin)

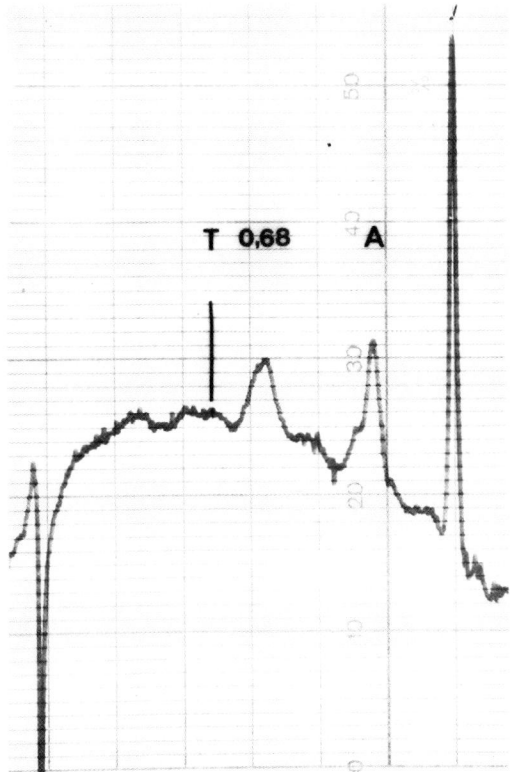

FIGURE 3. Electropherogram of homogenized isolated human tubal epithelium extracts. (A: albumin; T: transferrin)

REFERENCES

Beier, H.M., Petry, G., Kühnel, W.: Endometrial Secretion and early Mammalian development. In: 21. Coll. Ges. Biol. Chem. (H. Gibian & E.J. Plotz, EDS) pp. 264–285 (1970)

Beier, H.M., Beier-Hellwig, K.: Specific secretory protein of the female genital tract. Acta Endocr. (Kbh) (Suppl.) 180 : 404–425 (1973)

Davis, B.J.: Disc Electrophoresis II, Method and application to human serum proteins. Ann. N.Y. Acad. Sci. 121 : 404–427 (1964)

David, A., Serr, D.M., Czernobilsky, B.: Chemical composition of human oviduct fluid. Fert. Steril. 24 : 435–439 (1973)

Hafez, E.S.E., Blandau, R.J. (Eds): The Mammalian Oviduct. Univ. of Chicago Press, Chicago (1969)

Lippes, J., Enders, R.G., Pragay, D.A., Bartholomew, W.R.: Collection and analysis of human Fallopian tubal fluid. Contraception 5 : 85–103 (1972)

Lowry, O.H., Rosebrough, N.J., Farr, A.L., Randall, R.J.: Protein measurement with the Folin Phenol reagent. J. Biol. Chem. 193 : 265–275 (1951)

Maas, D.H.A.: Immunologie der Präimplantationsphase der Schwangerschaft-Proteingehalt und antigene Eigenschaften des Eileitersekretes beim Säugetier. Fortschr. Med. 94 : 1765–1770 (1976)

Moghissi, K.S.: Human Fallopian tube fluid, I. Protein composition. Fertil. Steril. 21 : 821–829 (1970).

Noske, I.G., Feigelson, M.: Immunological evidence of Uteroglobin (Blastokinin) in the male reproductive tract and in nonreproductive ductal tissue and their secretions. Biol. Reprod. 15 : 704–713 (1976)

Copyright 1979 by Elsevier North Holland, Inc.
F.K. Beller and G.F.B. Schumacher, eds.
The Biology of the Fluids of the Female Genital Tract

MAMMALIAN FERTILIZATION

D. P. Wolf

SUMMARY

The events comprising mammalian fertilization: sperm capacitation, the induction of an acrosome reaction, sperm incorporation into the egg and egg activation, are reviewed and evaluated in light of recent observations from the author's laboratory. The conditions commonly employed for *in vitro* fertilization in model mammalian systems are outlined, and attempts are made to relate the major conclusions derived from such studies to processes occurring naturally in the female reproductive tract. The probable importance of albumin in female reproductive tract fluids in the preconditioning of sperm is discussed. The nature of the sperm acrosome reaction and the mechanisms operative in its induction are considered, and cinemicrographs depicting capacitated sperm incorporation into zona-free mouse eggs are presented. Specific responses of the egg to penetration include cytoplasmic activation, as evidenced by the release of cortical granules, and nuclear activation when meiosis is resumed. The relationship of these events to the egg's block to polyspermy and subsequent developmental capabilities are examined.

Division of Reproductive Biology, Department of Obstetrics and Gynecology, University of Pennsylvania School of Medicine, Philadelphia, Pennsylvania, U.S.A.

INTRODUCTION

The term "fertilization", as commonly employed, encompasses a complex series of events which begins with the preconditioning of gametes in the female reproductive tract and includes: sperm penetration of egg investments, the cumulus matrix and the zona pellucida, fusion of sperm and egg plasma membranes, sperm incorporation into the ooplasm, male and female pronuclei formation and migration to the center of the egg, and finally, syngamy, the joining of haploid chromosomal complements. In mammals, fertilization usually occurs in the ampulla of the oviduct in the presence of tubal and follicular fluids which contain, among their principal constituents, plasma-derived and locally-secreted proteins, pyruvate, lactate, bicarbonate and various inorganic ions. Several recent reviews on various aspects of mammalian fertilization are available (Yanagimachi, 1977; Bedford and Cooper, 1978).

In considering the complex sequence of events that comprises fertilization, the necessity for simplification is obvious. Experimentally, one of the most rewarding approaches has involved the development and application of *in vitro* systems, and the prerequisite methodologies are now readily available in most common laboratory animals (Rogers, 1978). Accordingly, while it hasn't been demonstrated conclusively that *in vitro* conditions accurately reflect those *in vivo*, I would like to review the fertilization process as it occurs *in vitro* and attempt wherever possible to relate *in vitro* events and conditions to the processes occurring in the oviduct.

METHODOLOGY OF IN VITRO FERTILIZATION

Unfertilized tubal oocytes are usually recovered from superovulated animals and inseminated directly or after being freed from surrounding cumulus cells by exposure to the enzyme, hyaluronidase, in a Krebs-Ringer bicarbonate buffered medium, supplemented with lactate, pyruvate, glucose and serum albumin. When desired, zona-free eggs can be prepared by enzymatic or mechanical removal of zonae. Eggs are inseminated with caudal epididymal sperm (ejaculated sperm in the rabbit) at 10^4–10^6 sperm/ml and incubated for several hours at 37°C. Sperm are usually capacitated by preincubation in culture medium. All solutions are gassed routinely with 5% CO_2 in air and maintained at 37°C under a covering layer of silicone oil. Experiments are terminated by washing eggs free of adherent sperm, followed by transfer to a slide for mounting, fixing and staining with aceto-lacmoid. Eggs are considered penetrated when a sperm tail(s) and head remnants(s) are observed in the ooplasm. Fertilization of superovulated eggs with epididymal sperm is considered a normal process, since viable young are produced when transfers to foster mothers are made. In contrast, recent successful attempts at *in vitro* fertilization in the human have involved oocytes aspirated from mature ovulatory follicles and ejaculated sperm.

SPERM MOTILITY, CAPACITATION AND THE ACROSOME REACTION

Sperm motility, although of questionable importance when considering sperm transport through the female reproductive tract, still serves as a convenient indicator of fertility potential, as it is presumed necessary for successful sperm-egg interaction. The clinician often differentiates between normal and presumed subfertile semen specimens by motility measurements, and there are obvious differences in epididymal sperm preparations from the mouse in this regard. We are presently correlating motility scores with fertility in an effort to ascertain the importance of one for the other, thereby strengthening the diagnostic significance of motility testing. Motility can be measured by several methods; we use a turbidimetric technique that allows rapid, reproducible quantitation in 40 μl aliquots of semen and is applicable to the low sperm concentrations often associated with epididymal preparations (Sokoloski et al., 1977). So far, our experimental findings indicate that motility is a prerequisite for penetration, even of zona-free eggs in human sperm-hamster egg crosses or in the mouse system. The challenge, of course, in the human involves assigning significance to borderline semen specimens, such as those in the range of 5–20 $\times$ 10^6 cells/ml, and the turbidimetric method looks promising. Sperm motility is dependent upon an energy source, adequately provided by tubal fluid or the culture medium *in vitro*. Additionally, in the hamster, a motility stimulating factor of biological origin has been described.

Austin (1951) and Chang (1951) concluded independently that sperm must reside in the female reproductive tract before they are capable of penetrating the egg. This process, termed "capacitation", applies to both epididymal and ejaculated sperm, is a prerequisite for penetration of zona-free eggs and is probably ubiquitous among mammals. In some instances, capacitation can occur in the uterus or in the oviduct alone under the proper hormonal influence, although synergistic effects of the reproductive tract appear likely (Bedford and Cooper, 1978). At the molecular level, a destabilization of sperm membranes overlying the head, specifically the acrosome, is probably involved. *In vitro*, only capacitated epididymal sperm of the mouse bind to the zona in what is now seen as a calcium-dependent phenomenon (Saling et al., 1978). Capacitation of mouse, hamster, guinea pig and human sperm occurs in chemically defined medium containing albumin, and the latter has received notoriety as a possible natural capacitator. We have been interested in the ability of albumin to support mouse sperm capacitation. Epididymal sperm are preincubated under test conditions and then used for the insemination of zona-free eggs under non-capacitating conditions. A specificity for albumin can be demonstrated over proteins of similar molecular weight, and the requirement for albumin is concentration-dependent over the range of 2–20 mg/ml. Crystalline, fatty acid-free, heat-treated or acid-precipitated albumin is active, so it seems unlikely that the notorious chelating capacities of this protein are involved. In the hamster, even pepsin-digested albumin is active in inducing acrosome reactions (Meizel, 1978), but we do not yet fully appreciate the role of this important protein in mammalian fertilization.

Capacitation sets the stage for the occurrence of an acrosome reaction: multiple fusions of the sperm plasmalemma and the outer acrosomal membrane, producing extensive vesiculation and sloughing of the membranes limiting the acrosome (Yanagimachi, 1977). This process results in the exposure of lytic activity, presumably the trypsin-like enzyme, acrosin, which is implicated in sperm penetration of the zona pellucida and in sperm-egg fusion *per se*. Additionally, sperm hyaluronidase, which may be critical to cumulus dispersal, is released during capacitation or as a concomitant of the acrosome reaction. While reacted sperm can be recovered from throughout the female reproductive tract, a physiologic acrosome reaction is confined to capacitated sperm at or near the site of fertilization. *In vitro*, in the absence of a cumulus matrix, we think the acrosome reaction usually occurs only after sperm bind to the outer margin of the zona, and it may even be the rate-limiting step in the penetration process (Nicosia et al., 1977). Induction of the reaction is calcium-dependent, and it could involve: 1) specific factors of tubal, follicular or egg origin; 2) a spontaneous response to prevailing ionic conditions at the site of fertilization; or 3) a combination of these mechanisms. In vitro, it can be induced by a number of substances, including follicular fluid, cumulus cells and the divalent cation ionophore, A23187. Contrary to previous contentions, Moore and Bedford (1978) have demonstrated that follicular fluid and cumulus cells are not absolutely essential to sperm capacitation or to the occurrence of acrosome reactions either in vivo or in vitro. We have suggested that cortical granules which break down before sperm-egg fusion may play a role in inducing an acrosome reaction in the mouse (Nicosia et al., 1977). We are presently pursuing this and similar possibilities through the development of techniques for detecting morphologically and biochemically the occurrence of an acrosome reaction in living mouse sperm.

SPERM-EGG FUSION AND EGG RESPONSES TO PENETRATION

Cumulus cells surrounding the freshly ovulated oocyte are dispersed rapidly in the oviduct. Several factors have been implicated; namely, bicarbonate and the action of hyaluronidase either produced by the tubal epithelia or released by sperm. Preceding or during this process, capacitated sperm binding to the zona occurs followed by the acrosome reaction and zona penetration. Shortly after gaining access to the perivitelline space and the vitelline surface, binding between sperm and egg plasma membranes occurs. This interaction involves specifically that sperm plasma membrane covering the posterior region of the sperm head, the so-called equatorial segment, and microvilli-rich sites on the egg. In our studies on zona-free mouse eggs (Wolf and Armstrong, 1978), sperm incorporation occurred rather quickly after binding (Figure 1). As incorporation proceeded, the sperm sank into the egg cytoplasm, with the head becoming less refractile and its borders becoming less distinct. Engulfment of the sperm head is in progress in frame b of Figure 1, where vitelline particulate structures obscure the broad profile of the sperm head, and is probably complete by frame c or, at the latest, frame d, approximately 5 minutes later. Sperm head decondensation was seen initially in Figure 1, frame e, where a slight increase in head size is apparent. In frame f, decondensation has progressed substantially, and the head appears as a number of separated particulate structures. Subsequently, most of these structures disappeared, and a dramatic clearing occurred in the cytoplasm, radiating from the sperm insertion point, Figure 1, frame h.

Sperm penetration of the egg is associated with egg activation, early visible evidence of which includes: 1) the release of the egg's complement of cortical granules, and 2) the resumption of meiotic maturation in the "arrested" metaphase II oocyte. Activation does not result from the action of unique sperm contributions, since a number of different parthenogenetic treatments will also trigger the resumption of meiosis. Partly by analogy to marine invertebrate systems and partly due to mammalian investigations, we envision the molecular events of activation to involve initially changes in the egg plasma membrane's permeability, primarily to sodium, which in turn alters calcium uptake and culminates in increased intracellular free calcium levels. Microinjection of calcium into mouse

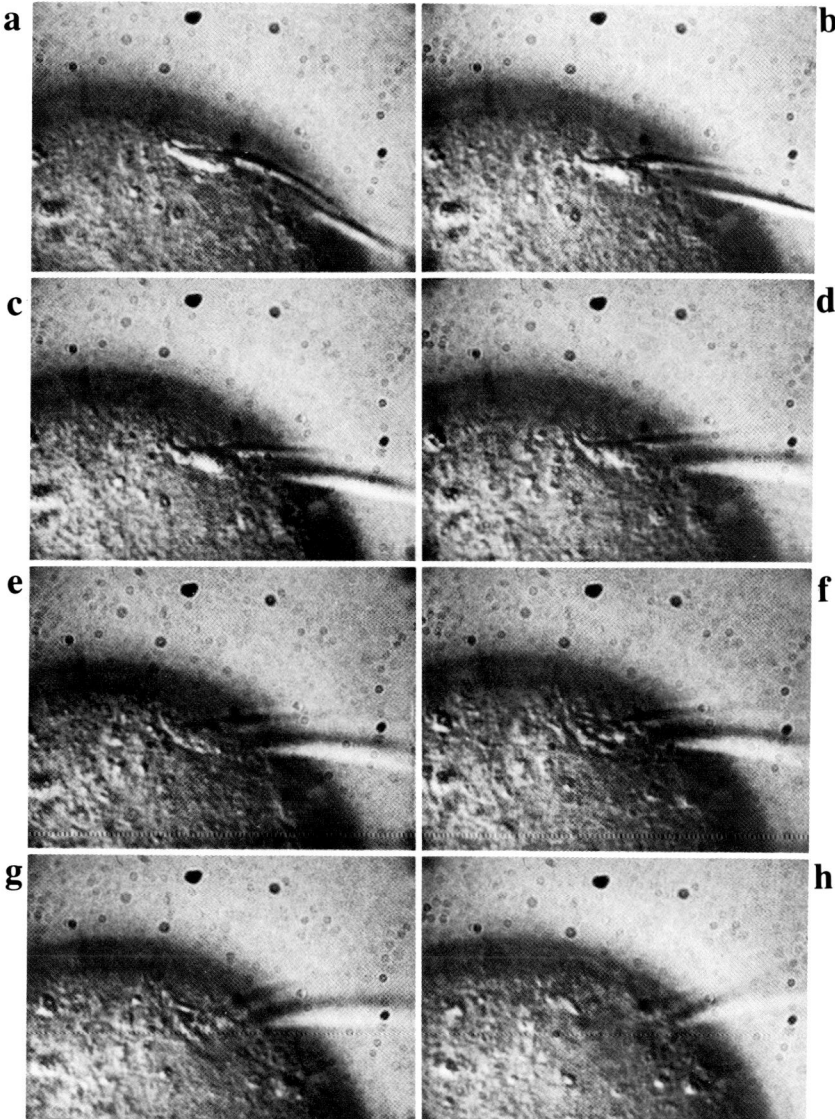

FIGURE 1. Capacitated epididymal sperm incorporation into the zona-free mouse egg. Focus was established initially at the egg surface and maintained throughout a filming time of 31 minutes. Times in each frame refer to the time after filming began. Insemination occurred 20 minutes before the filming started (one-second exposure; 20 frames/minute). Time after filming began: a) two minutes, 24 seconds; b) four minutes, 36 seconds; c) seven minutes; d) nine minutes, 48 seconds; e) 13 minutes, 30 seconds; f) 18 minutes, 42 seconds; g) 23 minutes, 45 seconds; h) 30 minutes, 33 seconds. (Reprinted from Wolf and Armstrong, 1978 with permission).

eggs elicits an activation response (Fulton and Whittingham, 1978), as does incubation of eggs in the divalent cation ionophore, A23187, in the absence of extracellular divalent cations (Steinhardt et al., 1974). Interestingly, calcium concentrations in postcoital ampullary fluid of the mouse are substantially reduced relative to serum levels (Borland et al., 1977). In the sea urchin egg, proton efflux and an elevation of intracellular pH is also an early response in egg activation (Epel, 1977). Activated ooplasm, in turn, controls nuclear events, the resumption of meiosis, sperm head decondensation and the formation of pronuclei through largely undefined mechanisms.

Egg activation is associated with establishment of a block to multiple sperm penetration. In mammals, multiple penetration leads to abnormal embryonic development and fetal wastage, hence its description as pathological polyspermy. Some interesting recent results from our laboratory indicate that the mouse egg may also be capable of physiological polyspermy; thus, the mean number of incorporated sperm recovered per inseminated zona-free egg reaches a plateau and then decreases as a function of time, concomitant with the extrusion or pinching off of cytoplasmic blebs containing sperm heads and pronuclei (Yu and Wolf, 1979). Several mechanisms are operative to prevent multiple sperm penetration. The female reproductive tract and the cumulus play a sieving role in restricting sperm access to the egg. Indeed, sperm reach the ampulla of the oviduct in a continuous progression, and their concentrations probably do not begin to approach those employed *in vitro*. The egg's block responses *per se* are twofold; a plasmalemma block and the zona reaction. The existence of a plasmalemma block is necessitated by the presence of perivitelline space sperm in monospermic embryos recovered from natural matings. In the rabbit, large numbers are always seen, while the rat and mouse show occasional supplemental sperm, and the hamster none (Austin, 1965). A block has been demonstrated in zona-free mouse eggs, and its temporal requirements (approximately 40 minutes post penetration) have been defined (Wolf, 1978). Although little definitive information exists concerning the mechanisms underlying this response, the masking or disappearance of sperm receptor sites on the egg plasmalemma is likely to be involved, and differences have been demonstrated in the sperm binding properties of unpenetrated and *in vivo* or *in vitro* penetrated eggs (Figure 2). Many mammalian eggs utilize a zona reaction to limit sperm penetration, a morphologically subtle change in the zona which has been correlated with alterations in zonae solubility, lectin binding and sperm binding properties. Cortical granules have been implicated as primary factors responsible for both of the egg's block responses (Austin, 1965). However, a cautionary note is warranted, since direct experimental evidence in mammalian systems is limited, apart from the observation that granules are absent in fertilized eggs. Crude cortical granule preparations have been isolated from activated zona-free eggs of the hamster and mouse. The subsequent incubation of zona-intact eggs in these preparations results in decreased levels of penetration, an activity which is susceptible to inhibition by synthetic and natural trypsin inhibitors. On this basis, a cortical granule trypsin-like activity has been implicated in the block response (Barros and Yanagimachi, 1972; Gwatkin et al., 1973; Wolf and Hamada, 1977). This activity has not yet been isolated or unequivocally associated with cortical granules. Moreover, in zona-free mouse eggs, premature loss of cortical granules does not influence subsequent egg penetrability by capacitated epididymal sperm (Wolf et al., 1979).

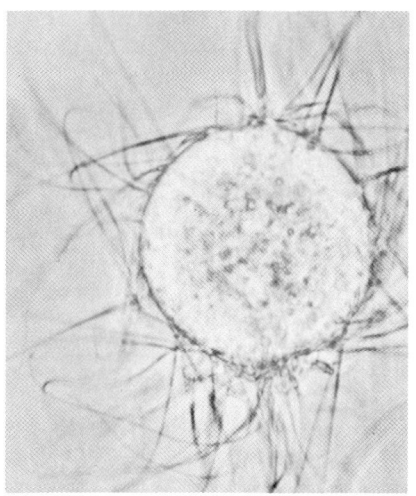 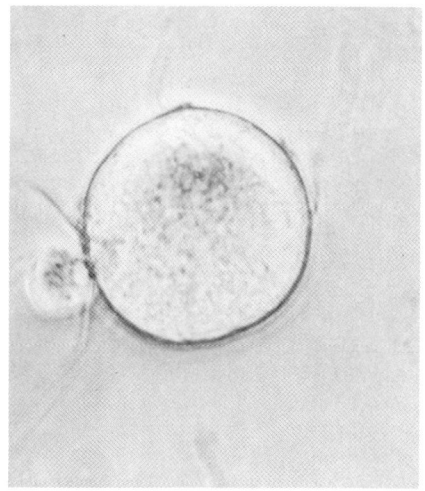

FIGURE 2. Capacitated sperm binding to zona-free mouse eggs. Whole mounts of living eggs. Left: Unpenetrated egg. Right: *In vitro* penetrated egg. Eggs were inseminated for 15 minutes with capacitated sperm (approximately 10^5 cells/ml), removed from the insemination dish, mounted on a slide and photographed without fixation or staining.

CONCLUDING COMMENTS

Based on pioneering studies conducted with gametes of lower vertebrates and marine invertebrates, substantial progress has been made at the molecular level in defining those events and mechanisms that comprise fertilization. Our understanding of mammalian fertilization has benefited immeasurably from these insights, while simultaneously appreciation for the uniqueness of the mammalian condition has accumulated. For instance, sperm capacitation, the occurrence of an acrosome reaction, and several aspects of sperm incorporation into the egg are relatively species-specific phenomena. On the other hand, the role of intracellular free calcium ion concentrations in triggering egg activation appears universal. The importance of a symbiotic relationship between mammalian and non-mammalian studies is especially notable when the biochemistry of fertilization is considered, for the size and availability of the mammalian egg are limiting. Extracorporeal fertilization, as in marine invertebrates, is, of course, relatively simplistic, as perhaps is *in vitro* fertilization of mammalian eggs when compared with the process as it occurs naturally. However, the present discussion attempts to make obvious the necessity of a coordinated approach involving, simultaneously, the characterization of the milieu in which fertilization occurs and the fertilization process *per se*.

ACKNOWLEDGEMENTS

The author expresses appreciation to all members of the laboratory who participated in the work described here and to Ms. Patricia Park for secretarial and editorial assistance. Supported by United States Public Health Service grant HD-06274.

REFERENCES

Austin, C.R.: Observations on the penetration of the sperm into mammalian egg. Austral. J. Biol. Sci. B4:581–596, 1951.

Austin, C.R.: Fertilization, Prentice-Hall, Englewood Cliffs, N.J., 1965.

Barros, C., Yanagimachi, R.: Polyspermy-preventing mechanisms in the golden hamster egg. J. Exp. Zool. 180:251–266, 1972.

Bedford, J.M., Cooper, G.W.: Membrane fusion events in the fertilization of vertebrate eggs. Cell Surface Reviews 5:65–125, 1978.

Borland, R.M., Hazra, S., Biggers, J.D., and Lechene, C.P.: The elemental composition of the environments of the gametes and preimplantation embryo during the initiation of pregnancy. Biol. Reprod. 16:147–157, 1977.

Chang, M.C.: Fertilizing capacity of spermatozoa deposited in the Fallopian tubes. Nature (London) 168:697, 1951.

Epel, D.: The egg surface in relation to metabolic activation at fertilization. In: Immunobiology of Gametes. Eds.: M. Edidin and M.H. Johnson, Cambridge University Press, Cambridge, 1977, pp. 235–254.

Fulton, B.P., Whittingham, D.G.: Activation of mammalian oocytes by intracellular injection of calcium. Nature (London) 273:149–151, 1978.

Gwatkin, R.B.L., Williams, D.T., Hartmann, J.F., and Kniazuk, M.: The zona reaction of hamster and mouse eggs: production *in vitro* by a trypsin-like protease from cortical granules. J. Reprod. Fert. 32:259–265, 1973.

Meizel, S.: The mammalian sperm acrosome reaction, a biochemical approach. In: Development in Mammals, Volume 3. Ed.: M.H. Johnson, North-Holland Publishing Co., Amsterdam, 1978, pp. 1–64.

Moore, H.D.M., Bedford, J.M.: An *in vivo* analysis of factors influencing the fertilization of hamster eggs. Biol. Reprod. 19:879–885, 1978.

Nicosia, S.V., Wolf, D.P., and Inoue, M.: Cortical granule distribution and cell surface characteristics in mouse ova. Develop. Biol. 57:56–74, 1977.

Rogers, B.J.: Mammalian sperm capacitation and fertilization: a critique of methodology. Gamete Res. 1:165–223, 1978.

Saling, P.M., Storey, B.T., and Wolf, D.P.: Calcium-dependent binding of mouse epididymal spermatozoa to the zona pellucida. Develop. Biol. 65:515–525, 1978.

Sokoloski, J.E., Blasco, L., Storey, B.T., and Wolf, D.P.: Turbidimetric analysis of human sperm motility. Fertil. Steril. 28:1337–1341, 1977.

Steinhardt, R.A., Epel, D., Carroll, E.J., and Yanagimachi, R.: Is calcium ionophore a universal activator for unfertilized eggs? Nature (London) 252:41–43, 1974.

Wolf, D.P.: The block to sperm penetration in zona-free mouse eggs. Develop. Biol. 64:1–10, 1978.

Wolf, D.P., Armstrong, P.B.: Penetration of the zona-free mouse egg by capacitated epididymal sperm: cinemicrographic observations. Gamete Res. 1:39–46, 1978.

Wolf, D.P., Hamada, M.: Induction of zonal and oolemmal blocks to sperm penetration in mouse eggs with cortical granule exudate. Biol. Reprod. 17:350–354, 1977.

Wolf, D.P., Nicosia, S.V., and Hamada, M.: Premature cortical granule loss does not prevent sperm penetration of mouse eggs. Develop. Biol. 71: 22–32, 1979.

Yanagimachi, R.: Specificity of sperm-egg interactions. In: Immunobiology of Gametes. Eds.: M. Edidin and M.H. Johnson, Cambridge University Press, Cambridge, 1977, pp. 255–295.

Yu, S.F., Wolf, D.P.: Zona-free mouse eggs are capable of disposing of supernumerary sperm. Proc. 12th annual meeting, Society for Study of Reproduction, August 1979, Quebec City, Canada p. 39A.

Copyright 1979 by Elsevier North Holland, Inc.
F.K. Beller and G.F.B. Schumacher, eds.
The Biology of the Fluids of the Female Genital Tract

PERITONEAL FLUID IN FEMALE FERTILITY AND STERILITY

P. R. Koninckx, I. A. Brosens, and W. H. Heyns

SUMMARY

Peritoneal fluid volume increases during the follicular phase of the cycle, and is highest during the luteal phase. The volume of peritoneal fluid is not influenced by pelvic varicosities, endometriosis, nor by the absence or occlusion of the fallopian tubes. Women taking oral contraceptives have low volumes of peritoneal fluid.

The concentrations of electrolytes in peritoneal fluid are comparable with those in serum. Protein concentration in peritoneal fluid is about 65 percent of that in serum except for prolactin and luteinizing hormone. During the luteal phase peritoneal protein concentration is significantly higher than during the follicular phase.

Free progestins and 17β-estradiol concentrations are always higher in peritoneal fluid than in serum. After ovulation a concentration for both hormones of 20 to 100 times higher than in serum is maintained for at least 1 week.

In women with an ovulation stigma the concentration of both progestins and 17β-estradiol are higher than in women with corpus luteum but without ovulation stigma (luteinized unruptured follicle syndrome).

The Unit for the Study of Human Reproduction, Department of Obstetrics and Gynecology, Katholieke Universiteit Leuven, Belgium

In conclusion, we suggest that peritoneal fluid is an ovarian transudate and that the progestins and 17β-estradiol concentrations could be used for the diagnosis of the luteinized unruptured follicle syndrome.

INTRODUCTION

Ovulation in the human is routinely estimated by basal body temperature, serum progesterone assay and endometrial biopsy.

These are however only secondary events associated with the formation of a corpus luteum but not with rupture of the Graafian follicle. Recently it was demonstrated in the human that a corpus luteum can be formed without ovulation: the so called luteinized unruptured follicle syndrome (Brosens et al., 1978; Koninckx et al., 1978; Marik et al., 1978).

The diagnosis of the luteinized unruptured follicle syndrome is, however, difficult to make in the individual patient since the rupture of the Graafian follicle cannot be demonstrated routinely.

We therefore investigated peritoneal fluid in order to ascertain whether steroid hormone assays could discriminate between a ruptured follicle with subsequent corpus luteum formation and a luteinized unruptured follicle.

MATERIALS AND METHODS

Patients and Peritoneal Fluid Collection

Women with regular menstrual cycles and women taking oral contraceptives were included in the present study. At laparoscopy a blood sample was taken and all the peritoneal fluid from the pouch of Douglas was aspirated and its volume measured. A sample of both blood and peritoneal fluid was assayed for hemoglobin; they were allowed to clot for 0.5 to 4 hours at room temperature, centrifuged for 20 minutes at 500 g, and the supernatant fluid was frozen until assayed.

During laparoscopy the ovaries were carefully inspected for the presence or absence of an ovulation stigma. Pelvic endometriosis was classified according to Acosta et al. (1973) and the presence of varicose veins in the parametria or in the infundibulo-pelvic ligaments was noted.

The day of the cycle was determined by basal body temperature (BBT) charts and by endometrial biopsy (Koninckx et al., 1977).

Assays

Sodium, potassium, chloride, carbon dioxide, calcium, phosphorous, urea, creatinine and total protein were assayed on a SMAC autoanalyzer (Technicon).

Transcortin was assayed by radial immuno-diffusion (Van Baelen et al., 1974) and sex hormones binding globulin (SHBG) by ammonium sulfate precipitation (Heyns et al., 1971). Prolactin, luteinising and follicle stimulating hormone (Koninckx et al., 1976), and 17β-estradiol (Verhoeven et al., 1979) were assayed by radio-immuno-assay.

Cortisol and progesterone were assayed by competitive protein binding (CPB). The extract was assayed for progesterone without prior chromatography as described by Johansson (1969). In later experiments we found in peritoneal fluid high concentrations of $20\alpha\beta$-pregn-4-en-3-one and of some unidentified Δ^4-3-keto steroid (unpublished results), which both compete actively with progesterone for transcortin. Therefore we will use "progestins" to designate the products measured in the progesterone CPB assay. Peritoneal fluids in which the concentration of progestins was higher than 100 ng/ml were not assayed for cortisol.

Standards

For LH, FSH and Prolactin, the MRC standards 68/40, 69/39 and 71/222 were used.

Statistics

Mean and standard deviations of hormone concentrations were calculated after logarithmic transformation. Means ±SD are indicated except when stated otherwise.

Statistical significance was evaluated according to Student's paired and unpaired t-test.

RESULTS

Volume

The volume of peritoneal fluid increased slightly during the follicular phase, but became much greater during the luteal phase of the cycle (Figure 1).

No correlation was found between the volume of the peritoneal fluid and presence or absence of pelvic endometriosis, the presence or absence of an ovulation stigma (Figure 1) or the presence of pelvic varicosities.

In two women without oviducts, 6 and 22 ml of peritoneal fluid was found on day 22 and 23 of the cycle respectively. In women taking oral contraceptives (combined pill) no variation was found during the cycle and the volume was uniformly low: 4.2 ±2.3 ml (n = 20).

Electrolytes

Differences between the concentrations of electrolytes in plasma and peritoneal fluid, although significant, were small (Table I).

No difference was found between women in the two phases of the cycle nor between the control group and the group with endometriosis.

Proteins

The concentration of proteins in peritoneal fluid was about 65 percent of the serum concentration except for LH and Prolactin (Table II). During the luteal phase protein concentration was significantly higher than in the follicular phase for total protein, transcortin and SHBG (Table III).

Contamination of peritoneal fluid with blood was estimated at 3 percent by hemoglobin assay: 14 ±4.4 g/dl (n = 11) in blood and 0.56 ±53 g/dl (n = 15) in peritoneal fluid.

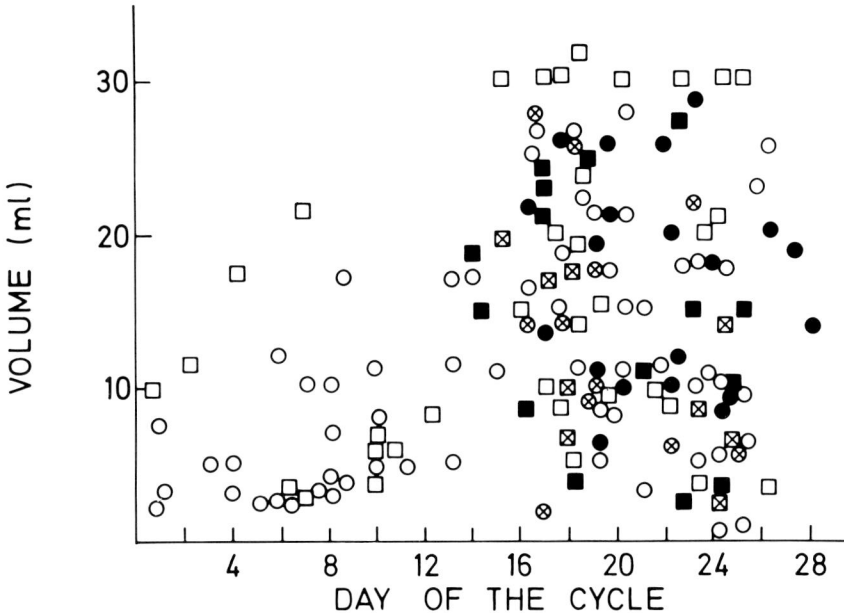

FIGURE 1. Peritoneal fluid volume in normal (○) women and in women with pelvic endometriosis (□). The presence (● ■), absence (○ □) or a doubtful (⊗ ⊠) ovulation stigma is indicated.

TABLE I. Electrolyte Concentrations in Peritoneal Fluid and in Plasma

	Plasma	Peritoneal Fluid	P Value
Sodium (mEq/l)	139.0 ± 3.2 [28]	136 ± 0.7 [36]	0.017
Potassium (mEq/l)	5.2 ± 0.7 [28]	3.9 ± 0.1 [36]	0.051
Chloride (mEq/l)	102.8 ± 1.4 [67]	110.6 ± 4.2 [86]	<0.001
Carbon Dioxide (mEq/l)	16.3 ± 0.3 [67]	22.4 ± 2.1 [86]	0.012
Calcium (mg/dl)	8.3 ± 0.2 [28]	7.4 ± 0.1 [36]	<0.001
Phosphorus (mg/dl)	2.9 ± 0.1 [67]	2.6 ± 0.1 [86]	0.003
Urea (mg/dl)	20.4 ± 0.7 [67]	21.1 ± 0.6 [86]	N.S.
Creatinine (mg/dl)	0.80 ± 0.02 [67]	0.70 ± 0.01 [86]	0.001

The mean ± SE and the number of determinations [ ] are indicated.

TABLE II. Protein Concentration in Peritoneal Fluid and in Plasma

	Plasma	Peritoneal Fluid	Percentage in Peritoneal Fluid
Total protein (g/dl)	6.4 ± 0.1 [67]	4.3 ± 0.1 [86]	68
Transcortin (mg/l)	34.2 ± 0.9 [53]	24.1 ± 0.7 [68]	71
SHBG (μg/l)	16.5 ± 0.7 [45]	11.2 ± 0.5 [61]	68
LH (mIU/ml)	4.8 ± 1.6 [28]	2.0 ± 0.4 [40]	42
FSH (mIU/ml)	3.0 ± 0.4 [41]	1.9 ± 0.1 [93]	63
Prolactin (mIU/ml)	3.4 ± 0.1 [41]	1.2 ± 0.1 [86]	34

The mean ± SE and the number of determinations [ ] are indicated.

Steroid Hormones

Total progestins and 17β-estradiol concentrations were much higher in peritoneal fluid than in serum during the luteal phase. During the follicular phase total progestin concentration was higher than in serum but the concentration of 17β-estradiol did not differ significantly (Figure 2).

After ovulation both the 17β-estradiol and the progestin concentration increased abruptly, remained elevated for several days and returned progressively to normal values after day 20 of the cycle (Figure 2).

The concentration of cortisol was 137.4 ±81 ng/ml in plasma (n = 52) and 53.7 ±33 ng/ml in peritoneal fluid (n = 36). No differences were found between the two phases of the cycle.

TABLE III. Concentration of Total Protein, Transcortin and Sex Hormone Binding Globulin (SHBG) in Peritoneal Fluid During the Cycle

	Total protein (mEq/l)	Transcortin (mg/l)	SHBG (μg/l)
Follicular phase	9.0 ± 0.3 [17]	20.3 ± 1.6 [19]	9.8 ± 1.4 [17]
Luteal phase day 14-20	10.9 ± 0.2^{ooo} [39]	25.1 ± 0.7^{oo} [29[	12.1 ± 0.5^{ooo} [29]
day 21-28	10.7 ± 0.2^{ooo} [29]	26.9 ± 1.5^{oo} [20]	11.1 ± 1.1 [15]

The mean ± SE and the number of determinations [ ] are indicated.
P versus follicular phase ^{oo} <0.005 ^{ooo} <0.001

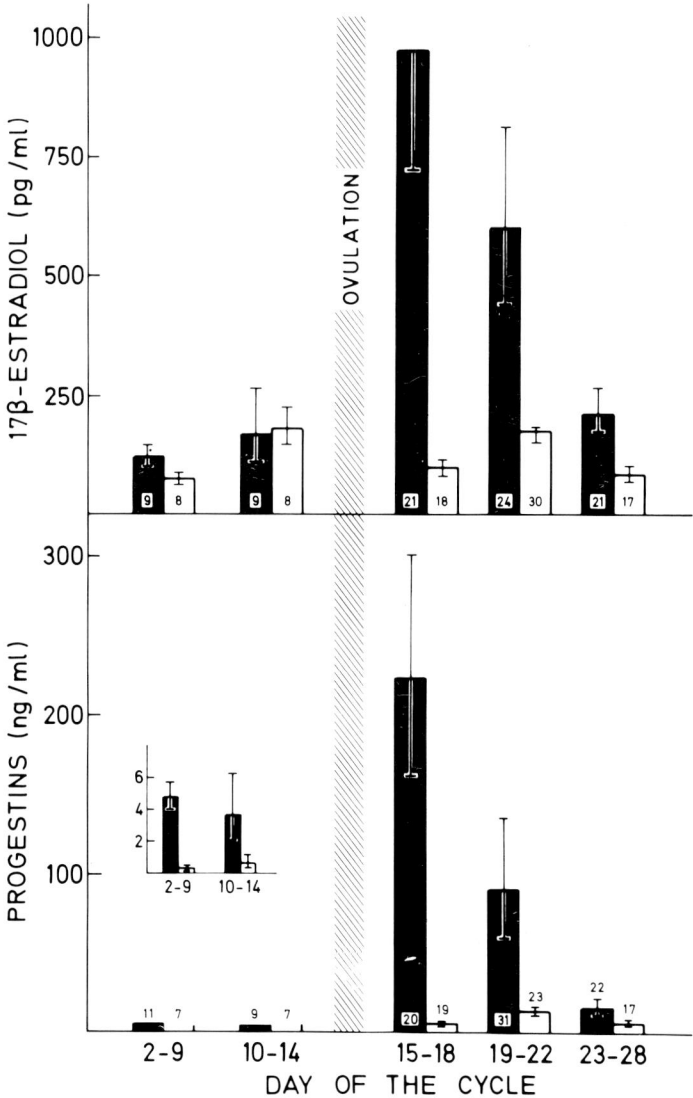

FIGURE 2. Progestins and 17β-estradiol concentrations in peritoneal fluid (closed bars) and in plasma (open bars) during the menstrual cycle. Mean ±SE and the number of experiments are indicated.

The Luteinized Unruptured Follicle Syndrome

Between days 14 and 20 of the cycle, the concentration of progestins (p = 0.022) and of 17β-estradiol (NS) were higher when an ovulation stigma was present (Table IV). The correlation between the presence of an ovulation stigma and the concentration of both progestins 17β-estradiol is significant (Table V).

DISCUSSION

Formation of Peritoneal Fluid

Our findings suggest that peritoneal fluid is predominantly a transudate of the hyperemic functioning ovary. In women using oral contraceptives, postmenopausal women, and men (Maathuis et al., 1978) only small amounts of peritoneal fluid are found. The volume of peritoneal fluid increases pari-passu with follicular development and is most abundant after the formation of the corpus luteum. In women without fallopian tubes the volume of peritoneal fluid is not notably lower suggesting that the peritoneal fluid is not predominantly a secretion of the tubes. These factors together with the finding that peritoneal fluid volume is not influenced by the presence of varicose veins also suggests that it is not merely due to peritoneal edema or transudation.

The hypothesis of an ovarian origin is strongly supported by the significantly higher concentrations of ovarian steroid hormones in the peritoneal fluid than in plasma during both phases of the cycle. Indeed when the lower (67%) concentration of SHBG is taken into account not only the progestins, but also the free 17β-estradiol concentrations are higher in peritoneal fluid than in plasma. The concentration of free cortisol, on the other hand, is very similar in

TABLE IV. Volume of Peritoneal Fluid and the Concentration of 17β-Estradiol, Progestins, Protein, Transcortin and SHBG (Day 14-20) in Women With and Without a Doubtful Ovulation Stigma

	Present	Absent	Doubtful
Volume (ml)	18.2 ± 2.1 [22]	20.1 ± 1.6 [32]	16.5 ± 2.5 [16]
17β-estradiol (pg/ml)	1497 (1020-2197) [11]	743 (512-1077) [18]	571 (389-838) [8]
Progestins (ng/ml)	316 (205-486) [11]	77 (53-113)° [18]	124 (61-250) [8]
Protein (mEq/l)	4.6 ± 0.2 [12]	4.5 ± 0.1 [17]	4.6 ± 0.1 [6]
Transcortin (mg/l)	24.4 ± 1.6 [9]	25.1 ± 0.6 [11]	25.0 ± 1.5 [6]
SHBG μg/l	12.6 ± 0.9 [9]	11.6 ± 0.9 [11]	12.1 ± 0.2 [6]

The mean ± SE or the mean (M−1SE, M+1SE) and the number of determinations [ ] are indicated.

TABLE V. Progestins and 17β-Estradiol Concentration in Women With and Without a Doubtful Ovulation Stigma

	Ovulation Stigma		
	Present n = 11	Absent n = 18	Doubtful n = 10
17β-estradiol concentration (pg/ml)			
>500	81.8%	44.4%°	60.0%
>1000	45.5%	16.7%	30.0%
>2000	45.5%	11.1%°	10.0%
Progestins concentration (ng/ml)			
>50	100.0%	55.6%°°	77.8%
>100	72.7%	27.8%°	66.7%
>200	54.5%	16.7%°	33.3%

P versus present   ° <0.05 °° <0.01

plasma and in peritoneal fluid: the total concentration of cortisol (60%) in peritoneal fluid is comparable with the transcortin concentration (67%).

Protein concentration in peritoneal fluid is about 65% of the plasma concentration. This suggests that peritoneal fluid is formed by transudation. The relatively low prolactin concentration in peritoneal fluid also suggests such a mechanism. The high plasma concentrations of prolactin are probably caused by stress and/or anaesthesia, and the equilibrium with peritoneal fluid was not yet reached at the moment of sampling.

The higher protein concentration in the luteal phase can be explained by increased vascular permeability in the hyperemic corpus luteum or to some degree of exudation after ovulation through the opened ovarian surface.

The Diagnosis of Ovulation

Concentrations of free 17β-estradiol and free progestins are some 20 to 100 times higher in peritoneal fluid than in plasma for at least 1 week following ovulation.

The concentration in peritoneal fluid of progestins measured by CPB are much higher than those of progesterone measured by radioimmuno-assay (Maathuis et al., 1978, and unpublished results). This discrepancy can be explained by the presence of steroid hormones cross-reacting in progesterone-CPB but not in progesterone-RIA. The progestin concentration has to be interpreted cautiously since the affinity of progesterone and of the interfering steroids for transcortin are not identical.

In order to maintain such a concentration gradient for several days, continuous steroid hormone secretion into the peritoneal cavity must be postulated. The very high steroid hormone concentrations found in the follicular fluid (McNatty et al., 1976) can only maintain high concentrations in the peritoneal fluid for a limited period of time after ovulation. When an ovulation stigma is present the concentrations in peritoneal fluid of both progestins and 17β-estradiol are elevated up to at least day 20 of the cycle. These data need careful interpretation since ovulation stigmas could have been overlooked at laparoscopy, or could have been reepithelialized. Indeed the life course of a normal ovulation stigma in the human is not known.

We therefore suggest that after ovulation some exudation takes place for several days through the ovulation stigma: this intercellular fluid derives from the corpus luteum and is laden with estrogens and progestins. When a luteinized unruptured follicle is formed only a lesser amount of transudation through the corpus luteum capsule occurs with consequent lower steroid hormone concentrations in the peritoneal fluid. Therefore we suggest that steroid hormone assays of peritoneal fluid could be used in the diagnosis of the luteinized unruptured follicle syndrome. High steroid hormone concentrations in the peritoneal fluid is direct evidence of the presence of a corpus luteum with stigma and therefore of ovulation sensu stricto.

ACKNOWLEDGEMENTS

We thank Prof. M. Renaer, Prof. P. De Moor, Prof. G. Dixon, Dr. G. Verhoeven, Dr. H. Van Baelen and Dr. Lissens for fruitful discussions and Miss V. Celis, Mr. B. Van Halewyck and Mrs. M.R. Van Gossum for excellent technical help. Our standards were a gift of the medical research council. This work was partly supported by a grant of the Fonds Derde Cyclus Catholic University of Leuven.

REFERENCES

Acosta, A.A., Buttram, V.C., Besch, P.K., Malinak, L.R., Franklin, R.R., and Vanderheyden, J.D.: A proposed classification of pelvic endometriosis. Obstet. Gynaecol. 42:19–25, 1973.

Brosens, I.A., Koninckx, P.R., and Corveleyn, P.A.: A study of plasma progesterone, oestradiol-17β, prolactin and LH levels, and of the luteal phase appearance of the ovaries in patients with endometriosis and infertility. Brit. J. Obstet. Gynaecol. 85:246–250, 1978.

Heyns, W., De Moor, P.: The binding of 17-hydroxy-5α-androstan-3-one to the steroid-binding β-globulin in human plasma as studied by means of ammonium sulphate precipitation. Steroids. 18:709–730, 1971.

Johansson, E.D.B., Wide, L.: Periovulatory levels of plasma progesterone and luteinizing hormone in women. Acta Endocrinol (Kbh). 62:82–88, 1969.

Koninckx, P., Bouillon, R., and De Moor, P.: Second antibody chemicaly linked to cellulose for the separation of bound and free hormone: an improvement over soluble second antibody in gonadotrophin radioimmuno-assay. Acta Endocrinol (Kbh) 81:43–53, 1976.

Koninckx, P., Goddeeris, P.G., Lauwereyns, J.M., De Hertogh, R.C., and Brosens, I.A.: Accuracy of endometrial biopsy dating in relation to the midcycle luteinizing hormone peak. Fertil. Steril. 28:443–445, 1977.

Koninckx, P.R., Heyns, W.J., Corveleyn, P.A., and Brosens, I.A.: Delayed onset of luteinization as a cause of infertility. Fertil. Steril. 29:266–269, 1978.

Maathuis, J.B., Van Look, P.F.A., and Michie, E.A.: Changes in volume, total protein and ovarian steroid concentrations of peritoneal fluid throughout the human menstrual cycle. J. Endocr. 76:123–133, 1978.

McNatty, K.P., Baird, D.T., Bolton, A., Chambers, P., Corker, C.S., and McLean, H.: Concentrations of estrogens and androgens in human ovarian venous plasma and follicular fluid throughout the menstrual cycle. J. Endocr. 71:77–85, 1976.

Marik, J., Hulka, J.: Luteinized unruptured follicle syndrome: a subtle cause of infertility. Fertil. Steril. 29:270–274, 1978.

Van Baelen, H., De Moor, P.: Immunochemical quantitation of human transcortin. J. Clin. Endocrinol. Metab. 39:160–163, 1974.

Verhoeven, G., Dierickx, P., and De Moor, P.: Stimulatory effect of neurotransmitters on the aromatization of testosterone by Sertoli-cell enriched cultures. J. Mol. Cell. Endocrinol. 13 (1979), 13:241–253.

Part IV:
SUMMARY AND CONCLUSIONS

SUMMARY AND CONCLUSIONS OF THE CONFERENCE *

R.M. Wynn

The first session was devoted to the oviduct and its secretions. The discussion was initiated by Dr. Pauerstein, who traced the history of tubal anatomy, crediting Fallopius with the first modern description of the fallopian tube. It was Fallopius who first pointed out that the tube did not originate from the ovary as do the homologous male organs from the testes. The regional anatomy of the tube was then described utilizing histologic and scanning electron microscopic techniques. The role of the inner longitudinal muscle in ovarian transport was elucidated. Dr. Pauerstein stated that the intrinsic muscle was not essential, nor was the ampullary-isthmic junction, at least in his experimental work in the rabbit. The complexity of the mucosal folds was described, as it increases from the cornua to the fimbriated ends; furthermore, the indistinct muscular layer in the ampulla was shown. He described a greater concentration of ciliated cells at the fimbriated end, although this observation has not been confirmed by all investigators. The anastomoses between the ovarian and the uterine arteries were emphasied with particular respect to tubal surgery. The nerve supply was then described. It was pointed out that the amine content varies with the hormonal state, although it was suggested that adrenergic innervation was not essential to ovum transport. Again, the implications with respect to tubal surgery were raised. A discussion ensued re-

---

* The following summary reflects the order in which the papers were presented at the conference. The sequence in the text proper was rearranged for more logical reference.

427

garding the relations of secretory, ciliated, and intercalary, or peg, cells in the oviductal epithelium. Dr. Pauerstein suggested that the peg cells were exhausted secretory cells and that there was not good evidence for estrogen-driven ciliogenesis. The question arose whether the cilia were crucial to the transport of the ovum. In this connection the clinical syndrome of immotile cilia, of which Kartagener's syndrome is an example, was mentioned. In this condition the cilia lack dynein arms and thus are therefore essentially functionless. Although the male has immotile sperm, the female is normally fertile.

The discussion continued with Dr. Blandau's presentation of mechanisms of tubal transport. He appropriately stressed the significant differences in mechanism among various species, using rodents, rabbits, and primates as examples. In the rat, for example, the ovary is surrounded by a periovarial sac, into which ovulation occurs freely. In addition, there is a ciliary crown on the spermatozoa in the rat. The spermatozoa apparently traverse the uterotubal junction one at a time. In the rabbit, the egg remains attached to the site of ovulation. As a result of dual ciliary action, deposition of a regular periovular coat occurs. In this species also, ciliary crowns are found. In the rabbit both ciliary current and muscular action appear important in tubal transport. Isoproterenol may paralyze the muscle but the egg is nevertheless propelled through the ampulla. In the human being there are no ciliary crowns and a longer period is required for transport of the ovum. Physical characteristics of the human egg have, in fact, not yet been quantified. Unlike Pauerstein, Blandau believes that ciliary action is important in human ovum transport. A technically superb motion picture of tubal transport of ova in the rat was then shown. Isthmic activity appears to vary with hormonal status. In the rabbit the ovum cannot be pulled easily from the site of ovulation even with forceps. In the rabbit the regularly deposited extracellular coats presumably reflect ciliary action and the rotation of the ovum in all directions. In the human being also, isthmic function depends on hormonal status. Again, the great interspecific differences in tubal function were stressed.

Dr. Wolf then presented data from Dr. Mastroianni's laboratory on tubal secretions. He showed that the fluids resulted from both secretion and transudation. Various methods of collection were described, emphasizing the influence of estrogen on the volume of fluid. Macromolecules that appeared in the fluid were mostly proteins, but no quantification of the unique proteins in tubal fluids was described. Trypsin-inhibiting activity in the oviduct did not reflect the plasma concentrations, implying that the responsible substances did not result entirely from transudation. The pH was recorded with in-situ probes, and microprobes were used also for measurement of oxygen tension and steroid concentrations in the tubes.

Dr. Spornitz studied the hormonal status of patients at the time of laparotomy and correlated these data with ultrastructural observations. He quantitated the ratios of ciliated to non-ciliated cells throughout the cycle but found that the ultrastructural appearance of the tube at the time of cesarean section did not correlate well with that of any particular phase. He found also a basal level of secretion in postmenopausal women. Finally, he reported the effect of a minipill (Exlutona) on oviductal fine structure.

Dr. Lippes presented his analysis of the constituents of the human tubal fluid, obtained through catheterization of the oviduct at the time of elective sterilization. Electrolytes and glucose were measured in the oviductal fluid and in the serum. Amylase was twice as high in the fluid as in the serum, and lactate dehydrogenase was ten times higher in the fluid. Constituents varied with the hormonal states. Xanthines and related compounds also varied according to endocrine status. If the catheter were left in situ for more than 72 hours, leukocytes appeared. The situation is different from that in certain experimental animals, in which a more nearly physiologic fluid was collected after several days of catheterization. Presumably these changes in xanthines and related substances reflect synthesis of nucleic acids for nourishment of the embryo.

During the ensuing discussion of the first few papers, opinions differed on the definitions of peg, or intercalarly, cells and reserve cells. The consensus was that the reserve cell was a monocyte and that the peg, or intercalary, cell was probably an exhausted secretory cell. The unavoidable effects of the experimental method, whether morphological or physiological, on the tissues under study were clearly brought to light. An important question was whether the hormones acted directly on the tube or indirectly through other mechanisms. Hormonal receptors were discussed as they appear during different phases of the cycle and in different portions of the female genital tract. It was pointed out that the presence of ovulation from one ovary and pregnancy in the contralateral tube does not necessarily reflect external migration of the ovum in the human being but rather pickup of the ovum by the contralateral tube.

Dr. Schumacher then spoke about specific antibodies. He showed that antibodies could be raised against T-4 phages in the Rhesus monkey and measured by phage neutralization techniques after antigens were applied vaginally and systemically. The implications of this technique for immunological control of fertility were suggested. Unfortunately, a high antibody level in the tube is required for this purpose. He found that the level of antibody in the tube was approximately ten times lower than that in the circulating serum. The antibody levels during treatment with gonadotropins decrease by a factor of five, with the minimum approximately two days after administration of HCG.

The next paper, by Dr. Wolf, dealt with fertilization. He showed the vesiculation of the plasma membranes of the capacitated sperm in relation to penetration of the zona pellucida. He showed also that the dispersal of the cumulus followed fertilization but was not a prerequisite to it. Apparently the loss of cortical granules is associated with the block to polyspermy. This block may occur either in the zona pellucida or in the vitellus and may vary according to species. The importance of scientific study of *in vitro* fertilization has become more obvious since the birth of the first alleged test-tube baby, which was an extraordinary example of fundamental scientific data following rather than preceding clinical application. The hamster may be a poor model for the study of *in vitro* fertilization because its egg accepts spermatozoa from a variety of unrelated mammalian species, including man. Practically, however, the creation of a premature block to polyspermy may be developed as a contraceptive technique.

The next paper, by Dr. Koninckx, concerned the biochemistry of peritoneal fluid. He described a low volume of peritoneal fluid in women who are postmenopausal and in women who are using oral contraceptives. Steroid hormone concentration always appears to be higher in the peritoneal fluid than in the plasma. He concluded that the peritoneal fluid was an ovarian transudate insofar as its volume was not affected by the absence of tubes or uterus. Assays of progesterone and 17-beta estradiol may help in the diagnosis of the luteinized unruptured follicle syndrome, which appears to be an important clinical entity in his clinic.

Dr. Maas continued the dicussion of the protein content of tubal fluids. In his experiments the tubes were flushed and the protein content was measured in the fluid. The content appears to be increased after ovulation but was still present in reduced amounts in the menopause.

In the discussion that followed these papers the question arose regarding the main function of the tube, that is, transportation or preparation for fertilization. It was pointed out that the survival of spermatozoa, that is, motility, is not equivalent to fertilizability. The question was asked whether the peritoneal fluid could arise from the peritoneum itself and steroids from the ovary. It was pointed out that in this connection the male has no peritoneal fluid.

The session on the vagina was appropriately introduced by Dr. Ferenczy, whose interest in that organ is well known. His morphological presentation included light microscopy, scanning and transmission electron microscopy, and radioautography. Emphasis was placed on the desmosomes, the hemidesmosomes, and the gap junctions. He pointed out that the sparseness of desmosomes in the superficial layers of the epithelium may be correlated with facilitation of desquamation. The synthesis and degradation of collagen were then described.

Dr. Moghissi described the constituents of the vaginal fluid. Very few studies have, in fact, been made of this fluid, which must be regarded as a transudate inasmuch as there are no vaginal glands. Sodium was low and potassium was high in this fluid compared with the respective values of these electrolytes in plasma, with the implication of active transport. Volatile acids and amino acids were also described. Many proteins present in the cervix were absent from the vaginal fluid although some were found in both locations. The presence of immune globulins was suggested in possible relation to infection.

The next paper, by Dr. Gorm Wagner, described in detail the fluids of the vagina in particular relation to sexual arousal. Oxygen and pH measurements in association with orgasm were described.

In the general discussion that followed these presentations, it was noted that vaginal lubrication was present even after construction of an artificial vagina but few quantifiable data were available.

The third session was devoted to postpartum fluids. In the first paper, Dr. Hirsch discussed the bacteriology. He pointed out, as expected, that there were fewer organisms recovered with transabdominal than with transcervical methods. The most common organisms found were T-mycoplasma, bacteroides species, diphtheroids, and anaerobic cocci. Growth of the anaerobes was greater when the anaerobic medium was supplemented with carbon dioxide. A sharp rise occurred at the time of delivery, particularly in *E. coli*. The organisms were similar in cervix, vagina, perineum, and amniotic fluid. He stated that the same organisms were found in febrile and afebrile patients after cesarean section. It was therefore suggested that postpartum colonization was less important in infection than was trauma incident to delivery. The bacteria causing the infections are usually endogenous organisms.

Dr. H. Wagner then described the morphology of the postpartum uterus, utilizing light and electron microscopic techniques. He differentiated the placental from the nonplacental portions of the endometrium. There was no difference in rate of endometrial regeneration in women who lactated as compared with those who did not. There appeared to be an inverse relation between the number of fibroblasts and typical decidual cells. He suggested that enzymes are related to this transformation and that regeneration of the placental site required a longer period. The events of regeneration were correlated with the appearance of the lochia.

Dr. Ebert then presented biochemical data on the lochia, with particular reference to clotting factors and she compared the proteins in the lochia with those in the serum. There appears to be high proteolytic activity of the lochia.

In the discussion of these papers it was suggested that a high concentration of T-mycoplasma (Ureaplasma) reflects greater sexual activity. It was pointed out that transcervical cultures were valueless in bacteriologic studies of patients with intrauterine devices. Perhaps the uterus with a foreign body behaves differently from the postpartum uterus with respect to its susceptibility to infection. The question was raised whether the differences in socioeconomic class reflect differences in the types and numbers of bacteria or rather a difference in host resistance. In a clarification of the relation of decidual cells to fibroblasts, it seemed that the decidual cells were replaced by fibroblasts rather than transformed into them.

The afternoon session concluded with another technically superb movie by Dr. Blandau, showing fertilization and polar body formation of the mouse egg *in vitro*.

The fourth session was devoted to the endometrium. The first paper, by Dr. Wynn, was devoted to morphology of the endometrium, in which classical cyclic histology was correlated with electron microscopy (scanning and transmission) and ultrastructural localization of enzymes. During this presentation, emphasis was placed on the origin and significance of the nucleolar channel system and of the possible role of glycogen, glycoproteins, and giant mitochondria. The relation of estrogens to ciliogenesis was again discussed.

Dr. Moyer's paper on the cellular elements of endometrial secretions followed. He flushed the uterus and counted the leukocytes, which were increased after IUD usage. As time passed after insertion of the foreign body, the proportion of polymorphonuclear leukocytes increased. Erythrocytes also passed through the endometrium and discharged their granules into the endometrial fluid. Phagocytosis of sperm by polymorphonuclear leukocytes was illustrated.

Dr. Flowers then presented a paper on enzymology of the endometrium. He reviewed histologic and ultrastructural data previously presented and elaborated on the histochemical demonstration of a variety of enzymes using PAS, alcian blue, and other stains. He attempted a close correlation of the electron microscopic and histochemical appearance of the endometrium with the clinical events of the menstrual cycle.

During the discussion of these papers, the question was raised whether progesterone acted on its own or primarily through estradiol. The consensus was that estradiol was required before the endocrine and morphologic effects of progesterone could be manifested. It was noted that the nucleolar channel system was not found in women on the minipill, despite their having ovulated. Nevertheless, this endometrium was considered to be not representative of normally responsive tissue. Further discussion ensued about the function of glycogen and, in fact, of the decidua itself. Again, the pitfalls of the comparative approach were stressed, with particular reference to the great variations in the implantation relation in even closely related species. Caution was expressed about teleologic approaches and overinterpretation of histochemical data obtained from endometrial studies. It was suggested that the appearance of red cells in the endometrium following insertion of an IUD probably represented breakdown in the capillary endothelium rather than diapedesis.

Continuing the discussion of endometrial secretions, Dr. Beier presented biochemical data derived from animal experimentation. He showed that it was possible, in animals, to ligate the genital tract and thereby collect large volumes of fluid. He found a large band of uteroglobins in the rabbit but, instead, a family of macromolecules in the rat and mouse. It appears that all of these proteins are steroid-dependent. The preuteroglobin and uteroglobin may be involved in formation of the coverings of the rabbit blastocyst. The human protein pattern appears to resemble that of the rodents more than it does that of the rabbit, in the sense that there is not one large macromolecular band. The maternal uterine proteins may be prerequisites to the establishment of early pregnancy. As a practical consideration with respect to *in vitro* fertilization, it was suggested that the developmental ages of egg and endometrium must closely approximate each other if implantation is to take place.

Dr. Schumacher, in presenting techniques of studying secretions, clearly pointed out the difficulties in obtaining human secretions in reasonably normal circumstances. Trauma or other conditions imposed by the experiment yield a fluid that is different from that in the natural state. He explained his method of obtaining tissue cylinders from the inner surface of the uterus and studying the enzymes by radial diffusion on agar. He also described the preparation of endometrial secretions from the surgically removed uterus. Immunoglobulins and complement components were found in both endometrial fluid and serum, as were proteinase inhibitors. Selective secretion rather than passive transudation was apparent. Fibrinolytic enzymes and fibrinogen-related antigens were also studied in the endometrial fluid and the serum.

Dr. Tauber continued the biochemical discussion of human endometrial secretions. He studied proteins of the proliferative, periovulatory, and secretory phases and came to the following conclusions: the proteins under consideration were present in highest concentrations in the periovulatory phase; the concentration was higher in the cervical mucosa than in the uterus; immunoglobulin IgG was found in greater concentration than was IgA; alpha$_1$-antitrypsin was present in higher concentrations than was alpha$_1$-antichymotrypsin; and plasminogen activator was highest in the fundus.

The final paper of this session was contributed by Dr. Denker, who discussed inhibitors of trophoblastic proteinases. He referred to this enzyme in the rabbit as blastolemmase, which acts like trypsin and may be involved with implantation in the rabbit.

In the discussion that followed it was pointed out that some of the material studied consisted not simply of uterine secretion but included uterine tissue itself, which therefore must have been contaminated with blood, at least from the subepithelial vessels. Again the problems of collection and the artifacts of preparation were stressed. Inhibiting implantation by interference with blastolemmase was considered in possible relation to control of fertility. Again, the limitations of the comparative approach were stressed, with elucidation of the unique anatomic properties of the implanting blastocyst of the rabbit. The exact details of implantation in the human being have never been adequately studied for obvious technical and perhaps ethical reasons.

The final session was devoted to morphology and biochemistry of menstruation. Dr. Taubert introduced the session with a clearly organized summary of relevant hormonal data, including steroid levels, binding proteins, and receptors. He concluded with a discussion of the role of prostaglandins and their clinical implications.

Dr. Ferenczy then presented convincing histologic and autoradiographic evidence bearing on current theories of endometrial regeneration. He summarized three current concepts: regeneration of the endometrium from stumps of basal glands and adjacent intact endometrium; conversion of residual spongiosa into proliferative endometrium; and conversion of stromal fibroblasts into proliferative endometrium. Ferenczy concluded that regeneration of the human endometrium occurred from areas peripheral to denuded zones, i.e., the tubal ostia and lower uterine segment, as well as from basal glands. He suggested also that in the rabbit the regeneration was essentially a process of healing, as in other injured tissues, and was not dependent on estrogen.

Dr. H. Wagner, studying hysterectomy specimens by electron microscopy, confirmed the findings of Ferenczy. He stated that stromal regeneration was not a significant factor. He showed a few islands of residual spongiosa and carefully pointed out the limitations of scanning electron microscopy in the study of a dynamic process such as menstruation. Perhaps the amount of residual functionalis is related to irregular shedding of the endometrium. Dr. Flowers presented additional histochemical and ultrastructural data relative to the menstrual endometrium.

Dr. Lindemann showed a series of hysteroscopic pictures of the endometrial surface throughout the menstrual cycle. He described changes in viscosity of mucus and depicted the gross appearance of superficial bleeding.

In the ensuing discussion, the question arose about the importance of studying the mechanism of menstruation. The answers related to understanding mechanisms of abnormal bleeding, for example, anovulatory dysfunctional bleeding and breakthrough bleeding with oral contraceptives. It was further questioned whether the breaks seen at hysteroscopy were artifacts, inasmuch as they were not seen in the freshly removed uterus. A final question concerned diurnal variations in mitotic activity in endometrial epithelium and stroma.

The last major topic addressed was the incoagulability of menstrual blood. Dr. Beller carefully traced the history of studies of menstrual bleeding. He mentioned the interesting differences in volumes of menstrual blood loss in various geographic regions. Most obviously, fibrinogen is absent from menstrual blood; prothrombin and Factor V are very low; but Factors VII and VIII are present. Factor IX is normal, but platelets number only about 10,000. Dr. Beller then addressed the crucial question of why menstrual blood does not coagulate. He stressed the importance of enzymatic breakdown of fibrinogen and local proteolytic activity. Menstrual blood, furthermore, has a high concentration of fibrinogen split products, which themselves prevent further coagulation. He suggested that the mechanism of incoagulability of intraperitoneal blood in cases of ruptured ectopic pregnancy was different.

Dr. Ebert then presented technical details of the enzymatic analysis of the clotting mechanism. She showed that fibrinogen was very rapidly dissolved by a variety of enzymes.

In the final general discussion the significance of the endocrine products of the blastocyst itself was addressed. Suggestions for future research included study of the fluids of the female genital tract in abnormal conditions. Some skepticism was raised about the need for preparation of fluid exactly like that of the oviduct as a requirement for *in vitro* fertilization. A lengthy argument then ensued regarding the basic nature of research and the conceptual construction of experiments, hypotheses, and theories. Dr. Wynn referred the group to the philosophical treatises of Ernst Mach and Jules Henri Poincaré as background for further discussion.

The group expressed its unanimous appreciation to Organon and Dr. Günther Weiland in particular for the extraordinary efficiency with which this conference had been organized. It voiced its hope that the published proceedings would be as valuable to the readership as the conference was to the participants.

INDEX

Entries in italic indicate tabular material; entries in bold-face indicate illustrations.

A

acid phosphatase, 11, 49, 55, 73, 75, 77, 78, 81
acrosome reactions, 408–410
acrylamide disc gel electrophoresis, 403
actinomycin D, 157
activation of plasminogen to plasmin, 255
adenocarcinoma, 62
advanced secretion, 103
aerobic cultures
  lactobacillus Döderlein's bacillus, 16
alanine, 18
albumin, 13, 19, 91, 104, 119, 124, 166, 281–283, **292**, 339, 401, 403, 407, 409
alcian blue, 73, 74, 76
  cell coat of, 207
aliphatic acids, 16
  nonproducers of, 16
  producers of, 16
alkaline phosphatase, 53, 73, 75–77, 80, 206–207, 282, 340
acid phosphatase, 206, 210, 213
α-amylase, 124, 126
α-antichymotropsin, 124, 131–134, **138**, 142, 340
α_1-antitripsin, 13, 19, 119, 124, 131–133, 137, 142, 146, 153–154, 156, 281–283, 340
α_2-haptoglobin, 13, 19–20
α_2-macroglobulin, 13, 19–20, 124, 153, 156, 247–248, 281–283, 295, 340
α_1-trypsin inhibitor, 247–248
amenorrhea, 266, 368, 371
amino acids, 18, 27
ampulla
  human, 302, **304**, 307, **315**, 320, 323, 325–326, 328, 340
  monkey, 326
anaerobic cocci, 259, 261
anaerobic cultures, 258
amylase, 429

antibodies, 390, 397, 429
anticlotting activity, 255
antithrombin III, 124, 247–248, 281–283
apical cytoplasm, 212
apical secretion, 191
apocrine secretion, 49, 52
aprotinin, 156, 284
arginine, 18
arginyl bonds, 152
arteries, spiral or coiled, 164
artifacts, 30
artificial coitus, 14
aspartic acid, 18

B

baboon, 105
bacteria, 60, 64, 257, 375
B. fragilis, 258
bartholin glands, 14
basal cytoplasm, 212
basalis, 207
basophils, 64, 81
β-galactosidase, 129
β-globulin, 337
β-glucorinadase, 6
β-glycoprotein, 104, 337
β-lipoprotein, 13, 19–20
biopsies, 74–75, 362–363
biosynthesis, 22
blastocyst, 89–91, 96, 100–105, 107, 109, 116, 147, 167
blastolemmase, 151–152, 154
  similarity to trypsin, 152
  nature of bond, 152
  subsite positions, 152
  residue, 152
  specificity pocket of, 152
blood flow, 25–26, 29, 31–32
blood perfusion rate, 32–33
blotting method, 119, 122, 129
boar seminal plasma trypsin-acrosin inhibitor, 154, 156, **158**
blood coagulation, 234–240, **239**

435

C

C¹q, 124, 133
C1r, 133
C¹3, 124, 131–132, 134, 141
C3–C6 acids, 16
C_3C, 281–283, 341
C¹3 activator, 124
C¹4, 124
CBG, 166
CO_2-hysteroscopy, 225
C-reactive protein (CRP), 19, 124, 396
CRP (*see* C-reactive protein)
calcium, 373, 379, 416
cannula, 29, 117, 336, 393
capacitated sperm, 410, **413**
capacitation, 338, 409–410
carbohydrates, 74–75
carbon dioxide, 416
carbonic anhydrase, 340
cardiac cycle, 30
cat, 324–325
cathepsin-D, 11, 124
cells, 310–311, 346, 363
  basal, 6
  decidual, 40, 49, 76, 86–87, 265–266, 268–269, 276
  endometrial, 43, 61–62, **98**, 171
  epithelial, 38, 43, 49, 60, 62, 76, 81, 85–86, 92, **98**, 177–178, 181, **350**, 354
  exfoliated, 60–62
  glandular, 60, 76, 87, 178
  immunocomponent, 22
  inflammatory, 60–61
  intercalated, 363
  intermediate, 6–7
  Langerhans, 9
  migrating, 60, 64–65
  mononuclear, 59, 61
  peg cells, (intercalated), 363
  plasma, 22
  red blood, 60, 64, **65**, 395
  stellate, 38
  stromal, 39–40, 60, 62, 75–77, 85, 87, 178
  superficial squamous, 6, **8–9**
  villous, 361, 363–364, **366–369**
  white blood, 60–61, 124, 146
cells containing foreign matter, 60
cells of menstrual tissue, 60
cells of the uterine fluid, 59–60
centrosomes, 363, 367
ceruloplasmin, 13, 19, 119, 124, 281–282, 295
cervical canal, 60–61, 279
cervical cap, 27
cervical cytology smears, 61–62
cervical fluid, 28
cervical mucus, 19–21, 60, 64–65, 107, 116, 119, 131, 148

cervical secretion, 14–15, 18, 20, 107, 117, 142
cervicitis, 19
cervico-anginal artery, 3
cervix, 8, 14, 19, 26, 29, 118, 129, 133, 142, 265
cervix uteri, 276, **277–278**, 279
chimpanzee (*see* monkeys)
chloride, 378, 416
  concentration, 28–29
chorionic gonadotropin (*see* gonadotropin)
chromogenic substrates, 248, 253, 282, 285
chymotrypsin, 124
cilia, 191
  cat, 324–325
  rabbit, 324–325
ciliogenesis, 53, 312, 354, 362, 368, 371
cinematography, 331
clitoris, 33
  clitoral stimulation, 32–33
coagulation factors, 237
collagen, 11
collagenase, 11, 124, 146–147
collecting chambers, refrigerated, 392
compacta, 207
complement components, 124, 131–134, 141, 147
complement system, 147
contamination,
  red cells, 395
  with blood constituents, 142
contraception, intrauterine, 132
contraceptives, oral, 16, 417
contractile activity, 331
cornification, 7
cornua uteri, 226, 300
corpus luteum, 118, 163–164, 166, 416
corpus mucosa, 133
corpus uteri, 129, 134, 142
cortical granules, 410, 412
cortisol, 416, 419
cow, 91, 105
creatinine, 383, 416
cumulus, 339, 408, 410, 412
cumulus matrix, 408
curet, 60
cylic changes in cervical mucus, 142
cyclic thrombocytopenia, 237
cytology smears, 61–62
cytoplasm, 6, 38–43, 49, **51**, 53, 60, 67, **70**, 81, 86, 167, 171, 179, 308–309
cytoplasmic vesicles, 62
cytosol binding sites, 167, **168**, **169**
cytosol receptors, 167, 169, 171

D

dating of the endometrium, 37
decidua parietalis, 269, **270**, **272**, **274–257**, 276

deer
    doe, 92
    roe, 91
defense system, 142, 147
delayed secretion, 103–104
desmosomes, 62
desquamation, 61, 163–164, 178, 189, 191, 196
    endometrial, **190**
    epithelial, **192**
    glandular openings, 190
dialysis sacs, 29
diagnosis of ovulation, 422
diaphragms, 26
direct measurement, 33
DNA-historadioautography, 5
DNA-synthesis, 6
DPNH-diaphorase, 6
dryness of vagina, 26

E

E. coli, 259, 261
edema, 38–39
egg activation, 410, 412
egg transport, 320–326
    ampullar, 324, 326
    fimbrial, 324
    monkeys and women, 326
    ovulated, 326
    rabbit and cat, 324–325
eggs, 323
elastase, 11, 124, 146–147
electrode, oxygen, 33
electrode, vaginal, 29, 31
electrolytes, 13, 25, 28, 373, 375, *378*, 415, 417
electron microscopy (*see also* scanning electron microscopy and transmission electron microscopy), 5–6, **63–64**, **68–69**, 362, 364
electrophoresis, 91, 104–105, 337
electrophoretic analysis, 400
electrophoretic protein separation, 400, 403
embryo, 339–340
    preimplantation, 60
embryoblast, 107
endocervical canal, 60, 62
endocervix, 52
endometrial
    cancer, 146
    cavity, 64, 117, 181, 257–261, *260*, 300
    degeneration, 177
    fluid, 59–60, 116, 118, 122, 124, 126, *127–128*, 129
    glands, 53
    mucosal shedding, 178
    nuclei, 42, 107
    secretion, 91, 115–117, *121*, 129, 148
    in vivo, 117
endometritis, 261
endometrium, 26, 37, **38–41**, 42, **44–47**, **50**, 52, **53**, **55–57**, 64, 73, 74, 78–91, 101, 105, 107, 116–119, 131–134, **143**, **144**, 146, 163–168, **177–182**, 265, 371
    activator activity in, **240**, **241**
    desquamation of, 225
    early, **228**
    destructed, 191, **200**
    human, 153
    luteal phase, 191, **194**
    menstruating, 187, **192**, 201, 203–222
    proteinase inhibitors in, 153
    re-epithelization of, 197
    regeneration, 187
    repaired, 191, **198**, **200**
    "shedding of" epithelial surface of, 196
    surface of, 225
endosalpinx, 300, **303**, 316, 336, 340
endothelial cells, 217–218
endothelial surface, 65
enzymatic activity, 234
enzymes, 6, 75, 84
    electrophoretically distinguishable, 154
enzyme technology, 248
eosin, 74–75
eosinophils, 64
epithelial reparation, 191
epithelium, 40, 42, 74, 299, 308, **310**, **347–349**, 354, 356, 362–363, **365**, 368
    acid phosphatase in, 210
    apical secretion of, **194**
    denudation of, 207
    denuded and intact, 191
    desquamation of, **192**
    endometrial, 38, 53
    endometrial surface, 195
    glandular, 39, **41**, 42–43, 55, 60–65, **63**, 167, 171
    regeneration of, 191, **199**
    squamous, 3, 5, 6
    superficial, 59–60, 62, 65
    surface, 61, 64, 79, 269
    vaginal, **4**, 5–6, 9, 14–15, 28–29, 33
    turnover time, 5
erythrocytes, **195**, 208
esterase, 6
estradiol, 17-β, 92, 100, 153, 181, 415–416, 419, 421–**422**
estradiol (E_2), 5, 92, 95, 163, 165–169, **170–171**, 172
estrogen, 6, 14, 16, 22, 26, 31–32, 52, 61–62, 81, 89, 91, 101, 115–117, 145, 164, 168, 173, 181, **184**, 313, 337–338, 340, 345, 362, 370–371, 375, 403, 423
Evaporimeter (probe), 27

F

Fallopian tubes, 60, 90, 299, 305, 308, 310, **358**, 374, 397, 427
  cornua of, 191
Fallopius, 427
fatty acids, 13, 16, **17–18**
fertilization, 37, 340, 408, 413, 429
fibrin, 19, 253, 255, 282
fibrin degradation products, 248, **252**, **285**
fibrinogen, 124, 247–248, 252, 255, 282–283, 295
  fibrin(ogen) breakdown products, 239
  degradation products, 255, 281, 285, 295
  split product D, 124
  split product E, 124
fibrinogenolysis, 248, 255
fibrinolysis, 124, 146, 237
filter papers, 28, 32–33, 116, 118–119, 122
fimbria, 319–321, 326
  ovarica, 300, **301**, 304
fluid protection, 32
Foley catheters, 374, **376–377**
follicle stimulating hormone, 204, 208
functionalis, 206
  endometrium layer, 177–178
fundus, 118, 129, 131, 133, 148, 181, **183**

G

gametes, 341, 408, 413
  transport, 320, 326, 390
γ-G.K. (Bence Jones), 13, 19
γ-detector, 32
γ-chains, 13
ganglia, 307–308
gelatin substrate film tests, 152
gestational endometrium, 74
globulin, 91
glucose, 373, 375, *378*, 379
glucose-6-phosphatase, 55
glycine, 18
glycogen, 6–7, 16, 42–43, 49, 53, 74, 76, 81–83, 85, 210
glycoproteins, 11, 74, 76, 84, 87, 106, 210, 281–283, 295, 339, 403
golgi, 309
  apparatus, 43, 49, 312, 354
  hypertrophy, 84–85
Gomori method, 210, **211**
gonadotropin, 74, 178, 181, **184**, 393, 396–397
  chorionic, 164
granular endoplasmic reticulum, 49

H

haptoglobin, 124
heat measurement, 33
heat method, 31
hematoxylin, 74–75
hemidesmosomes, 6
hemolytic complement, 395–396
hemorrhagic shock, 211–212
heparin, 232
heterophagocytosis, 11, 214
histidine, 18
hormonal profiles, **346**, **352–353**, **356–357**
hormonal status, 337–338
hormones, 320
human oviduct, 390–391
human oviductal fluid (HOF), 373–375, **376–377**, 378, 383, **384**, **385**, 390, 403
human chorionic gonadotropin (HCG), 389, 393–394, 397
human menopausal gonadotropin (HMG), 389, 393, 397
human tubal flushings, 400
hyaluronidase, 339, 408
hypermenorrhoea, 232
hyperplasia, 62
hypoxanthine, 379, 383
hysterectomy, post-partum, 266
hysterectomy specimens, 132, 142, 188
hysteroscope, 225

I

IgA, 124, 131–134, **136**, **141**, 142, 146, 281–282, 295, 340–341, 390–391
IgD, 124, 126
IgG, 112, 131–134, **135**, **141**, 142, 146, 281–282, 295, 341, 390–391
IgM, 19–20, 124, 126, 281–282, 295, 341, 390–391
ideopathic thrombocytopenic purpora, 232
iliac veins, 5
immune assays, 248
immunization, 391–392
immunocytes, 145
immunodiffusion, 20, 91, 118, 124
immunoelectrophoretic techniques, 19–20, 122
immunofluorescence, 379
immunoglobulins, 11, 13–14, 19–20, 22, 91, 107, 119, 124, 126, 129, 131, 133–134, 141–142, 145–146, 295, 341, 390, 397
immunological reactions, 105
implantation
  initiating factor, 152
  inhibiting factors, 157
incoagulability, 234, 237, 240
  proteolysis and digestion, 234
inflammatory processes, 146
inflammatory reactions, 396
inhibitors, 252

inhibitors of enzyme, 340
inorganic constituents, 15
inter-alpha-trypsin inhibitor, 124, 154
intercellular space, 9, 29, 33, 62, 116, 118
IUD (see intrauterine devices)
interstitium, 64
intrauterine devices, 59–61, *62*, 64–65, 116, 122, 147, 148, 255, 355–356
  menstrual blood loss associated with, 158
intraluminal secretion, 39, 49
introitus, 27–29
involution, 265
  of decidual, 266
ions, 29, 320
iron, 232
isoleucine, 18
isoproterenol, 325
isthmus, 302, **303**, **309**, 319, 326–329, **330**, **331**
  contractile activity, 327, 332
  motility, 329

K

KSCN extractable activators, 239
kallikrein, 124, 247, 249, 284
karyorrhexis, 209

L

lactate dehydrogenase, 429
lactating women, 364
lactation, 266
lactobacillus, 259, 261
  Döderlein's bacillus, 16
lactoferrin, 106–107, 119, 124, 126, 132–133
lamina propria, 14, 304, 379
laporotomy, 389, 391–393
leucine, 18
leukocytes, 13–14, *62*, 65, 268, 276, 295, 375
  polymorphonuclear, 40, 276
level of antibodies, 393
light microscopy, 363–364
lipid, 49, 73, 210–222, **212**, **213**
liposomes, 312
Lippes loop, 59, 61
liquid chromatography, 375
local immune system-uterine tissues, 145
lochiae 268, 279, 281–284, **286–295**
  flavae, 276
lumen, 80, 91, 208–216, 311, 335
  glandular, 39, 41, 62, **63**, **64**
  vaginal, 14–15, 34
luteal phase, 60, 311–312, 354, 417
luteinized unruptured follicle syndrome, 416, 421, 423

luteinizing hormone, **204**, 206
lymphatics, 307
lymphocytes, 9, 14, 40, 60–61, 64–65, 195, 276, 370, 391
lynestrenol, 354
lyophilization, 118
lysosomal acid phosphatase activity, 85
lysosomal activity, 255
lysosomes, 46, 55, 78, 81, 84, 118, 147, 213–214, **215**, 216, 268, 354, 356–357
lysozyme, 119, 124, 126, 131–134, **139**, 141–142, 147

M

mRNA (see Messenger Ribonucleic Acid)
Maccaque, 92
macrophages, 60–65, 214–215, 268–276
  in stroma, **217**
magnesium, 373
Marquiles spiral, 59
masturbation, 14
menopause, 316
menorrhagia 234
Menotoxin, 232
menstruation, 148, 163, 177
  hematological data, 232
  significance of, 232
menstrual bleeding, 231–242
menstrual blood,
  coagulation factor in, **239**
menstrual blood loss, 232, **233**
  cellularity, *238*
  enzyme activity, 234, *236*
  inorgacic substances in, *237*
  in surveyed population, **233**
  "normal value", 232
  organic substances in, *238*
  per day, *234*
  physical data, *236*
  review of literature, *233*
menstrual "plasma", 232
menstrual "serum", 232
mesosalpinx, 300, 307
Messenger Ribonucleic Acid (mRNA), 41, 93, 95, 171
metaplastic transformation, 178
microapocrine, 83
micrococcus luteus substrate, 132
microimmunodiffusion, 19
microphages, 269, 276
micro radial diffusion, 118, 122, 126
mid-cycle surge, 165
millipore filter, 61
mitochondria, 42–43, 49, 79, 82–83, 211–212, 309, 312, 363, 364, 369
mitotic figures, 39, 42

monkeys, 164, 166, 392
  chimpanzees, 166
  Maccaques, 92
mons pubis, 32
motility, oviductal, 341
mouse, 91, 92, **94**, 105
mucins, 74, 76, 90, 104
mucosal ultrastructure, 345
mucous membrane, 228
mycoplasma, 259
myometrium, 41

N

neutral proteinase, 124, 133
neuroanatomy, 307
neutrophils, 59–61, 64–65, 70, 146–147
nexus, 6
niacin, 383
nonproducers, of aliphatic acids, 16
non-nucleated, 60
nuclei, 214
nucleolar channel system, 46, **48**, 49

O

olfaction, 16
oocyte, 90, 408, 410
oophorectomy, 14, 173
  bilateral, 132
organelles, 6, 43, 49
orgasm, 32–33
orosomircoid, 13, 19–20
osmium tetroxide, **212**
ovarian cycle, 164, 310–311
ovarian follicles, 26, 118
ovarian steroids, 73
oviduct, 26, 52–53, **301**, 320, 331, 335, **351**, 354, 361–362, 368, 370–371
  epithelium, 363, *364*
  postmenopausal, 354
oviductal fluid, 335–341, 373, 389–390, 393, 396–397, 400, 403
  collection, 336, 392
  trace elements, 340
oviductal flushings, 400
oviductal motility, 341
oviductal secretion, rabbit, 390
oviductal sensors, 331
ovulation, 393
ovum, **305**, 339

P

PAS (*see* Periodic Acid Schiff)
paroophoron, 300
pelvic fascia, 3
Periodic Acid Schiff (PAS), 73–75, 209–210, 220

periodicity, loss of, 216
peritoneal cavity, 26
peritoneal fluid, 415–*421*, 429, 430
peritoneum, 375
phage neutralization, **394**, **395**
phagocytose vesicles, 212
phagocytosis, 67
phagosome, 67
phosphorus, 378, 416
phosphorylase, 49
photopletysmography
  vaginal, 30, 33
pinocytosis, 212
pinocytotic vesicles, 86
placenta
  insertion site, 268, 269, **271**, **273**, 276, 279, 285, 295
  site repair, 266, 276
plasma, 15, 28
  progesterone, 164, 166
  proteins, 65, 167, 234, 283
plasmin, 124, 147, 255
plasminogen, 124, **127**, 240, **255**, 281–284, **292**, 295
  to plasmin
    activation of, 255
plasminogen activator, 119, 124, 126, 129, 131–134, **140**, 141, 147, 148, 255
pleomorphic masses, **214**
plexus, 307, **308**
  mucosal, 5
  venous, 3, 14, 306
    hemorrhoidal, 3
    pudendal, 3
polyachrimide gels, 90
polyps, 62
polyspermy, 412
portio externa
  of cervix, 14
post partum fluid, 146
postalbumin, 403
postmenstrual endometrial repair, 181
posttransferrin, 106
posterior vaginal fornix, 61
postmenopausal oviduct, 354
postovulatory secretory phase, 38, 39, 52
potassium
  concentration of, *28*, *29*, 373, 378–379, 416
prealbumin, 106
predecidual cells, 207–209, 212, 219–220
preimplantation, 95
premarin
  oral, 32
producers, of aliphatic acids, 16
progestational agents, 117
progesterone, 16, 43, 49, 53, 74–75, 89–95, 99–103, 107, 115–117, 145, 153, 163–173, 266, 337–340, 345–346, 400, 416

plasma, 164, 166
progestins, 415, 419, 421, *422*, 423
progestogen, 89, 92, 167, 172, 362
prolactin, 422
proliferative phase, 42, 43, 52–54, 60–61, 73–81, 84, 87, 133–134, 145, 164, 166–168, 310, 314, 337, 371
 early, **226**
proliferation-maturation-desquamation, 5, 38, 179
proline, 18
prostoglandins, 11, 65, 172, 320, 341, 379
protease-inhibitors, 105
protein, 73, 81, 89–95, 97, 99–109, 118, 122, 126, 132, 141–145, 166, 247, **284**, 285, 390, 416, 417
 concentration of, 417
 content, 399–*401*, 403
 foreign, 60
 plasma, 65, 167, 234, 283
 tubal fluid, 337
 vaginal fluid, 19–20, 22
proteinase, 119, 124, 151–159
 activity associated with implantation, 152
proteinase inhibitors, 100, 119, 124, *126*, 129–134, 141–146, 153
 in rabbit blastocyst, *155*–**158**
prothrombin, 282, 283, **292**
proteolysis, 234
proteolytic activity, 239
 of menstrual blood, 249, 253, 255, 283, 285, 295
pseudomenstruation, 173
pseudopods, 62
pseudostratification, 38, 39, 42, 49
puerperal phase, 268
puerperal uterus, 259, 261
puerperium, 313, 362
pykinosis, **194**
pykinotic nuclei, 209

R

RER (*see* rough endoplasmic reticulum)
RNR (*see* ribonucleoprotein)
rabbit, 22, 61, 91–**93**, 99, 100, **102**, 104–105, 107, 167, 181, **324**, **325**, 331, 338, 390
radioimmunoassays, 74, 378, 422
radiometer (electrode), 31
radiothymidine, 181
rat, 91–92, **95**, 105, **322**, **323**
receptor-binding of steroids, 171
red blood corpuscles, 30
regression of decidua parietalis, 276
repair mechanism, 276
reserve cell, 310, 369
reticular stroma, 216

rhesus monkey, 16, 106, 124, 389, 391, 396
re-epithelialization, 207
ribonucleoprotein (RNA), 53, 73–76, 145, 383
ribosomes, 49, 81–82, 84, 171
rough endoplasmic reticulum (RER), 81–82

S

SEM (*see* scanning electron microscopy)
SGOT, 282
SGPT, 282
SHBG, 166, 167
scanning electron microscopy (SEM), 7, 34, 49, 52–53, 73–75, 79, 220–221, 248, 253, 255, 265, 268, 311
secretion advanced, 103
secretory activity, 355
secretory granules, 354, 356
secretory immune system, 22
secretory phase, 43, 61, 73–74, 76–78, **79–80**, 81, **84–86**, 87, 133, 134, 164, 227
 postovulatory, 38, 39, 52
secretory piece, 124, 133
secretory products, 354
semen, 90
sensors, **332**
serine, 18
sex organs
 female, 26
 male, 26
sex steroids, binding, *166*, 169
sexual dysfunction, 26
sexual stimulation, 32–34
sheep, 92, 105
sialomucins, 74–76, 80–81, 207
sigma technique, 210, **211**
skenes, 14
sodium, 373, 378, 416
 concentration, 28–29, 33
source of vaginal fluid protein, 20
sperm, 15, 67, 116, 331, 338, 408–410, 412
 capacitation, 337–338, 407–408
 fertilizing ability (mobility), 338–339
 motility, 338, 408–409
sperm-acrosin, 124
spermatozoa, 60, 67, 90, 117, 326, 335, 338, 340
spongiosa, 207
squamous cells, superficial, 6, 8–9
squamous vaginal mucous membrane, 7–8
steroid hormones, 341, 419, 421
 secretion, 422–423
"Stiftchenzelen" (peg cells), 363
stilbestrol, 362
stroke volume, 31
stroma, 38, 40–41, 64, 172, 208
 edema of, 189, **190**, 196

stroma [cont.]
  blood capillary of, **190**
  denuded, **193**, **196**
  fibroblast-like, **219**
  macrophages in, **217**
  reticular fibers of, **218**, **219**
stromal cells, 209–210, 217, **220**
  transformation, 191
stromal fibroblasts, 11
subnuclear vacuole, 42
succinate dehydrogenase, 73, 75, 78, 83, 206–207
sulfomucins, 74–76, 80, 207
superficial squamous cells, 6, 8–9
supernatant, 19
synthesis, 92–93, 96, 99
  of proteins, 81, 90, 92, 107

T

T-4 antibodies, level of, 393
T-4 coliphages, 391–393, 397
TEM (*see* transmission electron microscopy)
tampons, 25–28
taurine, 18
tenting effect, 30
testosterone, 166
thermistor, 31
threonine, 18
thrombin, 284, 295
thromboplastin, 234
thymidine, 5
tissue cyliner, 133
  method, 118, 141–142
tissue reaction, 396
tonofilaments, **4**, 6
topographical variations, 134
total protein content, 19
transferrin, 19, 107, 124, 337, 400–403
transmigration, 65
transmission electron microscopy (TEM), 41–43, 73–75, 81, 210–220, 248, 253, 255, 265, **313**, **315**
transport
  eggs (*see* egg transport)
  luminal contents, isthmus, 329
transudate, 20, 383, 416, 421
transudation, 14–15, 25–26, 33, 91–92, 107, 336, 341, 390, 422, 428
transuterine, 258
transvaginal potential difference, 29
tripeptide p-nitroanilide substrates, 151, 154
trophoblast, 87, 104–105, 107
  proteinases, 151–159
tropocollagen, 217
trypsin, 99, 124, 147, 249, 284, 340
  similarity to blastolemmase, 152

tryptophan, 18
tubal fluid, 390, 393, 395, 399
  composition of, 399
tubal function, 345
tubal transport, 428
tunica propria, 3
tupaia javanica, 164
tyrosine, 383

U

ultrastructure
  localization of enzymes, 53
  mucosal, 345
uracil, 383
urea, 15, 416
urethral meatus, 14
uric acid, 383
uridine, 383
urocanic acid, 383
urokinase, 132, 284, 295
uterine artery, 3
uterine cavity, 60–65, 90–91, 104, 109, 117, 178, 257–258
uterine colonization, 259
uterine fluid, 59–61, 64–65, 90–91, **101**
  presence of plasma protein inhibitors, 153
uterine mucosa, 133, *145*, 146–148
uterine mucus, 107
uterine secretion, 89–**97**, 102–**109**, 147
uteroglobin, 89, 92–105, 107, 153, 167
  trypsin-inhibiting activity, 153
uterotubal junction (UTJ), 300, **301**
uterus, 5, 14, 67, 90–92, 99–101, 117–122, 124, 131

V

vaginal formix, posterior, 61
vascularization, 228
vacuoles, 39, **40**, 49, 82, 84
vacuum aspiration, 266
vagina, 3, 8, 14–16, 22, 26–33
vaginal epithelium, (*see* epithelium)
vaginal fluid, 13–*16*, 18–22, 25–29, 34, 60
vaginal lubrication, 14, 26, 33
vaginal lumen, (*see* lumen, vaginal)
vaginal measurements, 31
vaginal mucosa, 14, 20, 22
vaginal mucous membrane, 5, 6
vaginal photopletysmography, (*see* photopletysmography, vaginal)
vaginal secretion, 19–*21*
vaginal stroma, **10**, 11
vaginitis, 19
valine, 18
vasodilatation, 15, 25
vascular anatomy, 305

442

vascular system, 3
vasculo-muscular layer, 305
venous plexus, 3, 14, 306
  hemorrhoidal, 3
  pudendal, 3
vestibular glands, 26
volatile acids, 16
volume pulse, 30, 31

X

xanthine, 379, 383, 429
xenon, 25
  method, 32, 33
xenon[133], 32

Z

zona basilis, 41, 181
zona compacta, 40
zona-free eggs, 408–410, 412, **413**
zona functionalis, 41
zona pellucida, 90, 104, 152, 339, 340, 408–409, 429
zona spongiosa, 38, 40, 42
zygote, 339, 340

17 α-hydroxyprogesterone, 166
20 α-hydroxyprogesterone, 166